DRUG DISCOVERY

Edited by **Hany A. El-Shemy**

Drug Discovery
http://dx.doi.org/10.5772/3388
Edited by Hany A. El-Shemy

Contributors

Melanie A. Jordan, Lourdes Rodriguez-Fragoso, Irina Piatkov, Elizabeth Hong-Geller, Sonia Lobo-Planey, Pawel Kafarski, Gluza Karolina, Malemud, Jolanta Natalia Latosińska, Magdalena Latosińska, Terry Smith, Luis Jesús Villarreal-Gómez, Irma E. Soria-Mercado, Ana Leticia Iglesias, Graciela Lizeth Perez-Gonzalez, Carsten Wrenger, Eva Liebau, Taosheng Chen, Asli Nur Goktug, Sergio C. Chai, Xin Liang, Jimmy Cui, Jonathan Low, Henning Ulrich, Claudiana Lameu, Gabriel Magoma, Samuel Constant, Christophe Mas, Song Huang, Ludovic Wiszniewski

Published by InTech

Janeza Trdine 9, 51000 Rijeka, Croatia

Publishing Process Manager Ana Pantar

Technical Editor InTech DTP team

Cover InTech Design team

First published November, 2013

Printed in Croatia

Additional hard copies can be obtained from orders@intechopen.com

Drug Discovery, Edited by Hany A. El-Shemy

p. cm.

ISBN 978-953-51-0906-8

For EU product safety concerns:
IN TECH d.o.o., Prolaz Marije Krucifikse Kozulić 3, 51000 Rijeka, Croatia,
info@intechopen.com or visit our website at intechopen.com.

Meet the editor

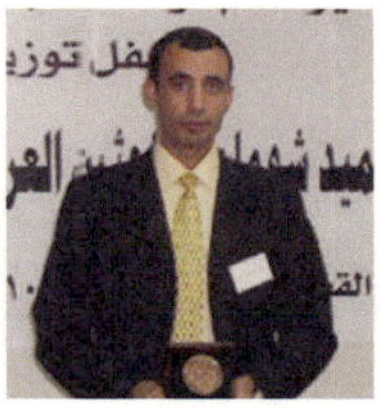

Prof. Hany A. El-Shemy received his two Ph.D. degrees in biochemistry and genetic engineering from the University of Cairo, Egypt and University of Hiroshima, Japan. He became an Assistant Professor at the Biochemistry Department of Cairo University, Egypt in September 1996, and advanced to Associate Professor in September 2002, as well as full Professor in March 2007. His research interests are in the fields of plant biotechnology and medicinal plants (Molecular Biology). He received 2 patents, wrote 7 international books, published more than 65 SCI Journal papers, and 30 conference presentations. He served as the technique committee member, chair in many international conferences and as editor including PLoS ONE journal, BMC Genomics. He also served as reviewer for more than 10 SCI cited journals. He received several awards, including State prize awarded from Academy of Science, Egypt (2004), Young Arab Researcher prize Awarded from Shuman Foundation, Jordan (2005), State Excellence prize from Academy of Science, Egypt (2011), Cairo University Prizes 2007, 2010.

Contents

Preface

Natural products are a constant source of potentially active compounds for the treatment of various disorders. The Middle East and tropical regions are believed to have the richest supplies of natural products in the world. Plant derived secondary metabolites have been used by humans to treat acute infections, health disorders and chronic illness for tens of thousands of years. Only during the last 100 years have natural products been largely replaced by synthetic drugs. Estimates of 200 000 natural products in plant species have been revised upward as mass spectrometry techniques have developed. For developing countries the identification and use of endogenous medicinal plants as cures against cancers has become attractive. Books on drug discovery will play vital role in the new era of disease treatment using natural products.

This book consists of 17 chapters and covers diverse topics from isolation, identification and validation and hit the drug cell interaction.

I would like to thank all contributors for their excellent effort regarding the drug discovery issues and I believe this book will provide significant knowledge to students and scientists.

Hany El-Shemy
Faculty of Agriculture
Cairo University, Egypt

Chapter 1

Fruit/Vegetable-Drug Interactions: Effects on Drug Metabolizing Enzymes and Drug Transporters

Lourdes Rodríguez-Fragoso and
Jorge Reyes-Esparza

Additional information is available at the end of the chapter

http://dx.doi.org/10.5772/48283

1. Introduction

Dietary habits are an important modifiable environmental factor influencing human health and disease. Epidemiologic evidence suggests that regular consumption of fruits and vegetables may reduce risk of some diseases, including cancer [1]. These properties have been attributed to foods that are rich sources of numerous bioactive compounds such as phytochemicals [2]. Modifying the intake of specific foods and/or their bioactive components seems to be a prudent, noninvasive, and cost-effective strategy for preventing some diseases in people who appear to be "healthy" [3]. As will be discussed in this chapter, potential problems occur when patients taking medicines regularly also consume certain fruits or vegetables.

Thousands of drugs are commercially available and a great percentage of the population takes at least one pharmacologically active agent on a regular basis. Given this magnitude of use and variability in individual nutritional status, dietary habits and food composition, there is a high potential for drug-nutrient interactions. However, there is a relatively short list of documented fruit-drug or vegetable-drug interactions, necessitating further and extensive clinical evaluation. Healthcare providers, such as physicians, pharmacists, nurses, and dietitians, have to be aware of important food-drug interactions in order to optimize the therapeutic efficacy of prescribed and over-the-counter drugs. Here, we review some of the most widely consumed fruits and vegetables to inform healthcare providers of possible nutrient-drug interactions and their potential clinical significance.

There are numerous patients who encounter increased risks of adverse events associated with drug-nutrient interactions. These include elderly patients, patients with cancer and/ or malnutrition, gastrointestinal tract dysfunctions, acquired immunodeficiency syndrome and chronic diseases that require the use of multiple drugs, as well as those receiving enteral nutrition or transplants. Therefore, the main reason for devoting a major review to nutrient-drug interactions is the enormous importance of fruits and vegetables used for their beneficial effects as nutrients and as components in folk medicine. There are currently few studies that combine a nutrient-based and detailed pharmacological approach [4], or studies that systematically explore the risk and benefits of fruit and vegetables [5-7].

2. Food-drug interactions

A drug-nutrient interaction is defined as the result of a physical, chemical, physiological, or pathophysiological relationship between a drug and a nutrient [8,9]. An interaction is considered significant from a clinical perspective if it alters the therapeutic response. Food-drug interactions can result in two main clinical effects: the decreased bioavailability of a drug, which predisposes to treatment failure, or an increased bioavailability, which increases the risk of adverse events and may even precipitate toxicities (See Figure 1) [4, 10,11].

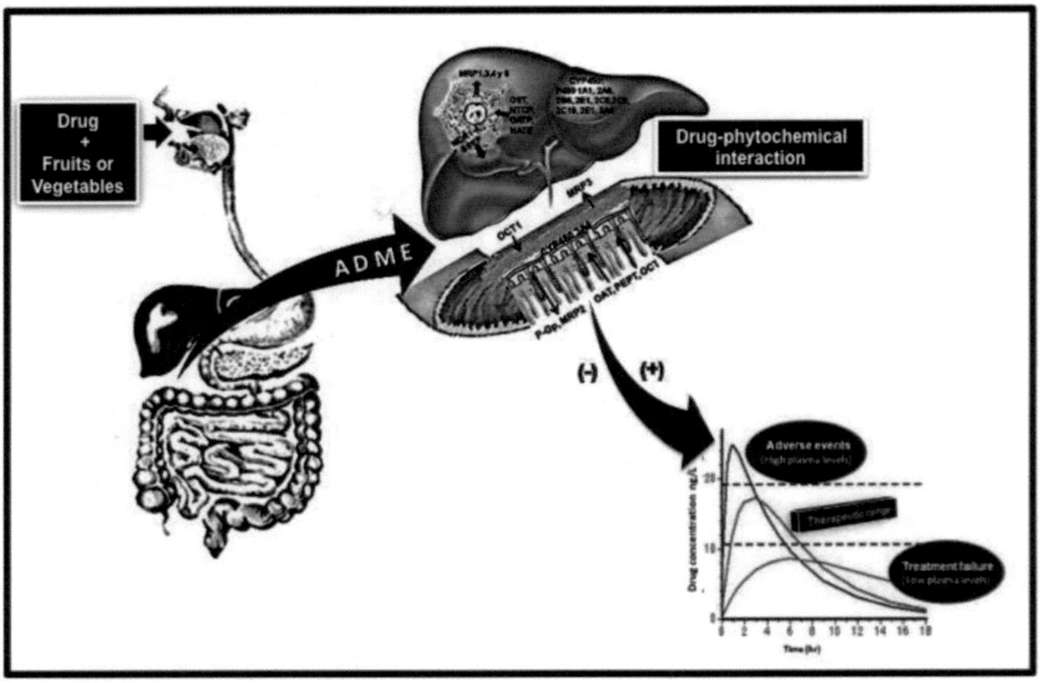

Figure 1. Drug-fruit/vegetable interaction and effects on bioavailability of drugs. During the consumption of drugs with fruits or vegetables the **ADME** properties of drug (**A**bsorption, **D**istribution, **M**etabolism and **E**xcretion) can be modified by drug-phytochemical interaction. As a result of this interaction can be increased or decreased plasma concentrations of a drug which can lead to the presence of adverse events or treatment failure.

Nutritional status and diet can affect drug action by altering metabolism and function. In addition, various dietary components can have pharmacological activity under certain circumstances [12]. For healthy-treatment intervention, it is necessary to understand how these drug-food interactions can induce a beneficial result or lead to detrimental therapeutic conditions (less therapeutic action or more toxicity). Drug-drug interactions are widely recognized and evaluated as part of the drug-approval process, whether pharmaceutical, pharmacokinetic, or pharmacodynamic in nature. Equal attention must be paid to food-drug interactions (Figure 2).

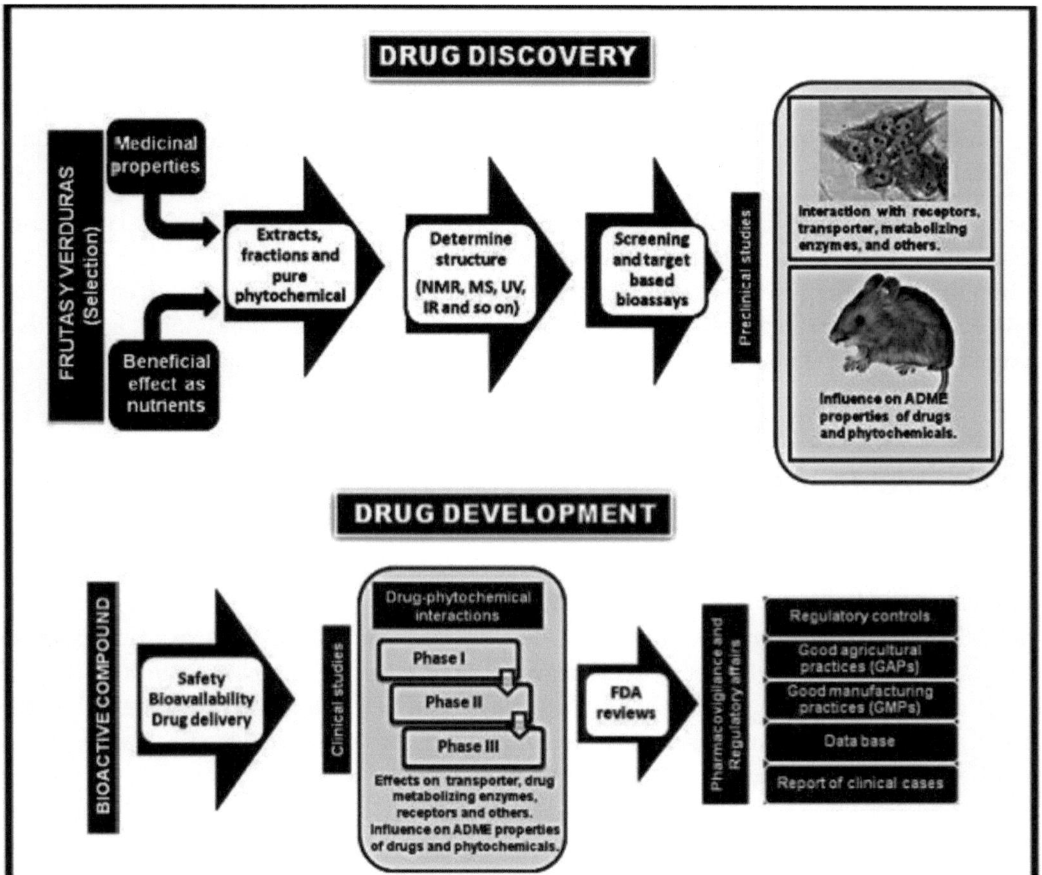

Figure 2. Bioassay models for studying drug-phytochemical interaction.

There are four types of accepted drug-food interactions based on their nature and mechanisms.

- Type I are *ex vivo* bioinactivations, which refer to interactions between the drug and the nutritional element or formulation through biochemical or physical reactions, such as hydrolysis, oxidation, neutralization, precipitation or complexation. These interactions usually occur in the delivery device.
- Type II interactions affect absorption. They cause either an increase or decrease in the oral bioavailability of a drug. The precipitant agent may modify the function of enzymes or transport mechanisms that are responsible for biotransformation.
- Type III interactions affect the systemic or physiologic disposition and occur after the drug or the nutritional element has been absorbed from the gastrointestinal tract and entered the systemic circulation. Changes in the cellular or tissue distribution, systemic transport, or penetration to specific organs or tissues can occur.
- Type IV interactions refer to the elimination or clearance of drugs or nutrients, which may involve the antagonism, impairment or modulation of renal and/or enterohepatic elimination [13].

Drug metabolizing enzymes and drug transporters play important roles in modulating drug absorption, distribution, metabolism, and elimination. Acting alone or in concert with each other, they can affect the pharmacokinetics and pharmacodynamics of a drug. The interplay between drug metabolizing enzymes and transporters is one of the confounding factors that have been recently shown to contribute to potential complex drug interactions [14].

3. Food and drug transporters

The oral administration of drugs to patients is convenient, practical, and preferred for many reasons. Oral administration of drugs, however, may lead to limited and variable oral bioavailability because of absorption across the intestinal barrier [15,16]. Drug absorption across the gastrointestinal tract is highly dependent on affinity for membrane transporters as well as lipophilicity [17]. On the other hand, the liver plays a key role in the clearance and excretion of many drugs. Hepatic transporters are membrane proteins that primarily facilitate nutrient and endogenous substrate transport into the cell via uptake transporters, or protect the cell by pumping out toxic chemicals via canalicular transporters [18]. Consequently, drug transporters in both the gut and the liver are important in determining oral drug disposition by controlling absorption and bioavailability [19]

The major uptake transporters responsible for nutrient and xenobiotic transport, both uptake and efflux transporters, belong to the two solute carrier (SLC and SLCO) superfamilies [20]. The SLC superfamily encompasses a variety of transporters, including the organic anion transporters (OAT, SLC22A), the organic cation transporters (OCT, SLC22A), the electroneutral organic cation transporters (OCTN, SLC22A), the equilibrative nucleoside transporters (ENT, SLC29), the concentrative nucleoside transporters (CNT, SLC28), the apical Na^{+}–dependent bile salt transporter (ASBT, SLC10), the monocarboxylate transporters (MCT, SLC16), and the peptide transporters (PEPT, SLC15) [21]. The SLCO family is made up of the organic anion transporting polypeptides (OATP) [22]. Efflux transporters expressed in the intestine and liver include P-glycoprotein (Pgp, ABCB1), bile salt export pump (BSEP, ABCB11), multidrug resistance proteins (MRP1- 6, ABCC1-6), and breast cancer resistance protein (BCRP, ABCG2), all members of the ATP-Binding Cassette superfamily (ABC transporters) [23]. Members of this superfamily use ATP as an energy source, allowing them to pump substrates against a concentration gradient. In the liver, uptake transporters are mainly expressed in the sinusoid, and excretion transporters are mainly expressed on the lateral and canalicular membranes. There are transporters on the lateral membrane the primary function of which is pumping drugs back into the blood circulation from the hepatocytes. Nowadays, a large amount of work has identified and characterized intestinal and hepatic transporters in regards to tissue expression profiles, regulation, mechanisms of transport, substrate and inhibitor profiles, species differences, and genetic polymorphisms. Given the circumstances outlined above, there is no doubt of the overall relevance of drug transport for clinical pharmacokinetics.

Until recently, little regard was given to the possibility that food and food components could cause significant changes to the extent of drug absorption via effects on intestinal and liver transporters. It is now well known that drug-food interactions might affect the pharmacokinetics of prescribed drugs when co-administered with food [24]. Common foods, such as fruits and vegetables, contain a large variety of secondary metabolites known as phytochemicals (Tabla 1), many of which have been associated with health benefits [25]. However, we know little about the processes through which these phytochemicals (and/or their metabolites) are absorbed into the body, reach their biological target, and are eliminated. Recent studies show that some of these phytochemicals are substrates and modulators of specific members of the superfamily of ABC transporting proteins [26]. Indeed, *in vitro* and preclinical data in rats suggest that a variety of foodstuffs [27,28], including herbal teas [29,30] and vegetables and herbs [31,32] can modulate the activity of drug transporters. It is not yet known whether these effects are predictive of what will be observed clinically.

4. Foods and drug-metabolizing enzyme

It has been shown that, before reaching the systemic circulation, the metabolism of orally ingested drugs ('first-pass metabolism' or 'presystemic clearance') has clinically relevant influences on the potency and efficacy of drugs. Both the intestine and liver account for the presystemic metabolism in humans. Drug metabolism reactions are generally grouped into 2 phases. Phase I reactions involve changes such as oxidation, reduction, and hydrolysis and are primarily mediated by the cytochrome P450 (CYP) family of enzymes. Phase II reactions use an endogenous compound such as glucuronic acid, glutathione, or sulfate, to conjugate with the drug or its phase I–derived metabolite to produce a more polar end product that can be more readily excreted [33].

The CYP enzymes involved in drug metabolism in humans are expressed predominantly in the liver. However, they are also present in the large and small intestine, lungs and brain [34]. CYP proteins are categorized into families and subfamilies and can metabolize almost any organic xenobiotic [35]. CYP enzymes combined with drug transport proteins constitute the first-pass effect of orally administered drugs [33]. On the other hand, the Phase II drug metabolizing or conjugating enzymes consist of many enzyme superfamilies, including sulfotransferases (SULT), UDP-glucuronosyltransferases (UGT), DT-diaphorase or NAD(P)H:quinone oxidoreductase (NQO) or NAD(P)H: menadione reductase (NMO), epoxide hydrolases (EPH), glutathione S-transferases (GST) and *N*-acetyltransferases (NAT). The conjugation reactions by Phase II drug-metabolizing enzymes increase hydrophilicity and thereby enhance excretion in the bile and/or the urine and consequently affect detoxification [36].

The metabolism of a drug can be altered by foreign chemicals and such interactions can often be clinically significant [37]. The most common form of drug interactions entail a foreign chemical acting either as an inhibitor or an inducer of the CYP enzyme isoform responsible for metabolizing an administered medicinal drug, subsequently leading to an unusually slow or fast clearance of said drug [38,39]. Inhibition of drug metabolism will result in a concentration elevation in tissues, leading to various adverse reactions, particularly for drugs with a low therapeutic index.

Often, influence on drug metabolism by compounds that occur in the environment, most remarkably foodstuffs, is bypassed. Dietary changes can alter the expression and activity of hepatic drug metabolizing enzymes. Although this can lead to alterations in the systemic elimination kinetics of drugs metabolized by these enzymes, the magnitude of the change is generally small [8, 40]. Metabolic food-drug interactions occur when a certain food alters the activity of a drug-metabolizing enzyme, leading to a modulation of the pharmacokinetics of drugs metabolized by the enzyme [12]. Foods, such as fruits, vegetables, alcoholic beverages, teas, and herbs, which consist of complex chemical mixtures, can inhibit or induce the activity of drug-metabolizing enzymes [41].

The observed induction and inhibition of CYP enzymes by natural products in the presence of a prescribed drug has (among other reasons) led to the general acceptance that natural therapies can have adverse effects, contrary to popular beliefs in countries with active ethnomedicinal practices. Herbal medicines such as St. John's wort, garlic, piperine, ginseng, and gingko, which are freely available over the counter, have given rise to serious clinical interactions when co-administered with prescription medicines [42]. Such adversities have spurred various pre-clinical and *in vitro* investigations on a series of other herbal remedies, with their clinical relevance yet to be established. The CYP3A4-related interaction based on food component is the best known; it might be related to the high level of expression of CYP3A4 in the small intestine, as well as its broad substrate specificity. If we consider that CYP3A4 is responsible for the metabolism of more than 50% of clinical pharmaceuticals, all nutrient-drug interactions should be considered clinically relevant, in which case all clinical studies of drugs should include a food-drug interaction screening [43].

5. Nutrient-drug interactions: examples with clinical relevance

Fruits and vegetables are known to be important components in a healthy diet, since they have low energy density and are sources of micronutrients, fiber, and other components with functional properties, called phytochemicals (See Figure 2). Increased fruit and vegetable consumption can also help displace food high in saturated fats, sugar or salt. Low fruit and vegetable intake is among the top 10 risk factors contributing to mortality. According to the World Health Organization (WHO), increased daily fruit and vegetable intake could help prevent major chronic non-communicable diseases [44]. Evidence is emerging that specific combinations of phytochemicals may be far more effective in protecting against some diseases than isolated compounds (Table 1 and 2). Observed drug-phytochemical interactions, in addition to interactions among dietary micronutrients, indicate possibilities for improved therapeutic strategies. However, several reports have examined the effects of plant foods and herbal medicines on drug bioavailability. As shown in Tables 3 and 4 and as discussed below, we have surveyed the literature to identify reports suggesting important food and phytochemical modulation of drug-metabolizing enzymes and drug transporters leading to potential important nutrient-drug interactions.

Fruit	Phytochemicals	Traditional Uses
Grapefruit *Citrus paradisi, Citrus reticulata*	Bergamottin, flavonoids (nobilein, tangeretin, quercetin, diosmin, naringenin, naringin and kaempferol), and furanocoumarins.	Insomnia, and anxiety or nervousness
Orange *Citrus sinensis, Citrus aurantium*	Flavonoids as tangeretin, nobiletin, diosmin and hesperetin.	Inflammatory ailments in respiratory tract, Arthritis, gastrointestinal tract ailments and others
Tangerine *Citrus reticulata, Citrus deliciosa*	Flavonoids as diosmin, tangeritin, nobilein and quercetin.	Inflammatory ailments in respiratory tract, arthritis, gastrointestinal tract ailments and others
Grapes *Vitis vinifera*	Stilbens (resverestrol, viniferin), and flavonoids,	Antianemic, Inflammatory ailments in respiratory tract and others
Cranberry *Vaccinium macrocarpon Vaccinum myrtillus*	Flavonoids as anthocyanidin (cyaniding and poenidin) and flavonols (quercetin); and carotenoids.	Genitourinary ailments, nephrolithiasis, wound healing and others
Pomegranate *Punica granatum*	Phenolic acids (punicalagin and tannins), flavonoids (anthocyanins) and pectin.	Inflammatory ailments in respiratory tract and others Gastrointestinal tract ailments and others
Apple *Malus domestica*	Phenolic acids (tannins), flavonoids (including quercetin), glycosylated xanthones (mangiferin) and Saponins.	Diuretic, genitourinary ailments, inflammatory ailments in respiratory tract and others
Mango *Mangifera indica*	Phenolic acids (tannins), flavonoids (anthocyanins), carotenoids, essential oils, fatty acids, lectins, phenols, saponins, alkaloids, and triterpenes.	Recommended to combat heart disease. It is also a laxative, and diuretic
Black raspberry *Rubus coreanus, Rubus idaeus, Rubus fruticosus*	Phenolic acids (ellagic acid, gallic acid), flavonoids (quercetin, anthocyanins, pelargonidins, Kaempferol and cyanidins), catechins and salicylic acid.	Antianemic, anti-infectious, inflammatory ailments in respiratory tract, gastrointestinal tract ailments and others
Black mulberry *Morus nigra*	2-arylbenzofuran derivative, flavones (mornigrol D, mornigrol G, mornigrol H, and norartocarpetin), flavonol (dihydrokaempferol), albanin A, albanin E, stilbenes (moracin M), and albafuran.	Genitourinary ailments, Inflammatory ailments in respiratory tract, gastrointestinal tract ailments and others
Guava *Psidium guajava*	Flavonoid as quercetin and phloretin.	Genitourinary ailments, hypertension
Papaya (*Carica papaya L.*)	beta-cryptoxanthin and benzyl isothiocyanates.	Abdominal discomfort, pain, malaria, diabetes, obesity, infections and oral drug poisonings

Data from: [26,52,53,55, 82, 111, 112]

Table 1. Commonly Consumed Fruits

Vegetable	Phytochemicals	Traditional Uses
Broccoli *Brassica oleracea var. italica*	Isothiocyanate sulforaphane, glucosinolate glucoraphanin, glucosinolates, phenolic acid, indol and dithiolthiones.	Antioxidant, Anti-cancer, Antiseptic, anti-ulcerous, hypoglycemic, anti-anemic, Gastrointestinal tract ailments and others
Cauliflower *Brassica oleracea var. botrytis*	Isothiocyanate, glucosinolate, indole-3-Carbinol, sulforaphane, indol,	Antioxidant
Spinach *Spinacia oleracea*	Flavonoids and *p*-coumaric acid derivatives, α-lipoic acid, poliphenols, lutein, zeaxantin, betaine	Diuretic, inflammatory ailments, gastrointestinal tract ailments, Inflammatory ailments in respiratory tract and others.
Watercress *Nasturtium officinale*	phenylethyl isothiocyanate (PEITC) and methylsulphinylakyl isothiocyanates (MEITCs), flavonoids such as quercetin, hydroxycinnamic acids, and carotenoids such as β-carotene and lutein	Antioxidants, diuretic, gastrointestinal tract ailments, Inflammatory ailments in respiratory tract and others.
Tomato *Lycopersicum esculentum*	Carotenoids phytofluene, phytoene, neurosporene, γ-carotene, and ζ-carotene lycopene, phytoene, phytofluene, quercetin, polyphenols, kaempferol	Antioxidant, hydratant, hypocholesterolemic
Carrot *Dactus carrota*	Polyphenols, α and β-carotene, quercetin, myrecetin and panaxynol	Constipation
Avocado *Persea americana*	Persin, carotenoids (zeaxanthin, α-carotene, and β-carotene), lutein, β-sitosterol, glutathione	Genitourinary ailments, inflammatory ailments in respiratory tract, gastrointestinal tract ailments and others
Red pepper *(Capsicum annuum L.)*	Capsaisin, lycopene, anthocyanins	Scarlatina, putrid sore throat, hoarseness, dyspepsia, yellow fiber, peals and snakebite

Data from: [26,105,114,126, 151]

Table 2. Commonly Consumed Vegetables

Fruit	Molecular Target	Drug Interactions in Humans and Others
Grapefruit	Inhibits CYP3A4, CYP1A2, MRP2, OATP-B and P-glycoprotein, [29, 45, 50, 53, 54, 65]	In humans: reports of more than 40 drug interactions: calcium channel antagonists [57], central nervous system modulators [58], HMG-CoA reductase [59], immunosuppressants [60], anti-virals [61], phosphodiesterases-5 inhibitor [62], antihistamines [63], antiarrythmics [62], and antibiotics [64].
Sevilla orange	Inhibits CYP3A4, P-glycoprotein, OATP-A, OATP-B [11, 29, 5469, 117]	*In vitro* system: vinblastine [55], fexofenadine [29], glibenclamida [53] In humans: atenolol, ciprofloxacine, ciclosporine, celiprolol, levofloxacin and pravastatin [54, 72]
Tangerine	Stimulates CYP3A4 activity and inhibits P-glycoprotein [52]	*In vitro* system: nifedipine [74], digoxina [52]
Grapes	Inhibits CYP3A4 and CYP2E1 [13]	In humans: cyclosporine [78],
Cranberry	Inhibits CYP3A and CYP2C9 [31, 81, 83]	In humans: Warfarin [81, 82] *In vitro* system: Diclofenac [83]
Pomegranate	Inhibits CYP3A and phenol sulfotransferase activity [56,89]	Animals: carbamacepine [56]
Mango	Inhibits CYP1A1, CYP1A2, CYP 3A1, CYP2C6, CYP2E1, P-glycoprotein (ABCB1) [97]	*In vitro* system: midazolam, diclofenac, chlorzoxazone [95, 96]; Verapamil [97].
Guava	Inhibits P- glycoprotein [23]	Not documented
Black raspberry	Inhibits CYP3A [49]	*In vitro* system: midazolam
Black mulberry	Inhibits CYP3A and OATP-B [49]	*In vitro* system: midazolam; glibenclamida [53]
Apple	Inhibits CYP1A1, OATP family (Oatp-1, Oatp-3 and NTCP) [63, 110]	*In vitro* system: fexofenadine [63]
Papaya	Inhibits CYP3A4 [114]	No documented

Table 3. Fruit-Drug Interactions

Vegetable	Molecular target	Drug Interactions in Humans and Others.
Broccoli	Inhibits: CYP1A1, CYP2B1/2, CYP3A 4, CYP2E1, hGSTA1/2, MRP-1, MRP-2, BCRP, UDP, Glucorosytransferases, Sulfotransferases, Quinone reductases phenolsulfotransferases [26, 120,121] Induces: UDPglucuronosyltransferases, (UGTs), sulfotransferases, (SULTs) and quinone reductases (QRs) [26]	Not documented
Cauliflower	Inhibits: CYP1A1, CYP2B1/2, CYP3A 4, CYP2E1, hGSTA1/2, MRP-1, MRP-2, BCRP, UDP, Glucorosytransferases, Sulfotransferases, Quinone reductases phenolsulfotransferases [26,120, 121] Induces: UDPglucuronosyltransferases, (UGTs), sulfotransferases, (SULTs) and quinone reductases (QRs) [26]	Not documented
Watercress	Inhibits: CYP2E1, P-glycoprotein, MRP1, MRP2 and BCRP [26, 126]	In humans: Chlorzoxazone
Spinach	Possible inhibition of CYP1A2 [1132]	*In vitro* system: heterocyclic aromatic amines
Tomato	Inhibits: CYP1A1, CYP1B1, UGP, [138] Increases: UGT and CYP2E1, [139]	In vitro system: diethylnitrosamine, N-methyl-N-nitrosourea, and 1,2-dimethylhydrazine
Carrot	Induces: phenolsulfotransferases and ethoxycoumarin O-deethylase ECD [123, 143] Inhibits: CPY2E1 [122]	Not documented
Avocado	Unknown	Humans: Warfarin
Red pepper	Inhibits CYP 1A2, 2A2, 3A1, 2C11, 2B1, 2B2 and 2C6 [154,155]	*In vitro* and *in vivo*

Table 4. Vegetable-Drug Intractions

5.1. Grapefruit (*Citrus paradisi*)

The interaction of grapefruit with certain drugs was unintentionally discovered two decades ago [45]. Since then, there have been numerous reports on the effects of grapefruit and its components on CYP450 drug oxidation and transportation [46,47]. Several findings showed that grapefruit juice had a major effect on the intestinal CYP system with a minor effect at the hepatic level [48]. The predominant mechanism for this interaction is the inhibition of cytochrome *P*-450 3A4 in the small intestine, which results in a significant reduction of drug presystemic metabolism. Grapefruit juice intake has been found to decrease CYP3A4 mRNA activity through a post transcriptional activity, possibly by facilitating degradation of the enzyme [49]. An additional mechanism may be the inhibition of P-glycoprotein and MRP2-mediated drug efflux, transporters that carry drugs from enterocytes back to the gut lumen, all of which results in a further increase in the fraction of drug absorbed and increased systemic drug bioavailability [50-52]. It has also been reported that the major constituents of grapefruit significantly inhibit the OATP-B function *in vitro* [53,54].

The interaction between grapefruit juice and drugs has been potentially ascribed to a number of constituents [27]. It has been suggested that flavonoids such as naringin, naringenin, quercetin, and kaempferol, major components in grapefruit, are responsible for drug interaction. Some of these chemicals are also found in other fruit juices. Pomegranate, for example, shares certain properties with grapefruit, suggesting that both could modify the bioavailability of drugs [55,56]. Another group of compounds that has been detected in grapefruit juice are the furanocoumarins (psoralens), which are known to be mechanism-based inactivators of CYP450. The major furanocoumarin present in grapefruit is bergamottin, which demonstrated a time- and concentration-dependent inactivation of CYP enzymes *in vitro* [49]. One interesting characteristic of this interaction is that grapefruit juice does not need to be taken simultaneously with the medication in order to produce the interaction. The bioavailability of drugs has been reported to be doubled by grapefruit juice, even when taken 12 h after ingestion. Colored grapefruit juice and white grapefruit juice are equally effective in producing drug interactions.

This inhibitory interaction should be kept in mind when prescribing drugs metabolized by CYP3A4. Examples of drugs affected by grapefruit or its components include: calcium channel antagonists such as felodipine, nisoldipine, amlodipines, verapamil, and diltiazem [57]; central nervous system modulators, including diazepam, triazolam, midazolam, alprazolam, carbamazepine, buspurone and sertraline [58]; HMG-CoA reductase inhibitors, such as simvastatin, lovastatin, atorvastatin, and pravastatin [59]; immunosuppressants such as cyclosporine [60]; anti-virals such as saquinavir [61]; a phosphodiesterases-5 inhibitor such as sildenafil [62]; antihistamines, including as terfenadine and fexofenadine [63]; antiarhythmics such as amiodarone [62]; and antibiotics such as eritromicine [64].

Epidemiologic studies reveal that approximately 2% of the population in the United States consumes at least one glass of regular strength grapefruit juice per day. This becomes pertinent if we consider that many people suffer from chronic metabolic diseases (including hypertension, hyperlipidemia, and cardiovascular diseases) and receive calcium channel antagonis therapy and HMG-CoA reductase inhibitors. Patients with mental disorders also chronically receive central nervous system modulators. In the case of many drugs, an increase in serum drug concentration has been associated with increased frequency of dose-dependent adverse effects [65-67]. In light of the wide ranging effects of grapefruit juice on the pharmacokinetics of various drugs, physicians need to be aware of these interactions and should make an attempt to warn and educate patients regarding the potential consequences of concomitant ingestion of these agents.

5.2. Orange (*Citrus sinensis*)

Consumption of most types of orange juice does not appear to alter CYP3A4 activity *in vivo* [55]. However, orange juice made from Seville oranges appears to be somewhat similar to grapefruit juice and can affect the pharmacokinetics of CYP3A4 substrates [68]. It has been previously shown that consumption of a single 240 mL serving of Sevilla orange juice resulted in a 76% increase in felodipine exposure, comparable to what is observed after grapefruit juice consumption [11]. Presumably, the mechanism of this effect is similar to that of grapefruit juice-mediated interactions, because Sevilla orange contains significant concentrations of flavonoids, mainly bergamottin and 6′,7′-dihydroxybergamottin [69]. Orange juice has also been shown to exert inhibitory effects on P-glycoprotein (P-gp)-mediated drug efflux. Takanaga and others showed that 3,3′,4′,5,6,7,8-heptamethoxyflavon and tangeretin were the major P-gp inhibitors present in orange juice and showed that another component, nobiletin, was also a P-gp inhibitor [55]. Therefore, the intake of orange juice might inhibit the efflux transporters by P-gp, which could enhance the bioavailability of drugs and thus lead to an increase in the risk of adverse events [52].

It has also been observed that components of orange juice -naringin in particular- are *in vitro* inhibitors of OATP transport activity [70]. Dresser et al., have previously reported that orange juice inhibits the function of human OATP-A (OATP1A2, gene symbol *SLC21A3/ SLCO1A2*) *in vitro* [29]. OATP-A, however, is predominantly expressed in the brain, but not in the intestine. On the other hand, Satoh et al. reported that OATP-B-mediated uptake of glibenclamide as well as estrone-3-sulfate was significantly inhibited by 5% orange juice [53]. Orange juice might reduce the intestinal absorption of substrates of OATP-B (e.g., digoxin, benzylpenicillin, and hormone conjugates), resulting in a decrease in concentration in the blood.

Previous studies in humans using fexofenadine as a probe showed that oral coadministration with orange juice decreased the oral bioavailability of fexofenadine [63]. Orange juice and its constituents were shown to interact with members of the OATP transporter family by reducing their activities. The functional consequences of such an interaction are reflected in a significant reduction in the oral bioavailability of fexofenadine, possibly by preferential direct inhibition of intestinal OATP activity. Other reports indicate that orange juice slightly reduced the absorption of ciprofloxacin, levofloxacin and celiprolol [65] A study of an interaction between orange juice and pravastatin showed an increase in AUC [54].Orange juice also moderately reduces the bioavailability of atenolol, which may necessitate a dose adjustment [71,72].

5.3. Tangerine (*Citrus reticulata*)

Early studies demonstrated the influence of tangeretin, a flavonoid found in high levels in tangerine juice, on drug metabolizing liver enzymes. It was demonstrated that tangeretin inhibits P450 1A2 and P450 3A4 activity in human liver microsomes [73]. Tangeretin is a potent regioselective stimulator of midazolam 1'-hydroxylation by human liver microsomes CYP3A4. Although, clinical studies have shown no influence on midazolam pharmacokinetics *in vivo*, further studies are needed to evaluate its effects on other drugs [74]. Diosmin is one of the main components of citrus fruits, such as tangerine. Diosmin may increase the absorption or bioavailability of co-administered drugs able to serve as P-gp substrates. As a result, some caution may be required with its clinical use [52].

5.4. Grapes (*Vitis vinifera*)

Grapes are one of the most valued conventional fruits worldwide. The grape is considered a source of unique and potentially useful medicinal natural products; they are also used in the manufacturing of various industrial products [75,76](Yadav and others 2009; Vislocky and Fernandez 2010). The main biologically active and well-characterized constituent from the grape is resveratrol, which is known for various medicinal properties in treating human diseases [75](Yadav and others 2009). Resveratrol was shown to be an irreversible (mechanism-based) inhibitor of CYP3A4 and a non-competitive reversible inhibitor for CYP2E1 in microsomes from rat liver and human liver cells containing cDNA-expressed CYPs [77,78] (Chan and Delucchi 2000; Piver and others 2001). Resveratrol is an electron-rich molecule with two aromatic benzene rings linked by an ethylene bridge. CYP3A-mediated aromatic hydroxylation and epoxidation of resveratrol are possible, resulting in a reactive p-benzoquinone methide metabolite which is capable of binding covalently to CYP3A4, leading to inactivation and potential drug interactions.

5.5. Cranberry (*Vaccinium macrocarpon*)

American cranberry is a fruit used as a prophylactic agent against urinary tract infections [79]. Drug interactions with cranberry juice might be related to the fact that the juice is rich in flavonol glycosides, anthocyanins, proanthocyanidins, and organic and phenolic acids [80]. Izzo [81] described a total of eight cases of interaction between cranberry juice and warfarin, leading to changes in international normalized ratio (INR) values and bleeding. The mechanism behind this interaction might be the inhibition by cranberry flavonoids of CYP3A4 and/or CYP2C9 enzymes, which are responsible for warfarin metabolism [31,82].

It has also been shown that cranberry juice inhibits diclofenac metabolism in human liver microsomes, but this has not been demonstrated clinically in human subjects [83]. Cranberry juice may increase the bioavailability of CYP3A4 substrates (e.g., calcium antagonists or calcineurin inhibitors) as was discussed [61]. Uesawa and Mohri have demonstrated that nifedipine metabolism in rat intestinal and human hepatic microsomes are inhibited by preincubation with cranberry juice. Furthermore, cranberry juice increased the nifedipine concentration in rat plasma. These findings suggest that cranberry juice might affect the plasma concentration of nifedipine in humans as well [84].

5.6. Pomegranate (*Punica granatum*)

Pomegranate is commonly eaten around the world and has been used in folk medicine for a wide variety of therapeutic purposes [85-86]. Pomegranate is a rich source of several chemicals such as pectin, tannins, flavonoids, and anthocyanins. It has been have reported that pomegranate juice influenced the pharmacokinetics of carbamazepine in rats by inhibiting enteric CYP3A activity. Such inhibition of the enteric CYP3A activity by a single exposure to pomegranate juice appears to last for approximately 3 days [56]. Nagata and others [88] found that pomegranate juice inhibited human CYP2C9 activity and increased tolbutamide bioavailability in rats. Recently, pomegranate juice was shown to potently inhibit the sulfoconjugation of 1-naphthol in Caco-2 cells. It has been suggested that some constituents of pomegranate juice, most probably punicalagin, may impair the metabolic functions of the intestine (specifically sulfoconjugation) and therefore might have effects upon the bioavailability of drugs [89].

5.7. Mango (*Mangifera indica*)

The beneficial effects of mango include anti-inflammatory and antimicrobial activities [90,91] Preliminary phytochemical screening revealed the presence of flavonoids, including quercetin and glycosylated xanthones such as mangiferin [92,93] Quercetin has been shown to possess antioxidant, antimicrobial, antitumor, antihypertensive, antiatherosclerosis, and anti-inflammatory properties [94]. In a series of studies, Rodeiro and others have shown the effects of mango on drug metabolizing enzymes and drug transporters [95, 96] They found that exposure of hepatocytes to mango extract produced a significant reduction (60%) in 7-methoxyresorufin-O-demethylase (MROD; CYP1A2) activity and an increase (50%) in 7-penthoxyresorufin-O-depentylase (PROD; CYP2B1) activity. This group also studied the effect of mangiferin on CYP enzymes and found that mangiferin reduced the activities of five P450s: POD (CYP1A2), midazolam 1'-hydroxylation (M1OH; CYP3A1), diclofenac 4'-hydroxylation (D4OH; CYP2C6), S-mephenytoin 4'-hydroxylation (SM4OH), and chlorzoxazone 6-hydroxyaltion (C6OH; CYP2E1). Recently, mango and mango-derived polyphenols have been shown to potentially affect the activity of the multidrug transporter P-gp ABCB1 [97]. These findings suggest that mango and its components inhibit the major human P450 enzymes involved in drug metabolism and some transporters. The potential for drug interactions with mango fruit should therefore be considered.

5.8. Guava (*Psidium guajava* L)

Guava is an important food crop and medicinal plant in tropical and subtropical countries; it is widely used as food and in folk medicine around the world [98, 99]. A number of metabolites such as phenolics, flavonoid, carotenoid, terpenoid and triterpene have been found in this fruit. Extracts and metabolites of this plant, particularly those from the leaves and fruit, possess useful pharmacological activities [100]. There is only one report about the effect of guava extracts on drug transport: guava extract showed a potent inhibitory effect on P-gp mediated efflux in Caco-2 cells. It was also found to inhibit efflux transport from serosal to mucosal surfaces in the rat ileum [101]. This means that guava could interact with P-gp substrates such as digoxin, fexofenadine, indinavir, vincristine, colchicine, topotecan, and paclitaxel in the small intestine. For this reason, this fruit should be consumed with caution by patients taking medicines.

5.9. Raspberry (*Rubus* spp.)

Berries have been shown to have a positive impact on several chronic conditions including obesity, cancer, and cardiovascular and neurodegenerative diseases [102-104]. Like other fruits, raspberries contain micro- and macronutrients such as vitamins, minerals, and fiber. Their biological properties, however, have been largely attributed to high levels of various phenolic compounds, as well as the interactive synergies among their natural phytochemical components (e.g., ellagic acid, quercetin, gallic acid, anthocyanins, cyanidins, pelargonidins, catechins, kaempferol and salicylic acid). Raspberry or raspberry constituents have antioxidant and anti-inflammatory properties, and inhibit cancer cell growth [105-107]. Black raspberries (*Rubus coreanus)* have been called the "king of berries" for their superior health benefits, whereas black mulberry (*Morus nigra)* is most commonly used for its antioxidants properties and for its high bioactive content of phenolics, anthocyanins, and gallic acid. It has been shown that black raspberry and black mulberry are able to inhibit the human

CYP3A-catalyzed midazolam 1-hydroxylation activity in liver microsomes, and the inhibitory effects are somewhat greater than those of pomegranate [49, 56]. It has also been reported that black mulberry extract potently inhibits OATP-B function at concentrations that seem to be physiologically relevant *in vitro* [53]. These results suggest that black raspberry and black mulberry may decrease the plasma concentrations of concomitantly ingested OATP-B substrate drugs or increase the plasma concentration levels of concomitantly ingested CYP3A-substrate drugs. *In vivo* studies on the interaction between black mulberry and black raspberry and CYP3A substrates are needed to determine whether inhibition of CYP3A activity by fruit juices is clinically relevant.

5.10. Apple (*Malus domestica*)

Apple and its products contain high amounts of polyphenols, which show diverse biological activities and may contribute to beneficial health effects such as protecting the intestine against inflammation due to chronic inflammatory bowel diseases [108, 109]. It has been found that apple juice extract inhibits CYP1A1 at levels of CYP1A1 mRNA, protein, and enzymatic activity [110]. On the other hand, it has also been reported that apple juice and its constituents can interact with members of the OATP transporter family (OATP-1, OATP-3 and NTCP) by reducing their activities *in vitro*. The functional consequence of such an interaction was a significant reduction in the oral bioavailability of fexofenadine in human plasma levels, possibly by preferential direct inhibition of intestinal OATP activity [29]. These findings suggest that apple might interact with OATP substrates (e.g., estrone-3-sulfate, deltorphin II, fexofenadine, vasopressin, and rosuvastatin).

5.11. Papaya (*Carican papaya* L.)

Papaya is prized worldwide for its flavor and nutritional properties. An ethno-botanical survey showed that papaya is commonly used in traditional medicine for the treatment of various human diseases, including abdominal discomfort, pain, malaria, diabetes, obesity, infections, and oral drug poisoning [111,112]. Papaya leaves and seeds are known to contain proteolytic enzymes (papain, chymopapain), alkaloids (carpain, carpasemine), sulfurous compounds (benzyl iso- thiocyanate), flavonoids, tannins, triterpenes, anthocyanins, organic acids and oils. Papaya fruit is a good source of nutrients and some phytochemicals such as beta-cryptoxanthin and benzyl isothiocyanates [113]. Hidaka et al. found that *papaya* produced an inhibition of CYP3A activity in human microsomes [114]. So far, there has been no clinical report suggesting adverse food-drug interaction caused by the intake of papaya. Accordingly, the inhibition of CYP3A by papaya may not be observed in vivo. However, the results obtained by others raised the hypothesis that papaya extracts were capable of altering the pharmacokinetics of therapeutic drugs coadministered via CYP3A inhibition, as in the case of grapefruit. Thus, the possibility of adverse food-drug interaction involving papaya and medicine acting via CYP3A metabolism should be examined in vivo. The empirical evidence regarding the wide use of fermented papaya preparation (FPP), especially by elderly people, has indicated an unknown collateral effect, i.e., drops in blood sugar levels, especially in the afternoon. Those findings have been corroborated by a clinical study that shows that FPP use can induce a significant decrease in plasma sugar levels in both healthy subjects and type 2 diabetic patients [115]. Therefore, patients consuming papaya and taking antidiabetic therapy could suffer from potential drug-food interaction.

5.12. Leafy vegetables

Broccoli (*Brassica oleracea var. italica)* and cauliflower (*Brassica oleracea var. botrytis)* are unique among the common cruciferous vegetables that contain high levels of the aliphatics glucosinolate and glucoraphanin [116]. Upon hydrolysis, glucoraphanin produces several products that include the bioactive isothiocyanate sulforaphane. The percentage of isothiocyanate sulforaphane present in these vegetables may vary depending on conditions of hydrolysis, food handling, and preparation procedures [117, 118]. In animal studies, dietary freeze-dried broccoli was found to offer protection against several cancers [119]. However, broccoli, cauliflower and their glucosinolate hydrolysis products have been shown to induce phase I and phase II drug-metabolizing enzymes in intact liver cells from both rats and humans. The isothiocyanate sulforaphane decreased the enzyme activities hepatocytes associated with CYP1A1 and 2B1/2, namely ethoxyresorufin-O-deethylase and pentoxyresorufin-O-dealkylase, respectively, in a dose-dependent manner [120]. An increase in hGSTA1/2 mRNA has been observed in isothiocyanate sulforaphane-treated human hepatocytes, whereas the expression of CYP3A4, the major CYP in the human liver, markedly decreased at both mRNA and activity levels [121]. Conversely, it was recently shown that sulforaphane induces mRNA levels of MRP1 and MRP2 in primary hepatocytes and Caco-2 cells [122]. It has been additionally reported that broccoli is able to induce the activity of phenolsulfotransferases [123]. These results suggest that other vegetables with a high content of isothiocyanates, such as those of the family *Cruciferae* (e.g., cabbage, cauliflower, Brussels sprouts, watercress, broccoli, and kale) and the genus *Raphanus* (radishes and daikons) may have pharmacological and toxicological implications in humans.

Watercress is another important member of the cruciferous vegetables, an excellent source for glucosinolates and other bioactive phytochemicals [124]. Watercress (*Nasturtium officinale)* is an exceptionally rich dietary source of beta-phenylethyl isothiocyanate (PEITC) [125]. Previous studies have shown that a single ingestion of watercress inhibits the hydroxylation of chlorzoxazone, an *in vivo* probe for CYP2E1, in healthy volunteers [126]. It has also been shown that watercress is a bifunctional agent with the ability to induce both phase I (CYP450) and II enzymes. Adding watercress juice to human liver cells induced the activity of CYP450 1A and ethoxyresorufin-O-deethylase and NAD(P)H-quinone reductase [127]. According to reports, PEITC also has several anti-carcinogenic effects given that it can inhibit phase I enzymes and/or activate phase II enzymes. Watercress juice can increase the enzymes *SOD* and *GPX* in blood cells *in vitro* and *in vivo* [128]. Isothiocyanates also interact with ATP-binding cassette (ABC) efflux transporters such as P-glycoprotein, MRP1, MRP2 and BCRP, and may influence the pharmacokinetics of substrates of these transporters [26]. According to current data, watercress and isothiocyanate may have clinical repercussions by inducing changes in the bioavailability of some drugs.

Spinach (*Spinacia oleracea)* is an important antioxidant vegetable usually consumed after boiling the fresh or frozen leaves [129]. Freshly cut spinach leaves contain approximately 1,000 mg of total flavonoids per kilogram, and the occurrence of at least 10 flavonoid glycosides has been reported [130]. These are glucuronides and acylated di-and triglycosides of methylated and methylene dioxide derivatives of 6-oxygenated flavonols [131]. While epidemiological and preclinical data support the nutritional benefits of spinach and the safety of its consumption there are no publications about its effects on drug metabolizing enzymes and drug transporters. Little is currently known about the *in vivo* effects these compounds have on the bioavailability of xenobiotics the clearance and/or tissue distribution of which is determined by active transport and biotransformation. Platt and others [132] reported the protective effect of spinach against the genotoxic effects of 2-amino-3-methylimidazo[4,5-f]quinoline (IQ) by interaction with CYP1A2 as a mechanism of anti-genotoxicity. Its high isothiocyanate and flavonoid content demands additional research to evaluate possible nutrient-drug interactions.

5.13. Vegetable fruits

Tomatoes (*Lycopersicon esculentum)* and tomato-based products are a source of important nutrients and contain numerous phytochemicals, such as carotenoids, that may influence health (carotenoids such as phytofluene, phytoene, neurosporene, γ-carotene, and ζ-carotene) [133,134]. Tomatoes are also a source of a vast array of flavonols (e.g., quercetin and kaempferol), phytosterols, and phenylpropanoids [135]. Lycopene is the most important carotenoid present in tomatoes and tomato products, and their dietary intake has been linked to a decreased risk of chronic illnesses such as cancer and cardiovascular disease [136,137]. Studies performed on human recombinant CYP1 showed that lycopene inhibits CYP1A1 and CYP1B1. Lycopene has also been shown to slightly reduce the induction of ethoxyresorufin-*O*-deethylase activity by 20% by DMBA in MCF-7 cells [138]. It appears to inhibit bioactivation enzymes and induce detoxifying enzymes. It has been suggested that lycopene might have a potential advantage over other phytochemicals by facilitating the elimination of genotoxic chemicals and their metabolites [138]. Recent *in vitro* evidence suggests that high dose lycopene supplementation increases hepatic cytochrome P4502E1 protein and inflammation in alcohol-fed rats [139].

Carrots (*Daucus carrota)* are widely consumed as food. The active components of carrots, which include beta-carotene and panaxynol have been studied by many researchers [140-142]. Carrots induce phenolsulfotransferase activity [123] and decrease CYP1A2 activity [122]. It has been reported that a carrot diet increased the activity of ethoxycoumarin O-deethylase ECD activity in a mouse model [143].

Avocado (*Persea americana*) is a good source of bioactive compounds such as monounsaturated fatty acids and sterols [144]. Growing evidence on the health benefits of avocadoes have led to increased consumption and research on potential health benefits [145, 146]. Phytochemicals extracted from avocado can selectively induce several biological functions [147,148]. Two papers published in the 1990's reported avocados interact with warfarin, stating that the fruit inhibited the effect of warfarin. They, however, did not establish the cause of such inhibition [149, 150].

Red pepper (*Capsicum annuum* L.) is used as a spice that enhances the palatability of food and drugs such as the counterirritant present in stomach medicines across many countries [151]. The pungencyof red pepper is derived from a group of compounds called capsaicinoids, which possess an array of biological properties and give it its spicy flavor. Two major capsaicinoids, dihydrocapsaicin (DHC) and capsaicin (CAP) are responsible for up to 90% of the total pungency of pepper fruits. Red pepper has several uses as a fruit stimulant and rubifacient in traditional medicine; it is also used in the treatment of some diseases such as scarlatina, putrid sore throat, hoarseness, dispepsia, yellow fever, piles and snakebite [152]. Capsaicin (8-methyl-N-vanillyl-6-nonenamide) is a fundamental component of *Capsicum* fruits. Capsaicin is known to have antioxidant properties and has therefore been associated with potent antimutagenic and anticarcinogenic activities [153]. Early studies have reported that capsaicin strongly inhibited the constitutive enzymes CYP 2A2, 3A1, 2C11, 2B1, 2B2 and 2C6 [154]. There is also a report indicating that capsaicin is a substrate of CYP1A2 [155]. Pharmacokinetic studies in animals have shown that a single dose of *Capsicum* fruit could affect the pharmacokinetic parameters of theophylline, while a repeated dose affected the metabolic pathway of xanthine oxidase [156]. Therefore, a potential interaction may occur when is taken along with some medicines that are CYP450 substrates. Recently, it has been evidenced that red pepper induces alterations in intestinal brush border fluidity and passive permeability properties associated with the induction of increased microvilli length and perimeter, resulting in an increased absorptive surface for the small intestine and an increased bioavailability not only of micronutrients but also of drugs [157]. Cruz et al. have shown that pepper ingestion reduces oral salicylate bioavailability, a likely result of the gastrointestinal effects of capsaicin [158]. On the other hand, Imaizumi et al. have reported capsaicinoid-induced changes of glucose in rats. Therefore, there is a possible interaction risk between red pepper and hypoglycemic drugs in diabetic patients [159]. Patients consuming red pepper and taking antidiabetic therapy could suffer potential drug-food interaction.

5.14. Other vegetables

Yeh and Yen have reported that asparagus, cauliflower, celery and eggplant induced significant phenol sulfotransferase –P (PST-P) activity, whereas asparagus, eggplant and potato induced PST-M activity [123]. It has been have also reported that a diet supplemented with apiaceous vegetables (dill weed, celery, parsley, parsnip) resulted in a 13-15% decrease in CYP1A2 activity [122]. The authors speculate that furanocumarins present in the apiaceous vegetables were responsible for the inhibitory effects on CYP1A2 ^115 [117,160].

Vegetables such as cabbage, celery, onion and parsley are known to have a high content of polyphenols. It has been reported that polyphenols can potentially affect phase I metabolism either by direct inhibition of phase I enzymes or by regulating the expression of enzyme levels *via* their interactions with regulatory cascades. Several studies have directly and indirectly shown that dietary polyphenols can modulate phase II metabolism [161]. In addition, polyphenols have been shown to interact with ABC drug transporters involved in drug resistance and drug absorption, distribution and excretion [32].

6. Drug-food interaction in specific diets with high content of fruits and vegetables

Weight-reduction diets, vegetarian diets, hospitalization, or post-operative regimes all lead to dietary modifications. These diets are often maintained for long periods of time and are likely to result in metabolic changes due to subsequently administered drugs or exposure to environmental chemicals. Several epidemiologic, clinical, and experimental studies have established that certain types of diet may have beneficial effects on health. For example, the traditional Mediterranean diet has been shown to reduce overall mortality and coronary heart disease events [162]. This diet, however, varies across at least 16 countries bordering the Mediterranean Sea. Cultural, ethnic, religious, economic and agricultural differences in these regions account for variations in dietary patterns, which are widely characterized by the following: daily consumption of fruits, vegetables, whole grain breads, non-refined cereals, olive oil, and dairy products; moderate weekly consumption of fish, poultry, nuts, potatoes, and eggs; low monthly consumption of red meat, and daily moderate wine consumption [163]. Increasing evidence suggests that a Mediterranean-style diet rich in fruits, vegetables, nuts, fish and oils with monounsaturated fat and low in meat promotes cardiovascular health and aids cancer prevention because of its positive effects on lipid profile, endothelial function, vascular inflammation, insulin resistance, and its antioxidant properties [164,165].

Vegetarians, on the other hand, exhibit a wide diversity of dietary practices often described by what is omitted from their diet. When a vegetarian diet is appropriately planned and includes fortified foods, it can be nutritionally suitable for adults and children and can promote health and lower the risk of major chronic diseases [166]. A vegetarian diet usually provides a low intake of saturated fat and cholesterol and a high intake of dietary fiber and many health-promoting phytochemicals. This is achieved by an increased consumption of fruits, vegetables, whole-grains, legumes, nuts, and various soy products. As a result of these factors, vegetarians typically have a lower body mass index, low-density lipoprotein cholesterol levels, and lower blood pressure; a reduced ischemic heart disease death rate; and decreased incidence of hypertension, stroke, type 2 diabetes, and certain cancers that are more common among non-vegetarians [167]. The vegan dietary category may be more comparable across countries and cultures because avoiding all animal products leaves little choice but to include large quantities of vegetables, fruit, nuts, and grains for nutritional adequacy. Admittedly, vegetable and fruit variety may also vary widely according to location [168].

Due to their high content of fruits and vegetables, all these diets contain a large proportion of antioxidant vitamins, flavonoids, and polyphenols [169]. Phenolic compounds may help protect the gastrointestinal tract against damage by reactive species present in foods or generated within the stomach and intestines. However, they may be beneficial in the gut in correct amounts. The overall health benefits of polyphenols are uncertain, and consumption of large quantities of them in fortified foods or supplements should not yet be encouraged [170].

Flavonoids have been known as plant pigments for over a century and belong to a vast group of phenolic compounds that are widely distributed in all foods of plant origin. Unfortunately, the potentially toxic effects of excessive flavonoid intake are largely ignored. At higher doses, flavonoids may act as mutagens, pro-oxidants that generate free radicals, and as inhibitors of key enzymes involved in hormone metabolism [171]. It has been shown that phenol ring-containing flavonoids yield cytotoxic phenoxyl radicals upon oxidation by peroxidases; co-oxidize unsaturated lipids, GSH, NADH, ascorbate, and nucleic acids; and cause ROS formation and mitochondrial toxicity [172]. In high doses, the adverse effects of flavonoids may outweigh their beneficial ones, and caution should be exercised when ingesting them at levels above those which would be obtained from a typical vegetarian diet [173]. Moreover, it is possible that people ingesting a vegetarian or Mediterranean diet may be taking medication and thus have drug-food interaction.

Inhibition of CYP enzymes, which are necessary for carcinogen activation, is a beneficial chemopreventive property of various flavonoids but may be a potential toxic property in flavonoid-drug interactions. Inhibition of CYP activities by flavonoids has been extensively studied because of their potential use as blocking agents during the initial stage of carcinogenesis [174]. The general conclusion after an analysis of available data on CYP-flavonoid interactions is that flavonoids possessing hydroxyl groups inhibit CYP activity, whereas those lacking hydroxyl groups may induce the metabolizing enzyme [175]. Flavonoids can either inhibit or induce human CYP enzymes depending on their structure, concentration, or experimental conditions [176]. The interaction of flavonoids with CYP3A4, the predominant human hepatic and intestinal CYP responsible for metabolizing 50% of therapeutic agents as well as the activation of some carcinogens, is of particular interest [177].

The simultaneous administration of flavonoids present in fruits or vegetables and clinically used drugs may cause flavonoid-drug interactions by modulating the pharmacokinetics of certain drugs, which results in an increase in their toxicity or a decline in their therapeutic effect, depending on the flavonoid structure [178]. Additional reasons for concern regarding mega flavonoid supplements include potential flavonoid-drug interactions, since flavonoids have been shown to both induce and inhibit drug-metabolizing enzymes [38, 39]. Further research regarding the potential toxicities associated with flavonoids and other dietary phenolics is required if these plant-derived products are to be used as therapy.

It is a fact that diets based on fruits and vegetables may have a variety of phytochemicals, as was mentioned earlier, so the possibility of developing a drug-food interaction is high. While dietary polyphenols may be beneficial in the correct amount, but too much may not be good and combining them with medication should be avoided.

7. Conclusion

WHO and the Food and Agriculture Organization of the United Nations (FAO) recommend a daily intake of at least 400 grams or five servings of fruits and vegetables to aid in the prevention of chronic illnesses such as heart disease, cancer, diabetes, and obesity. As a consequence, there is an increased global consumer demand for fruits and vegetables, and some consumers purchase organic foods with the understanding that they are healthy. The use of natural products for improving human health has evolved independently in different regions of the world and production, use, attitudes, and regulatory aspects vary globally. Although modern medicine may be available in most countries for the treatment of many chronic degenerative diseases, folk medicine (phytomedicine) has remained popular for historical and cultural reasons. Although the significance of interactions between drugs is widely appreciated, little attention has been given to interactions between drugs and nutrients. Most of the documented information about the effects of fruit and vegetables on metabolizing enzymes and drug transporters comes from preclinical studies. However, the possibility that these effects could occur in humans should not be ignored. Several clinical studies on the interactions of grapefruit juice and drugs have been conducted with impressive results. Most of the fruits and vegetables examined in this review contain a similar phytochemical mix to that of grapefruit juice. *In vitro* models and animal models have shown that many of these agents influence drug metabolizing enzymes and drug transporters. It is possible that other fruits and vegetables could have the same potential for fruit and drug interactions, and this should be taken into account. This review shows evidence of the influence of fruit, vegetables or their components (phytochemicals) on the CYP3A4 enzyme, which metabolizes most drugs used by the human population. A more consistent approach to the evaluation of nutrient-drug interactions in human beings is therefore needed. Said approach must be systematic in order to a) assess the influence of nutritional status, foodstuffs, or specific nutrients on a drug's pharmacokinetics and pharmacodynamics, and b) evaluate the influence of a drug on overall nutritional status or the status of a specific nutrient. In addition to all this, we must account for the fact that we live in an era of very varied lifestyles. Some people are vegetarians, others take high doses of flavonoids or antioxidants as supplements, some ingest large amounts of bottled water from plastic bottles, or use chlorinated disinfectants. In industrialized countries, fruits and vegetables tend have been subjected to some sort of processing (e.g., refrigeration, acidification, fermentation, and thermal, high pressure, chemical, or physical processing) that might have an effect on the bioactive compound. All of these factors could have an impact on the metabolism or transport of drugs in a individual, potentially altering pharmacological responses. Our knowledge regarding the potential risk of nutrient-drug interactions is still limited. Therefore, efforts to elucidate potential risk of food-drug interactions should be intensified in order to prevent undesired and harmful clinical consequences.

http://dx.doi.org/10.5772/48283

Author details

Lourdes Rodríguez-Fragoso* and Jorge Reyes-Esparza

*Address all correspondence to: mrodriguezf@uaem.mx

Universidad Autónoma del Estado de Morelos, Facultad de Farmacia, Cuernavaca, México

References

[1] Liu RH (2004) Potential synergy of phytochemicals in cancer prevention: mechanism of action. J. Nutr. 134:3479S-3485S.

[2] Milner JA (2004) Molecular targets for bioactive food components. J. Nutr. 134: 2492s-2498s.

[3] Liu RH (2003) Health benefits of fruit and vegetables are from additive and synergistic combinations of phytochemicals. Am. J. Clin. Nutr. 78: 517S-5120S.

[4] Custodio JM, Wu CY, Benet LZ (2008) Predicting drug disposition, absorption/elimination/transporter interplay and the role of food on drug absorption. Adv. Drug Deliv. Rev. 60:717-733.

[5] Franco OH, Bonneux L, de Laet C, Peeters A, Steyerberg EW, Mackenbach JP (2004) The Polymeal: a more natural, safer, and probably tastier (than the Polypill) strategy to reduce cardiovascular disease by more than 75%. BMJ 329:1447-1450.

[6] Ortega RM (2006) Importance of functional foods in the Mediterranean diet. Public Health Nutr. 9(8A):1136-1140.

[7] Dangour AD, Lock K, Hayter A, Aikenhead A, Allen E, Uauy R (2010) Nutrition-related health effects of organic foods: a systematic review. Am. J. Clin. Nutr. 92:203-210.

[8] Santos CA, and Boullata JI (2005) An Approach to Evaluating Drug-Nutrient Interactions. Pharmacother. 25: 1789-1800.

[9] Genser D (2008) Food and Drug Interaction: Consequences for the Nutrition/Health Status. Ann. Nutr. Metab. 52: 29-32.

[10] Singh BN, Malhotra BK (2004) Effects of food on the clinical pharmacokinetics of anticancer agents: underlying mechanisms and implications for oral chemotherapy. Clin. Pharmacokinet. 43:1127-1156.

[11] Malhotra S, Bailey DG, Paine MF, Watkins PB (2001) Seville orange juice-felodipine interaction: comparison with dilute grapefruit juice and involvement of furocoumarins. Clin. Pharmacol. Ther. 69: 14-23.

[12] Schmidt LE, Dalhoff K (2002) Food-drug interactions. Drugs 62:1481-1502.

[13] Chan LN (2006) Drug-Nutrient Interactions; in Shils ME, Shike M, Ross AC, Caballero B, Cousins RJ (eds) In: Modern Nutrition in Health and Disease. Lippincott Williams & Wilkins, 1540 p.

[14] Muntané J (2009) Regulation of drug metabolism and transporters. Curr. Drug Metab. 10: 932-995.

[15] Sai Y (2005) Biochemical and molecular pharmacological aspects of transporters as determinants of drug disposition. Drug Metab. Pharmacokinet. 20: 91-99.

[16] Zhang L, Zhang YD, Strong JM, Reynolds KS, Huang S M (2008). A regulatory viewpoint on transporter based drug interactions. Xenobiotica 38: 709-724.

[17] Ayrton A, Morgan P (2001) Role of transport proteins in drug absorption, distribution and excretion. Xenobiotica 8: 469-497.

[18] Li P, Wang GJ, Robertson TA, Roberts MS (2009) Liver transporters in hepatic drug disposition: an update. Curr. Drug Metab. 10:482-498.

[19] Kohl C (2009) Transporters--the view from industry. Chem. Biodivers. 6: 1988-1999.

[20] The International Transporter Consortium (2010) Membrane transporters in drug development. Drug Discovery. Macmillan Publishers Limited , 215 p.

[21] VanWert AL, Gionfriddo MR, Sweet DH (2010) Organic Anion transporters: Discovery, Pharmacology, Regulation and Roles in Pathophysiology. Biopharm. Drug Dispos. 31: 1-71.

[22] Hagenbuch B, Gui C (2008) Xenobiotic transporters of the human organic anion transporting polypeptides (OATP) family. Xenobiotica 38: 778–801.

[23] Schinkel A H, Jonker J W (2003) Mammalian drug efflux transporters of the ATP binding cassette (ABC) family: an overview. Adv. Drug Deliv. Rev. 55: 3-29.

[24] Huang SM, Strong JM, Zhang L, Reynolds KS, Nallani S, Temple R, Abraham S, Habet SA, Baweja RK, Burckart GJ, Chung S, Colangelo P, Frucht D, Green MD, Hepp P, Karnaukhova E, Ko HS, Lee JI, Marroum PJ, Norden JM, Qiu W, Rahman A, Sobel S, Stifano T, Thummel K, Wei XX, Yasuda S, Zheng JH, Zhao H, Lesko LJ (2008). New era in drug interaction evaluation: US Food and Drug Administration update on CYP enzymes, transporters, and the guidance process. J Clin. Pharmacol. 48: 662–670.

[25] Wink M (2008) Evolutionary Advantage and Molecular Modes of Action of Multi-Component Mixtures Used in Phytomedicine. Curr Drug Metab 9: 996-1009.

[26] Telang U, Ji Y, Morris ME (2009) ABC Transporters and Isothiocyanates: Potential for Pharmacokinetic Diet–Drug Interactions. Biopharm. Drug Dispos. 30: 335-344.

[27] Huang SM Hall SD, Watkins P, Love LA, Serabjit-Singh C, Betz JM, Hoffman FA, Honig P, Coates PM, Bull J, Chen ST, Kearms GL, Murray MD (2004). Drug interac-

tions with herbal products & grapefruit juice: a conference report. Clin. Pharmacol. Ther. 75: 1-12.

[28] Tomlinson B, Hu M, Lee VW (20089 In vivo assessment of herb-drug interactions: Possible utility of a pharmacogenetic approach? Mol. Nut. Food Res. 52: 799-809.

[29] Dresser GK, Bailey DG, Leake BF, Schwarz UI, Dawson PA, Freeman DJ, Kim RB (2002). Fruit juices inhibit organic anion transporting polypeptide-mediated drug uptake. Clin. Pharmacol. Ther. 71: 11-20.

[30] Meijerman I, Beijnen JH, Schellensa JH (2006) Herb–Drug Interactions in Oncology: Focus on Mechanisms of Induction. Oncol. 11: 742-752.

[31] Zhou S, Lim LY, Chowbay B (2004) Herbal modulation of P-glycoprotein. Drug Metab. Rev. 36: 57-104

[32] Alvarez AI, Real R, Perez M, Mendoza G, Prieto JG, Merino G (2010) Modulation of the activity of ABC transporters (P-glycoprotein, MRP2, BCRP) by flavonoids and drug response. Pharm. Sci. 99: 598-617.

[33] Rushmore TH, Kong AN (2002). Pharmacogenomics, Regulation and Signaling Pathways of Phase I and II Drug Metabolizing Enzymes. Curr. Drug Metab. 3: 481- 490.

[34] Watkins PB (1992) Drug metabolism by cytochromes P450 in liver and small bowel. Gastrointerol. Clin. North Am. 21: 511-526.

[35] Rendic S (2002) Summary of information on human CYP enzymes: human P450 metabolism data. Drug Metab. Rev. 34: 83-448.

[36] Iyanagi T (2007) Molecular mechanism of phase I and phase II drug-metabolizing enzymes: implications for detoxification. Int. Rev. Cytol. 260: 35-112.

[37] [37] Xu C, Li CYL and Kong ANT (2005) Induction of Phase I, II and III Drug Metabolism/Transport by Xenobiotics. Arch. Pharm. Res. 28: 249-268.

[38] [38] Saxena A, Tripathi KP, Roy S, Khan F, Sharma A (2008) Pharmacovigilance: Effects of herbal components on human drugs interactions involving Cytochrome P450. Bioinformation 3: 198-204.

[39] Foti RS, Wienkers LC, Wahlstrom JL (2010). Application of Cytochrome P450 Drug Interaction Screening in Drug Discovery. Comb Chem High Throughput Screen 13:145-158.

[40] Walter-Sack I, Klotz U (1996). Influence of diet and nutritional status on drug metabolism. Clin. Pharmacokinet. 31: 47-64.

[41] Mandlekar S, Hong JL, Kong AN (2006) Modulation of Metabolic Enzymes by Dietary Phytochemicals: A Review of Mechanisms Underlying Beneficial Versus Unfavorable Effects. Curr. Drug Metab. 7: 661-675.

[42] Nahrstedt A, Butterweck V (2010) Lessons learned from herbal medicinal products: the example of St. John's Wort (perpendicular). J. Nat. Prod. 28: 1015-1021.

[43] Kimura Y, Ito H, Ohnishi R, Hatano T (2010) Inhibitory effects of polyphenols on human cytochrome P450 3A4 and 2C9 activity. Food Chem. Toxicol. 48: 429-435.

[44] World Health Organization (2003) Diet, nutrition, and the prevalence of chronic diseases. Geneva, Switzerland: World Health Organization. Contract No.: WHO Technical Report Series No. 916.

[45] Flanagan D (2005) Understanding the grapefruit-drug interaction. Gen. Dent. 53: 282-285.

[46] Cuciureanu M, Vlase L, Muntean D, Varlan I, Cuciureanu R (2010) Grapefruit juice--drug interactions: importance for pharmacotherapy. Rev. Med. Chir. Soc. Med. Nat. Iasi 114:885-891.

[47] Hanley MJ, Cancalon P, Widmer WW, Greenblatt DJ (2011). The effect of grapefruit juice on drug disposition. Expert Opin. Drug Metab. Toxicol. 7: 267-286.

[48] Bressler R (2006) Grapefruit juice and drug interactions. Exploring mechanisms of this interaction and potential toxicity for certain drugs. Geriatrics 61:12-18.

[49] Kim H, Yoon YJ, Shon JH, Cha IJ, Shin JG, Liu KH (2006). Inhibitory effects of fruit juices on CYP3A activity. Drug Metab. Dispos. 34: 521-523.

[50] Honda Y, Ushigome F, Koyabu N, Morimoto S, Shoyama Y, Uchiumi T, Kuwano M, Ohtani H, Sawada Y (2004) Effects of grapefruit juice and orange juice components on P-glycoprotein- and MRP2-mediated drug efflux. Br. J. Pharmacol. 143: 856-864.

[51] Konishi T, Satsu H, Hatsugai Y, Aizawa K, Inakuma T, Nagata S, Sakuda SH, Nagasawa H, Shimizu M (2004) Inhibitory effect of a bitter melon extract on the P-glycoprotein activity in intestinal Caco-2 cells. Br. J. Pharmacol. 143: 379-387.

[52] Yoo HH, Lee M, Chung HJ, Lee SK, Kim DH (2007) Effects of diosmin, a flavonoid glycoside in citrus fruits, on P-glycoprotein-mediated drug efflux in human intestinal Caco-2 cells. J. Agric. Food Chem. 55: 7620-7625.

[53] Satoh H, Yamashita F, Tsujimoto M, Murakami H, Koyabu N, Ohtani H, Sawada Y (2005) Citrus juices inhibit the function of human organic anion-transporting polypeptide OATP-B. Drug Metab. Dispos. 33. 518-523.

[54] Greenblatt DJ (2009) Analysis of drug interactions involving fruit beverages and organic anion-transporting polypeptides. J. Clin. Pharmacol. 49: 1403-1407.

[55] Takanaga H, Ohnishi A, Yamada S, Matsuo H, Morimoto S, Shoyama Y, Ohtani H, Sawada Y (2000) Polymethoxylated flavones in orange juice are inhibitors of P-glycoprotein but not cytochrome P450 3A4. J. Pharmacol. Exp. Ther. 293: 230-236.

[56] Hidaka M, Okumura M, Fujita K, Ogikubo T, Yamasaki K, Iwakiri T, Setoguchi N, Arimori K (2005) Effects of pomegranate juice on human cytochrome p450 3A

(CYP3A) and carbamazepine pharmacokinetics in rats. Drug Metab. Dispos. 33: 644-648.

[57] Sica DA (2006) Interaction of grapefruit juice and calcium channel blockers. Am. J. Hypertens. 19: 768-773.

[58] Pawełczyk T, Kłoszewska I (2008) Grapefruit juice interactions with psychotropic drugs: advantages and potential risk. Przegl Lek. 65: 92-95.

[59] Reamy BV, Stephens MB (2007) The grapefruit-drug interaction debate: role of statins. Am. Fam. Phys. 76: 190-192.

[60] Paine MF, Widmer WW, Pusek SN, Beavers KL, Criss AB, Snyder J, Watkins PB (2008) Further characterization of a furanocoumarin-free grapefruit juice on drug disposition: studies with cyclosporine. Am. J. Clin. Nutr. 87: 863-871.

[61] Van den Bout-Van den Beukel CJ, Koopmans PP, van der Ven AJ, De Smet PA, Burger DM (2006) Possible drug-metabolism interactions of medicinal herbs with antiretroviral agents. Drug Metab. Rev. 38: 477-514.

[62] Bailey DG, Dresser GK. (2004) Interactions between grapefruit juice and cardiovascular drugs. Am. J. Cardiovasc. Drugs 4: 281-297.

[63] Dresser GK, Kim RB, Bailey DG (2005) Effect of grapefruit juice volume on the reduction of fexofenadine bioavailability: possible role of organic anion transporting polypeptides. Clin. Pharmacol. Ther. 77: 170-177.

[64] Amory JK, Amory DW (2005) Oral erythromycin and the risk of sudden death. N. Engl. J. Med. 352: 301-304.

[65] Saito M, Hirata-Koizumi M, Matsumoto M, Urano T, Hasegawa R (2005) Undesirable effects of citrus juice on the pharmacokinetics of drugs: focus on recent studies. Drug Saf. 28: 677-694.

[66] Kiani J, Imam S (2007) Medicinal importance of grapefruit juice and its interaction with various drugs. Nutr. J. 6: 33-35.

[67] Pillai U, Muzaffar J, Sen S, Yancey A (2009) Grapefruit juice and verapamil: a toxic cocktail. South Med. J. 102: 308-309.

[68] Ho PC, Saville DJ, Coville PF, Wanwimolruk S (2000) Content of CYP3A4 inhibitors, naringin, naringenin and bergapten in grapefruit and grapefruit juice products. Pharm. Acta Helv. 74:379-385.

[69] Kamath AV, Yao M, Zhang Y, Chon S (2005) Effect of fruit juices on the oral bioavailability of fexofenadine in rats. J. Pharm. Sci. 94: 233-239.

[70] Farkas D, Greenblatt DJ (2008) Influence of fruit juices on drug disposition: discrepancies between in vitro and clinical studies. Expert Opin. Drug Metab. Toxicol. 4: 381-393.

[71] Lilja JJ, Juntti-Patinen L, Neuvonen PJ (2004) Orange juice substantially reduces the bioavailability of the beta-adrenergic-blocking agent celiprolol. Clin. Pharmacol. Ther. 75: 184-190.

[72] Lilja JJ, Raaska K, Neuvonen PJ (2005) Effects of orange juice on the pharmacokinetics of atenolol. Eur. J. Clin. Pharmacol. 61: 337-340.

[73] Obermeier MT, White RE, Yang CS (1995) Effects of bioflavonoids on hepatic P450 activities. Xenobiotica 25: 575-584.

[74] Backman JT, Maenppa J, Belle DJ, Wrighton SA, Kivisto KT, Neuvonen PJ (2000) Lack of correlation between in vitro and in vivo studies on the effects of tangeretin and tangerine juice on midazolam hydroxylation. Clin. Pharmacol. Ther. 67, 382–390.

[75] Yadav M, Jain S, Bhardwaj A, Nagpal R, Puniya M, Tomar R, Singh V, Parkash O, Prasad GB, Marotta F, Yadav H (2009) Biological and medicinal properties of grapes and their bioactive constituents: an update. J. Med. Food 12: 473-484.

[76] Vislocky LM, Fernandez ML (2010) Biomedical effects of grape products. Nutr. Rev. 68:656-670.

[77] Chan WK, Delucchi BA (2000) Resveratrol, a red wine constituent, is a mechanism-based inactivator of cytochrome P450 3A4. Life Sci. 67: 3103-3112.

[78] Piver B, Berthou F, Dreano Y, Lucas D (2001) Inhibition of CYP3A, CYP1A and CYP2E1 activities by resveratrol and other non volatile red wine components. Toxicol. Let. 125: 83-91.

[79] Rossi R, Porta S, Canovi B (2010) Overview on cranberry and urinary tract infections in females. J. Clin. Gastroenterol. 44:S61-S62.

[80] Côté J, Caillet S, Doyon G, Sylvain JF, Lacroix M (2010) Bioactive compounds in cranberries and their biological properties. Crit. Rev. Food Sci. Nutr. 50:666-679.

[81] Izzo AA (2005) Herb–drug interactions: an overview of the clinical evidence. Fundam. Clin. Pharmacol. 19:1–16.

[82] Pham DQ, Pham AQ (2007) Interaction potential between cranberry juice and warfarin. Am. J. Health Syst. Pharm. 64: 490-494.

[83] Ushijima K, Tsuruoka S, Tsuda H, Hasegawa G, Obi Y, Kaneda T, Takahashi M, Maekawa T, Sasaki T, Koshimizu TA, Fujimura A (2009) Cranberry juice suppressed the diclofenac metabolism by human liver microsomes, but not in healthy human subjects. Br. J. Clin. Pharmacol. 68: 194-200.

[84] Uesawa Y, Mohri K (2006) Effects of cranberry juice on nifedipine pharmacokinetics in rats. J. Pharm. Pharmacol. 58: 1067-1072.

[85] Shabtay A, Eitam H, Tadmor Y, Orlov A, Meir A, Weinberg P, Weinberg ZG, Chen Y, Brosh A, Izhaki I, Kerem Z (2008) Nutritive and antioxidative potential of fresh and

stored pomegranate industrial byproduct as a novel beef cattle feed. J. Agric. Food Chem. 56:10063-10070

[86] Ross SM (2009) Pomegranate: its role in cardiovascular health. Holist Nurs. Pract. 23:195-197.

[87] Oliveira RA, Narciso CD, Bisinotto RS, Perdomo MC, Ballou MA, Dreher M, Santos JE (2010) Effects of feeding polyphenols from pomegranate extract on health, growth, nutrient digestion, and immunocompetence of calves. J. Dairy Sci. 93:4280-4291

[88] Nagata M, Hidaka M, Sekiya H, Kawano Y, Yamasaki K, Okumura M, Arimori K (2007) Effects of pomegranate juice on human cytochrome P450 2C9 and tolbutamide pharmacokinetics in rats. Drug Metab. Dispos. 35:302-305.

[89] Saruwatari A, Okamura S, Nakajima Y, Narukawa Y, Takeda T, Tamura H (2008) Pomegranate juice inhibits sulfoconjugation in Caco-2 human colon carcinoma cells. J. Med. Food 11: 623-628.

[90] Knodler M, Conrad J, Wenzig EM, Bauer R, Lacorn M, Beifuss U, Carle R, Schieber A (2008) Anti-inflammatory 5-(11′Z-heptadecenyl)- and 5-(8′Z,11′Z-heptadecadienyl)-resorcinols from mango (Mangifera indica L.) peels. Phytochemistry 69: 988-993.

[91] Engels C, Knodler M, Zhao YY, Carle R, Ganzle MG, Schieber A (2009) Antimicrobial activity of gallotannins isolated from mango (Mangifera indica L.) kernels. J. Agric. Food Chem 57: 7712– 7718.

[92] Schieber A, Berardini N, Carle R (2003) Identification of flavonol and xanthone glycosides from mango (Mangifera indica L. Cv. "Tommy Atkins") peels by high-performance liquid chromatography-electrospray ionization mass spectrometry. J. Agric. Food Chem. 51: 5006-5011.

[93] Berardini N, Fezer R, Conrad J, Beifuss U, Carle R, Schieber A (2005) Screening of mango (Mangifera indica L.) cultivars for their contents of flavonol O- and xanthone C-glycosides, anthocyanins, and pectin. J. Agric. Food Chem. 53: 1563-1570

[94] Bischoff SC (2008) Quercetin: potentials in the prevention and therapy of disease. Curr. Opin. Clin. Nutr. Metab. Care 11: 733-740

[95] Rodeiro I, Donato MT, Lahoz A, Garrido G, Delgado R, Gómez-Lechón MJ (2008) Interactions of polyphenols with the P450 system: possible implications on human therapeutics. Mini Rev. Med. Chem. 8: 97–106.

[96] Rodeiro I, Donato MT, Jimenez N, Garrido G, Molina-Torres J, Menendez R, Castell JV, Gómez-Lechón MJ (2009) Inhibition of human P450 enzymes by natural extracts used in traditional medicine. Phytother. Res. 23: 279-282.

[97] Chieli E, Romiti N, Rodeiro I, Garrido G (2009) In vitro effects of Mangifera indica and polyphenols derived on ABCB1/P-glycoprotein activity. Food Chem. Toxicol. 47: 2703-2710.

[98] Jouad H, Haloui M, Rhiouani H, El Hilaly J, Eddouks M (2001) Ethnobotanical survey of medicinal plants used for the treatment of diabetes, cardiac and renal diseases in the North centre region of Morocco (Fez-Boulemane). J. Ethnopharmacol. 77:175-182.

[99] De Wet H, Nkwanyana MN, van Vuuren SF (2010) Medicinal plants used for the treatment of diarrhoea in northern Maputaland, KwaZulu-Natal Province, South Africa. J. Ethnopharmacol. 130:284-289.

[100] Qian H, Nihorimbere V (2004) Antioxidant power of phytochemicals from Psidium guajava leaf. J. Zhejiang Univ. Sci. 5:676-683.

[101] Junyaprasert VB, Soonthornchareonnon N, Thongpraditchote S, Murakami T, Takano M (2006) Inhibitory effect of Thai plant extracts on P-glycoprotein mediated efflux. Phytother. Res. 20: 79-81.

[102] Patel AV, Rojas-Vera J, Dacke CG (2004) Therapeutic constituents and actions of Rubus species. Curr. Med. Chem. 11:1501-1512.

[103] Zafra-Stone S, Yasmin T, Bagchi M, Chatterjee A, Vinson JA, Bagchi D (2007) Berry anthocyanins as novel antioxidants in human health and disease prevention. Mol. Nutr. Food Res. 51:675-683.

[104] Del Rio D, Borges G, Crozier A (2010) Berry flavonoids and phenolics: bioavailability and evidence of protective effects. Br. J. Nutr. 104:S67-S90.

[105] Wang SY, Lin HS (2000) Antioxidant activity in fruits and leaves of blackberry, raspberry, and strawberry varies with cultivar and developmental stage. J. Agric. Food Chem. 48:140-146.

[106] Juranic Z, Zixack Z (2005) Biological activities of berries: from antioxidant capacity to anti-cancer effects. BioFactors 23: 207-211.

[107] Seeram NP, Adams LS, Zhang Y, Lee R, Sand D, Scheuller HS, Heber D (2006) Blackberry, black raspberry, blueberry, cranberry, red raspberry, and strawberry extracts inhibit growth and stimulate apoptosis of human cancer cells in vitro. J. Agric. Food Chem. 54:9329-9339.

[108] Lewis N, Ruud J (2004) Apples in the American diet. Nutr. Clin. Care 7:82-88.

[109] Gerhauser C (2008) Cancer chemopreventive potential of apples, apple juice, and apple components. Planta Med. 74:1608-1624.

[110] Pohl C, Will F, Dietrich H, Schrenk D (2006) Cytochrome P450 1A1 Expression and Activity in Caco-2 Cells: Modulation by Apple Juice Extract and Certain Apple Polyphenols. J Agric Food Chem 54: 10262-10268.

[111] Nakasone HY, Paull RE. The production of papain—an agri- cultural industry for tropical America. In: Tropical Fruits. CAB International, Wallingford, UK, 1998, pp. 62–79.

[112] Adeneye AA, Olagunju IA (2009) Preliminary hypoglycemic and hypolipidemic activities of the aqueous seed extract of Carica papaya Linn. in Wistar rats. Biol Med, 1: 1–10.

[113] Chavez-Quintal P, Gonzalez-Flores T, Rodriguez-Buenfil I, Gallegos-Tintore S (2011) Antifungal Activity in Ethanolic Extracts of Carica papaya L. cv. Maradol Leaves and Seeds. Indian J Microbiol 51:54–60.

[114] Hidaka M, Fujita K, Ogikubu T, Yamasaki K, Iwakiri T, Okumura M, Arimori K. (2004) Potent inhibition by star fruit of human cytochrome p450 3a (cyp3a) activity. DMD 32:581-583.

[115] Danese C, Esposito D, D'Alfonso V, Cirene M, Ambrosino M, Colotto M (2006) Plasma glucose level decreases as collateral effect of fermented papaya preparation use. Clin Ter 157:195-198

[116] Cartea ME, Francisco M, Soengas P, Velasco P (2010) Phenolic compounds in Brassica vegetables. Molecules 16:251-280.

[117] Tian Q, Rosselot RA, Schwartz SJ (2005) Quantitative determination of intact glucosinolates in broccoli, broccoli sprouts, Brussels sprouts, and cauliflower by high-performance liquid chromatography-electrospray ionization-tandem mass spectrometry. Anal. Biochem. 343:93-99.

[118] Vasanthi HR, Mukherjee S, Das DK (2009) Potential health benefits of broccoli- a chemico-biological overview. Mini Rev. Med. Chem. 9:749-759.

[119] Velasco P, Francisco M, Moreno DA, Ferreres F, García-Viguera C, Cartea ME (2011) Phytochemical fingerprinting of vegetable Brassica oleracea and Brassica napus by simultaneous identification of glucosinolates and phenolics. Phytochem. Anal. 22: 144-152

[120] Anwar-Mohamed A, El-Kadi AO (2009) Sulforaphane induces CYP1A1 mRNA, protein, and catalytic activity levels via an AhR-dependent pathway in murine hepatoma Hepa 1c1c7 and human HepG2 cells. Cancer Lett. 275: 93-101.

[121] Fimognari C, Lenzi M, Hrelia P (2008) Interaction of the isothiocyanate sulforaphane with drug disposition and metabolism: pharmacological and toxicological implications. Curr. Drug Metab. 9: 668-678.

[122] Harris KE, Jeffery EH (2008) Sulforaphane and erucin increase MRP1 and MRP2 in human carcinoma cell lines. J. Nutr. Biochem. 19: 246-254.

[123] Yeh CT, Yen GC (2005) Effect of vegetables on human phenolsulfotransferases in relation to their antioxidant activity and total phenolics. Free Radic. Res. 39: 893-904.

[124] Getahun SM, Chung FL (1999) Conversion of glucosinolates to isothiocyanates in humans after ingestion of cooked watercress. Cancer Epidemiol. Biomarkers Prev. 8:447-451.

[125] Palaniswamy UR, McAvoy RJ, Bible BB, Stuar JD (2003) Ontogenic variations of ascorbic acid and phenethyl isothiocyanate concentrations in watercress (Nasturtium officinale R.Br.) leaves. J. Agric. Food Chem. 51: 5504-5509.

[126] Leclercq I, Desager JP, Horsmans Y (1998) Inhibition of chlorzoxazone metabolism, a clinical probe for CYP2E1, by a single ingestion of watercress. Clin. Pharmacol. Ther. 64: 144-149.

[127] Lhoste EF, Gloux K, De Waziers I, Garrido S, Lory S, Philippe C, Rabot S, Knasmüller S (2004) The activities of several detoxication enzymes are differentially induced by juices of garden cress, water cress and mustard in human HepG2 cells. Chem. Biol. Interact. 150: 211-219.

[128] Hofmann T, Kuhnert A, Schubert A, Gill C, Rowland IR, Pool-Zobel BL, Glei M (2009) Modulation of detoxification enzymes by watercress: in vitro and in vivo investigations in human peripheral blood cells. Eur. J. Nutr. 48: 483-491.

[129] Schirrmacher G, Skurk T, Hauner H, Grassmann J (2010) Effect of Spinacia oleraceae L. and Perilla frutescens L. on antioxidants and lipid peroxidation in an intervention study in healthy individuals. Plant Foods Hum. Nutr .65:71-76

[130] Bergquist SA, Gertsson UE, Knuthsen P, Olsson ME (2005) Flavonoids in baby spinach (Spinacia oleracea L.): changes during plant growth and storage. J. Agric. Food Chem. 53:9459-9464.

[131] Lomnitski L, Bergman M, Nyska A, Ben-Shaul V, Grossman S (2003) Composition, efficacy, and safety of spinach extracts. Nutr. Cancer 46: 222-231.

[132] Platt KL, Edenharder R, Aderhold S, Muckel E, Glatt H (2010) Fruits and vegetables protect against the genotoxicity of heterocyclic aromatic amines activated by human xenobiotic-metabolizing enzymes expressed in immortal mammalian cells. Mutat. Res. 703: 90-98.

[133] Heber D (2004) Vegetables, fruits and phytoestrogens in the prevention of diseases. J. Postgrad. Med. 50:145-149

[134] Tan HL, Thomas-Ahner JM, Grainger EM, Wan L, Francis DM, Schwartz SJ, Erdman JW Jr, Clinton SK (2010) Tomato-based food products for prostate cancer prevention: what have we learned? Cancer Metastasis Rev. 29:553-568.

[135] Ellinger S, Ellinger J, Stehle P (2006) Tomatoes, tomato products and lycopene in the prevention and treatment of prostate cancer: do we have the evidence from intervention studies? Curr. Opin. Clin. Nutr. Metab. Care 9: 722-727.

[136] Riccioni G, Mancini B, Di Ilio E, Bucciarelli T, D'Orazio N (2008) Protective effect of lycopene in cardiovascular disease. Eur. Rev. Med. Pharmacol. Sci. 12:183-190.

[137] Waliszewski KN, Blasco G (2010) Nutraceutical properties of lycopen]. Salud Publica Mex. 52:254-265

[138] Wang H, Leung LK (2010) The carotenoid lycopene differentially regulates phase I and II enzymes in dimethylbenz[a]anthracene-induced MCF-7 cells. Nutrition 26: 1181-1187.

[139] Veeramachaneni S, Ausman LM, Choi SW, Russell RM, Wang XD (2008) High dose lycopene supplementation increases hepatic cytochrome P4502E1 protein and inflammation in alcohol-fed rats. J. Nutr. 138: 1329-1335.

[140] Surles RL, Weng N, Simon PW, Tanumihardjo SA (2004) Carotenoid profiles and consumer sensory evaluation of specialty carrots (Daucus carota, L.) of various colors. J. Agric. Food Chem .52:3417-3421

[141] Sikora M, Hallmann E, Rembiałkowska E (2009) The content of bioactive compounds in carrots from organic and conventional production in the context of health prevention. Rocz. Panstw. Zakl. Hig. 60:217-220

[142] Sun T, Simon PW, Tanumihardjo SA (2009) Antioxidant Phytochemicals and Antioxidant Capacity of Biofortified Carrots (Daucus carota L.) of Various Colors. J Agric. Food Chem. 57: 4142-4147.

[143] Bradfield CA, Chang Y, Bjeldanes LF (1985) Effects of commonly consumed vegetables on hepatic xenobiotic-metabolizing enzymes in the mouse. Food Chem. Toxicol. 23: 899-904.

[144] Duester KC (2001) Avocado fruit is a rich source of beta-sitosterol. J. Am. Diet Assoc. 101:404-405.

[145] Whiley AW, Schaffer B (2002) History, distribution and uses. In The Avocado: Botany, Production, and Uses; CABI Publishing: New York, Chapter 1, p 1-30.

[146] Ernst E (2003) Avocado–soybean unsaponifiables (ASU) for osteoarthritis—A systematic review. Clin. Rheumatol. 22: 285-288.

[147] Lu QY, Arteaga JR, Zhang Q, Huerta S, Go V L, Heber D (2005) Inhibition of prostate cancer cell growth by an avocado extract: Role of lipid-soluble bioactive substances J. Nutr. Biochem. 16: 23-30.

[148] Plaza L, Sánchez-Moreno C, de Pascual-Teresa S, de Ancos B, Cano MP (2009) Fatty acids, sterols, and antioxidant activity in minimally processed avocados during refrigerated storage. J. Agric. Food Chem. 57:3204-3209

[149] Blickstein D, Shaklai M, Inbal A (1991) Warfarin antagonism by avocado. Lancet 337: 914-915.

[150] Wells PS, Holbrook AM, Crowther NR, Hirsh J (1994) Interactions of warfarin with drugs and food. Ann. Intern. Med. 121: 676-683.

[151] Watanabe T, Sakurada N, and Kobata K (2001) Capsaici-, resiniferatoxin-, and olvanil-induced adrenaline secretion in rats via the vanilloid receptor. Biosci Biotechnol Biochem 65: 2443-2447.

[152] Ishtiaq M, Hanif W, Khan MA, Ashraf M, Butt AM (2007) An ethnomedicinal survey and documentation of important medicinal folklore food phytonims of flora of Samahni Valley (Azad Kashmir) Pakistan. Pak J Biol Sci 10: 2241-2256.

[153] Materska M, Perucka I (2005) Antioxidant activity of the main phenolic compounds isolated from hot pepper fruit (Capsicum annuum L.). J Agric Food Chem 53:1750-1756.

[154] Zhang Z, Hamilton SM, Stewart C, Strother A, Teel RW (1993) Inhibition of liver microsomal cytochrome P450 activity and metabolism of the tobacco-specific nitrosamine NNK by capsaicin and ellagic acid. Anticancer Res 13:2341-2346.

[155] Oikawa S, Nagao E, Sakano K, Kawanishi S (2006) Mechanism of oxidative DNA damage induced by capsaicin, a principal ingredient of hot chili pepper. Free Radic Res 40(9):966-973.

[156] Bouraoui A, Brazier JL, Zouaghi H, Rousseau M (1995) Theophylline pharmacokinetics and metabolism in rabbits following single and repeated administration of Capsicum fruit. Eur J Drug Metab Pharmacokinet 20:173-178.

[157] Prakash UN, Srinivasan K (2010) Beneficial influence of dietary spices on the ultrastructure and fluidity of the intestinal brush border in rats. Br J Nutr 104: 31–39.

[158] Cruz L, Castañeda-Hernández G, Navarrete A (1999) Ingestion of chilli pepper (Capsicum annuum) reduces salicylate bioavailability after oral asprin administration in the rat. Can J Physiol Pharmacol 77:441-446.

[159] Imaizumi K, Sato S, Kumazawa M, Arai N, Aritoshi S, Akimoto S, Sakakibara Y, Kawashima Y, Tachiyahiki K (2011) Capsaicinoids-induced changes of plasma glucose, fre fatty acids and glicerol concentrations in rats. J Toxicol Sci 36: 109-116.

[160] Lampe JW, King IB, Li S, Grate MT, Barale KV, Chen C, Feng Z, Potter JD (2000) Brassica vegetables increase and apiaceous vegetables decrease cytochrome P450 1A2 activity in humans: changes in caffeine metabolite ratios in response to controlled vegetable diets. Carcinogenesis 21: 1157-1162.

[161] Lambert JD, Sang S, Lu AY, Yang CS (2007) Metabolism of dietary polyphenols and possible interactions with drugs. Curr. Drug Metab. 8: 499-507.

[162] Pauwels EK (2011) The protective effect of the Mediterranean diet: focus on cancer and cardiovascular risk. Med. Princ. Pract. 20:103-111.

[163] Bach-Faig A, Berry EM, Lairon D, Reguant J, Trichopoulou A, Dernini S, Medina FX, Battino M, Belahsen R, Miranda G, Serra-Majem L; Mediterranean Diet Foundation Expert Group (2011) Mediterranean diet pyramid today. Science and cultural updates. Public Health Nutr. 14:2274-2284

[164] Trichopoulou A, Lagiou P, Kuper H, Trichopoulos D (2000) Cancer and Mediterranean Dietary Traditions. Cancer Epidemiol. Biomark. Prevent. 9: 869-873.

[165] Nadtochiy SM, Redman EK (2011) Mediterranean diet and cardioprotection: the role of nitrite, polyunsaturated fatty acids, and polyphenols. Nutrition 27(7-8):733-744.

[166] Craig WJ (2010) Nutrition Concerns and Health Effects of Vegetarian Diets. Nutr. Clin. Pract. 25:613-620.

[167] Fraser GE (2009) Vegetarian diets: what do we know of their effects on common chronic diseases? Am. J. Clin. Nutr. 89:1607S-1612S

[168] Li D (2011) Chemistry behind Vegetarianism. J. Agric. Food Chem. 59:777-784.

[169] Halliwell B (2007) Dietary polyphenols: Good, bad, or indifferent for your health? Cardiovascular Res. 73: 341-347

[170] Skibola CF. and Smith TS (2000) Potential health impacts of excessive flavonoid intake. Free Radical Biol. Med. 29: 375-383.

[171] Galati G. O'Brien PJ (2004) Potential toxicity of flavonoids and other dietary phenolics: significance for their chemopreventive and anticancer properties. Free Radical Biol. Med. 37: 287-303.

[172] Chan T. Galati G. O'Brien PJ (1999) Oxygen activation during peroxidase catalysed metabolism of flavones or flavanones. Chem. Biol . Interact. 122:15-25.

[173] Galati, G. Sabzevari O. Wilson J X. O'Brien PJ (2002) Prooxidant activity and cellular effects of the phenoxyl radicals of dietary flavonoids and other polyphenolics. Toxicology 177:91-104.

[174] Oostdar H. Burke MD. Mayer RT (2000) Bioflavonoids: selective substrates and inhibitors for cytochrome P450 CYP1A and CYP1B1. Toxicology 144:31-38.

[175] Hodek P, Trefil P, Stiborova´M (2002) Flavonoids-potent and versatile biologically active compounds interacting with cytochromes P450. Chem. Biol. Interact. 139:1-21.

[176] Doostdar H. Burke MD. Mayer RT (2000) Bioflavonoids: selective substrates and inhibitors for cytochrome P450 CYP1A and CYP1B1. Toxicology 144:31-38.

[177] Tang W. Stearns RA (2001) Heterotropic cooperativity of cytochrome P450 3A4 and potential drug – drug interactions. Curr. Drug Metab

Chapter 2

Anticancer Drug Discovery — From Serendipity to Rational Design

Jolanta Natalia Latosińska and
Magdalena Latosińska

Additional information is available at the end of the chapter

http://dx.doi.org/10.5772/52507

1. Introduction

Cancer is nowadays used as a generic term describing a group of about 120 different diseases, which can affect any part of the body and defined as the state characterized by the uncontrolled growth and invasion of normal tissues and spread of cells [1]. According to WHO reports cancer is a leading cause of premature death worldwide, accounting for 7.6 million deaths (around 13% of all deaths) only in 2008 [2]. The deaths from cancer worldwide are projected to continue rising, reaching an estimated 13.1 million in 2030 (WHO 2012). The number of all cancer cases around the world reached 12.7 million in 2008 and is expected to increase to 21 million by 2030. Approximately one in five people before age 75 will suffer from cancer during their lifetime, while one in ten in this age range is predicted to die due to cancer [2]. About 70% of all cancer deaths occurred in low- and middle-income countries. Cancer statistics indicate that most common new cancer cases (excluding common non-melanoma skin cancer) include lung, breast, colorectum, stomach, prostate and liver. These statistics are affected by a few factors including the increase in the number of carcinogens in daily life conditions (food, alcohol, tobacco etc.; high levels of chemicals and pollutants in environment, exposure to UV and ionizing radiation and viruses), genetic disposition [1] but also higher effectiveness of the treatment regimes. The number of recognized carcinogens (agents, mixtures, oncoviruses, environmental factors) increased from 50 in 1987 to 108 in 2012. Although it seems small, this number increases continually with the evidence of new (probably and possibly) carcinogens (64 and 271 in 2012) to humans [3]. What is significant only one compound is listed as probably not carcinogenic - caprolactam. Moreover, since not all chemicals have been tested yet, the number of human carcinogens is undervalued and will increase in the near future. Although mortality rates for some cancers (e.g. leukaemia, testicular or ovarian cancer) are reduced and the overall survival time increased significantly, especially in high-developed countries, but in fact the metastases, not the cancer itself, are the major cause of death. In 1971, only 50% of people diagnosed with the cancer went on to live at least five years, while nowadays, the five-year survival rate is 63% [2]. However if a cancer has spread the chances of survival are only scarcely better than in the 1970s. These numbers indicate that although the knowledge about cancer in the last two decades raised, even to a larger degree than in all preceding centuries, but the problem of cancer diseases persists and our knowledge is still insufficient to solve it. Despite the remarkable progress in cancer prevention, early detection, and treatment, made during the last few decades, the methods of cancer diagnosis and treatment are still not sufficiently specific and effective thus cancer still takes a heavy toll.

Not so long ago in the beginning of 20th century, neither carcinogens nor cellular targets were identified while the treatment was carried out exclusively by surgeries or natural products selected by trial and error. Modern cancer therapy based on the so-called holistic approach - the combined use of surgical methods, radiotherapy, chemotherapy, hormonal therapy and immunotherapy - is applied in the treatment of cancer at most stages. In fact this approach originated from the ancient Sumerian, Akkadian, Babylonian, Assyrian and Egyptian medicine, and was largely influenced by the Roman and Greek ideas concerning anatomy, physiology as well as the achievements of practical medicine and natural science. The chemotherapy, hormonal therapy, immunotherapy and radiotherapy as the methods of cancer treatment joined to the oldest surgical one only in the 20th c. An important component of the combined therapy, but sometimes when cancer had already metastasised, the only available therapeutic method, is chemotherapy using natural or synthetic anticancer drugs and treated as curative, palliative, adjuvant or neoadjuvant. Over the centuries anticancer drugs evolved from natural products, discovered mainly from green plants and minerals to fully chemically synthesized chemotherapeutic agents. However, even today drugs of natural origin play an important role in the treatment of cancer as 14 of them were on the list of the top 35 drugs worldwide sales [4]. The process of anticancer drug discovery leading from natural products to chemotherapeutic agents, often illicitly limited only to cytostatic and antiproliferative, has evolved from serendipity to rational design based on advances in chemistry, physics and biology in a long and complicated process. Nowadays both cancer itself and anticancer drugs are investigated at the molecular level thus methods of drug discovery have changed diametrically. The dominant direction of contemporary aniticancer drug discovery is the search for the possibilities to influence the pathogenetic mechanisms specific of the tumour structures at the cellular and molecular levels, which require the knowledge of cancer origins.

This chapter will focus on the factors which influenced the direction of anticancer drug discovery methods from guessing to the targeted search i.e. from serendipity to rational design.

2. Cancer origins

Cancer (proper medical name - malignant neoplasm) commonly considered to be a civilization disease, has in fact been traced to occur even before the ancestral species of man [5]. The oldest

http://dx.doi.org/10.5772/52507

evidence of cancer dates back to several million years ago and has been found in fossilized remains (bones) of a dinosaur in Wyoming. The oldest specimens of cancer, a hominid malignant tumour (probably Burkitt's lymphoma) and bone cancer - were found in the remains of a body of either Homo erectus or an Australopithecus and in the remains of a female skull dating to the Bronze Age (1900-1600 B.C.), respectively. Bone cancers have been also discovered in mummies in the Great Pyramid of Giza and in mummified skeletal remains of Peruvian Incas. The earliest written records differentiating between benign and malignant cancers date back to ancient times (3000-1500 B.C., Mesopotamia and Egypt). Seven Egyptian Papyruses including the Edwin Smyth (2500 B.C.), Leyde (1500 B.C.), and George Ebers (1500 B.C.) described not only the symptoms but also the first primitive forms of treatment, i.e. the removal of a malignant tissue. The Hindu epic, the Ramayana (500 B.C.), mentioned not only cancer cases but also the first medicines in the form of arsenic pastes, for treatment of cancerous growth. Ancient Greek physician Hippocrates of Kos (ca. 460-370 B.C.) described many different types of cancer (breast, uterus, stomach, skin, and rectum) recognised the difference between benign and malignant tumours and formulated the humoral theory of cancer genesis. As the veins surrounding the tumour resembled the crab claws, he named the disease after the Greek word *carcinos*. Cornelus Celsus (ca. 25 B.C.-50 A.D.), who described the first surgeries on cancers, translated Greek carcinos into now commonly used Latin term cancer. Claudius Galen (129-216 A.D.), the most famous Roman Empire physician, who wrote about 500 medical treatises, left a comprehensive descriptions of many neoplasms. He introduced the Greek word *oncos* (swelling) to describe tumours. Nowadays the use of Hippocrates and Celsus term is limited to describe malignant tumours, while Galen's term is used as a part of the name of the branch of medicine that deals with cancer - that is oncology. Followers of his works in Constantinople, Alexandria, Athens explained the appearance of cancer as a result of an excess of black bile. This idea prevailed through up to the 16th century.

The intensive studies in the field of anatomy and physiology during the Renaissance, resulted in advancement of surgery and development of rational therapies based on clinical observations. Based on autopsies William Harvey (1578-1657) described the systemic circulation of blood through the heart and body. Although cancers were still incurable, their temporary inhibition was often observed thanks to complementary remedies including the most common arsenic-based creams and pastes. In the beginning of the 16th c. Zacutus Lusitani (1575-1642) and Nicholas Tulp (1593–1674) formulated the contagion theory and proposed isolation of patients in order to prevent the spread of cancer. Throughout the 17th and 18th centuries, this theory was so popular that the first cancer hospital founded in Reims, France, was forced to move outside the city. Nowadays, we know that their certain viruses, bacteria, and parasites can increase a risk of developing cancer. Gaspare Aselli (1581-1625), who discovered the lymphatic system, suggested a connection between the lymphatic system and cancer. Georg Ernst Stahl (1660-1734) and Friedrich Hoffman (1660-1742) proposed a concept that tumours grow from degenerating lymph constantly excreted by the blood. This idea was accepted by John Hunter (1728-1793), who described methods to identify surgically removable tumours. At that time the so-called humoral theory of cancer was replaced by the lymph theory. Claude-Deshasis Gendron (1663-1750) was convinced that cancer arises as a solid and growing mass untreatable with drugs, and must be completely removed. The discovery of a microscope by

Antonie van Leeuwenhoek (1632-1723) in the late 17th century extended the knowledge about the cancer formation process and accelerated the search for the origin of cancer. It was realised that the progress in cancer treatment critically depends on the ability to distinguish between normal and malignant cells. Giovanni Battista Morgagni (1682-1771), father of pathomorphology, related the illness to pathological changes that laid the foundation for scientific oncology. This observation in connection with discovery of anaesthesia in 1844 by Horace Wells (1815-1848) enabled development of precise diagnosis of cancer and modern radical cancer surgery. In 1838, Johannes Peter Muller (1801-1858) indicated cells as basic units of tumours and proposed the blastema theory that cancer cells developed from budding elements (blastema) between normal tissues. In 1860, Karl Thiersch (1822-1895), showed that cancers metastasize through the spread of malignant cells and described establishment of secondary cancer as a result of their spread by lymph. Rudolf Virchow (1821-1902), the founder of cellular pathology, recognized leukaemia cells. He showed that cancer cells can be differentiated from surrounding normal cells from which they originated and the stage of cancer can be determined using microscopic images. Virchow also properly recognized chronic irritation as one of the factors favouring cancer development. Nowadays, we are aware that cancers arise from sites of infection, chronic irritation and inflammation. The next key step in understanding the mechanism of cancer development was the discovery of chromosome and mitosis credited to German botanist Wilhelm Hofmeister (1824-1877). In 1902 Theodor Boveri (1862-1915) reasoned that a cancerous tumour begins with a single cell, which divided uncontrollably, while David Paul von Hansemann (1858–1920), included multipolar mitoses among the factors responsible for the arise of abnormal chromosome numbers in cells leading to tumour formation. In fact Hansemann formulated chromosomal theory of cancer, while Boveri proposed the existence of cell-cycle checkpoints, tumour suppressor genes, and oncogenes and speculated that uncontrolled growth might be caused by physical (radiation), chemical (some chemicals) or biological (microscopic pathogens) factors. Thomas Hunt Morgan (1866-1945) made a key observations of chromosomal changes and demonstrated in 1915 the correctness of this theory. But still the carcinogens like chemical agents or irradiation could not explain the fact that sometimes cancer seemed to run in families. Already in the 17th c. Lusitani and Tulp observed the appearance of breast cancer in whole families.

A rapid progress in understanding the cancer origins was possible thanks to the scientific progress and appearance of instruments required to solve complex interdisciplinary problems of chemistry and biology. The turning points in the research on cancer were the mapping of locations of the fruit fly (Drosophila melanogaster) genes by Alfred Sturtevant (1891-1970), the discovery that DNA is the genetic material by Oswald Avery (1877-1955), Colin Munro MacLeod (1909-1972) and Maclyn McCarty (1911-2005) and the resolution of the exact chemical structure of DNA, the basic material in genes, by James Watson and Francis Crick (1916-2004). Their results indicated that DNA was the cellular target for carcinogens and that mutations were the key to understanding the mechanisms of cancer. In 1970 the first oncogene (SRC, from sarcoma) a defective proto-oncogene i.e. gene which after mutation, predispose the cell to become a cancerous (stimulate cell proliferation) was discovered by G. Steve Martin in a chicken retrovirus. One year later, but long before the human genome was sequenced, Alfred George Knudson identified first tumour suppressor gene, the Rb gene, located on a region of

http://dx.doi.org/10.5772/52507

long arm of chromosome 13 at position 14.2 in humans. Its mutation results in retinoblastoma juvenile eye tumour. On the basis of the earlier (dated to 1953) findings of Carl Nordling, he has formulated the accepted till now "two-hit hypothesis" which assumes that both alleles coding a particular protein must be affected before an effect is manifested. Knudson provided an explanation of the relationship between the hereditary and non-hereditary origins of cancer and predicted the existence of tumor suppressor genes that can suppress cancer cell growth. It was later discovered that both classes of genes proto-oncogenes and tumor-suppressor genes encode many kinds of proteins controlling cell growth and proliferation and the mutations in these genes can contribute to carcinogenesis.

In 1976 John Michael Bishop and Harold Elliot Varmus discovered the presence of oncogenes in many organisms including humans. Nowadays, after human genome sequencing in 2004, we know that human DNA contains approximately 20,500 genes [6]. About 50 of them are known to be proto-oncogenes, while 30 tumour suppressor genes. The proto-oncogenes (*c-onc*) initiate the process of cell division and code enzymes which control grows and division of cells. Proto-oncogenes can be activated to oncogenes by many factors including chromosome rearrangements, gene duplication, mutation or overexpression. For example, a chromosome rearrangement results in formation of BCR-ABL gene which leads to chronic myeloid leukaemia [7], acquired mutation activate the KIT gene which results in gastrointestinal stromal tumour [8], while inheritance of BRCA1 or BRCA2 increase the risk of breast, ovarian, fallopian tube, and prostate cancers [9]. To cause cancer most oncogenes require an additional step, for example mutations in another gene or introduction of foreign DNA (e.g. by viral infection). Infection and inflammation significantly contribute to about 25% of cancer cases. During the inflammatory response to viral infection the free radicals - reactive oxygen and nitrogen species - are generated as a physiological protective response. During chronic inflammation the mechanism is different - free radicals induce genetic and epigenetic changes including somatic mutations in cancer-related genes and posttranslational modifications in proteins involved in DNA repair or apoptosis. However, irrespective of the origins, the tumour microenvironment created by inflammatory cells, is an essential factor in the whole neoplastic process. It facilitates proliferation and survival of malignant cells, promotes angiogenesis and metastasis, subverts adaptive immune responses, and alters responses to chemotherapeutic agents. If a cell accumulates critical mutations in a few of these proto-oncogenes (five or six), it will survive instead of undergoing apoptosis, will proliferate and become capable of forming a tumour. The protecting mechanism involves the tumour suppressor genes, "anti-oncogenes", which protect from developing or growing cancer by repairing DNA damages (mutations), inhibiting cell division and cell proliferation or prevent reproduction by stimulating apoptosis. Mutation of these genes may lead to cessation of the inhibition of cell division. As a result the cell will divide uncontrollably, and produce daughter cells with the same defect. For example, mutation in the TP53 gene (initially after discovery in 1979 by Arnold Levine, David Lane and William Old incorrectly believed to be an oncogene), one of the most commonly mutated tumour suppressor genes which encoding tumour protein - so called p53 protein, a key element in stress-induced apoptosis, is involved in the pathophysiology of leukaemias, lymphomas, sarcomas, and neurogenic tumours [10,11]. Homozygous loss of p53 is found in 70% of colon cancers, 50% of lung cancers and 30–50% of breast cancers. Other important tumour suppressor genes include p16, BRCA-1, BRCA-2, APC or PTEN [12]. Mutation of these genes may lead to melanoma (p16), breast and ovarian cancer in genetically related families (BRCA), colorectal cancer (APC) or glioblastoma, endometrial cancer, and prostate cancer (PTEN).

In general cancerogenesis is a multistep process thus it is usually a combination of proto-oncogene activation and tumour suppressor gene loss or inactivation is required. However, in a few cases (only 5-10% of cancer cases) this abnormal change in gene can be inherited, passed from generation to generation, in most cases it is a result of sporadic or somatic mutation acquired during a person's lifetime. Although cancer is generally believed to arise as a result of slow accumulation of multiple mutations, but in some cases (2-3%) massive multiple mutation can also arise in a single event. Thus cancer is described as a disease of abnormal gene function, genetically caused by the interaction of two factors: genetic susceptibility and environmental mutagens and carcinogens. Of key importance for the recognition of the molecular mechanism underlying cancer treatment - cell apoptosis - was the discovery of telomeres and telomerase. In the early 1970s, Alexei Olovnikov, on the basis of the Leonard Hayflick's concept of limited somatic cell divisions (Hayflick limit), suggested that chromosomes cannot completely replicate their ends. In 1978 Elizabeth Blackburn discovered the unusual nature of stretches of DNA in the ends of the chromosomes of protozon *Tetrahymena* - the so-called telomeres. The sequence of human telomere was established 10 years later, in 1988, by Robin Allshire. Blackburn described telomere-shortening mechanism which limits cells to a fixed number of divisions and protect chromosomes from fusing each other or rearranging that can lead to cancer. Shortened telomeres have been found in many cancers, including pancreatic, bone, prostate, bladder, lung, kidney, and head and neck. In 1985, Carol Greider isolated the enzyme telomerase, controlling the elongation of telomeres. Four years later, in 1989, Gregg B. Morin reported the presence of telomerase in human tumour cells and linked its activity with the immortality of these cells (inability to apoptosis), while Greider discovered the lack of active telomerase in normal somatic cells apart from stem cells, keratinocytes, intestines, and hair follicle. It was discovered that deactivation of telomerase prompts the apoptosis of human breast and prostate cancer cells. These results indicated the important role of telomerase in the process of oncogenesis.

Carcinogenesis have been found a complex and multi-step (preinitiation, initiation, promotion and metastasis) biological process characterised by independence from growth factors, insensitivity to inhibitors of growth, unlimited potential for replication (reactivation of telomerase), invasiveness, the ability to metastasis and to sustain angiogenesis, and resistance of apoptosis [13]. DNA mutation inherited and caused by exposure to carcinogens (chemical: compounds including drugs, physical: radiation, or biological: the introduction of new DNA sequences by viruses) have been found to be the true origin of uncontrolled growth of cells coupled with malignant behaviour: invasion and metastasis (Fig. 1).

The knowledge of the molecular mechanisms involving the above mentioned factors, especially apoptosis and cancer resistance to it, can improve cancer therapy through resensitization of tumour cells. Fundamental method of cancer treatment - classical chemotherapy (and radiotherapy) which is harmful also to normal cells, act primarily by inducing cell apoptosis either locally, in tumour, or globally, when cancer metastasize. Any disturbance in apoptosis

http://dx.doi.org/10.5772/52507

results in a decrease in the effectiveness of the therapy. The recent targeted therapies instead of interfering with rapidly dividing cells, interfere with selected targets in the cell and use small molecules to interfere with abnormal proteins (required for carcinogenesis and tumour growth) or cell receptors, or use monoclonal antibodies, which destroy malignant tumour cells and prevent tumour growth by blocking specific receptors. Targeted cancer therapy, which may be more effective and less harmful than classical chemotherapy but still are based on the use of chemical compounds is perceived as modern chemotherapy or chemotherapy of the future.

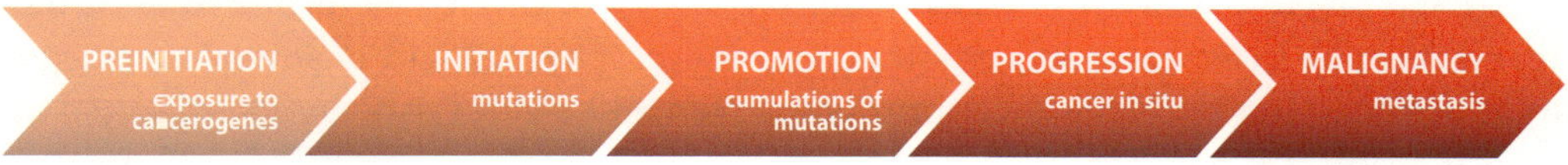
PREINITIATION
exposure to cancerogenes
INITIATION
mutations
PROMOTION
cumulations of mutations
PROGRESSION
cancer in situ
MALIGNANCY
metastasis

Figure 1. Multi-step process of carcinogenesis.

3. Cancer risk — Carcinogens and co-carcinogens

Currently we are aware that apart of inherited mutations, an important role in carcinogenesis play the factors connected with the expression to carcinogens [14]. This includes environmental factors (pollutions), lifestyle factors (tobacco smoking, diet, alcohol consumption, obesity, sedentary life), occupational factors (e.g. synthesis, dyes, fumes) and other factors (excessive exposure to sunlight, radiation, viruses, etc). Carcinogens (of chemical, physical or biological origin) include chemicals or non-chemical agents, which under certain conditions are able to induce cancer. Co-carcinogens, are not carcinogenic themselves but with other chemicals or non-chemical carcinogens, such as for example UV or ionizing radiation, promote the effects of a carcinogen in carcinogenesis. Carcinogens as well as co-carcinogens can be of natural or synthetic origins. In general, their carcinogenic action relay on direct or indirect action in the cellular DNA. Carcinogens acting directly can initiate the carcinogenesis by yielding highly reactive species that bind covalently to cellular DNA, while those acting indirectly can induce mutations to cellular DNA. Thus carcinogens are able to distort the conformation or function (replication/transcription) of DNA, which results not only in oncogene activation but also DNA amplification, gene transposition or chromosome translocation. Carcinogens may induce carcinogenesis directly by mutational activation of protooncogenes and/or inactivation of tumour suppression genes. Indirect action is realised through the mechanisms that generate chemical species (free radicals, reactive oxygen species, carcinogenic metabolites) which are capable of entering the nucleus of the cell.

Over 80% of carcinogenic substances are of environmental origins [15]. Restriction of the exposition to carcinogens can substantially reduce the risk of cancers also those of occupational type, which make approximately 4-5% of all human cancers. Thus evaluation and classification of the carcinogens is required from the cancer prevention point of view. Although there are many international and national organizations that classify carcinogens, but only a few are highly influential, the oldest and setting the standards, World Health Organization of the United Nations (WHO) International Agency for Research on Cancer (IARC) headquartered in Lyon, France, established in 1965; United Nations initiative from 1992 called Globally Harmonized System of Classification and Labelling of Chemicals (GHS), National Toxicology Program of the U.S. Department of Health and Human Services established in 1978, professional organization American Conference of Governmental Industrial Hygienists, founded in 1938 in Washington and reorganized in 1946, European Union directives Dangerous Substances Directive (67/548/EEC) and the Dangerous Preparations Directive (1999/45/EC) and Safe Work Australia (Independent Statutory Agency) which evolved from National Occupational Health and Safety Council (NOHSC) established in 1985. One of the prime roles of these organizations is to evaluate and classify the chemical, physical and biological carcinogens targeted to develop strategies for cancer prevention and control used by international and national health and regulatory agencies to protect public health. Since 1971 IARC evaluated the carcinogenicity of approximately 400 and collected data about 900 agents and published them in a series (101 till 2012) of Monographs on the Evaluation of Carcinogenic Risks to Humans [3]. Up to now IARC has identified 108 definitely, 66 probably, 284 possibly carcinogens, 515 not classifiable as carcinogens and 1 probably not carcinogenic, Table 1. Alternative to IARC, a complex GSH classification system, collects data from tests, literature, and practical experience [16]. Since 2003 four editions of GHS have been published, but only most recent one, dated to 2011, has the form convenient for worldwide implementation. GSH delivers a global system of classification of chemicals (substances, alloys, mixtures) divided into three groups of hazards: physical (16 classes), health and environmental (12 and 2 classes, respectively) and a unique system of labelling and collecting the information in the form of safety data sheets (SDS). GSH requires the use of the harmonized classification scheme and the harmonized label elements for any carcinogenic chemical. Within the GSH system, the class of carcinogens was clearly separated as health hazard risk factor and divided to two categories: known and presumed carcinogens (subcategories 1A and 1B, respectively) and suspected carcinogens (category 2), Table 2. Irrespective of the classification system, the epidemiological evidence indicates that many drugs, including antineoplastic, sex hormones, antithyroid, antibacterial, antiparasitic, immunosuppressive ones used as single agents or in combinations as well as radiation (γ, X or UV) are known carcinogens.

3.1. Carcinogens of chemical/environmental origins

As early as in 16th c. Phillippus Aureolus Theophratus Bombastus von Hohenheim (1493-1541) known as Paracelsus suggested that the "wasting disease of miners" might be linked to exposure to realgar (tetra-arsenic tetra-sulphide). Since the 17th c. cancer was associated with the presence of some chemicals. For example John Hill (1716-1775) linked tobacco use with nasal cancer, while Percivall Pot (1814-1788) described occupational risk of epithelial cancer of the scrotum connected with soot, in chimney sweepers. In 1795 Samuel Thomas von Soemmerring (1755-1830) cautioned that pipe smokers were excessively prone to cancer of the lip. Since then epidemiological evidence has been important in detecting carcinogens. In 1858, a Montpellier surgeon Etienne-Frédéric Bouisson (1813-1884) found that 63 of his 68 patients suffering from oral cancer were pipe smokers. Shortly after replacement of natural dyes by

http://dx.doi.org/10.5772/52507

synthetic aromatic amine dye in German industry, Ludwig Rehn (1849-1930) reported an increased incidence of bladder cancer in workers exposed to it. Many years later exact carcinogen, 2-naphthylamine, was recognized. In the 1930s the first company in American dye industry, DuPont, reported first cases of occupational cancer connected with the use of dyes, bladder cancer, at the Chambers Works plant. In 1935, Takaoki Sasaki and Tomizo Yoshida (1903-1973) induced malignant tumours (hepatoma) in a digestive organ by feeding rats by one of the azo dyes - *o*-aminoazotoluene.

IARC classification	Effect	Criteria	No	Agents and groups of agents/mixtures/ the exposure circumstance
Group 1	definitely carcinogenic	sufficient evidence of carcinogenicity to humans, epidemiologic evidence, occupational exposure, and animal studies; strong evidence that the agent acts through relevant mechanisms of carcinogenicity to humans	108	chlorambucil, cyclophosphamide, chlornaphazine, melphalan, tamoxifen5, thiotepa, sulfur mustard ultraviolet radiation (UV-A, UV-B, UV-C), X-radiation, γ-radiation, radiation, radionuclides, neutron radiation, solar radiation
Group 2A	probably carcinogenic	limited evidence of carcinogenicity to humans, but sufficient evidence of carcinogenicity in experimental animals; strong evidence that the carcinogenesis is mediated by mechanisms that are also operate in humans	66	azacitidine, cisplatin, nitrogen mustard, doxorubicin
Group 2B	possibly carcinogenic	limited evidence in humans; less than sufficient evidence in experimental animals; inadequate evidence in humans but sufficient or limited in experimental animals	284	aziridine, dacarbazine, daunomycin, thiouracil, bleomycin
Group 3	not classifiable as carcinogenic	inadequate evidence in humans; inadequate or limited to experimental animals; mechanisms of carcinogenesis in animals does not operate in humans.	515	ifosfamide, isophosphamide, actinomycin D
Group 4	probably not carcinogenic	negative evidence of carcinogenicity, not used	1	caprolactam

Table 1. Classification of carcinogens according to IARC, 2012

But the first chemical carcinogen - coal tar - was identified as early as in 1915 by Katsusaburo Yamagiwa (1863-1930) and Koichi Ichikawa (1888-1948) who induced cancer in laboratory animals by prolonged application of coal tar to rabbit skin. Inflammation accompanying the coal tar application and cancer formation was in a good agreement with Virchow findings. The search for specific chemical carcinogens led to the discovery of pure carcinogenic chemicals including polycyclic aromatic hydrocarbons PAHs (e.g. benzo[a]pyrene, 1,2,5,6-dibenzanthracene) by Ernest Lawrence Kennaway (1881-1958) and Izrael Hieger (1901-1986), which were shown to be carcinogenic in mouse skin by Hieger et al. in 1933 [17]. Nowadays, we know that PAHs, mainly benzo[a]pyrene and heterocyclic amines (HCAs) belong to definite carcinogens which appear in smoke as a result of incomplete combustion [18] and thus are present not only in tobacco smoke but also in a fried/smoked meat as well as barbeque. PAHs often induce stomach cancer.

Category	Effect	Criteria	Signal word	Hazard statement	Symbol/Pictogram
1A	known human carcinogen	known to have carcinogenic potential for humans – largely based on human evidence	Danger	may cause cancer	
1B	presumed human carcinogen	presumed to have carcinogenic potential for humans – largely based on animal evidence	Danger	may cause cancer	
2	suspected human carcinogen	evidence from animal and/or human studies is limited	Warning	suspected of causing cancer	

Table 2. Classification of carcinogens according to GSH, 2011

Although cancer-causing substances are often considered to be exclusively synthetic, there are numerous natural carcinogens, chemical compounds that occur in environment, and in food plants [19]. Isaac Berenblum (1903-2000) discovered the potent inflammatory agent, croton oil extracted from *Croton Tiglium* L. native or cultivated in Asia (India, Ceylon, China), Malay Argipelago and Africa (Zanzibar, Tanzania), and its most active ingredient, 12-*O*-tetradecanoylphorbol-13-acetate (TPA) in 1941 [20]. Both agents now belong to classic tumour promoters. In 1956, John Barnes (1913-1975) and Peter Magee, reported an example of synergistic interaction of chemical carcinogens with proinflammatory agents. i.e. liver tumors in rats induced by N-nitrosdimethylamine (NDMA) [21]. In 1972, another case, the influence of chronic respiratory infection with influenza virus on the development of lung cancer in rats induced by carcinogenic N-nitrosamine was reported [22], which occurs in some foodstuffs, latex, cosmetics. Since then about 90% of nitrosamine derivatives including hydrazines from raw mushrooms *Agaricus bisporus* (Lange) Imbach and *Gyromitra* (Pers.) Fr. have been deemed to be carcinogenic and promoters of benign hepatomas, liver cell carcinomas, angiomas and angiosarcomas of blood vessels, adenomas and adenocarcinomas of lungs.

One of the most potent naturally occurring microbial carcinogen is Aflatoxin B_1, which is produced as secondary metabolite by the fungi *Aspergillus flavus* and *Aspergillus parasiticm* [23] growing on stored grains, nuts and peanut butter and found worldwide as a contaminant in food. The discovery of Alfatoxin B_1 followed upon "Turkey X Disease" (a liver disease) which killed over 100,000 turkeys in the UK in the early 1960s. The major metabolite of Aflatoxin B1, Aflatoxin B1-8,9-epoxide, exerts hepatotoxic effect, but synergistic interaction between Aflatoxin B1 and hepatitis B virus results in hepatocellular carcinoma. Another fungal contaminant is mycotic toxin Ochratoxin-A (OTA) produced by *Penicillium viridicatum* discovered during laboratory studies in the mid-1960s and encountered as a natural contaminant in maize in 1969 in the USA [24]. Large group of carcinogens are tannins and tannic acid, which occur widely in plants (tea, coffee, and cocoa) but in concentrated doses reveal hepatocarcinogenic properties in both animals and humans. They have been found capable of causing liver tumours in experimental animals and oesophageal, throat & mouth cancers in humans. Cycads, important food sources in tropical regions, contain unique toxines cycasin and macrozamin that cause liver and kidney tumours in rats [25]. Safrole, 5-Allyl-1,3-benzodioxole found in sassafras tea, cinnamin, cocoa, nutmeg, black pepper, and other herbs and spices as well as isosafrole, 1,2-(Methylenedioxy)-4-propenylbenzene belong to liver carcinogens in rats, they produce liver tumours following their oral administration [26]. Dihydrosafrole is also carcinogenic in rats and mice, in which it produces tumours of the oesophagus, and liver tumours in males and lung tumours in both males and females, respectively. There is an evidence of the carcinogenic properties of estragole from anise, star anise, basil, bay, tarragon, fennel, marjoram or American wood turpentine oil, which proceeds through a genotoxic mechanism identical to that of safrole and also induce liver cancer in mice [27]. Black pepper (*Piper nigrum* L.), apart of tannic acid and safrole contains secondary amines pyperadine and alpha-methylpyrroline, which can be nitrosated to N-nitroso-piperidine, a strong carcinogen, carcinogenic to experimental mice. It has been known since the 1960s that Comfrey (*Symphytum officinale* L.) contains carcinogenic hepatoxines belonging to pyrrolizidine alkaloids (PAs) e.g. lasiocarpine and symphatine, which can interfere with RNA and DNA synthesis within the liver cells and cause liver damage, cancer, and death [28].

Some chemical carcinogens have been discovered as a result of industrial or environmental accidents. For example in 1976, notoriety was gained by Seveso disaster - an explosion occurred in a TCP (2,4,5-trichlorophenol) reactor at the ICMESA chemical plant located about 20 km north of Milan, Italy. A mixture of different chemicals including dioxin was released into the atmosphere. This industrial accident caused the highest known exposure to 2,3,7,8-tetrachlorodibenzo-p-dioxin (TCDD) in residential populations and linked dioxin exposure to chloracne, genetic impairments and excessive risk of lymphatic and hematopoietic tissue [29-32]. Another environmental disaster related to dioxines was contamination of a landfill of Love Canal in the Niagara Falls, New York, USA. This region was turned in 1920 to municipal and industrial chemical dumpsite by Hooker Chemica and in 1942-1953 it was contaminated by eleven highly toxic carcinogens including TCDD. In 1978 a record amount of rainfall in Love Canal resulted in leaching the chemicals from corroding waste-disposal drums in this area which caused environmental disaster, a drastic increase in birth defects, nervous disorders, high white-blood-cell counts in residents, a possible precursor of leukaemia and cancers [33-35]. Many years later probable carcinogenic action of triclosan, an antibacterial agent added to soaps, toothpastes etc., has been linked to its degradation to TCDD in chlorinated water [36]. In the early 1980s the high risk of lung, skin, kidney and bladder cancer due to chronic low level arsenic poisoning of water in different countries (Bangladesh, Vietnam, Cambodia, Tibet, Argentina, Chile, China, India, Mexico, Thailand, and US) caused by contamination of water by pesticides and various alloys containing arsenic, which resemble and thus substitute phosphorus in chemical reactions, was discovered [37]. In 1980 it was realized that exposure to formaldehyde (a hazard in embalming and production of plastics and vinyl chloride, from which PVC is manufactured) could cause nasal cancer in rats [38]. In the early 1970s, the carcinogenicity of vinyl chloride was linked to occupational angiosarcoma cancers in workers in industry. A few years later PVC was classified as a carcinogen [39-41]. Since then specific substances: aniline and benzidine, asbestos, wool/wood/leather dust have been linked to different types of cancer in humans bladder cancer, sinuses and lung cancer, mesothelioma, nasal sinuses, respectively [3]. Many drugs, including chemotherapeutic anticancer agents, diuretics, hormones have been recognized as a source of secondary cancers and thus classified as definite carcinogens. Most of anticancer drugs is classified as group 1 agents in IARC classification [3].

3.2. Carcinogens of biological origins (Oncogenic viruses/bacteria/parasites)

The hypothesis that cancer can originate from a virus comes from Danish scientists Oluf Bang (1881-1937) and Vilhelm Ellerman (1871-1924), who was the first to show, in 1908, that avian erythroblastosis (chicken leukaemia) can be transmitted by cell-free extracts. In 1911, Francis Peyton Rous (1879-1970), American pathologist, described a solid cancer, sarcoma, in domestic chickens caused by exposing the healthy bird to a cell-free filtrate containing retrovirus later became known as the *Rous sarcoma virus* [42]. Abbie Lathrop (1868-1918) and Leo Loeb (1869-1959) described breast cancer in mice caused by a transmissible agent as early as in 1915 [43]. Since then several oncoviruses have been linked to different types of cancer [44]. In 1933 Richard Edwin Shope (1901-1966) discovered the first mammalian tumour caused in cottontail rabbit by fibroma virus and papilloma virus (*Shope papilloma virus*). Shortly later, in 1936, a geneticist and cancer biologists John Joseph Bittner (1904-1961) discovered a mouse mammary tumour virus (MMTV), the so-called Bittner virus, causing a breast cancer, which is a promoter in models of human breast cancer [45]. In 1957, Sarah Elizabeth Stewart (1905-1976) and Berenice E. Eddy (1903-1989), pioneers in the field of viral oncology research, discovered the Stewart-Eddy polyoma virus, which produced several types of cancer in a variety of small mammals [46]. John J. Trentin (1908-2005) and others were the first to report of cancer (sarcoma) produced in animals (hamsters) by inoculation of virus of human origin (*Adenovirus*) [47]. Michael Anthony Epstein, Bert Achong (1928-1996) and Yvonne Barr identified the first human cancer virus (Epstein-Barr Virus or EBV) from Burkitt lymphoma cells in 1964 [48]. Baruch Blumberg (1925-2011) isolated Hepatitis B virus (HBV), a cause of hepatitis, and suggested that it contributed to liver cancer hepatocellular carcinoma. It was confirmed to be an oncovirus in the 1980s. Hepatitis C virus (HCV) was shown to be a major contributor to liver cancer (hepatocellular carcinoma) by Michael Houghton and Daniel W. Bradley in 1987. The first human retroviruses, Human T-lymphotropic virus 1 (HTLV I) and 2 (HTLV 2), linked to T-cell lymphoma/T-cell leukaemia and Hairy-cell leukaemia, respectively, were discovered by Bernard J. Poiesz, Robert Charles Gallo and Mistuaki Yoshida. In 1984 Harald zur Hausen and Lutz Gissman discovered that the human papillomaviruses HPV16 and HPV18 were responsible for approximately 70% of cervical cancers, while Alan Storey, Kit Osborn and Lionel Crawford in 1990 indicated that HPV types 6 and 11 were responsible for 90% of genital warts. Valerie Beral, Thomas A. Peterman, Harold W. Jaffe related Kaposi's sarcoma-associated herpesvirus (KSHV) with AIDS [49], which prompted Patrick S. Moore, Yuan Chang, Frank Lee and Ethel Cesarman to isolate Kaposi sarcoma-associated herpesvirus (KSHV or HHV8) in 1994 [50]. Very recently in 2008, Chang and Moore developed a new method to identify oncoviruses called digital transcriptome subtraction (DTS) and isolated DNA fragments of Merkel cell polyomavirus from a Merkel cell carcinoma, considered to be responsible for 70–80% of these cancers [51].

There is also evidence of a link between the bacteria Helicobacter pylori (HP) responsible for development of gastric and duodenal ulcers and cancer risk [52,53]. The human oncogenic viruses, which include HBV, HCV, HIV, HPVs, EBV, KSHV, HTLV-I and HTLV-II and HP are associated with nearly 20% of the human cancer cases. The elimination of these pathogens would decrease by 23.6% the cases of cancer in developing countries and by 7.7% in developed countries [54]. The commonly omitted advantage of the discovery of oncoviruses was the possibility of transplantation of carcinogen-induced tumour systems in mice, which delivered models for the studies on anticancer drugs.

Rare source of cancer are also parasitic diseases caused by *Clonorchis sinensis* (Japan, Korea, Vietnam) and *Opisthorchis viverrini* (Thailand, Laos, and Malaysia) or *Schistosomas species* (Africa, Asia). All of them are known to be carcinogenic and linked with biliary tract cancer (cholangiocarcinoma) and bladder cancer, respectively [55]. Most of the biological carcinogens are classified as group 1 agents in IARC classification [3].

3.3. Carcinogens of physical origins (Radiation)

Shortly after the discovery of chemical carcinogens, i.e. factors that suppress and activate the cell growth and division, the first physical carcinogens were identified. After discovery of X-rays by Wilhelm Roentgen (1845-1923) in 1895 and radioactive radiation by Henri Becquerel (1852-1908) in 1896, the exposure to radiation has been identified as one of the causes of cancer. Working with early X-ray generators resulted in the acute skin reactions and the first radiation-induced cancer arising in an ulcerated area of the skin was reported in 1902. In 1910 to 1912, Pierre Marie, Jean Clunet and Gaston Raulot-Lapointe reported the induction of sarcoma in rats by the application of X-irradiation. As early as in 1911 the first report of leukaemia in radiation workers appeared [56]. The 20th century pioneers in X-Ray/radium studies fell victims to their work; surgeon Robert Abbe (1851-1928), physicist Marie Skłodowska-Curie (1867-1934) and physician Jean Bergonie (1857-1925) died due to leukaemia. The use of uranium/plutonium based bombs against Hiroshima/Nagasaki during World War II revealed that ionising radiation irrespective of its origin is a cause of cancer [57]. Increased incidence of cancer of bone marrow and essentially all organs was noted in Japan years to decades later. Some physical carcinogens have been discovered as a result of nuclear disasters. In 1957, the cooling system failed and the radioactive wastes chemical explosion of at Mayak nuclear fuel reprocessing plant, Ozyorsk/Mayak, Russia caused radiation contamination which spread over hundred kilometres and pollution of the Techa River. This accident called Kyshtym disaster belongs to three most serious nuclear accidents ever recorded, although it was revealed only in 1976 [58]. The scarce epidemiological studies suggest very different numbers of cancer deaths among residents associated to radiation exposure. In 1979 the cooling system of Three Mile Island nuclear power plant near Harrisburg, Pennsylvania failed and the reactor core was partially melted. Radiation from the reactor contributed to the premature deaths and cancers in local residents, but the disaster was relatively small [59]. There is still vivid discussion about the carcinogenic effects of nuclear power plant explosion in 1986 in Chernobyl located 80 miles from Kiev, Ukraine, which was the greatest source of long-lived radioactive plutonium and short-lived radioactive caesium (^{137}Cs), iodines (particularly ^{131}I) and strontium (^{90}Sr). The major health effect of Chernobyl was an elevated thyroid-cancer incidence due to iodine absorption by the thyroid gland in adolescents and children some of whom were not yet born at the time of the accident, and drastic increase in leukaemia cases caused by distribution the strontium incorrectly recognized by the body as calcium throughout the bone structure [60]. Radioactive isotopes of barium, caesium, iodine and tellurium were detected in a radiation plume released by damaged nuclear reactors at the nuclear plant in Fukushima, Japan in 2011. Fukushima Daiichi disaster was the most serious accident in global scale. As the prolonged exposure to radiation in the air, ground and food can result in leukaemia and other cancers thus about 160,000 people were evacuated from the region surrounding the plant. According to theoretical 3-D global atmospheric models this nuclear disaster may cause as many as 2,500 cases of cancer, mostly in Japan. Only recently, in the 1990s, much-less energetic UV radiation has been also recognized as carcinogen causing not only genetic mutations but also melanoma or non-melanoma cancers. In 2011 WHO/IARC classified radiofrequency electromagnetic fields as possibly carcinogenic to humans (Group 2B), on the basis of an increased risk of glioma, a malignant type of brain cancer, associated with wireless phone use [3]. Nowadays we are aware that exposure to radiation can be incidental like in Hiroshima, Nagasaki, Chernobyl, Fukushima [1,61] or systematic due to repeated doses of radiation like UV during sun-bathing or MW during phone-cell use. Anyway the most common radiation induced cancers are basal cell carcinoma and squamous carcinoma of the skin, leukaemia and thyroid cancer. The first two can arise from excessive exposure to UV radiation, while the other are mainly result of ionising radiation e.g. γ, X-Ray [1]. The controlled use of ionising radiation in medicine and industry and annual limits of doses for each individual [62] has reduced the risk connected with ionising radiation but the awareness of UV or MW related risk is still low. Common feature of cancers induced by physical factor is late onset and long period of risk persisting. Most of the physical carcinogens are classified as group 1 or 2 agents in IARC classification [3].

4. Chemotherapeutical agents

4.1. Drugs of natural origin

In the second half of the 20th century, one more type of cancer therapy was added to surgery, irradiation and hormonotherapy, which was chemotherapy. Nowadays this term primarily refers to the treatment of cancer with an antineoplastic drug or a combination of drugs, but when it was introduced in 1909 by Paul Ehrlich (1854-1915) it had a broader meaning as it referred as well to antibacterial chemotherapy and treatment of autoimmune diseases, in general use of chemicals to treat disease. Chemotherapy, generally assumed as the youngest method of cancer treatment, is in fact rooted in ancient times. Although cutting out the cancer changed tissue was early found as the main treatment, it was not always effective. Thus various substances of natural origin were applied as complementary medications. Many even ancient cultures had proposed theories explaining the cause of cancer. These theories influenced the search for medicaments. For example Egyptians believed that natural substances similar in look or function to human organs can be used to treat ailments in those organs, thus the use of mixtures of pigs eyes or ears was popular.

Although the products of animal and mineral origin had made an important contribution to drug development, the main source of drugs for millennia have been green plants. The most frequently used included castor oil plant (*Ricinus communis* L.), exploding cucumber (*Ecballium elateritum* L.), belladonna (*Atropa belladonna* L.), myrrh (dried sap from trees *Commiphora Myrcha L.*), incense (dried sap from trees *Boswellia thurifera L., Boswellia frereana Birdw., Boswellia bhawdajiana* Birdw.), stinging nettle (*Urtica dioica* L.), gingers (*Zingiber Boehm.* L.), red clover (*Trifolium pratense* L.) and autumn crocus (*Colchicum autumnale* L.). Although, in nature most of them cause sickness, but in small doses or after chemical modifications, they revealed therapeutic effects. Some of them were rediscovered by modern medicine. For example from *Colchicum autumnale* L. described by Pedanius Dioscorides (40-90 A.D.) in De Materia Medica a toxic alkaloid colchicine was extracted in 1820 by Pierre Joseph Pelletier (1788-1842) and Joseph Bienaimé Caventou (1795–1877). Albert Pierre Dustin (1914-1993), described its antymitotic properties in 1934 [63]. In 2009 it was accepted by Food and Drug Administration (FDA) as a drug for gout and Familial Mediterranean Fever. Another interesting case described by Dioscorides is red viscous sap called the dragon's blood mostly collected from *Dracaena cinnabari* Balf. f or *Croton lechleri* L. and used as a dye and anti-inflammatory, antimicrobial and anticancer folk remedy not only by ancient Greek but also Romans and Arabs. Recently methanolic extract of *Croton lechleri* was shown to exert cytotoxic effects on HeLa (Human epithelial carcinoma cell line) cells and its antitumor effect in HeLa tumour in mice was documented [64]. Two other commonly used antileukemic drugs, vinblastine and vincristine, were extracted in 1950 from the species of Madagascar periwinkle (*Catharanthus roseus* L.), for centuries known as folk remedy, and shortly after approved by FDA. Nowadays vinblastine, which binds tubulin, thereby inhibiting the assembly of microtubules, is an important component of a number of chemotherapy regimens, including ABVD for Hodgkin lymphoma, advanced testicular cancer, breast and lung cancers, and Kaposi's sarcoma [65]. Realgar widely used in Chinese traditional medicine because of its anti-inflammation, antiulcer, anticonvulsion, and anti-schistosomiasis activity was recently found capable to induce cell apoptosis and thus effective in the treatment of hematological malignant diseases [66]. As early as in 1021, Avicenna described the medicinal use of *Taxus baccata* L. (Zarnab) as cardiac remedy in The Canon of Medicine. Various parts of *Taxus brevifolia* Peattie, *Taxus Canadensis* Marshall, *Taxus baccata* L. have been used by several Native American Tribes mainly for the treatment of non-cancerous diseases [65] but the use for the treatment of cancer was noted only in the Hindu Ayurvedic medicine. Paclitaxel (Taxol®), used in treatment for breast, ovarian, small and non-small cell lung cancer and Kaposi sarcoma, was isolated in 1967 by Monroe E. Wall and

Mansukh C. Wani from the bark of the 200-years old Pacific yew (*Taxus brevifolia* Nutt.) tree [67]. Its structure was elucidated in 1971 [67,68]. Its cytostatic mechanism of action (mitosis inhibition) was discovered by Susan B. Horowitz in the late 1970s, but only the discovery of total chemical synthesis of Paclitaxel in 1994 by Robert A. Holton widespread its use [69]. Camptothecin isolated from the Chinese and Tibetan ornamental joy tree Decne (*Camptotheca acuminata* var. rotundifolia B. M. Yang & L. D. Duan), *Nyssaceae* Arnott family, was discovered in 1966 by Wall and Wani in systematic screening of natural products [70]. Although it is a potent topoisomerase inhibitor, it was dropped in the 1970s from clinical trials because of severe bladder toxicity [71]. But two of its semi-synthetic derivatives - topotecan and irinotecan are used for the treatment of ovarian and small cell lung and colon-rectal cancers, respectively [72,73]. Epipodophyllotoxines also belong to active anti-tumour agents derived from plants. Podophyllotoxin and deoxypodophyllotoxin were obtained from the roots of American mandrake or May apple (*Podophyllum peltatum* L.), Himalayan mayapple (*Podophyllum emodi* Wallich ex Hook. f. & Thomson) and Chinese or Asian Mayapple (*Podophyllum pleianthum* L.), respectively [74], all belongs to *Berberidaceae* Juss. family. *Podophyllum peltatum* and *Podophyllum emodii* were used by the Native American Tribes for the treatment of cancer including skin-cancers. Podophyllotoxin was isolated from the rhizome in 1880 by V. Podwyssotski [75]. More cytotoxic 4-deoxypodophyllotoxin was isolated from Cow Parsley (*Anthriscus sylvestris* L.) and Korean pasque flower (*Pulsatilla koreana* Y.Yabe ex Nakai). Although native epipodophyllotoxines are not used but its synthetic analogues - etoposide and teniposide, which belongs to topoisomerase II inhibitors, are effective in the treatment of lymphomas and bronchial and testicular cancers [65,76]. Another example is bruceantin isolated from a tree, *Brucea antidysenterica* Mill from *Simaroubaceae* DC family, used traditionally for the tumour treatment in Ethiopia [77]. Recently it was discovered that bruceantin can be an effective agent for the treatment of hematological malignancies (leukaemia, lymphoma and myeloma). Its activity has been linked with the down-regulation of a key oncoprotein. Omacetaxine mepesuccinat (Homoharringtonine), alkaloid isolated from the Cowtail Pine called Japanese Plum Yew (*Cephalotaxus harringtonia* Koch), is one more example of plant-derived anticancer agent [78,79]. Its racemate (harringtonine mixed with homoharringtonine) which induces apoptosis by inhibition of protein synthesis, particularly Mcl-1 (induced myeloid leukemia cell differentiation protein), is used for the treatment of chronic leukaemia - acute lymphoblastic leukaemia and chronic myelogenous leukaemia [65]. Elliptinium acetate, a derivative of ellipticine, which was isolated from a Fijian plant *Bleekeria vitensis* A.C. Sm., is used for the treatment of breast cancer [65]. Recently numerous potential anticancer compounds have been isolated from different plants. A few of them are currently in clinical or preclinical trials but most require further investigation. A case of considerable interest is indirubine extracted from Mu Lan (*Indigofera tinctoria* L.) from *Leguminosae* Lindl. family called Indigo plant a main component of traditional Chinese herbal remedy called Dang Gui Long Hui Wan used to treat chronic myelogenous leukaemia. Synthetic agents flavopiridol derived from the indirubins - plant alkaloid rohitukine, which was isolated from *Dysoxylum binectariferum* Hook. f. (*Meliaceae* Juss.) [80] and roscovitine derived from olomucine, which was isolated from *Raphanus sativus* L. (*Brassicaceae* Burnett), are respectively in Phase I and II of clinical trials [65,81] against a broad range of cancers including leukaemia, lymphomas and solid tumours [82]. Both are belongs to inhibitors of cyclin-dependent kinases (Cdks), key regulatory proteins in the cell cycle. Most recent studies indicate that drugs of the indirubin family may block brain tumour and thus improve survival in glioblastoma. Other synthetic derivatives of indirubins (3'-monooxime and 5-bromo) reveal comparable activity to other Cdk inhibitors and thus are promising for drug development [83]. Unique source of indirubines are gastropod molluscs: *Bolinus brandaris* L. and *Hexaplex trunculus* L. (*Muricidae* L.) used for over 2,500 years to obtain purplish red dye known as "Tyrian Purple". The 6-bromoindirubine treated as impurity to indigo dye and its synthetic derivative show selective inhibition of glycogen synthase kinase-3 (GSK-3) [81]. The discovery of GSK-3 functions resulted in the search for its inhibitors as potential drugs against neurodegenerative diseases, inflammation and cancer. Combretastatin isolated from the bark of the South African "bush willow", tree *Combretum caffrum* (Eckl. & Zeyh.) Kuntze (*Combretaceae* Loefl. familly) [84] belongs to the most cytotoxic phytomolecules isolated so far [85,86] and is promising in the treatment of colon, lung cancers, lymphomas and leukaemias. Combretastatins belongs to stilbenes, which are anti-angiogenic agents, causing vascular shutdown resulting in tumour necrosis. *Combretum* was widely used in African and Hindu medicine for the treatment of a variety of diseases, but *Terminalia* L. flowering plant from the same family *Combretaceae* Loefl., have been used traditionally for cancer treatment. Another promising stilbene is trans-Resveratrol natural phenol produced by several plants (eg. *Vitis vinifera* L., *Vitis labrusca* L., *Vitis rotundifolia* Michx.), when under attack by pathogens (bacteria or fungi like Botrytis cinerea (De Bary) Whetzel). It was extracted from False Helleborine (*Veratrum Album* L.) by Michio Takaoka in 1939. More than 60 years later in 1997, Ming-Hua Jang reported that trans-Resveratrol prevented skin cancer development in mice treated with a carcinogen, which gain attention to its potential anticancer applications. It was shown that trans-Resveratrol acts on all steps of the process of carcinogenesis [87]. It triggered apoptosis in uterine, colon cancer cell line, colon, human breast, prostate, lung cancer and pancreatic cancer cell lines in vitro, but is also able to arrest the cell cycle or to inhibit kinase pathways. The inhibition in the development of oesophageal, intestinal, and breast cancer after oral administration of resveratrol was revealed in studies on animal models. The human clinical trials for cancer have not been reported. A few promising substances betulinic acid, lupeol have been obtained from white part of *Betula species* (*Betulaceae* Gray) bark. The alcohol precursor of betulinic acid - betulin - was isolated as long ago as in 1788 by Tobias Lowitz (1757-1804). Betulinic acid, a pentacyclic triterpene, is a common secondary metabolite of plants, it was isolated also from *Ziziphus zizyphus* L. H. Karst. species, e.g. *Ziziphus Mauritiana* Lam., *Ziziphus Rugosa* Lam. and *Ziziphus Oenoplia* (L.) Mill. [88,89], while lupeol was found in a variety of plants, including mango *(Mangifera L.)* and acacia visco *(Acacia visite* Griseb.). All of them are potent anti-inflammatory agents and displayed selective cytotoxicity against human melanoma cell lines [90]. A case of considerable interest is birch polypore fungus Chaga (*Inonotus obliquus* Pers. Pill.), which belongs to *Basidiomycetes* R.T. Moore. It forms black perennial woody growth called a conk on birch trees. It is traditionally used in Russia for the treatment of a number of conditions including cancer, gastritis and ulcers. Two phenolic compounds, hispidin and hispolon extracted from Chaga but also from Japan, Chinese and Korean medicinal fungus *Phellinus linteus* (Japanese *meshimakobu*, Chinese *song gen*, Korean *sanghwang*) were reported to be cytotoxic against human cell line HeLa [91], while the polysaccharides ß (1→3)-D glucopyrans and ß (1→6)-D-glucosyl, found also in ornamental plant *Pteris ensiformis* Burm., originating from tropical Africa, Asia and Pacific region, have promising anticancer activity against a number of different cell lines.

Claims for another efficient plant derivative - *Tabebuia* Gomes (*Bignoniaceae* Juss.) used traditionally by the indigenous people in the Amazonian region for the treatment of variable diseases, appeared in the 1960s. Numerous bioactive compounds including naphthaquinones, particularly lapachol and ß-lapachone have been isolated from the stem bark and wood of *Tabebuia impetiginosa* (Mart. Ex DC.) Standl., *Tabebuia rosea* Bertol., and *Tabebuia serratifolia* (Vahl) Nicholson. Lapachol revealed potent in vivo anti-tumour activity, but was dropped out because of unacceptable level of toxicity [92]. ß-lapachone was recently found active against breast cancer, leukaemia, prostate tumour and several multidrug resistant (MDR) cell lines and more promising than lapachol [93]. It is a potent inhibitor of Cdc25 phosphatases enzyme that play a key role in cell cycle progression [83]. Another potent and promising in the field of MDR is pervilleine A, aromatic ester tropane, selectively cytotoxic against oral epidermoid cancer cell line which was isolated from the roots of the Madagascar tree *Erythroxylum pervillei* Baill. from *Erythroxylaceae* Kunth family [94,95]. In the early 1970s another plant originated substance, maytansine was isolated from the Ethiopian plant, *Maytenus serrata* (Hochst. Ex A. Rich.) Wilczek from *Celastraceae* R. Br. family. Although the results of preclinical animal tests were very promising but the lack of efficacy in clinical trials in the early 1980s resulted in dropping it out from further study. However, related compounds, the ansamitocins, isolated from actinomycete *Actinosynnema pretiosum* shed some light on its possible microbial origin [96]. Its synthetic derivative - cytotoxic Mertansine is a component of humanized monoclonal antibodies: Cantuzumab mertansine, Bivatuzumab mertansine, Lorvotuzumab mertansine and Trastuzumab emtansine effective in colorectal, squamous cell carcinoma, small-cell lung or ovarian cancer and breast cancer, respectively. Another case of considerable interest is thapsigargin isolated from the umbelliferous plant, *Thapsia garganica* L. (*Apiaceae* Lindl.) from Mediterranean island of Ibiza [97]. Thapsigargin, induces apoptosis in prostate cancer cells and synthetic prodrug derived from it called "G-202" is in Phase II clinical trials. Silvestrol isolated from the fruits of *Aglaila sylvestre* Roemer from *Meliaceae* Juss. family [98], exhibit cytotoxicity against lung and breast cancer cell lines [65]. Its synthetic analogue 4'-desmethoxyepisilvestrol is cytotoxic against lung and colon cancer cell lines. Two alkaloids, schischkinnin and montamine isolated recently from the seeds of *Centaurea schischkinii* Tzvelev and *Centaurea montana* L. [99,100] exhibit significant cytotoxicity against HCCLs (human colon cancer cell lines). The essential oil of *Salvia officinalis* L., most popular folk remedy in Middle East known for its antitumor effects, which contains monoterpenes thujone, β-pinene, and 1,8-cineol was shown to be cytotoxic against squamous human cell carcinoma cell line of the oral cavity [101]. There are many other natural substances like extracts of unknown composition from *Colubrina macrocarpa* (Cav.) G. Don., *Hemiangium excelsum* (Kunth) A.C. Sm, *Acacia pennatula* (Schltdl. & Cham.) Benth., *Commiphora opobalsamum* Jacq., *Astragalus* L., *Paris polyphylla* Sm., *Teucrium polium* L., *Pistacia lentiscus* L. used as anticancer remedies on folk medicine in China, Israel, Plestina, Saudi Arabia etc.

In general, over 120 currently prescribed drugs including anticancer ones being the basis of modern chemotherapy were first extracted from plants. About 60% of the anticancer drugs available prior to 1983 were of natural origin [65]. As much as 40% of anticancer drugs developed from 1940 to 2002 had natural or natural-product origins, while another 8% were natural-product mimics. Although nowadays about 300,000 different plant species are known but less than 5,000 have been studied for their potential drug usefulness. Since 1989, the National Cancer Institute (NCI) has screened up to 10,000 potential anticancer agents per year including minerals, exotic plants from tropical rain forests and animal venoms and toxins.

Animal venoms and toxins which has been used as therapeutics in ancient Ayurvedic, Unani, Chinese folk medicine as well as in Homeopathy are also screened. Venoms of snakes, scorpions, toads, frogs and their derivatives protein or non-protein toxins, peptides, enzymes are promising and show some potential in cancer treatment. Léon Charles Albert Calmette (1863-1933) a French physician, bacteriologist and immunologist, was the first to describe an antitumor effect of the venom of Indian cobra Naja naja sp. on adenocarcinoma cells. Thereafter many reports have established the anticancer potential of venoms of different species of Elapidae, Viperidae, Crotalidae snakes [102-107] and Hydrophis spimlis sea snake [108,109] and assigned it to phospholipase activity. Scorpions venom has been used by traditional and folk medicine in India, China, Africa and Cuba. Chinese red scorpion (Buthus martensi Karsch) venom and skin extracts, known as Chan Su in China and Senso in Japan, have been used by traditional Chinese medicine for as long as 2000 years also as anti-leukaemia agents. 4',6-diamidino-2-phenylindole extracted from Buthus martensi Karsch induced cell apoptosis in malignant glioma cells in vitro [110], while serine proteinase and hylauronidase have promising anticancer activity against a number of different cell lines including breast ones [111]. Bengalin protein isolated from Hindu black scorpion is suspected to have anti-leukemic properties [112]. Chlorotoxin and Charybdotoxin, 36- and 37-amino acid peptides, respectively isolated from the venom of death stalker scorpion (Leiurus quinqestriatus Hebraeus) are promising for the treatment of several types of cancers including glioma and human breast cancer [113,114]. The anticancer effect of the venom of Cuba red scorpions (Rhopalurus junceus) was discovered 20 years ago in Guantanamo, but after 15 years of studies Vidatox drug was announced in 2011. The skin extract from Hindu toads (Bufo melanostictus, Bufo gargarizans Cantor), Chan Su used by Chinese traditional medicine, was discovered to contain a few bufadineolides showing specific activity against human leukemic, liver carcinoma and melanoma cell lines. Species belonging to the families Bufonidae (toads), Lampyridae (fireflies) and Colubridae (snakes) as well as mammalian tissues contain bufadienolides, but the richest source of them are toad species. Although all the bufadienolides showed potent cytotoxicity in vitro, but the evidence of their activity in vivo is limited to human hepatocellular carcinoma and HeLa human cancer cells in mice and require further investigation.

Some hope rises with the use of minerals as a source of anticancers drugs. Most important example is sodium bicarbonate, $NaHCO_3$, which was originally derived from Nahcolite (thermokalite) carbonate mineral. The ancient Egyptians used natural natron, a mixture of sodium carbonate decahydrate, and sodium bicarbonate as a soap and embalming tool. Recently it has been shown that sodium bicarbonate administered orally causes a selective increase in the pH of tumour and reduces the formation of spontaneous metastases in mouse models of metastatic breast cancer [115,116]. Another interesting case is selenite known since ancient times but recently revealed as a promising anticancer agent capable of inducing apoptosis in malignant mesothelioma and sarcoma cells [117].

As yet none of the new natural venom, toxin or minerals derived anticancer agents have reached the status of the clinical drug, but a number of agents are still in study or in preclinical development.

4.2. Synthetic drugs

The first steps toward chemical synthesis of drugs were undertaken by iatrochemistry, a branch of chemistry and medicine concerned with seeking chemical solutions to diseases and ailments. Paracelsus pioneered the use of chemicals and minerals in medicine. He introduced alcohol, arsenic, copper, lead and silver salts into medicine, and developed rules for drug administration and dosages of drugs. Paracelsus also devised methods of extracting the arcanum (active ingredient) from plant materials. For this reason he is considered to be the father of phytochemistry and pharmacognosy. Ehrlich, the father of chemotherapy, developed the animal model to screen a series of chemicals for their potential activity against diseases, which had a major influence on the direction of cancer drug development. He also studied the usability of aniline dyes and the first primitive alkylating agents in cancer treatment. The first overall cancer treatment programme was the work of another pioneer of modern chemotherapy - George Clowes (1915-1988). He developed the first transplantable carcinogen-induced tumour systems in mice, which allowed the standardization of models for cancer drug testing. These early model systems including Sarcoma 37 (S37), Sarcoma 180 (S180), Walker 256, and Ehrlich's ascites tumour have been used for several decades [118]. In 1935 Murray Shear developed the most organized program for cancer drug screening. About 3,000 compounds including natural ones, were screened with S37 as a model system. The reason for the failure of this first systematic attempt to search for anticancer drugs - only two drugs have been subjected to clinical trials, but finally dropped because of unacceptable toxicity - was the lack of knowledge on how to test cytotoxic effects in humans. An extension of the number of tumour systems available for studies by the Yoshida's ascites sarcoma model and a murine leukaemia induced by a carcinogen, Leukaemia 1210, described by Lloyd Law allowed fast progress.

4.3. Cell Cycle Non Specific Agents (CCNSA)

4.3.1. Alkylating agents

The first real breakthrough in the search for chemotherapeutics was the chemical synthesis of nitrogen mustards [4,119]. Sulphur mustard was synthesised much earlier, in 1822, but its harmful effects were not known until 1860. It was first used as chemical warfare weapon agent during the latter part of the First World War but its therapeutic activity against squamous cell carcinoma was discovered by accident. In fact most of the first so-called true synthetic chemotherapeutics, were discovered by serendipity, the special term *Serendipity* for accidental discoveries was introduced by Horace Walpole (1717-1797) in the 18th c. Nitrogen mustard, an

http://dx.doi.org/10.5772/52507

analogue of the highly toxic sulphur mustard gas, was introduced in 1942 as the first alkylating agent and a true chemotherapeutic. Alfred G. Gilman, Louis S. Goodman and Thomas Dougherty, examined the potential therapeutic effects of nitrogen mustard in rabbits and mice bearing a transplanted lymphoid tumour, while Gustaf E. Lindskog (1903-2002), a thoracic surgeon, administered it to patients with non-Hodgkin's lymphoma. Many cases of cancer regression succeed intensive screening of related alkylating compounds and discovery of busulphan by L.A. Elson, G.M. Timmis, and David A. G. Galton (1922-2006) in 1951, Chlorambucil by James Everatt in 1953, melphalan by Frank Bergel and John Stock in 1954, Cyclophosphamide by Herbert Arnold, Friedrich Bourseaux and Norbert Brock in 1956, Lomustine and Carmustine by John A. Montgomery, George S. McCaleb, Thomas P. Johnston in 1966. While many different classes of alkylating agents (nitrogen mustards, nitrosoureas, alkyl sulphonates, triazines, and ethylenimines) are known, the chemical mechanism of their action is common and based on three different mechanisms all of which achieve the same end result - disruption of DNA function and apoptosis. The first mechanism of DNA alkylation results in its fragmentation by repair enzymes to prevent DNA synthesis and RNA transcription from the affected DNA. The second mechanism is the formation of intrastrand or interstrand cross-links by an alkylating agent, which prevents DNA from being separated for synthesis or transcription. The third mechanism of action is the induction of mispairing of the nucleotides, which leads to mutations, even permanent ones.

Alkylating agent acts on a cancer cell in every phase of its life cycle, Fig. 2, thus can be used in the treatment of a wide range of cancers from various solid tumours to leukaemia. However strong adverse effect is their ability to induce secondary cancers, which is reflected by their classification as definite carcinogens by IARC [3].

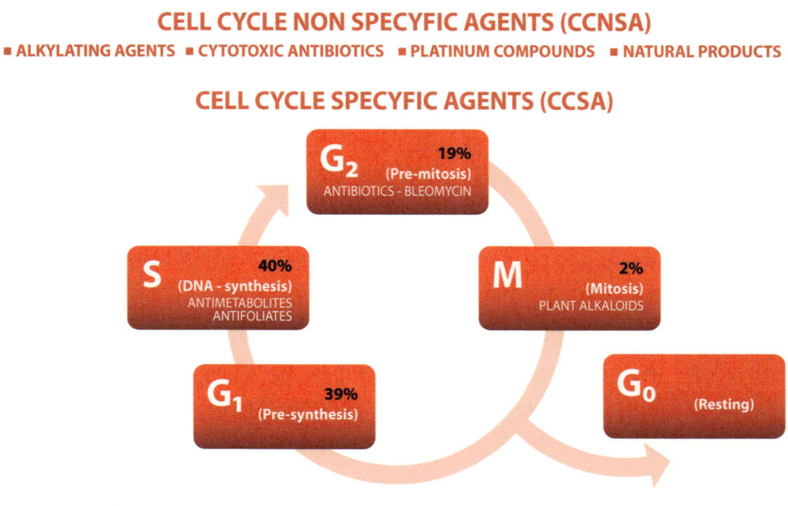

Figure 2. Cell replication occurs in the cell cycle (G_0, G_1, S, G_2 and M). The cell cycle nonspecific agents (alkylating agents, platinum compounds, cytotoxic antibiotics) are able to kill a cell during any phase of the cycle, while cell cycle specific (antimetabolites, antifoliates, planta alkaloids, some cytotoxic antiniotics line bleomycin) are only able to kill only during a specific phase.

4.3.2. Cytotoxic antibiotics

A number of cytotoxic antibiotics that have been derived from natural sources such as gram-positive bacteria in soil and water, belonging to genus *Streptomyces* (phylum *Actinobacteria*) [4,119]. They produce secondary metabolites, many of which have been successfully isolated and used as antifungals, antibiotics and anticancer drugs. The large-scale screening of fermentation products by the pharmaceutical industry which resulted in the discovery of antibiotics to treat wound infections is one more example of finding anticancer drugs by serendipity. Although penicillin, which was the basic compound for the above mentioned studies has no antitumor properties itself, but the chromo oligopeptide actinomycin D, isolated from *Streptomyces antibioticus* by Selman Abraham Waksman (1888-1973) and Boyd Woodruff in the 1940s as a result of search for drugs to treat tuberculosis, has significant antitumor properties and was applied in the 1950/1960s in paediatric oncology. This antibiotic was approved by the U.S. Food and Drug Administration (FDA) in 1964. In 1950, the search for anticancer compounds from soil-based microbes in the area of Castel del Monte, Italy, resulted in the discovery of an antibiotic - Daunorubicin (red pigment) - independently by Aurelio di Marco, Arpad Grein and Celestino Spalla from bacterium *Streptomyces peucetius* and by M. Dubost from *Streptomyces caeruleorubidus.* It was found to be active against murine tumours (Yoshida sarcoma). Although clinical trials which began in the 1960s suggested its significant activity against acute leukaemia and lymphoma, but shortly after, in 1967, it was recognized that daunorubicin had significant cardiac toxicity. In general, many antibiotics produced by *Streptomyces* are too toxic for use as antibiotics in humans, but their activity towards specific cells lines makes them useful in chemotherapy. The search for more effective antitumor antibiotics over 2,000 analogues of slightly modified structures yielded in a series of compounds, some of which are in common use till today. In 1969, Federico Arcamone developed a derivative of Doxorubicin which in the same year was tested against animal tumours by di Marco. Daunroubicin and Doxorubicin belongs to inhibitors of the topoisomerase II, one of two enzymes that regulate overwinding/underwinding of DNA. Inhibition of the topoisomerase II block cleavage of both strands of the DNA which ultimately leads to cell death. An important antibiotic of a wide spectrum of anticancer activity is Mitomycin C isolated from *Streptomyces caespitosu* in 1955 and *Streptomyces lavendulae* in 1958 and clinically used since the first successful trials against childhood leukaemia reported by Charlotte Tan in 1965. Mitomycin C belongs to bifunctional alkylating agents, whose biological activity mode is DNA alkylation and cross-linking. It has a broad activity against a range of tumours. In 1966 Hamao Umezawa discovered an important unique antibiotic in this group - bleomycin - a glycopeptide showing anticancer activity, while screening a culture filtrates of *Streptomyces verticullus.* Bleomycin is used to treat many types of cancer, including testicular cancer, non Hodgkin's lymphoma, Hodgkin's lymphoma and cancers of the head and neck. Anticancer antibiotics, apart from Bleomycin, act on a cancer cell in every phase of its life cycle and prevent cell divisions, but Bleomycin is considered as cell cycle agent specifically working in G2 and M phase, Fig. 2. However, the risk connected with the use of cytotoxic antibiotics classified as group 2 or 3 agent in IARC classification is smaller than that related to alkylating agents [3].

http://dx.doi.org/10.5772/52507

4.3.3. Platinum compounds

Cisplatin was synthesized in 1845 but its potential as an antitumour agent was not recognized until 1965 when its capabilities were discovered by Barney Rosenberg, Loretta van Camp and Thomas Krigas. The inhibition of growth caused by platinum complex of ammonia and chloride (Peyrone's salt i.e. Cis-platinum) was discovered by serendipity during the studies of the influence of electric current on bacterial growth. The positive result during the studies of murine tumours in vivo confirmed its antitumor activity and prompted the studies of other compounds from this class [4,56,119]. It was introduced into clinical practice one decade later in the 1970s [120]. By 1978 about 1,000 platinum complexes had been screened, but only seven were selected for detailed pharmacological evaluation on rats and only two - Carboplatin and Oxaliplatin - were non-toxic at effective antitumour dose. Although Cisplatin belongs to three most commonly used chemotherapeutics, progress made to improve its use since its discovery is in fact limited. The mechanism of action of Cisplatin and other platinum compounds resemble that of the alkylating agents. They interact covalently with DNA and form intrastrand (within the same DNA molecule; >90%) or interstrand (between two different DNA molecules; <5%), cross links between adjacent guanine molecules [121]. The formation of DNA adducts results in an inhibition of DNA synthesis and transcription. Platinum compounds act on a cancer cell in every phase of its life cycle, Fig.2. Their use is widespread and includes the treatment of bladder and colorectal cancer, upper gastrointestinal disease, germ cell tumours, head and neck malignancies, lung and ovarian cancer. Their ability to induce secondary cancers reflected by their classification as definite carcinogens by IARC is high [3].

4.4. Cell Cycle Specific Agents (CCSA)

4.4.1. Antifolates

Antimetabolites (folic acid, pyrimidine or purine analogues), which structurally resemble naturally occurring molecules necessary for DNA and RNA synthesis and either inhibit enzymes needed for nucleic acid production or induce apoptosis during the S phase of cell growth, Fig. 2, were among the first effective chemotherapeutics discovered. In the early 1940s, Sidney Faber (1903–1973) studied the effect of folic acid (pteroylglutamic acid; Vitamin B9) first isolated from spinach leaves. In 1945, Rudolf Leuchtenberger reported that folic acid inhibited tumour growth in mice, while Richard Lewisohn reported complete regression of spontaneous breast in mice observed with folic acid. Farber, Robert D. Heinle, and Arnold D. Welch tested folic acid in leukaemia and concluded spuriously that deficiency of Vitamin B9 accelerates leukaemia cell growth. Efforts to treat leukaemia resulted in pharmacological folic acid analogues with effects antagonistic to those of Vitamin B9. Shortly after Sidney Farber and Harriet Kilte developed a series of foliate antagonists including highly active aminopterin (4-amino-pteroylglutamic acid). Its analogue 4-amino-4-deoxy-10-*N*-methyl-pteroylglutamic acid, known nowadays as Methotrexate, was discovered by Yellapragada Subbarao (1895-1948) and successfully applied by Sidney Farber in 1947 to induce remissions in children with leukaemia. In 1958 Min Chiu Li, reported fully effective treatment of a very rare tumour of the placenta, choriocarcinoma with Methotrexate, which was the first-ever intentionally discovered synthetic anticancer drug i.e. first true chemotherapeutic. Starting from the 1950s, Methotrexate has replaced the more toxic aminopterin and is still in widespread clinical use. In general folate antagonists mechanism of action is linked with competing with folates for uptake into cells and inhibition of the formation of folate co-enzymes or reactions that are mediated by them. Only one of those mechanisms is clinically important, it is the prevention of formation of tetrahydrofolate by inhibition of the enzymes: dihydrofolate reductase (DHFR) or thymidylate synthase (TS). Methotrexate inhibits only DHFR, while a new-generation antifolate Pemetrexed developed by Edward C. Taylor in 1992 inhibits DHFR, TS and also transformylases (GAR and AICAR), but primarily acts as a TS inhibitor. Thus both act similarly by hindering enzymes needed for de novo synthesis of the thymidine and purine nucleotides but show different spectrum of activity. Methotrexate is effective mainly in the treatment of leukaemia, lymphoma and choriocarcinoma but also cancers of breast, head and neck, colorectal, osteosarcoma and bladder, while Pemetrexed is approved for the treatment of mesothelioma and non–small cell lung cancer, active in solid tumours treatment, especially those drug resistant. The risk connected with the use of Methotrexate classified as group 3 agent in IARC classification is smaller than that of alkylating agents [3].

4.4.2. Antimetabolites

The discovery of nitrogen mustard and Methotrexate and their success in medical applications was a breakthrough and stimulated the search for the other antimetabolites as well as new classes of cell cycle specific synthetic anticancer drugs [4,56,119]. In 1944, Richard O. Roblin and James W. Clapp synthesised 8-azaguanine (8-AZA), while 5 years later George W. Kidder and Virginia C., reported that 8-AZA was a guanine antagonist in the metabolism of *Tetrahymena geleii* (S) (*Colpidium campylum* L.) and inhibited the growth of transplanted mammary adenosarcoma in mice. Since 1944, George Herbert Hitchings (1905-1998) and Gertrude Belle Elion (1918-1999) have investigated the role of purines in nucleic acid metabolism and methods to prevent them from being incorporated to DNA synthesis along the metabolic pathway that would lead to interruption of cell reproduction. By the early 1950s, Hitchings & Elion synthesized more than 100 purine analogues including 2,6-diaminopurine, 6-thioguanine (6-TG), 6-mercaptopurine (6-MP) and Azathioprine (AZA) as a result of their rational approach to drug development. 6-TG, 6-MP and AZA although categorized as growth inhibitory antimetabolites, exert their functions more like a genotoxic methylating agents, such as alkylating drug Temozolomide, which methylates DNA. 6-MP, one of the early analogues, is widely used not only for acute leukaemias but also in gout and herpes viral infections, and as immunosuppressive agents in the organ transplantations, 6-TG is predominantly used as antileukaemic agent, while AZA as an immunosuppressive. The discovery of a few purine analogues Fludarabine (FLU), Cladribine (2CDA), and Pentostatin (DCF) was a result of further targeted studies performed within a NIH programme. Fludarabine discovered by John Montgomery and Kathleen Hewson in 1968 was the first halogenated ribonucleotide reductase inhibitor, a new-generation pro-drug of the purine class successfully used in treating refractory chronic lymphocytic and chronic B cell leukaemias, non-Hodgkin's lymphoma and T-cell lymphoma. Cladribine, resembling deoxyadenosine and remarkably active in hairy cell leukaemia was synthesised in 1972 by L.F. Christensen, A. Broom, M.J. Robins, and A.J. Bloch and in 1978 selected by Dennis A. Carson as the most potent enzyme adenosine deaminase (ADA) inhibitor from many candidate congeners. Pentostatin, which also inhibits ADA and similarly to 2CDA is active in hairy cell leukaemia and chronic lymphocytic leukaemia was synthesised by Hollis D.H. Showalter and David C. Baker in 1983. Recently, three new purine antimetabolites nerlabine, clofarabine, and forodesine have been found highly promising. Although these compounds belong to purine antimetabolites and reveal activity against specific types of leukaemia, they differ in metabolic properties and mechanism of action. As long ago as in 1964 Elmer Reist and Leon Goodman synthesized 9-β-Darabinofuranosyl guanine (ara-G), which despite of its antitumor properties in in-vitro canine leukaemia models evaluated by Elion & Kurtzberg was rejected because of inadequate solubility. In 1988, nelarabine, the 6-methoxy derivative of Ara-G, which is 10-fold more soluble than Ara-G, was synthesized by Thomas A. Krenitsky. In 2012, 48 years after synthesis of Ara-G, Nelarabine entered phase II of clinical studies with indication to T-cell acute lymphoblastic leukaemia or T-cell lymphoblastic lymphoma treatment. Clofarabine, a hybrid of Fludarabine and Cladribine, was synthesised by Mongomery in 1992. It also recently entered phase II of clinical studies with indication as antileukemic agent active in acute lymphoblastic leukaemia as well as in myeloid disorders in paediatrics. The third intensively studied purine antimetabolite is forodesine, synthesised by Peter C. Tyler and Vern L. Schramm in 1998. Forodesine, which is not incorporated into DNA and has unexplored mechanism of action is effective for the treatment of relapsed B-cell chronic lymphocytic leukaemia.

In the 1950s Robert Duschinsky synthesised the first pyrimidine analogue, 5-fluorouracil (5-FU). His discovery was based on the observation of the role of greater uptake of uracil in rat hepatoma metabolism, thus it was the first known case of "targeted" studies. 5-FU introduced into the clinic in 1957 by Charles Heidelberger has broad-spectrum activity against non-hematologic cancers, thus is now widely applied for treatment of many kinds of solid tumours of breast, head and neck, adrenal, pancreatic, gastric, colon, rectal, oesophageal, liver and G-U (bladder, penile, vulva, prostate). Even nowadays, 5-FU apart of its analogue Floxuridine, remains a fundamental drug in the treatment of colorectal cancer. Discovery of 5-FU was not only the first example of targeted studies but also the first targeted therapy, which later attracted much attention in current cancer drug development. However, the target in this case was understood not as a molecular target but as a biochemical pathway. In 1950 two spongo-nucleosides (spongouridine and spongothymidine) were isolated by Werner Bergman and Robert Feeney from a Caribbean sponge *Cryptotethya crypta*. It inspired Richard Walwick, Walden Roberts, and Charles Dekker to synthesise Cytarabine and Vidarabine in 1959. In 1964, John Evans tested activity of Cytarabine using in-vitro murine S180 model while four years later Rose Ruth Ellison introduced it into clinic for the B-cell leukaemia treatment. Cytarabine is effective in acute non-lymphocytic, lymphocytic, myelogenous, chronic myelocytic leukaemias, as well as leptomininingeal carcinomatosis and non-Hodgkin's lymphoma, Other pyrimidine antagonists include Capecitabine, which is an oral 5-FU pro-drug adjuvant in colon and breast metastasis therapy, Gemcitabine which is a prodrug of Cytarabine, effective in pancreatic, metastatic breast, bladder, ovarian and non-small cell lung cancers and Decitabine, used in myeloplastic syndrome. The antimetabolites of purines and pyrimidine compounds acts on a cancer cell in S phase of its life cycle, Fig.2 and are classified as a group 3 agents in IARC classification.

4.4.3. Plant alkaloids

A true breakthrough in chemotherapeutics came by in the 1950s as the discovery of the activity of plant alkaloids from Madagascar periwinkle plant *Vinca rosea* (*Catharanthus roseus* (L.) G. Don) by Canadian scientists Robert Laing Noble, Charles T. Beer and Gordon Sloboda [56]. The vinca alkaloids extracted from *Vinca rosea* consist of a subset of structurally similar compounds comprising two multiringed units, vindoline and catharanthine. Initially, they were investigated because of putative hypoglycaemic properties, but strong marrow suppression observed in rats and significant antileukaemic effects *in vitro* decided about their clinical use shortly after the discovery of their properties, in 1959. Nowadays, vinca alkaloids are produced synthetically and only four major ones - Vinblastine, Vincristine, Vinorelbine and Vindesine - are in the oncological clinical use. Vinblastine is most often applied in Hodgkin's disease, non-Hodgkin's lymphoma, breast cancer, and germ cell tumours, Vincristine is effective against leukaemia and Hodgkin's, Vinorelbine has significant antitumor activity in patients with breast cancer and antiproliferation effects on osteosarcoma, while Vindesine is used in the treatment of leukaemia, lymphoma, melanoma, breast cancer, and lung cancer. All vinca alkaloids have a unique mechanism of action; they bind to the microtubular proteins of the mitotic spindle, which leads to crystallization of the microtubule and mitotic arrest or apoptosis.

Another group of novel cytotoxic agents from plant alkaloids, taxane diterpenes, was discovered during long-term screening in the 1970s. The main compound in this class, Paclitaxel, was the first taxane introduced into clinical practice for the treatment of recurrent ovarian cancer metastatic, breast cancer, often in combination with Cisplatin. Nowadays, Paclitaxel is totally synthesized, but less popular than vinca because of its poor solubility. Both plant alkaloids vinca and taxanes are mitotic inhibitors M phase specific, Fig. 2, but they act in different ways. Their principal mechanism of action is the disruption of microtubule function, but in contrast to the vinca alkaloids, taxanes do not destroy mitotic spindles. The plant alkaloids are classified as a group 3 agents in IARC classification [3].

4.4.4. Combination regimens

In 2005, conventional chemotherapeutics still made the majority of the Top 20 Cancer Therapeutics. Their popularity was dictated not only by wide spectrum of activity and also long history of use in oncology but also their key role in the multidrug treatment programs. In the early 1960s, single alkylating agents were basic for all cancer treatment programmes. Although the remissions were observed for example up to 25% in advanced Hodgkin's disease but they were still incomplete and temporary. Increasing resistance of the cancer cells to classical drugs and numerous side effects forced new strategies. After Jacob Furth and Morton Kahn discovery that a single leukemic cell was sufficient to cause the death of an animal, Howard E. Skipper formulated "Cell Kill" hypothesis, according to which a given dose of drug is able to kill only a constant fraction of tumour cells. This hypothesis favoured search for more aggressive

http://dx.doi.org/10.5772/52507

chemotherapeutics but also resulted in the use of drug combinations. In 1965 Emil Frei and Emil J. Freireich developed the new treatment program for children leukaemia known as "VAMP" (Nethotrexate, 6-MP, Vincristine and Prednisone). The use of multiple drugs: Methotrexate, which disrupt folic-acid uptake, 6-MP which inhibits synthesis of purine, both critical in cell division, Vincristine which interfered with cell division by binding to spindle protein and Prednisone, anti-inflammatory steroid resulted in the remission rate level as high as 60%. Further modifications like "MOMP" (nitrogen mustard, Vincristine, Methotrexate, and Prednisone), "MOPP" (Procarbazine, nitrogen mustard, Vincristine, and Prednisone) and C-MOPP (Procarbazine, Cyclophosphamide, Vincristine, and Prednisone) resulted in the 80% complete remission rate in advanced Hodgkin's disease in the 1970s. On the basis of the above mentioned first programs dedicated exclusively to leukaemias many modifications - e.g. four drug EBVP (Epirubicin, Bleomycin, Vinblastine, Prednisone) and ABVD (Adriamycin, Bleomycin, Vinblastine and Dacarbazine) and six-drug STANFORD-V (Cyclophosphamide/Mechlorethamine/Ifosfamide, Doxorubicin, Vinblastine, Vincristine, Bleomycin, Etoposide) - have been developed. Nowadays, some cancer diseases like Hodgkin's or acute lymphocytic leukaemia are curable in 90% within the modern protocols using aggressive chemotherapy programs. Despite the reasonable position of classical chemotherapeutics in multidrug combined regimens, their capabilities inevitably decrease because of multidrug resistance (a major factor in the failure of many forms of treatment) and secondary effects (adverse or paradoxically carcinogenic). Significant limitation is also the need for multiple chemotherapy in long-term, sequential multidrug regimens and in-hospital administration.

4.4.5. Modern chemotherapeutics

At the beginning of the 20th c., Paul Ehrlich postulated the idea of a "Magic Bullet" (Zauberkugel) i.e. drugs that reach directly intended cell-structural targets. To some extent this idea is the driving force behind the development of modern targeted chemotherapeutics. Conventional chemotherapeutics are cytotoxic, but affect all cells and work in the so-called statistical manner. Because cancer cells multiply faster than normal, the cancerous cells are killed by the drug with a higher ratio than the normal ones, which are not spared. Therefore the principal criterion applied in the modern anticancer drug design is the principle of selective toxicity, which require activity restricted exclusively to the cancer cells. From the point of view of selective activity directed on tumour cells and mechanisms of carcinogenesis, a few different classes of modern drugs can be distinguished: inhibitors of cytokine stimulating cell proliferation, dissociation, motility; cytokine receptor blockers; intracellular kinases inhibitors; transcription factors inhibitors; cell cycle inhibitors; cell adhesion inhibitors and proteasome inhibitors.

Short-lived hopes were raised in the 1990s at the discovery of the inhibitors of angiogenesis, which hold back the growth of capillary vessels in cancer. Avastin, humanized monoclonal antibody, discovered by Napoleone Ferrara in 1997 was the first drug from this class approved by FDA in 2004 to use for several types of metastatic cancer, but the approval of the breast cancer indication was revoked in 2011. Two other inhibitors of angiogenesis include Cetuximab inverted by Joseph Schlessinger, Michael Sela in 1988, approved for by FDA in 2009 to use in colorectal cancer therapy and Sunitinib discovered by Joseph Schlessinger and Axel Ullrich approved by FDA in 2006 to use for renal cell carcinoma and gastrointestinal stromal tumour. Recent progress in genetic sequencing has led to the discovery of Vemurafenib by Fritz Hoffmann, approved by FDA in 2011. It targets the B-Raf gene that signals the growth of new blood cells in melanoma tumours, which are extremely difficult to treat.

Recently widespread attention has been given to inhibitors of protein kinases, enzymes that catalyze phosphorylation reactions, a principal mechanism of signal transduction governing various cellular processes including growth, division, migration and apoptosis. Imatinib, developed in the late 1990s by Nicholas Lydon, introduced to clinic by Brian Druker and approved to treat chronic myelogenous leukaemia by FDA in 2001 was the first drug of this new class of small active molecules. It inhibits the oncogene BCR-ABL1 and blocks the signals for cell proliferation, controlling tumour growth. Many imatinib analogues: including Nilotnib, Dasatinib, Bosutinib, Ponatinib, Bafetinib were obtained further by rational drug design. Gefitinib invented by ASTRA/ZENECA (approved by FDA in 2003 but withdrawn in 2005) and Erlotinib invented by OSI (approved by FDA in 2004), were the first selective inhibitors of epidermal growth factor receptor among the kinase inhibitors used for treatment of lung cancer.

Monoclonal antibodies that allow the cytotoxin to reach a target required to kill the malignant cells (induce apoptosis), without harming normal cells belong to the unique class of chemo-immunotherapeutics. In contrast to small molecule drugs which have a direct impact on their targets, the monoclonal antibodies stimulate the immune system i.e. re-direct targets to the immune system. Most popular includes: Gemtuzumab ozogamicin invented by Wyeth Ayerst and used for the treatment of acute myelogenous leukaemia, but withdrawn from the market in 2010 due to its toxicity, Ibritumomab tiuxetan developed by IDEC Pharmaceuticals used for the treatment of non-Hodgkin's lymphoma, but known to cause serious side effects, Panitumumab used for the treatment of colon cancer but ineffective, Rituximab developed by IDEC Pharmaceuticals and still used for the treatment of B-cell non-Hodgkin's lymphoma and tositumomab developed by Mark Kaminski and Richard Wahl used for the treatment of non-Hodgkin's lymphoma (mainly follicular lymphoma), currently in the clinical trials.

Although modern targeted therapies provide a new approach to cancer therapy and similarly to conventional ones are able to suppress tumour growth, but they also have drawbacks and limitations, while true cancer treatment is still a challenge for oncology.

5. Summary

Throughout history of medicine the process of new drug discovery has been based on natural sources and drugs have been discovered by serendipity (sheer luck) or in a trial-and-error process. While until the mid-1980s new drugs were discovered mainly by serendipity, over the next decade, till mid-1990s, the knowledge of structure was the basis for research, then the starting point was to identify a target and a relationship between structure and function [122]. Nowadays a few major classes of drugs useful in cancer treatment have been defined: (1)

http://dx.doi.org/10.5772/52507

General Chemotherapy Drugs (the alkylating agents, anti-neoplastics, anti-metabolites), (2) Steroids, (3) Bisphosphonates, (4) Hormone therapies and (5) Biological therapies/Immunotherapy. This modern classification reflects the fact that anticancer drugs evolved from classical chemotherapeutics discovered mostly by serendipity to drugs acting directly against abnormal proteins in cancer cells designed by rational drug design. All of them have remarkable influence on the growth of cancer cells and on the mechanisms whereby cells replicate, transmit, and translate genetic information.

Current research are so multidirectional that it is impossible to discuss all of them in a short chapter. New directions in this field include the search for the improved pharmaceutical forms, new analogues of currently used drugs, new chemical compounds (natural or synthetic) of anticancer activity, selective anticancer agents (acting on the basis of pathophysiological mechanisms), the search for drugs among old-known drugs currently used for other indications than cancer, search for the methods of precise delivering the anticancer drugs to cancer tissue and stroma or to stimulate the immune system to generate anti-tumor immune responses and protect against cancer.

Even nowadays precursors or generic drugs are frequently discovered by serendipity, while their analogues are developed by purely rational design. Often the newly synthesised drug proved effective in quite different than expected applications. For example Aminoglutethimide was found to be effective in breast cancer treatment instead of being an antiepileptic, Cisplatin, an electrolysis product, was discovered to be cytotoxic or Tamoxifen antiestrogenic activity of *cis*-isomer was discovered as unexpected bonus in the search for drugs to treat mania in bipolar disorder. Sometimes surprisingly a new field of activity is revealed for a long known drug. For example potassium-sparing diuretic Amiloride is effective in glioma; sedative Thalidomide, linked to birth defects, slows the propagation prostate cancer; Tebrophen, antiviral drug, slows the propagation of breast cancer; S-dimethylarsin-gluthathione, an organic form of arsenic, slow solid tumours expansion; anti-epileptic Valproic and Rapamycin, immunosuppressor in organ transplantation are valuable in antitumor therapy; Gossypol, potential male contraceptive overcome resistance to Cisplatin; antimalarial chloroquine may address a critical cell nutrition issue with proliferating cancer cells while insecticide benzoylphenylurea helps understand the microtubule assembly process important for growth of the pancreatic cancer cell. Anticancer properties have been ascertained to be shown by aspirin used commonly as analgesic, antipyretic and an anti-inflammatory medication, 9-aminoacridine used as an antiprotozoa and antibacterial agent and Quinacrine commonly used antimalarial drug. The use of long know drugs fasten modern process of drug discovery, which involves the identification of candidates, synthesis, characterization, screening, and assays for therapeutic efficacy and proceeds through many stages including discovery, product characterisation, formulation, pharmacokinetics, preclinical toxicology testing and IND (Investigational New Drug) application, bioanalytical testing and clinical trials. The new drugs (new completely or a long known one) often have many adverse effects. Sometimes in the final step the new drug proves toxic, ineffective or even carcinogenic. Many widely applied chemotherapeutic anticancer agents (nitrogen mustards, HN2 and HN3, treatamine, Chlorambucil,

Sacrolysin, Melphalan, and Busulphan), have been recognized as a source of secondary cancers and thus classified as definite carcinogens.

Sometimes known carcinogens have became invaluable drugs widely applied in clinical oncology. The most impressive example is arsenic - a component of the well known Poison of Kings (As_2O_3). It was used in traditional Chinese medicine in the treatment of promyelocytic leukaemia and acute myelogenous leukaemia. Reaglar containing arsenic was used by Hipocrates as a component of antitumor liniment. Avicenna in the 11th c. recommended it for cancer, both internally and topically. In the 16th century Paracelsus used it as a drug but linked with a cancer disease. In 1786 Thomas Fowler discovered Fowler's Solution (a 1% aqueous solution of potassium arsenite, KAsO2),which was applied as first chemotherapeutic in chronic myeloid leukaemia treatment in 1865 by Lissauer and persisted till the introduction of the first modern cytotoxic drugs in the 1940s. In 1931, its use in chronic myeloid leukaemia was described. In the late 1960s in China, an arsenic containing liniment was rediscovered for use as an effective anticancer treatment in melanoma. First reports of the intravenous administration of Fowler's Solution in acute promyelocytic leukaemia appeared in the 1990s, also in China. But in the 1990s IARC classified arsenic compounds as definite carcinogens. Despite this, in 2001 Fowler's Solution was accepted by FDA for the treatment of relapsed or refractory acute promyelocytic leukaemia in children. After being abandoned for decades, arsenic trioxide in the 21st c started to be prescribed as a drug for acute promyelocytic leukaemia, and still it is classified as definite anticancer. Recently some hope rises with realgar as well as new arsenic-based compounds (e.g. C-glycosides), which have been intensively studied. On the other hand, a very recent studies performed by Peter S. Nelson et al. indicated that chemotherapy can damage healthy cells which secrete a protein WNT16B that sustains tumour growth and results in a resistance to further treatment [123]. This proves that chemotherapy itself can boost cancer growth. The paradox drug/carciogen concerns not only chemotherapeutics but also the methods, which revolutionized the treatment of cancer, being on the other hand carcinogenic, like X-Ray widely used in the diagnosis of cancer cells, cancer treatment and anticancer drug design, UV radiation being a basis of the photodynamic therapy. Paracelsus, father of toxicology already wrote "*All substances are poisons: there is none which is not a poison. The right dose differentiates a poison and a remedy.*" Paraphrasing him - the method and conditions of the use differentiates a carcinogen and anticancer drug. Thus the search for new drugs among carcinogens seems quite reasonable, while the protection against contact with or exposure to a carcinogen is a necessity.

The recent advances in genomics and proteomics deliver a promise of understanding the true internal mechanisms of cancerogenesis - a basis for cancer diseases. They cover the knowledge of genes alteration caused by cancer, its influence on the proteins encoded by them, the interaction of these proteins with each other in living cells, the resulting changes in the specific tissues and finally the effect on the entire body. The achievements in this field delimit new fully rational directions in anticancer drug discovery and development of drugs addressing the specific needs (targeted drugs).

Author details

Jolanta Natalia Latosińska* and Magdalena Latosińska

*Address all correspondence to: jolanta.latosinska@amu.edu.pl

Faculty of Physics, Adam Mickiewicz University, Poznań, Poland

References

[1] Yarbro C.H.; Goodman M.; Frogge M.H. (Eds.) (2005). Cancer Nursing Principles and Practice (6th edition); Boston, Jones & Bartlett Publishers. pp. 1879. ISBN 0815169906.

[2] Ferlay J.; Shin H.R.; Bray F.; Forman D.; Mathers C.; Parkin (2010). D.M. GLOBOCAN 2008 v1.2. Cancer Incidence and Mortality Worldwide: IARC CancerBase No. 10. Lyon, France: International Agency for Research on Cancer, Available from: http://globocan.iarc.fr, accessed on day/month/year.

[3] IARC monographs on the evaluation of carcinogenic risks to humans, vol. 100 (A,B,C,D,E,F) 2012, Available from: http://monographs.iarc.fr/ENG/Classification. ISBN 9283213297.

[4] Olson J.S. (1989). The History of Cancer: An Annotated Bibliography (Bibliographies and Indexes in Medical Studies), Greenwood Press, Inc. pp. 434. ISBN 0313258899.

[5] Butler M.S. (2004). The role of natural product chemistry in drug discovery. *Journal of Natural Products*. 67:2141-2153. *ISSN 0163-3864*.

[6] Ensemble Human Genome. Available from: http://www.ornl.gov/sci/techresources/Human_Genome/project/hgp.shtml

[7] Morris C.; Kennedy M.; Heisterkamp N.; Columbano-Green L.; Romeril K.; Groffen J.; Fitzgerald P. (1991). A complex chromosome rearrangement forms the BCR-ABL fusion gene in leukemic cells with a normal karyotype. Genes Chromosomes Cancer. 3:263-71. ISSN 1098-2264

[8] Hirota S.; Isozaki K.; Moriyama Y.; Hashimoto K.; Nishida T.; Ishiguro S.; Kawano K.; Hanada M.; Kurata A.; Takeda M.; Muhammad Tunio G.; Matsuzawa Y.; Kanakura Y.; Shinomura Y.; Kitamura Y. (1998). Gain-of-function mutations of c-kit in human gastrointestinal stromal tumors. Science. 279:577-580. ISSN 1095-9203.

[9] Burke W.; Daly M.; Garber J. (1997). Recommendations for follow-up care of individuals with an inherited predisposition to cancer. II. BRCA1 and BRCA2. The Journal of the American Medical Association. 277:997-1003. ISSN 0002-9955.

[10] Haupt S.; Haupt Y. (2006). Importance of p53 for cancer onset and therapy. Anticancer Drugs. 17:725–32. ISSN 1473-5741.

[11] Vazquez A.; Bond E.E.; Levine A.J.; Bond G.L. (2008). The genetics of the p53 pathway, apoptosis and cancer therapy. *Nature Reviews Drug Discovery*.7:979–87. *ISSN 1474-1776.*

[12] Jorde L.B.; Carey J.C.; Bamshad M.J.; White R.L. (2000). Cancer genetics. In: Schmitt W. (ed.), Medical Genetics, 2nd ed. St Louis: Mosby, pp. 221–238. ISBN 9780323040358.

[13] Hanahan D.; Weinberg R.A. (2000). The hallmarks of cancer. *Cell* 100: 57–70. ISSN 0969-2126

[14] Pohanish R.P. (2011). Sittig's Handbook of Toxic and Hazardous Chemicals and Carcinogens, William Andrew, 6 edition. pp. 3096. *ISBN 1437778690.*

[15] Baba A.I.; Câtoi C. (2007). Comparative Oncology. Bucharest: The Publishing House of the Romanian Academy. ISBN 9732714573.

[16] United Nations (UN) (2003) Globally harmonized system of classification and labelling of chemicals (GHS). New York and Geneva. Available from: http://www.unece.org/trans/danger/publi/ghs/ghs_rev00/00files_e.html

[17] Cook J.W.; Hewett C.L.; Hieger, I. (1933). Isolation of A Cancer-producing Hydrocarbon from Coal Tar II. Isolation of 1,2- and 4,5-Benzopyrenes, Perylene, and 1,5-Benzoanthracene, Journal of the Chemical Society. 396-8. ISSN 0368-1769.

[18] Pott F.; Stöber W. (1983). Carcinogenicity of airborne combustion products observed in subcutaneous tissue and lungs of laboratory rodents. Environmental Health Perspectives. 47: 293–303. ISSN 0091-6765.

[19] Concon, J.M. (1988). Food Toxicology, Parts A and B. Marcel Dekker, New York. ISBN: 0824777360.

[20] Berenblum I. (1941). The mechanism of carcinogenesis. A study of significance of cocarcinogenic action and related phenomena. *Cancer Research.* 1:807-814. *ISSN 0008-5472.*

[21] Magee P.N.; Barnes J.M., (1956). The production of malignant primary hepatic tumours in the rat by feeding dimethylnitrosamine, British Journal of Cancer. 10:114-22. ISSN 0007-0920.

[22] Schreiber, H.; Nettesheim, P.; Lijinsky W.; Richter, C. B.; Walburg, H. E., Jr. (1972). Induction of lung cancer in germ-free specific-pathogen-free, and infected rats by N-nitrosoheptamethyleneimine: Enhancement by respiratory infection. Journal of the National Cancer Institute. 49: 1107-1114. ISSN 0027-8874.

[23] Dvorackova, I. (1990). Aflatoxins and Human Health. Boca Raton, FL: CRC Press. *ISBN 0849346282.*

[24] van Walbeek W.; Scott P.M.; Harwig J.; Lawrence J.W. (1969). Penicillium viridicatum Westling: a new source of ochratoxin A. Canadian Journal of Microbiology. 11:1281–1285. ISSN 1480-3275.

[25] Laqueur G. L.; Mickelsen O.; Whiting M. G.; Kurland L. T. (1963). Carcinogenic Properties of Nuts from Cycas Circinalis L. Indige nous to Guam. Journal of the National Cancer Institute. 31: 919-951. ISSN 0027-8874.

[26] Homburger F.; Boger E. (1968). The Carcinogenicity of Essential Oils, Flavors, and Spices: A Review. *Cancer Research*. 28: 2372-2374. ISSN 0008-5472.

[27] McDonald T.A. (1999). Evidence on the carcinogenicity of estragole, Environmental Protection Agency. Available from: http://oehha.ca.gov/prop65/pdf/estragf.pdf

[28] Mei N.; Guo L.; Fu P.P.; Fuscoe J.C.; Luan Y.; Chen T. (2010). Metabolism, genotoxicity, and carcinogenicity of comfrey. *Journal of Toxicology and Environmental Health*. 13:509-26. ISSN 1528-7394.

[29] Caramaschi F.; del Corno G.; Favaretti C.; Giambelluca S.E.; Montesarchio E.; Fara G.M. (1981). Chloracne following environmental contamination by TCDD in Seveso, Italy. *International Journal of Epidemiology*. 10:135–43. ISSN 1464-3685.

[30] Bertazzi P.A.; Bernucci I.; Brambilla G.; Consonni D.; Pesatori A.C. (1998). The Seveso studies on early and long-term effects of dioxin exposure: a review. Environmental Health Perspectives. 106: 625–633. ISSN 0091-6765.

[31] Pesatori A.C.; Consonni D.; Rubagotti M.; Grillo P.; Bertazzi P.A. (2009). Cancer incidence in the population exposed to dioxin after the "Seveso accident": twenty years of follow-up. *Environmental Health*. 47, 8:39. ISSN 1476-069X.

[32] Viluksela M.; Bager Y.; Tuomisto J.T. (2000). Liver tumor-promoting activity of 2,3,7,8-tetrachlorodibenzo-p-dioxin (TCDD) in TCDD-sensitive and TCDD resistant rat strains. *Cancer Research*. 60:6911–20. *ISSN 0008-5472.*

[33] Gibbs L. M. The Citizen's Clearinghouse for Hazardous Wastes (Arlington Va.) (1995). Dying from dioxin : a citizen's guide to reclaiming our health and rebuilding democracy. Boston, MA, South End Press. ISBN 049608-187-7.

[34] Paigen B.; Goldman L.R.; Magnant M.M.; Highland J.H.; Steegmann A.T. (1987). Growth of children living near the hazardous waste site, Love Canal. Human Biology. 59: 489-508. ISSN 1520-6300.

[35] Rahill A. A. (1989). The effects of prenatal environmental toxin exposure (dioxin): A case study. Psychosocial effects of hazardous toxic waste disposal on communities. D. L. Peck. Springfield, Illinois, Charles C. Thomas, Publisher.

[36] Canosa P.; Morales S.; Rodríguez I.; Rubí E.; Cela R.; Gómez M.(2005). Aquatic degradation of triclosan and formation of toxic chlorophenols in presence of low concentrations of free chlorine. Analytical and Bioanalytical Chemistry 383:1119-26. ISSN 1618-2650.

[37] Ravenscroft P.; Brammer H.; Richards K. (2009). Arsenic Pollution: A Global Synthesis Wiley. *ISBN 9781405186025.*

[38] Infante, P.F. (1976). Oncogenic and Mutagenic Risks in Communities with Polyvinyl Chloride Production Facilities. Annals of the New York Academy of Sciences. 271:49 - 57. ISSN 1749-6632.

[39] Hathway, D.E. (1977). Comparative Mammalian Metabolism of Vinyl Chloride and Vinylidene Chloride in Relation to Oncogenic Potential. Environmental Health Perspectives. 21:55 - 59. ISSN 0091-6765.

[40] Emmerich K.H.; Norpoth K. (1981). Malignant Tumors after Chronic Exposure to Vinyl Chloride. Journal of Cancer Research and Clinical Oncology. 102:1 - 11. ISSN 1432-1335.

[41] Allsopp M.W.; Vianello G. (2012). Poly(Vinyl Chloride): Ullmann's Encyclopedia of Industrial Chemistry, 2012, Wiley-VCH, Weinheim. ISBN 9780494193815.

[42] Rous F.P. (1911). Transmission of a malignant new growth by means of a cell-free filtrate. Journal of the American Medical Association. 56:198. ISSN 1538-3598.

[43] Lathrop A.E.; Loeb L. (1915). Further Investigations On The Origin Of Tumors In Mice : I. Tumor Incidence And Tumor Age in Various Strains of Mice. The Journal of Experimental Medicine. 22:646–673. ISSN 1540-9538.

[44] Brower V. (2004). Connecting Viruses to Cancer: How Research Moves from Association to Causation. Journal of the National Cancer Institute. 96:4. ISSN 1540-9538.

[45] Bittner J.J. (1942). The Milk-Influence of Breast Tumors in Mice. Science. 95:462–463. ISSN 0036-8075.

[46] Eddy B.E.; Stewart S.E. (1959). Characteristics of the SE Polyoma Virus. American Journal Public Health Nations Health. 49:1486–1492. ISSN 0090-0036.

[47] Trentin J.J., Yabe Y., Taylor G. (1962). The quest for human cancer viruses. Science .137: 835-841. ISSN 0036-8075.

[48] Epstein M.A., Achong B.G., Barr Y.M. (1964). Virus Particles in Cultured Lymphoblasts from Burkitt's Lymphoma. Lancet. 7335:702–3. ISSN 0140-6736.

[49] Beral, V., Peterman T., Berlelman R., Jaffe H. (1990). Kaposi's sarcoma among persons with AIDS: a sexually transmitted infection? Lancet. 335:123–127. ISSN 0140-6736.

[50] Chang Y.; Cesarman E.; Pessin M.S.; Lee F.; Culpepper J.; Knowles D.M.; Moore P.S. (1994). Identification of herpesvirus-like DNA sequences in AIDS-associated Kaposi's sarcoma. Science. 266:1865-9. ISSN 0036-8075.

[51] Feng H.; Shuda M.; Chang Y.; Moore P.S. (2008). Clonal integration of a polyomavirus in human Merkel cell carcinoma. Science. 319:1096–100. ISSN 0036-8075.

[52] Caruso M.L.; Fucci L. (1990). Histological identification of Helicobacter pylori in early and advanced gastric cancer. Journal of Clinical Gastroenterology. 12:601-2. ISSN 0192-0790.

[53] Ruggiero P. (2012). Helicobacter pylori infection: what's new. Current Opinion in Infectious Diseases. 25:337-44. ISSN 1473-6527.

[54] Parkin, D.M. (2006). The Global Health Burden of Infection-Associated Cancers in the Year 2002. International Journal of Cancer. 118:3030-3044. ISSN 1097-0215.

[55] Samaras V.; Rafailidis P.I.; Mourtzoukou E.G.; Peppas G.; Falagas M.E. (2010). Chronic bacterial and parasitic infections and cancer: a review. Journal of Infection in Developing Countries. 4:267-281. ISSN 19722680.

[56] Upton, A.C. (1986). Historical perspectives on radiation carcinogenesis. In Upton A.C.; Albert R.E.; Burns F.J. and Shore R.E. (Eds) Radiation Carcinogenesis. Elsevier, New York, 1–10. ISBN 0444008594.

[57] Goodman M.T.; Mabuchi K.; Morita M.; Soda M.; Ochikubo S.; Fukuhara T.; Ikeda T.; Terasaki M. (1994). Cancer incidence in Hiroshima and Nagasaki, Japan, 1958-1987. The European Journal of Cancer. 30A:801-7. ISSN 09615423.

[58] Gyorgy, A. (1980). No Nukes: Everyone's Guide to Nuclear Power. South End Press. *ISBN 0896080064.*

[59] Parenti Ch. (2011). After Three Mile Island: The Rise and Fall of Nuclear Safety Culture, The Nation, March 22, 2011, http://www.thenation.com/article/159386/after-three-mile-island-rise-and-fall-nuclear-safetyculture.

[60] Brenner A.V.; Tronko M.D.; Hatch M.; Bogdanova T.I.; Oliynik V.A.; Lubin J.H.; Zablotska L.B.; Tereschenko V.P.; McConnell R.J.; Zamotaeva G.A.; O'Kane P.; Bouville A.C.; Chaykovskaya L.V.; Greenebaum E.; Paster I.P.; Shpak V.M.; Ron E. (2011). I-131 Dose-Response for Incident Thyroid Cancers in Ukraine Related to the Chornobyl Accident. Environmental Health Perspectives. 119:933-9. ISSN 0091-6765.

[61] Walter J. (1977) Radiation hazards and protection: Cytotoxic chemotherapy. In: Walter J. (Ed.), Cancer and Radiotherapy: A short guide for nurses and medical students. London: Churchill Livingstone. ISBN 0443015333.

[62] Palmer A. (2001). Understanding radiotherapy and its applications. In: Gabriel J. (Ed.), Oncology Nursing in Practice. London: Whurr, pp. 30-51. ISBN 9780470057599.

[63] Dustin, A. P. (1934). Action de la colchicine sur le sarcome greffe de la souris. Bulletin et Académie Royale de Médecine de Belgique, 14:487-502. ISSN 0377-8231.

[64] Alonso-Castro A.J.; Ortiz-Sánchez E.; Domínguez F.; López-Toledo G.; Chávez M.; De Jesús Ortiz-Tello A.; García-Carrancá A. (2012). Antitumor effect of Croton lechleri Mull. Arg. (Euphorbiaceae). Journal of Ethnopharmacology .140:438-442. ISSN 0378-8741.

[65] Cragg G.M.; Newman D.J. (2005). Plants as source of anticancer agents. Journal of Ethnopharmacology. 100:72-79. ISSN 0378-8741.

[66] Chen S.; Zheng L.; Liu J.; Li J.; Zhang L.; Gu J.; Li X.; Shen W.; Ma F.; Yao Y.; Wu G.; Chen Q. (2011). Effects of realgar (tetra-arsenic tetra-sulfide) on malignant tumor cells. Journal of Clinical Oncology 29: e13525. ISSN 0732-183X.

[67] Wani M.C.; Taylor H.L.; Wall M.E.; Coggon P.; McPhail A.T. (1971). Plant anti-tumor agents. VI. The isolation and structure of taxol, a novel anti-leukemic and anti-tumor agent from Taxus brevifolia. Journal of the American Chemical Society. 93:2325-27. ISSN 0002-7863.

[68] Rowinsky E.K.; Onetto N.; Canetta R.M.; Arbuck S.G. (1992). Taxol-the 1st of the texanes, an important new class of anti-tumor agents. Seminars in Oncology.19: 646-62. ISSN 0093-7754.

[69] Holton R.A.; Somoza C.; Hyeong Baik Kim; Feng Liang; Biediger R.J.; Douglas Boatman P.; Mitsuru Shindo; Smith C. C.; Soekchan Kim (1994). First total synthesis of taxol. 1. Functionalization of the B ring. Journal of the American Chemical Society.116:1597–1598. ISSN 0002-7863.

[70] Wall, M.E.; Wani M.C.; Cook C.E.; Palmer K.H.; McPhail A.T.; Sim G.A. (1966). Plant antitumor agents. 1. The isolation and structure of camptothecin, a novel alkaloidal leukemia and tumor inhibitor from Camptotheca acuminata. Journal of the American Chemical Society. 88:3888-3890. ISSN 0002-7863.

[71] Potmesil M.; Pinedo H. (1995). Camptothecins: new anticancer agents. Boca Raton, Florida, CRC Press. 149-150. ISBN 0849347645.

[72] Creemers G.J.; Bolis G.; Gore M.; Scarfone G.; Lacave A.J.; Guastalla J.P.; Despax R.; Favalli G.; Kreinberg R.; VanBelle S.; Cuendet M.; Pezzuto J.M. (2004). Antitumor activity of Bruceantin. An old drug with new promise. Journal of Natural Products. 67:269–272. ISSN 0163-3864.

[73] Bertino J.R. (1997). Irinotecan for colorectal cancer. Seminars in Oncology. 24:S18-S23. ISSN 0093-7754.

[74] Stahelin H. (1973). Activity of a new glycosidic lignan derivative (VP 16-213) related to podophyllotoxin in experimental tumors. *The European Journal of Cancer.* 9:215-21. *ISSN 0959-8049.*

[75] Podwyssotski V. (1880). Pharmakologische Studien uber Podophyllum peltatum. Archiv für Experimentelle Pathologie und Pharmakologie. 13:29–52. ISSN 0028-1298.

[76] Harvey A.L. (1999). Medicines from nature: are natural products still relevant to drug discovery. Trends in Pharmacological Sciences. 20:196-98. ISSN 01656147.

[77] Creemers G.J.; Bolis G.; Gore M.; Scarfone G.; Lacave A.J.; Guastalla J.P.; Despax R.; Favalli G.; Kreinberg R.; VanBelle S.; Cuendet; M.; Pezzuto J.M. (2004). Antitumor activity of Bruceantin. An old drug with new promise. Journal of Natural Products. 67:269–272. ISSN 0163-3864.

[78] Itokawa H.; Wang X.; Lee, K.H. (2005). Homoharringtonine and related compounds. In: Cragg, G.M., Kingston, D.G.I., Newman, D.J. (Eds.), Anticancer Agents from Natural Products. Brunner-Routledge Psychology Press, Taylor & Francis Group, Boca Raton, FL, pp. 47–70. ISBN 1439813825.

[79] Powell R.G.; Weisleder D.; Smith C.R. Jr; Rohwedder W.K. (1970). Structures of harringtonine, isoharringtonine, and homoharringtonine. *Tetrahydron Letters*. 11:315-818. *ISSN 0040-4039.*

[80] Kelland L. R. (2000). Flavopiridol, the first cyclic-dependent kinase inhibitor to enter the clinic: current status. *Expert Opinion on Investigational Drugs*. 9: 2903-11. ISSN 1354-3784

[81] Meijer L.; Skaltsounis A.L.; Magiatis P.; Polychronopoulos P.; Knockaert M.; Leost M.; Ryan X.P.; Vonica C.A.; Brivanlou A.; Dajani R.; Crovace C.; Tarricone C.; Musacchio A.; Roe S.M.; Pearl L.; Greengard P. (2003). GSK-3-selective inhibitors derived from Tyrian purple indirubins. Chemistry & Biology. 10:1255-66. ISSN 1074-5521.

[82] Christian M.C.; Pluda J.M.; Ho P.T.; Arbuck S.G.; Murgo A.J.; Sausville E.A. (1997). Seminars in Oncology 24:219-40. ISSN 0093-7754.

[83] Newman D.J.; Cragg G.M.; Holbeck S.; Sausville E.A. (2002). Natural products as leads to cell cycle pathway targets in cancer chemotherapy. Current Cancer Drug Targets. 2:279–308. ISSN 1873-5576.

[84] Pettit G.R.; Singh S.B.; Boyd M.R.; Hamel E.; Pettit R.; Schmit J.M.; Hogan F. (1995). Antineoplastic agents. 291. Isolation and synthesis of combretastatins A-4, A-5 and A-6. The Journal of Medicinal Chemistry. 38: 1666-72. ISSN 0022-2623.

[85] Ohsumi K.; Nakagawa R.; Fukuda Y.; Hatanaka T.; Morinaga Y.; Nihei Y.; Ohishi K.; Suga Y.; Akiyama Y.; Tsuji T. (1998). New combretastatin analogues effective against murine solid tumors: design and structure-activity relationship. The Journal of Medicinal Chemistry .41: 705-06. ISSN 0022-2623.

[86] Pettit G. R.; Herald C. L.; Hogan F. (2002). In *Anticancer Drug Development*. B. C. Baguley and D. J. Kerr (Eds.), pp. 203–235, Academic Press, San Diego

[87] Delmas D.; Lançon A.; Colin D.; Jannin B.; Latruffe N. (2006). Resveratrol as a Chemopreventive Agent: A Promising Molecule for Fighting Cancer.*Current Drug Targets. 7* ISSN 1389-4501

[88] Pisha E.; Chai H.; Lee I.S.; Chagwedera T.E.; Farnsworth N.R.; Cordell G.A.; Beecher C.W.; Fong H.H.; Kinghorn A.D.; Brown D.M.; Wani M.C.; Wall M.E.; Hieken T.J.; Das Gupta T.K.; Pezzuto J.M. (1995). Discovery of betulinic acid as a selective inhibitor of human melanoma that functions by induction of apoptosis. *Nature Medicine*.1: 1046-51. ISSN 1078-8956.

[89] Nahar N.; Das R.N.; Shoeb M.; Marma M.S.; Aziz M.A.; Mosihuzzaman M. (1997). Four triterpenoids from the bark of Zizyphus rugosa and Z. oenoplia. Journal of Bangladesh Academy of Sciences. 21: 151-56. ISSN 0378-8121.

[90] Balunas M.J.; Kinghorn A.D. (2005). Drug discovery from medicinal plants. *Life Sciences*. 78: pp. 431-41. *ISSN 0024-3205.*

[91] Rzymoska J. (1998). The effect of aqueous extracts from Inonotus obliquus on the mitotic index and enzyme activities. *Bollettino Chimico Farmaceutico.* 137:13-5. ISSN. 0006-6648

[92] Suffness M.; Douros J. (1980). Miscellaneous natural products with antitumor activity. In: Cassady, J.M., Douros, J.D. (Eds.), Anticancer Agents Based on Natural Product Models. Academic Press, New York, p. 474 (Chapter 14). *ISBN* 0121631508.

[93] Ravelo A.G.; Estevez-Braun A.; Chavez-Orellana H.; Perez-Sacau E.; Mesa-Siverio D. (2004). Recent studies on natural products as anticancer agents. Current Topics in Medicinal Chemistry. 4:241–265. ISSN 0929-8673.

[94] Silva G.L.; Cui B.; Chavez D.; You M.; Chai H.B.; Rasoanaivo P.; Lynn S.M.; O'Neill M.J.; Lewis J.A.; Besterman J.M.; Monks A.; Farnsworth N.R.; Cordell G.A.; Pezzuto J.M.; Kinghorn A.D. (2001). Modulation of the multidrug-resistance phenotype by new tropane alkaloid aromaticesters from Erythroxylum pervillei. Journal of Natural Products. 64,1514–1520. ISSN 0163-3864.

[95] Mi Q.; Cui B.; Silva G.L.; Lantvit D.; Reyes-Lim E.; Chai H.; Pezzuto J.M.; Kinghorn A.D.; Swanson S.M. (2003). A new tropane alkaloid aromatic ester that reverses multidrug resistance. Anticancer Research. 23:3607–3616. ISSN 0250-7005.

[96] Yu T.W.; Floss, H.m(2005). The ansamitocins. In: Cragg, G.M., Kingston, D.G.I., Newman, D.J. (Eds.), Anticancer Agents from Natural Products. Brunner-Routledge Psychology Press, Taylor & Francis Group, Boca Raton, FL, pp. 321–338. ISBN 1439813825.

[97] Denmeade S.R.; Jakobsen C.M.; Janssen S.; Khan S.R.; Garrett E.S.; Lilja H.; Christensen S.B.; Isaacs J.T. (2003). Prostate-specific antigen-activated thapsigargin prodrug as targeted therapy for prostate cancer. *Journal of the National Cancer Institute.* 95: 990–1000. ISSN 0027-8874.

[98] Hwang B.Y.; Lee J.H.; Koo T.H.; Kim H.S.; Hong Y.S.; Ro J.S.; Lee K.S.; Lee J.J. (2001). Kaurane diterpenes from Isodon japonicus inhibit nitricoxide and prostaglandin E2 production and NF-nB activation in LPS-stimulated macrophage RAW264.7 cells. Planta Medica. 67:406–410. ISSN 0032-0943.

[99] Shoeb M.; Celik S.; Jaspars M.; Kumarasamy Y., MacManus S., Nahar L., Kong T.L.P., Sarker S.D. (2005). Isolation, structure elucidation and bioactivity of schischkiniin, a unique indole alkaloid from the seeds of *Centaurea schischkinii*. *Tetrahedron.* 61: 9001-06. *ISSN 0040-4020.*

[100] Shoeb M.; MacManus S.M.; Jaspars M.; Trevidadu J.; Nahar L.; Thoo-Lin P.K.; Sarker S.D. (2006). Montamine, a unique dimeric indole alkaloid, from the seeds of *Centaurea montana* (Asteraceae), and its in vitro cytotoxic activity against the CaCo2 colon cancer cells. *Tetrahedron.* 62:11172-77. *ISSN 0040-4020.*

[101] Sertel S.; Eichhorn T.; Plinkert P.K.; Efferth T. (2011). Cytotoxicity of Thymus vulgaris essential oil towards human oral cavity squamous cell carcinoma. Anticancer Research. 31:81-7. ISSN 1791-7530.

[102] Tu A.T.; Giltner J.B. (1974). Cytotoxic effects of snake venoms on KB and Yoshida sarcoma cell. Research Communications in Chemical Pathology and Pharmacology. 9:783–786. ISSN 0034-5164.

[103] Iwaguchi T.; Takechi M.; Hayashi K. (1985). Cytolytic activity of cytotoxin isolated from Indian cobra venom against experimental tumor cells. Biochemistry International. 10:343–349. ISSN 0158-5231.

[104] Chaim-Matyas A.; Ovadia, M. (1987). Cytotoxic activity of various snake venoms on melanoma, B16F10 and chondrosarcoma. *Life Sciences.* 40:1601–1607. *ISSN 0024-3205.*

[105] Zhong X.Y.; Liu G.F.; Wang Q.C. (1993). Purification and anticancer activity of cytotoxin-14 from venom of Naja naja atra. Zhongguo Yao Li Xue Bao. 14:279–282. ISSN 0253-9756.

[106] Lipps B.V. (1999). Novel snake venom proteins cytolytic to cancer cells in vitro and in vivo systems. Journal of Venomous Animals and Toxins including Tropical Diseases. 5:173–183. ISSN 16789199.

[107] Jokhio R.; Ansari A.F. (2005). Cobra snake venom reduces significantly tissue nucleic acid levels in human breast cancer. The Journal of the Pakistan Medical Association. 55:71–73. ISSN 0030-9982.

[108] Araya C.; Lomonte B. (2007). Antitumor effects of cationic synthetic peptides derived from Lys49 phospholipase A2 homologues of snake venoms. Cell Biology International. 31: 263-268. ISSN 1065-6995.

[109] Karthikeyan R.; Karthigayan S.; Sri Balasubashini M.; Vijayalakshmi S.; Somasundaram S.T.; Balasubramanian T. (2007). Inhibition of Cancer Cell Proliferation in vitro and Tumor Growth in vivo by Hydrophis spiralis Sea Snake Venom. International Journal of Cancer Research. 3:186-190. ISSN 1811-9727.

[110] Wang W.X.; Ji Y.H. (2005). Scorpion venom induces glioma cell apoptosis in-vivo and inhibits glioma tumor growth in-vitro. The Journal of Neuro-Oncology. 73:1-7. ISSN 1573-7373.

[111] Gao R.; Zhang Y.,;Gopalakrishnakone P. (2008). Purification and N-terminal sequence of a serine proteinase-like protein (BMK-CBP) from the venom of the Chinese scorpion (Buthus martensii Karsch). Toxicon. 52:348-53. ISSN 0041-0101.

[112] DasGupta S.; Debnath A.; Saha A.; Giri B.; Tripathi G.; Vedasiromoni J.R.; Gomes A.; Gomes A. (2007). Indian black scorpion (*Heterometrus bengalensis Koch*) venom induced antiproliferative and apoptogenic activity against human leukemic cell lines U937 and K562. *Leukemia Research.* 31:817-82. *ISSN 0145-2126.*

[113] DeBin J.A.; Maggio J.E.; Strichartz G.R. (1993). Purification and characterization of chlorotoxin, a chloride channel ligand from the venom of the scorpion. American Journal of Physiology. 264:361–369. ISSN 0363-6119.

[114] Lyons S.A.; O'Neal J.; Sontheimer H. (2002). Chlorotoxin a scorpion-derived peptide, specifically binds to gliomas and tumors of neuroectodermal origin. *Glia* 39:162–173. *ISSN 0894-1491.*

[115] Robey I.F.; Martin N.K. (2011). Bicarbonate and dichloroacetate: Evaluating pH altering therapies in a mouse model for metastatic breast cancer BMC Cancer. 11:235. ISSN 1471-2407.

[116] Robey I.F.; Baggett B. K.; Kirkpatrick N.D.; Roe D.J.; Dosescu J.; Sloane B.F.; Hashim A.I.; Morse D.L.; Raghunand N.; Gatenby R.A.; Gillies R.J.(2009). Bicarbonate Increases Tumor pH and Inhibits Spontaneous Metastases. *Cancer Research.* 69:2260–8. ISSN 0008-5472.

[117] Nilsonne G.; Olm E.; Szulkin A.; Mundt F.; Stein A.; Kocic B.; Rundlöf A.K.; Fernandes A.P.; Björnstedt M.; Dobra K. (2009). Phenotype-dependent apoptosis signalling in mesothelioma cells after selenite exposure. Journal of Experimental & Clinical Cancer Research. 28:92. ISSN 0392-9078.

[118] DeVita V.T.; Chu E. (2008). A History of Cancer Chemotherapy. (AACR Centennial series). *Cancer Research.* 68: 8643-8653. ISSN 0008-5472.

[119] Holland-Frei Cancer Medicine. (2000). 5th edition. E.D. Bast R.C. Jr, Kufe D.W., Pollock R.E., et al., Hamilton (ON): BC Decker. ISBN 1607950146.

[120] Cisplatin Chemistry and Biochemistry of a Leading Anticancer Drug (1999). Ed. B.Lippert, Verlag Helvetica Chimica Acta, Zürich. ISBN 3906390209.

[121] Muggia F.M.; Fojo, T. (2004). Platinums: extending their therapeutic spectrum. Journal of chemotherapy. 16:77-82. ISSN 1120-009X.

[122] Latosińska J.N., Latosińska M. (2011). Towards Understanding Drugs on the Molecular Level to Design Drugs of Desired Profiles. In Drug Discovery and Development - Present and Future, Eds. Kapetanovic I.M. Intech. ISBN 9789533076157.

[123] Sun Y.; Campisi J.; Higano C.; Beer T.M.; Porter P.; Coleman I.; True L.; Nelson P.S. (2012) Treatment-induced damage to the tumor microenvironment promotes prostate cancer therapy resistance through WNT16B. *Nature Medicine.* 18: 1359–1368. ISSN: 1078-8956.

Chapter 3

Drug Interactions, Pharmacogenomics and Cardiovascular Complication

Irina Piatkov, Trudi Jones and Mark McLean

Additional information is available at the end of the chapter

http://dx.doi.org/10.5772/48423

1. Introduction

Early identification of patients who will be at a higher risk for the development of adverse side effects and who will need dosage adjustment has the potential to help the clinician to limit a patient's exposure to drug side effects. When on multiple medications and complex regimens, cardiac patients are at increased risk and particularly vulnerable to drug interactions. A rational and informed approach to drug interactions, based on scientific knowledge, can reduce the chance of adverse effects and improve patient outcomes.

Cardiovascular drugs are used to treat various forms of illnesses, but there are often large differences between individual patients in drug response and dosage requirement. Treatment that has been proven effective for one person can be ineffective or even dangerous for another.

A drug produces its therapeutic effect when it reaches its target concentration in the bloodstream. Whether a steady therapeutic concentration is obtained largely depends on the balance between the dose administered and the rate at which the body metabolises the drug. An individual patient's response to a drug is not totally predictable. Below the target therapeutic range, a drug may be ineffective or, when it is higher, the drug may cause adverse reactions or become toxic. To ensure the safe and effective action of many drugs, the concentration in the bloodstream and their clinical effects are monitored. If necessary, the dose can be adjusted or the medication changed to achieve the best possible outcome.

To avoid unintended and untoward adverse drug reactions, the prescriber should use the fundamental principles of pharmacology and pharmacogenetics. Several drugs are metabolised through the same pathways and knowledge of the potential pathway capacity could help to predict treatment success. Variability in the reaction to medication may be due to age, gender, morbidity, co-medication, food components, smoking and environmental factors. However, polymorphisms present in genes, are responsible for most of the variation. Pharmacogenetic research and candidate gene approaches have succeeded in the identification of several genetic factors influencing treatment response. In particular, associations between variants in CYP enzymes and transporter genes have been repeatedly associated with different response and treatment--associated side effects [1-6]. Knowledge of pharmacogenomics is providing a key to understanding fundamentals of the drug interaction process.

A specific genotype might differ in its frequency in different ethnic populations, leading to differences in drug response. However, gene combination between ethnic groups makes it impossible for the practitioner to simply predict if a drug will be efficient or not. There is no specific genetic definition of ethnicity and ethnicity does not sufficiently separate those for whom a given therapy will be effective.

In contrast, the pharmacogenetics potentially presents a more effective way of identifying responders, nonresponders and potential adverse drug reactions. Pharmacogenetics provides defined clinical biomakers for individualised therapy [7].

Personalised medicine can be defined as a form of medicine that uses information about a person's genes, proteins and environment to prevent, diagnose and treat diseases, including predicting therapeutic response, nonresponse and likelihood of adverse reactions. Diagnostic biomarkers are necessary to successfully select patients for therapy, distinguish likely responders from nonresponders, identify patients at high risk for adverse events, or select an appropriate dose for safe and efficacious use of the therapy.

The human genome consists of approximately 3 billion base pairs (NCBI database) and the sequence of these varies among individuals. These variations can change the function of proteins that interact with a drug and hence, the response to a drug may differ among individuals. Sequence variations in drug-disposition genes can alter the pharmacokinetics of a drug and those in drug-target genes can change the pharmacodynamics of a drug.

When a genetic polymorphism alters the function of a protein that is involved in the absorption, metabolism, distribution and excretion of a drug, the concentrations of the parent drug or its active metabolites may be affected. For example, *CYP2D6**4 polymorphism leads to lower activity of a metabolising enzyme and the plasma concentrations of the parent drug metabolised by cytochrome P-450 isoenzyme 2D6 may increase and concentration of metabolites may decrease (some antidepressants). As a result, it could lead to the development of toxicity. For prodrugs, when metabolites have pharmacologic activity, the genetic polymorphism may reduce the drug response (some analgesics). Genetic polymorphisms that change the activity of the drug target (pharmacodynamics) may also alter the drug response. For example, vitamin K epoxide reductase complex subunit 1 gene polymorphisms influence warfarin response and β_1-adrenergic receptor gene polymorphisms after β-blocker response. Therefore, drugs can compete for binding sites on the receptors or be metabolised by the same enzyme, consequently create dug-drug interaction problem.

The information about pharmacogenetic terms and recourses is presented in the Appendix.

http://dx.doi.org/10.5772/48423

Early identification of patients who will be at a higher risk for the development of adverse side effects and who will need dosage adjustment has the potential to help the clinician to limit a patient's exposure to drug side effects. Characterisation of drug metabolising polymorphisms has been shown to be useful for identifying individuals who are poor drug metabolisers and at risk of developing adverse reactions, and several genotyping methods are already being used in clinical settings (Table1). The evidence provided by pharmacogenetics and pharmacogenomics can be successfully used for drug interaction interpretation.

Drugs	Tests of polymorphisms	Affected WSLHD Population*
Wafarin Phenytoin	CYP2C9	1% - Poor Metabolisers, 15% - Intermediate
Warfarin	VKORC1	11% with altered function
Clopidogrel	*CYP2C19*	4% - Poor Metabolisers, 13% - Intermediate, 20% - Ultra fast metabolisers
Carvedilol Metoprolol Propafenone Propranolol Quinidine	CYP2D6	5% - Poor Metabolisers, 27% - Intermidiate, 1% - Ultra fast metabolisers
Isosorbide Hydralazine	NAT1, NAT2	10-90%
Warfarin	Protein C Deficiencies	1/200 population, 2-5% Patients with Venous Thromboembolism
Atorvastatin	LDLR	1-5% Familial Cholesterolemia Patients
Statins	SINM PhyzioType (50 genes)	10-30% Patients on statin (multi-gene biomarker system manufacture results, no data available)

Table 1. Available Pharmacogenetics tests for cardiovascular medication. (*Western Sydney Population combined data. WSLHD population is a mix of Caucasians, Asians and Africans.)

2. Hypertensive drugs

Hypertension is a common condition associated with increased risk of stroke, heart failure, ischemic heart disease, and chronic renal failure. Thiazide diuretics, β-blockers, ACE inhibitors, angiotensin receptor blockers (ARBs) and calcium channel blockers (CCBs) are a common first line treatment for hypertension [8].

Despite availability of many effective agents, only about 40 percent [9] of treated hypertensive patients have their blood pressure controlled, mostly due to the unpredictable individual responses to treatment. Blood pressure responses to monotherapy vary widely within ethnic and gender subgroups [10].

Numerous studies have tried to establish associations between genetic polymorphisms and response to antihypertensive drugs. New developments in pharmacogenetics and pharmacogenomics already offer in pharmacogenetics and pharmacogenomics already offers the opportunity to provide individualised drug therapy on the basis of a person's genetic makeup for some drugs, despite varied approaches in study designs and methodology. These tests are provided by several laboratories and available at some hospitals; pharmacogenetic methods will not only help to achieve treatment goals and limit adverse effects, but also avoid drug interactions.

2.1. β-blockers

β-blockers through binding to β-adrenergic receptors (BAR) antagonise the binding of endogenous agonists. Variations in the gene encoding the β1-adrenergic receptor probably influence the treatment outcome. Two single nucleotide polymorphism (SNPs), resulting in Ser49Gly and Arg389Gly were identified and these variants demonstrate altered biological function in vitro, including enhanced agonist induced adenylyl cyclase activation by Gly49 compared to Ser49 and by Arg389 compared to Gly389 [11].

Some studies have shown that the Arg389Arg genotype and Ser49/Arg389 haplotype are associated with a greater response to blood pressure-lowering metoprolol [12].

The differential survival of Acute Coronary Syndrome (ACS) patients treated with β-blockers was associated with patients' β-adrenergic receptors 2 variant Gly16Arg and Gln27Glu genotypes; however, β-adrenergic receptors 1 variants showed no significant associations [13, 14].

No significant correlation has been found for outcomes of death, MI or stroke in coronary artery disease patients on atenolol treatment and β-adrenergic receptors variants or haplotypes [15] and β-adrenergic receptors 2 variants in MI and stroke outcomes. However, the case-control study found significant interaction with two SNPs in β-adrenergic receptors variant and cardiovascular complications [16, 17].

Angiotensin-converting enzyme (ACE) genes variations were also associated with β-blockers therapy outcome. In heart failure, patients survival without a transplant, has been associated with the angiotensin-converting enzyme I/D genotype (insertion/deletion).

http://dx.doi.org/10.5772/48423

Patients with the D allele may derive greater benefits from pharmacologic interventions with Beta-blocker treatment, probably through the decrease of sympathetic nervous system activity [18].

The effects of the CYP450 enzyme systems has been studied intensively during the last years and its role in the metabolism of drugs and other endogenous and exogenous chemicals is well defined. Numerous publications confirm the association of these enzymes with drug-drug, drug-toxins and drug-food interactions. Polymorphisms in the gene coding for the CYP2D6 isoenzyme, which catalyses the metabolism of β-blockers such as metoprolol, carvedilol, timolol, and propranolol, may also affect blocker response. It has been demonstrated that the clearance of the R(+) enantiomer of carvedilol was 66% lower and the area under the concentration-versus-time curve 156% higher among poor metabolizers than extensive metabolizers [19-22].

Some studies showed association with other genes. Genes involved in calcium signalling - CACNA1C, CACNB2, and KCNMB1- were found to be associated with myocardial infarction or stroke with β-blockers versus calcium channel blockers [23-25]. Variable stroke risk by genotype was described for an MMP3 promoter polymorphism in patients treated with lisinopril [26] and different treatment-related outcomes with thiazides and β-blockers, but not diltiazem, by NEDD4L (protein reduce renal tubular expression of epithelial Na+ channel) genotype [27].

Finally, the two studies by Schelleman et al reported no β-blocker interactions (for outcomes MI or stroke) variants of angiotensin receptor II type 1 (AGTR1) and ACE [28, 29].

2.2. Diuretics

Diuretics may act at a number of sites, including the proximal tubule, the Loop of Henle, and the distal and collecting tubules. Diuretics are thought to indirectly activate the renin-angiotensin-aldosterone system and block sensitivity of blood vessels to catecholamines. Thiazide diuretics are the drug of choice for initial therapy, but genes responsible for renal sodium reabsorption can affect the patient's responsiveness to diuretic therapy.

Antihypertensive response in black African Americans is found to be associated with locus at chromosome12q15 [30, 31] where the FRS2 gene is located, which is involved in fibroblast growth factor signalling. FRS2 plays a role in vascular smooth muscle cell regulation.

Genome-wide association (GWA) studies are aimed at identifying common genetic variants modulating disease susceptibility, physiological traits and variable drug responses. These studies also provide further evidence for the large effects that single gene variants may exert for some drugs. GWA has explained relatively large proportions of variability compared to studies of traits such as disease susceptibility or physiological measurements. GWAS demonstrated that SNPs in lysozyme and Yeats domain-containing protein 4 (YEATS4) were associated with response to diuretic [30].

Lynch et al. found that C carriers of the NPPA T2238C variant, which codes for the precursor of atrial natriuretic polypeptide, had more favourable clinical outcomes when treated with a diuretic, whereas individuals homozygous for the T allele responded better to a calcium channel blocker [32].

Patients with SNP of T594M gene (epithelial sodium channel) variant responded more favourably to amiloride therapy for BP control than to thiazide-based drugs. In cases of severe hypokalemia, potassium-sparing diuretics such as amiloride or triamterene should be used according to serum sodium and potassium levels [33, 34].

NEDD4L is also a candidate gene with a documented functional SNP, a role in sodium reabsorption, and several studies have found an association between this SNP and blood pressure response with thiazides [27, 35].

A common functional polymorphism resulting in Gly460Trp in the α-adducin gene ADD1 has been associated with response to thiazides. This finding led to the development of a novel antihypertensive drug class targeting adducin [36, 37]. Manunta et al. performed single SNP association analysis and combination analysis on ADD1 (Gly460Trp), NEDD4L, WNK1 in a 4-week diuretic trial. They found ADD1 460Trp carriers had significantly greater BP reduction than Gly460 homozygotes. When considered together, there was a significant trend in decreases of systolic blood pressure (SBP) (ranging from −3.4 mm Hg to −23.2 mm Hg) for different combinations of genotypes [35].The ADD1 Gly460Trp polymorphism has been associated with an increased risk of myocardial infarction or stroke during thiazide diuretic treatment [38] In contrast, these findings were not confirmed by other studies [39, 40].

The 825T allele in the G-protein is probably associated with a sodium-sensitive form of hypertension. Blood pressure declines for both the C/T and T/T genotypes were significantly greater than for the C/C genotype. The study revealed that the decreases in blood pressure varied on the basis of genotype and even after multiple regression analysis, genotype remained a significant predictor of blood pressure lowering [41].

2.3. Renin-angiotensin system inhibitors

Numerous genes from the renin-angiotensin system (RAS) pathway have been shown to play a key role in the regulation of blood pressure and influence the cardiovascular system. Several pharmacogenetic studies of the RAS were conducted. However, due to the complexity of RAS, associations between drug efficiency and polymorphisms are not consistent [42-45].

Angiotensin-converting enzyme (ACE) inhibitors prevent the conversion of angiotensin I to angiotensin II in plasma and tissue and prevent the degradation of bradykinin. Clinically, ACE inhibitors reduce peripheral vascular resistance and pulmonary capillary wedge pressure and increase cardiac output and renal blood flow. Treatment with ACE inhibitors in hypertension has been associated with improvements in vascular compliance, regression of left ventricular hypertrophy, improved systolic and diastolic function, and improvements in insulin sensitivity [46]. One study showed that ACE DD polymorphism is associated with poor collateral circulation (PCC). PCC in patients carrying the D allele may be associated with endothelial dysfunction and elevated blood ACE levels in these patients [47].

http://dx.doi.org/10.5772/48423

The insertion/deletion (I/D) in the angiotensin I-converting enzyme (ACE) gene is one of the candidates for studies. The D allele has been associated with more improvement in coronary endothelial dysfunction with ACE inhibitor therapy than the I allele [48]. Reductions in systolic and diastolic blood pressures were significantly greater for patients with the D/D genotype than for patients with the I/D and I/I genotypes [49].

Diastolic blood pressure tended to decrease more for the ACE I/I genotype than for other ACE genotypes and the I/I genotype was also predictive of greater diastolic blood pressure decline [50]. Decline in renal function during ACE inhibitor treatment tended to be greater in heart failure patients with the ACE I/I genotype [51]. The I/I genotype has also been associated with increased susceptibility to the development of cough during ACE inhibitor therapy. After four weeks of therapy with an ACE inhibitor in healthy volunteers, the threshold for cough was significantly reduced for the I/I genotype but not the D/D genotype [52].

Another gene of interest is the angiotensinogen (AGT) gene. It was reported that the angiotensinogen 235Met/Thr polymorphism is also associated with RAS activity and drug responses. In subjects on ACE inhibitor monotherapy with 235Thr allele the response is higher than in the control group. Systolic and diastolic blood pressures were higher and the likelihood of using two or more antihypertensive medications was 2.1 times higher with the 235Thr polymorphism [53].

An association with polymorphisms in the angiotensin AT1 receptor (AGT1R) gene and ACE inhibitors' efficiency are found in some studies. The AGT1R mediates some negative effects of angiotensin II, such as vasoconstriction, cardiac remodelling, and aldosterone secretion. Angiotensin II blockers bind to angiotensin II receptors, thereby antagonizing the effect of angiotensin II, a potent vasoconstrictor [54]. The 1166C allele of AGT1R has been associated with increased arterial responsiveness to angiotensin II in ischemic heart disease and increased aortic stiffness in hypertension. During ACE inhibitor treatment, reductions in aortic stiffness were reported to be three times greater in carriers of the 1166C allele than in 1166A homozygotes [55, 56]. AGTR1 (C573T) and ACE (ID) association between ACE inhibitor therapy and increased MI risk for carriers of the AGTR1 C573 allele were reported; however, no significant interaction between ACE inhibitor treatment and ACE (ID) alleles for either stroke or MI were found [28]. One research group found no associations between BP response and ACE (ID), AGTR1 (A1166C), CYP11B2 (-344 C/T), AGT (-6 A/G) [57].

After 12 weeks of treatment with irbesartan (Angiotensin II Blocker), plasma concentration of the drug was related to change in systolic BP in TT homozygotes of AGTR1 (C5245T) but not for other genotypes [58].

3. Calcium Channel Blockers (CCBs)

Drugs in this class block voltage-gated calcium channels in the heart and vasculature, thereby reducing intracellular calcium. Calcium channel blockers drugs vary in their effect on cardiac versus vascular calcium channels. CCBs fall into three subclasses: phenylalkylamines, which are selective for the myocardium; dihydropyridines which mostly affecting smooth muscle and benzothiazepines with a broad range.

A few studies describe some association; three SNPs in CACNA1C had significant associations with treatment in a study of BP lowering with calcium channel blockers [59]; between CYP3A5*3 and *6 variants and verapamil treatment for BP and hypertension risk outcomes in blacks and Hispanics [60]; individuals that are homozygous for the T allele of NPPA T2238C had more favourable clinical outcomes when treated with a calcium channel blocker whereas C carriers responded better to a diuretic [32]. Beta Adrenergic Receptor 1 (BAR1) Ser49-Arg389 haplotype carriers had higher death rates than those with other haplotypes when treated with verapamil [15].

4. Anticoagulants

4.1. Warfarin

Warfarin is a widely used anticoagulant in the treatment and prevention of thrombosis. It was initially marketed as a pesticide against rats and mice and is still used for this purpose. It was approved for use as a medication in the early 1950s and is widely prescribed. Despite its common use, warfarin therapy can be associated with significant bleeding complications. Achieving a safe therapeutic response can be difficult because of warfarin's narrow therapeutic index and great individual variability in the dose required, which is mostly a consequence of individual genetic variants. This fact is well known among clinicians and the wide range, from 1 mg/day to 20 mg/day, of warfarin maintenance doses are observed across the population. To maintain a therapeutic level of anti-thrombosis and to minimise the risk of bleeding complications, warfarin therapy requires intensive monitoring via the International Normalized Ratio (INR) to guide its dosing. The INR is used to monitor the effectiveness of warfarin and measures the pathway of blood coagulation. It is used to standardize the results for a prothrombin time. INR is the ratio of a patient's prothrombin time to a control sample, raised to the power of the index value for the analytical system used.

Several factors increase the risk of over-anticoagulation: genetic polymorphisms affecting the metabolising enzymes, impaired liver function, drug interactions, congestive heart failure, diarrhoea, fever, and diets rich in vitamin K [61] [62]. Nevertheless, genetic factors and drug interactions mostly account for the risk of over-anticoagulation. Warfarin metabolism involves primarily the cytochrome P450 (CYP) enzymes. Some loss-of-function CYP2C9 and vitamin K epoxide reductase complex subunit 1 (VKORC1) polymorphisms are known to be associated with decreased enzymatic activity and as a result, with an increased risk of haemorhage. These are CYP2C9*2 (Cysl44/Ile359), CYP2C9*3 (Argl44/Leu359) and VKORC1 (-1639G>A) [63-65].

Warfarin-induced haemorrhage is an important complication of anticoagulation therapy. A review of many studies shows average yearly rates of warfarin-related bleeding as high as 0.8%, 4.9%, and 15%, for fatal, major and minor bleeding complications respectively [66].

Vitamin K is required by proteins C and S, together with clotting factors II, VII, IX, and X, to allow assembly of the procoagulant enzyme complexes necessary to generate fibrin. Warfarin as an anticoagulant agent has the ability to interfere with the recycling of vitamin K in the liver. The pharmacologic effect of warfarin is mediated by the inhibition of vitamin K epoxide reductase complex subunit 1 (EC 1.1.4.1) [67].

Warfarin consists of (R)- and (S)-warfarin enantiomers. (R)- and (S)-warfarins differ in their relative plasma concentrations, in their antithrombotic potency and in the specific isoenzymes responsible for their metabolism. (S)-warfarin has a 3 to 5 times greater anticoagulant effect than the (R)-enantiomer and accounts for 60% to 70% of warfarin's overall anticoagulant activity. (S)-warfarin is metabolised almost exclusively by CYP2C9 [68-70].

The activity of the CYP2C9 enzyme has a significant impact on the clearance of (S)-warfarin and as a consequence on anticoagulant effect. In the presence of genetic variations where the activity of CYP2C9 is reduced, clearance of (S)-warfarin is also reduced. Activity of CYP2C9 between individuals can vary by more than 20-fold. (R)-warfarin is metabilised by multiple different CYP enzymes [71].

While several single-nucleotide polymorphisms of CYP2C9 have been reported, the CYP2C9*2 (Cysl44/Ile359) and CYP2C9*3 (Argl44/Leu359) polymorphisms have been identified as clinically relevant [72]. Both of these variants are associated with decreased enzymatic activity [24, 73-78].

Homozygous CYP2C9*3 variant genotypes have only 5% to 10% metabolic efficiency compared to the wild-type genotype. As a result, compared to wild-type CYP2C9*1*1 controls, enzyme activity and the median maintenance warfarin dose for CYP2C9*3*1 heterozygotes was reduced by 40%, and by approximately 90% for CYP2C9*3*3 homozygotes [72-74].

Furuya [79] and Steward [75] showed that the CYP2C9*2 variant is also associated with reduced warfarin elimination. Heterozygotes demonstrate 40% and homozygotes 15% of the wild-type enzyme activity, causing dose adjustment for heterozygote CYP2C9*2 individuals down to 20% less than the standard dose.

Margaglione [76] has also demonstrated bleeding rates as high as 27.9 per 100 patient-years in carriers of CYP variants. In this study, findings were adjusted for other common variables associated with increased bleeding risk, such as increased age, drug interactions and abnormal liver function.

Several studies of the *2 and *3 CYP2C9 polymorphisms consistently show that patients with at least one CYP2C9 allele polymorphism have reduced warfarin requirements [76, 80-84]. Freeman [85] reported reduced warfarin weekly dosages for carriers of CYP2C9*2 or CYP2C9*3 alleles compared with patients who were homozygous for the wild-type allele (0.307 mg/kg/wk and 0.397 mg/kg/wk, respectively). Taube [83] compared warfarin maintenance dosages in 683 patients carrying different CYP2C9 genotypes. Mean warfarin maintenance dosages were 86% in patients with CYP2C9*1*2, 79% in patients with CYP2C9*1*3, 82% in compound heterozygotes CYP2C9*2/*3, and 61% in patients homozygous for CYP2C9*2. Furthermore, Aithal [80] warns that even when warfarin dosages are decreased, carriers of CYP2C9 poor metaboliser alleles experience a rate of major bleeding that is 3.68-fold higher than the rate seen in patients with the wild type genotype.

The frequency of CYP2C9 alleles is ethnically related [82, 86]. Approximately 20% of the Caucasian population carries one of the loss-of-function CYP2C9 alleles, and it is estimated that 1% of Caucasian carry two such alleles [71]. The frequency of the CYP2C9*2 allele reportedly ranges from 8-13% in different Caucasian populations. CYP2C9*2 is present in 4% of African-Americans and is rare among Japanese individuals [87, 88]. The frequency of CYP2C9*3 is 6-10% among Caucasian populations and 3.8% in Japanese populations [88, 89]. This data suggests that a substantial fraction of the Caucasian patient population may carry at least one defective CYP2C9 allele. In this group, the usual prescription dosage of warfarin may lead to major or even life-threatening haemorrhage.

Warfarin is commonly prescribed in combination with selective serotonin reuptake inhibitors (SSRIs), as depression often coexists with cardiovascular disease. Case reports suggest that some SSRIs can interact with warfarin to increase the likelihood of bleeding [90]. SSRIs cause adverse effects in isolation [91, 92] and can interact with other medications by inhibiting various isoenzymes of the CYP450 enzyme group [93, 94]. It has been shown that metronidazole and cimetadine increase the prothrombin time in patients on warfarin therapy. Chloramphenicol enhances warfarin's effect by inhibiting the action of the hepatic P450 system [71]. Some authors [95], [96] have warned that antidepressants with a known or predictable interaction with warfarin, such as fluoxetine and fluvoxamine, should be avoided in patients receiving warfarin because of the risk of adverse outcomes.

Drug-drug interaction is a main concern in adverse drug reactions. The primary complication occurring with warfarin treatment is bleeding. SSRIs may increase the risk of bleeding during warfarin therapy by hindering platelet aggregation through depletion of platelet serotonin levels [97-99]. Some SSRIs may also inhibit the oxidative metabolism of warfarin by CYP 2C9 [95].

It has been shown that concurrent use of selective serotonin reuptake inhibitors and warfarin increases the risk of hospitalisation due to haemorrhage [90, 98]. Drugs which affect serotonin may have a detrimental effect on platelet function, as drugs which inhibit the reuptake of serotonin may decrease platelet serotonin levels leading to a reduction in serotonin-mediated platelet aggregation. Potential drug interactions can involve modification in either of these mechanisms and may result in pharmacodynamic interference or enhancement of warfarin's action.

It was shown that major and moderate drug-drug interactions with warfarin are very common in inpatients and are associated with INR results outside the therapeutic range. The most common drugs involved in the increase of anticoagulation effect were enoxaparin, simvastatin, omeprazole and tramadol. Multivariate analysis showed that age, length of hospital stay, exposure to >/=4 major or moderate drug interactions, and refusal of pharmacist recommendations contribute significantly to the patient's INR result >5 [100].

One study demonstrated that acetaminophen, at 2 g/day or 3 g/day, enhanced the anticoagulant effect of warfarin in stable patients, thus requiring close INR monitoring in the clinical setting [101].

4.2. Heparin

One of the preventative treatments of thromboembolic disease in patients is a prescription of heparin. However, heparin induced thrombocytopenia (HIT) is one of the most serious adverse reactions. HIT consequences can include thromboembolic complications and death.

An association between the Fc receptor gene and the risk for HIT has been found in some studies and it was demonstrated that the homozygous 131Arg/Arg genotype occurred significantly more often in patients with HIT than in the healthy volunteers' group [102] [103] ; however, another group have found no association [104]. Results are very preliminary and more evidence are needed before it may be possible to genotype candidates for heparin therapy to identify those at risk for drug-induced thromboembolic complications.

5. Statins

Hydroxymethylglutaryl-coenzyme A reductase inhibitors (statins) have reduced coronary and cerebrovascular events and overall mortality when used for both primary and secondary prevention of ischemic heart disease [105]. Several known gene polymorphisms are associated with the treatment progress [106, 107].

Some studies examined polymorphism in the gene encoding cholesteryl ester transfer protein (CETP), which is involved in the metabolism of high-density lipoprotein (HDL). Pravastatin-treated patients with either the B1/B1 or B1/B2 genotype (B1 presence and B2 absence of polymorphism) had significantly less atherosclerotic progression than patients receiving a placebo. Placebo-treated patients with the B2/B2 genotype had the least progression. However, pravastatin-treated patients with the B2/B2 genotype (16% of the study population) derived no benefit from pravastatin [108, 109].

The substitution (-455G/A) of the fibrinogen gene was found to be associated with an increased risk of myocardial infarction and stroke. During follow-up, placebo-treated patients homozygous for the -455A genotype had the greatest disease progression; although, no association was found with benefit in disease progression in patients on pravastatin therapy [110].

A five year study of pravastatin therapy in patients with a history of myocardial infarction and hypercholesterolemia showed that the largest benefit of pravastatin treatment in reducing these events occurred in patients with the platelet GP IIIa PlA1/A2 genotype who also carried at least one D allele of the ACE gene [111, 112].

An effect of polymorphism in the alloprotein gene was found on simvastatin therapy in a Scandinavian study. Among patients who received the placebo and had at least one apolipoprotein e4 allele, the relative risk of death from all causes was higher than in simastatin patients with the same polymorphism [113]. This study demonstrates the potential clinical value of the alloprotein APOE genotype as a robust marker for low-density lipoprotein (LDL) responses to statin drugs, which might contribute to the identification of a particularly drug-resistant subgroup of patients [114].

Genetic variants in CYP3A4, which metabolises simvastatin, atorvastatin and lovastatin, have been associated with variability in statin efficacy. Both a nonsynonymous polymorphism (M445T) as well the CYP3A4*4 haplotype have been associated with lower LDL cholesterol levels with atorvastatin. However, in carriers of either a CYP3A4 promoter polymorphism (A290G) or the CYP3A4*1G haplotype the lipid-lowering effect of statins is not demonstrated [115-117].

Variation in Hydroxymethylglutaryl-coenzyme A reductase (HMGCR) and low-density lipoprotein receptor (LDLR) genes are associated with the LDL-lowering effect of statins. The H7 haplotype within HMGCR, defined by the presence of three intronic SNPs, has been associated with an 11% to 19% reduction in LDL cholesterol with statin treatment in multiple independent populations as well as ethnically diverse population-based cohorts [107, 114, 118]. The H7 haplotype has been shown to interact with other genetic variants, including a second HMGCR haplotype, H2, as well as the LDLR L5 haplotype, defined by six SNPs within the LDLR 3′ untranslated region. Ethnic variations in LDL cholesterol-lowering with statin treatment is also demonstrated in African-Americans who carry multiple copies of these haplotypes versus any haplotype alone [106, 118, 119].

Statin-related myotoxicity, especially rhabdomyolysis, is the subject of medical concerns as it requires changes in medications and treatment discontinuation. It was found that variants in CYP3A5 and solute carrier organic anion transporter family (SLCO1B1) gene can be potential predictors of myotoxicity [120-123].

Increased risk of coronary artery disease, coronary heart disease and myocardial infarction are associated in some studies with a missense SNP, Trp719Arg, in the KIF6 gene (kinesin family member 6). Statin treatment significantly reduce coronary events in carriers of Trp719Arg, and SNPs in high linkage disequilibrium with it, whereas no benefit of statin treatment is reported in noncarriers [124].

The differences in drug-drug interaction profiles among available statins offer the possibility of reducing the risk of myotoxicity among high-risk patients. The risk of developing the rhabdomyolysis condition with statin therapy increases at higher therapeutic doses. This effect is increased by combination with certain other medications due to drug-drug interactions. Co-administration of drugs that inhibit the cytochrome P450 (CYP) enzymes responsible for metabolizing statins, or that interact with the organic anion-transporting polypeptides (OATPs) responsible for statin uptake into hepatocytes, substantially increases the risk of developing myotoxicity. Pitavastatin, a novel statin approved for the treatment of hypercholesterolemia and combined (mixed) dyslipidemia, is not catabolized by CYP3A4, unlike other lipophilic statins, and may be less dependent on the OATP1B1 transporter for its uptake into hepatocytes before clearance [125].

6. Antiarrhythmic

Many antiarrhythmic agents have antagonistic effects on sodium ion and potassium ion channels in the heart. A risk of proarrhythmic effects of antiarrhythmic drugs and its mechanism is associated with genetic variations. Some evidence indicates that polymorphisms in genes encoding components of cardiac ion channels have been associated with congenital arrhythmia syndromes, such as long-QT and idiopathic ventricular fibrillation syndromes [126].

The fact that the risk of drug-induced arrhythmia usually increases with increasing drug concentrations also indicates the involvement of liver enzyme polymorphisms. The CYP2D6 gene regulates cytochrome P450 metabolic pathways and some evidence shows an association between poor metaboliser phenotype and antiarrhythmic drug toxicity {127}.

A number of polymorphisms in the N-acetyltransferace 2 gene contribute to different acetylator phenotypes. Rapid acetylators have increased conversion of procainamide by N-acetyltransferase 2 to N-acetylprocainamide (NAPA) consequently leading to the QT-interval prolongation, and life-threatening ventricular arrhythmias. Slow acetylators will attain an increased concentration of procainamide levels with normal procainamide dosages, which can lead to a procainamide- induced lupus-like syndrome [128].

Sotalol, dofetilide and quinidine increase the chances of QT interval prolongation, polymorphic ventricular tachycardia and torsades de pointes. Several genes encoding ion channels or function-modifying subunits were associated with these syndromes [129],[130-132].

One study suggested that a NOS1AP variant in the gene encoding an accessory protein for neuronal nitric oxide synthase, was associated with total and cardiovascular mortality during treatment with dihydropyridine calcium channel blockers. Variants in NOS1AP also have been reported to modulate the risk of arrhythmias, at equivalent QT interval durations, in patients with the congenital long QT syndrome and to modulate risk for sudden death in the general population [133-135].

7. Antiplatelet agents

7.1. Aspirin

Pharmacogenetic studies of aspirin response to date have found associations with a few genes. It was reported that PLA2 (Leu59Pro) carriers, the variant in platelet glycoprotein IIIa, have impaired aspirin responses. After seven days of aspirin therapy in healthy volunteers, plasma prothrombin fragment concentrations in bleeding-time wounds were reduced in 23 of 25 PLA1 homozygotes, compared with 9 of 15 PLA2 carriers [136]. A meta-analysis [137] of 50 polymorphisms in 11 genes reported in 31 studies with a combined sample size of 2834 subjects suggested that the common PLA1/2 polymorphism does confer aspirin resistance (odds ratio in healthy subjects=2.36; P=0.009); however, when combining both healthy subjects and those with cardiovascular disease, the odds ratio was 1.14 (P=0.40). The PLA2 allele occurs with a frequency of approximately 15% in humans and has been associated with increased platelet activation and aggregation in vitro [138].

Associations between the PLA polymorphisms and subacute thrombosis after coronary intervention have been described in some reports [139-141] and it was shown that an increased risk of subacute thrombosis is associated with the PLA2 allele. In one study, the risk of subacute thrombosis after coronary angioplasty and stent placement was five times greater in coronary artery disease patients with the PLA2 polymorphism than in patients homozygous for the PLA1 allele, despite similar antiplatelet therapy and similar clinical, angiographic and procedural characteristics [139].

7.2. Clopidogrel

The obvious candidates for pharmacogenetic analysis are genes involved in clopidogrel metabolism. Clopidogrel is a prodrug and its active form, thiol, is formed during the biotransformation in the liver. CYP2C19, CYP3A4/5, CYP1A2, and CYP2B6 are involved in this process [142].

P2Y12 belongs to the G protein-coupled purinergic receptor for adenosine diphosphate (ADP). The P2Y12 protein is found mainly, but not exclusively, on the surface of blood platelets, and is an important regulator in blood clotting. The active clopidogrel metabolite irreversibly binds to platelet ADP P2Y12 receptors. ADP P2Y12 receptors and loss-of-function CYP2C19*2 was identified as the single major genetic determinant of biochemical response to clopidogrel, accounting for approximately 12% of the variation in ADP-stimulated platelet aggregation during drug treatment [143]. CYP2C19*2 carriers treated with clopidogrel have an increased risk for major adverse cardiovascular events compared to noncarriers and increased risks of stent thrombosis [144].

Loss-of-function CYP2C19*2 allele has been reproducibly shown to be associated with a decreased conversion of clopidogrel into its active metabolite, reduced antiplatelet effect and increased risk for cardiovascular events in patients using clopidogrel [4, 145].

The frequency of CYP2C19*2 polymorphism varies in different populations: in Caucasian, African American, and Mexicans it presence is 18% to 33% (2%–3% homozygotes) and the allele frequency is higher in Asians. The loss-of-function *3 variant is also associated with poorer response and is highly prevalent in Asians [146, 147].

P-glycoprotein, also known as multidrug resistance protein 1 (MDR1) or ATP-binding cassette sub-family B member 1 (ABCB1) or cluster of differentiation 243 (CD243), is a glycoprotein that in humans is encoded by the ABCB1 gene. ABC transporters are transmembrane proteins that utilize the energy of adenosine triphosphate hydrolysis to carry out certain biological processes including translocation of various substrates across membranes and non-transport-related processes such as translation of RNA and DNA repair. Contradicting results have been reported for variants in ABCB1 and Gln192Arg allele in paraoxonase 1, which have been implicated in clopidogrel responsiveness. These associations need further confirmation [148-150].

8. Conclusion

Adverse drug reactions (ADRs) have been reported to be the cause for drug withdrawal after marketing, hospital admissions, death in hospitalised patients and to be the fourth leading cause of death in developed countries. The costs associated with ADRs may radically escalate the cost for healthcare.

There is an increasing use of multiple medications to treat patients with chronic illnesses. Drug-drug interactions are common and growing in frequency due to increasing numbers of medications available and the number of patients on multiple medications. The knowledge of the pharmacodynamics and pharmacokinetics of the drugs helps to avoid unintended and problematic drug interactions. Several web sites, books, and cards are available for the clinician. The web sites are updated on a regular basis and are useful tools for prescribers.

The necessity to understand drug combination pharmacokinetics and pharmacodinamics in drug interactions is illustrated by the following example: a patient who is taking a drug equally cleared by CYP2D6 and CYP3A. That patient may not be at substantial risk for toxicity when treated with either a CYP2D6 or CYP3A inhibitor alone, but may be if treated with both inhibitors at the same time [151]. Pharmacodynamic or pharmacokinetic drug interaction is a complex process and includes understanding of individual variations in drug metabolism.

Pharmacogenetics has a potential role in reducing ADRs at the pre-marketing and post-marketing stages of drug development and in clinical care. A priori identification of individuals at risk of developing ADRs for a given drug will help develop strategies to reduce the risk for ADRs in these patients. It can also be used to identify individuals at risk of developing serious ADRs and to treat these individuals with alternative therapy, thus converting ADRs that are traditionally considered unavoidable to avoidable ADRs.

Although pharmacogenetics is a highly complex and ever-evolving science, it has amassed knowledge that can readily be used to provide efficient care to patients. It has been shown that gene variants that play a role in drug metabolism pathways can alter a patient's response or increase toxicity at normal dosage range, especially in combinational drug treatments. Pharmacogenetics seeks to understand the nature of variable drug responses. Several pharmacogenetics tests are already available for cardiovascular medications in biomedical laboratories (Table 1).

Pharmacogenetic findings may help to explain ethnic differences in drug response. The accumulated facts of ethnic differences in cardiovascular drug responses and the fact that many genetic polymorphisms differ in frequency on the basis of ethnicity (example in the Western Sydney population, Fig. 1) will undoubtedly support future development of pharmacogenetics in patient care and in drug interaction interpretation.

It is possible that use of genetic and other patient-specific information, including environmental factors will help guide drug therapy decisions for certain drugs and drug combinations.

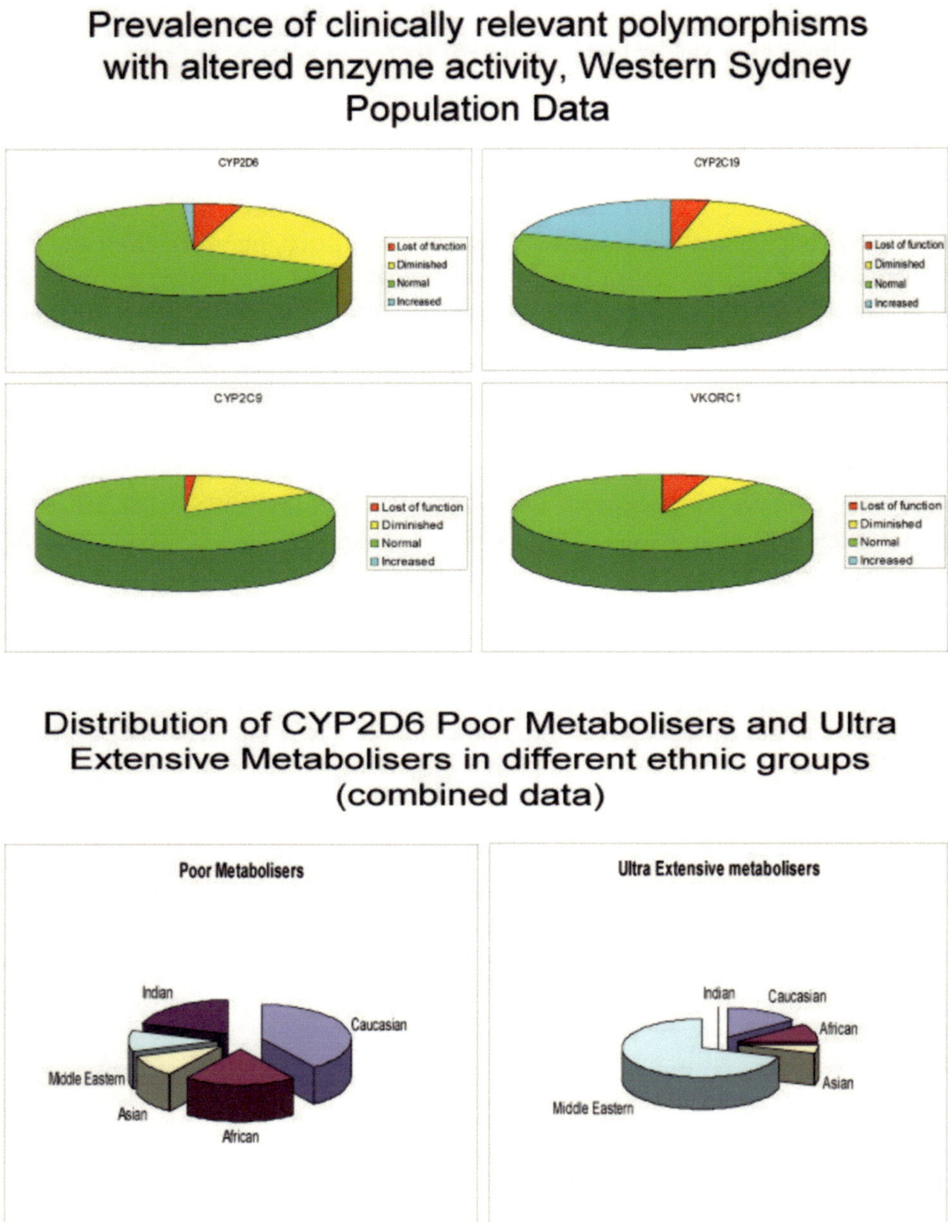

Figure 1. Example of diversity in prevalence of clinically relevant polymorphisms. (*Western Sydney Population combined data. WSLHD population is a mix of Caucasians, Asians and Africans.)

http://dx.doi.org/10.5772/48423

Appendix

Glossary of some Pharmacogenetic Terms

- **Allele:** An alternative form of a gene at a given locus.
- **Genetic polymorphism:** Minor allele frequency of ≥1% in the population.
- **Genome:** The complete DNA sequence of an organism. Sum total of the genetic material included in every cell of the human body, apart from the red blood cells.
- **Genomewide association study (GWAS):** A genetic association study in which the density of genetic markers and the extent of linkage disequilibrium are sufficient to capture a large proportion of the common variation in the human genome in the population under study, and the number of specimens genotyped provides sufficient power to detect variants of modest effect.
- **Genotype:** The alleles at a specific locus an individual carries. The genetic constitution of an individual, i.e. the specific allelic makeup of an individual.
- **Haplotype:** A group of alleles from two or more loci on a chromosome; inherited as a unit.
- **Heterozygote:** A person who has two copies of an allele that are different.
- **Homozygote:** A person who has two copies of an allele that are the same.
- **Pharmacogenetics:** A study of genetic causes of individual variations in drug response. In this review, the term "pharmacogenetics" is interchangeable with "pharmacogenomics."
- **Pharmacogenomics:** Genomewide analysis of the genetic determinants of drug efficacy and toxicity. Pharmacogenetics focuses on a single gene while pharmacogenomics studies multiple genes.
- **Phenotype:** Observable expression of a particular gene or genes.
- **Single nucleotide polymorphism (SNP):** is a DNA sequence variation occurring when a single nucleotide in the genome differs between members of a biological species or paired chromosomes in an individual.

Useful Internet Resources and databases:

- OMIM (Online Mendelian Inheritance in Man), National Centre for Biotechnology Information (NCBI): www.ncbi.nlm.nih.gov/sites/entrez?db=omim
- PharmGKB (The Pharmacogenetics and Pharmacogenomics Knowledge Base): www.pharmgkb.org/#public
- NCBI, Individual SNP information, such as genetic location, nucleotide and amino acid changes, and allele frequencies in diverse populations, can be obtained from dbSNP: www.ncbi.nlm.nih.gov/sites/entrez?db=snp

- Databases: ensembl (www.ensembl.org/index.html) and HapMap (www.hapmap.org/cgi-perl/gbrowse/hapmap_B35)
- FDA: http://www.fda.gov/Drugs/ScienceResearch/ResearchAreas/Pharmacogenetics
- FDA: Table of Pharmacogenomic Biomarkers in Drug Labels: http://www.fda.gov/Drugs/ScienceResearch/ResearchAreas/Pharmacogenetics/ucm083378.htm

Author details

Irina Piatkov*, Trudi Jones and Mark McLean

*Address all correspondence to: irina.piatkov@swahs.health.nsw.gov.au

University of Western Sydney, Blacktown Clinical School and Research Centre,, Blacktown Hospital, Western Sydney Local Health District, Blacktown, Australia

References

[1] Verschuren JJ, Trompet S, Wessels JA, Guchelaar HJ, de Maat MP, Simoons ML, Jukema JW (2012) A systematic review on pharmacogenetics in cardiovascular disease: is it ready for clinical application? Eur Heart J 33:165-175

[2] Scheen AJ (2011) Cytochrome P450-mediated cardiovascular drug interactions. Expert Opin Drug Metab Toxicol 7:1065-1082

[3] Rodriguez Arcas MJ, Garcia-Jimenez E, Martinez-Martinez F, Conesa-Zamora P (2011) Role of CYP450 in pharmacokinetics and pharmacogenetics of antihypertensive drugs. Farm Hosp 35:84-92

[4] Roden DM, Johnson JA, Kimmel SE, Krauss RM, Medina MW, Shuldiner A, Wilke RA (2011) Cardiovascular pharmacogenomics. Circ Res 109:807-820

[5] Masca N, Sheehan NA, Tobin MD (2011) Pharmacogenetic interactions and their potential effects on genetic analyses of blood pressure. Stat Med 30:769-783

[6] Howe LA (2011) Pharmacogenomics and management of cardiovascular disease. Nursing 41 Suppl:1-7

[7] PharmGKB d (2011) http://www.pharmgkb.org/. Stanford University

[8] Chobanian AV, Bakris GL, Black HR, Cushman WC, Green LA, Izzo JL, Jr., Jones DW, Materson BJ, Oparil S, Wright JT, Jr., Roccella EJ (2003) The Seventh Report of the Joint National Committee on Prevention, Detection, Evaluation, and Treatment of High Blood Pressure: the JNC 7 report. Jama 289:2560-2572

[9] Egan BM, Zhao Y, Axon RN (2010) US trends in prevalence, awareness, treatment, and control of hypertension, 1988-2008. Jama 303:2043-2050

[10] AHA (2008) Heart Disease and Stroke Statistics - 2008 Update. American Heart Association

[11] Brodde OE (2008) Beta-1 and beta-2 adrenoceptor polymorphisms: functional importance, impact on cardiovascular diseases and drug responses. Pharmacol Ther 117:1-29

[12] Liu J, Liu ZQ, Tan ZR, Chen XP, Wang LS, Zhou G, Zhou HH (2003) Gly389Arg polymorphism of beta1-adrenergic receptor is associated with the cardiovascular response to metoprolol. Clin Pharmacol Ther 74:372-379

[13] Lanfear DE, Jones PG, Marsh S, Cresci S, McLeod HL, Spertus JA (2005) Beta2-adrenergic receptor genotype and survival among patients receiving beta-blocker therapy after an acute coronary syndrome. Jama 294:1526-1533

[14] Lanfear DE, Spertus JA, McLeod HL (2006) Beta2-adrenergic receptor genotype predicts survival: implications and future directions. J Cardiovasc Nurs 21:474-477

[15] Pacanowski MA, Gong Y, Cooper-Dehoff RM, Schork NJ, Shriver MD, Langaee TY, Pepine CJ, Johnson JA (2008) beta-adrenergic receptor gene polymorphisms and beta-blocker treatment outcomes in hypertension. Clin Pharmacol Ther 84:715-721

[16] Lemaitre RN, Heckbert SR, Sotoodehnia N, Bis JC, Smith NL, Marciante KD, Hindorff LA, Lange LA, Lumley TS, Rice KM, Wiggins KL, Psaty BM (2008) beta1- and beta2-adrenergic receptor gene variation, beta-blocker use and risk of myocardial infarction and stroke. Am J Hypertens 21:290-296

[17] Lemaitre RN, Siscovick DS, Psaty BM, Pearce RM, Raghunathan TE, Whitsel EA, Weinmann SA, Anderson GD, Lin D (2002) Inhaled beta-2 adrenergic receptor agonists and primary cardiac arrest. Am J Med 113:711-716

[18] Hunt SA, Baker DW, Chin MH, Cinquegrani MP, Feldman AM, Francis GS, Ganiats TG, Goldstein S, Gregoratos G, Jessup ML, Noble RJ, Packer M, Silver MA, Stevenson LW, Gibbons RJ, Antman EM, Alpert JS, Faxon DP, Fuster V, Jacobs AK, Hiratzka LF, Russell RO, Smith SC, Jr. (2001) ACC/AHA guidelines for the evaluation and management of chronic heart failure in the adult: executive summary. A report of the American College of Cardiology/American Heart Association Task Force on Practice Guidelines (Committee to revise the 1995 Guidelines for the Evaluation and Management of Heart Failure). J Am Coll Cardiol 38:2101-2113

[19] Marez D, Legrand M, Sabbagh N, Lo Guidice JM, Spire C, Lafitte JJ, Meyer UA, Broly F (1997) Polymorphism of the cytochrome P450 CYP2D6 gene in a European population: characterization of 48 mutations and 53 alleles, their frequencies and evolution. Pharmacogenetics 7:193-202

[20] Relling MV, Cherrie J, Schell MJ, Petros WP, Meyer WH, Evans WE (1991) Lower prevalence of the debrisoquin oxidative poor metabolizer phenotype in American black versus white subjects. Clin Pharmacol Ther 50:308-313

[21] Zhou HH, Wood AJ (1995) Stereoselective disposition of carvedilol is determined by CYP2D6. Clin Pharmacol Ther 57:518-524

[22] Wang B, Wang J, Huang SQ, Su HH, Zhou SF (2009) Genetic Polymorphism of the Human Cytochrome P450 2C9 Gene and Its Clinical Significance. Curr Drug Metab 10:781-834

[23] Beitelshees AL, Gong Y, Wang D, Schork NJ, Cooper-Dehoff RM, Langaee TY, Shriver MD, Sadee W, Knot HJ, Pepine CJ, Johnson JA (2007) KCNMB1 genotype influences response to verapamil SR and adverse outcomes in the INternational VErapamil SR/Trandolapril STudy (INVEST). Pharmacogenet Genomics 17:719-729

[24] Beitelshees AL, Navare H, Wang D, Gong Y, Wessel J, Moss JI, Langaee TY, Cooper-DeHoff RM, Sadee W, Pepine CJ, Schork NJ, Johnson JA (2009) CACNA1C gene polymorphisms, cardiovascular disease outcomes, and treatment response. Circ Cardiovasc Genet 2:362-370

[25] Niu Y, Gong Y, Langaee TY, Davis HM, Elewa H, Beitelshees AL, Moss JI, Cooper-Dehoff RM, Pepine CJ, Johnson JA (2010) Genetic variation in the beta2 subunit of the voltage-gated calcium channel and pharmacogenetic association with adverse cardiovascular outcomes in the INternational VErapamil SR-Trandolapril STudy GENEtic Substudy (INVEST-GENES). Circ Cardiovasc Genet 3:548-555

[26] Sherva R, Ford CE, Eckfeldt JH, Davis BR, Boerwinkle E, Arnett DK (2011) Pharmacogenetic effect of the stromelysin (MMP3) polymorphism on stroke risk in relation to antihypertensive treatment: the genetics of hypertension associated treatment study. Stroke 42:330-335

[27] Svensson-Farbom P, Wahlstrand B, Almgren P, Dahlberg J, Fava C, Kjeldsen S, Hedner T, Melander O (2011) A functional variant of the NEDD4L gene is associated with beneficial treatment response with beta-blockers and diuretics in hypertensive patients. J Hypertens 29:388-395

[28] Schelleman H, Klungel OH, Witteman JC, Breteler MM, Hofman A, van Duijn CM, de Boer A, Stricker BH (2008) Interaction between polymorphisms in the renin-angiotensin-system and angiotensin-converting enzyme inhibitor or beta-blocker use and the risk of myocardial infarction and stroke. Pharmacogenomics J 8:400-407

[29] Schelleman H, Klungel OH, Witteman JC, Breteler MM, Yazdanpanah M, Danser AH, Hofman A, van Duijn CM, de Boer A, Stricker BH (2007) Angiotensinogen M235T polymorphism and the risk of myocardial infarction and stroke among hypertensive patients on ACE-inhibitors or beta-blockers. Eur J Hum Genet 15:478-484

[30] Turner ST, Bailey KR, Fridley BL, Chapman AB, Schwartz GL, Chai HS, Sicotte H, Kocher JP, Rodin AS, Boerwinkle E (2008) Genomic association analysis suggests

chromosome 12 locus influencing antihypertensive response to thiazide diuretic. Hypertension 52:359-365

[31] Duarte JD, Turner ST, Tran B, Chapman AB, Bailey KR, Gong Y, Gums JG, Langaee TY, Beitelshees AL, Cooper-Dehoff RM, Boerwinkle E, Johnson JA (2012) Association of chromosome 12 locus with antihypertensive response to hydrochlorothiazide may involve differential YEATS4 expression. Pharmacogenomics J

[32] Lynch AI, Boerwinkle E, Davis BR, Ford CE, Eckfeldt JH, Leiendecker-Foster C, Arnett DK (2008) Pharmacogenetic association of the NPPA T2238C genetic variant with cardiovascular disease outcomes in patients with hypertension. Jama 299:296-307

[33] Hollier JM, Martin DF, Bell DM, Li JL, Chirachanchai MG, Menon DV, Leonard D, Wu X, Cooper RS, McKenzie C, Victor RG, Auchus RJ (2006) Epithelial sodium channel allele T594M is not associated with blood pressure or blood pressure response to amiloride. Hypertension 47:428-433

[34] Swift PA, Macgregor GA (2004) Genetic variation in the epithelial sodium channel: a risk factor for hypertension in people of African origin. Adv Ren Replace Ther 11:76-86

[35] Manunta P, Lavery G, Lanzani C, Braund PS, Simonini M, Bodycote C, Zagato L, Delli Carpini S, Tantardini C, Brioni E, Bianchi G, Samani NJ (2008) Physiological interaction between alpha-adducin and WNK1-NEDD4L pathways on sodium-related blood pressure regulation. Hypertension 52:366-372

[36] Lanzani C, Citterio L, Glorioso N, Manunta P, Tripodi G, Salvi E, Carpini SD, Ferrandi M, Messaggio E, Staessen JA, Cusi D, Macciardi F, Argiolas G, Valentini G, Ferrari P, Bianchi G Adducin- and ouabain-related gene variants predict the antihypertensive activity of rostafuroxin, part 2: clinical studies. Sci Transl Med 2:59ra87

[37] Vormfelde SV, Sehrt D, Bolte D, Pahl S, Tzvetkov M, Brockmoller J (2006) Hydrochlorothiazide efficacy and polymorphisms in ACE, ADD1 and GNB3 in healthy, male volunteers. Eur J Clin Pharmacol 62:195-201

[38] Psaty BM, Smith NL, Heckbert SR, Vos HL, Lemaitre RN, Reiner AP, Siscovick DS, Bis J, Lumley T, Longstreth WT, Jr., Rosendaal FR (2002) Diuretic therapy, the alpha-adducin gene variant, and the risk of myocardial infarction or stroke in persons with treated hypertension. Jama 287:1680-1689

[39] Davis BR, Arnett DK, Boerwinkle E, Ford CE, Leiendecker-Foster C, Miller MB, Black H, Eckfeldt JH (2007) Antihypertensive therapy, the alpha-adducin polymorphism, and cardiovascular disease in high-risk hypertensive persons: the Genetics of Hypertension-Associated Treatment Study. Pharmacogenomics J 7:112-122

[40] Gerhard T, Gong Y, Beitelshees AL, Mao X, Lobmeyer MT, Cooper-DeHoff RM, Langaee TY, Schork NJ, Shriver MD, Pepine CJ, Johnson JA (2008) Alpha-adducin polymorphism associated with increased risk of adverse cardiovascular outcomes: results

from GENEtic Substudy of the INternational VErapamil SR-trandolapril STudy (INVEST-GENES). Am Heart J 156:397-404

[41] Poch E, Gonzalez-Nunez D, Compte M, De la Sierra A (2002) G-protein beta3-subunit gene variant, blood pressure and erythrocyte sodium/lithium countertransport in essential hypertension. Br J Biomed Sci 59:101-104

[42] Brugts JJ, Isaacs A, de Maat MP, Boersma E, van Duijn CM, Akkerhuis KM, Uitterlinden AG, Witteman JC, Cambien F, Ceconi C, Remme W, Bertrand M, Ninomiya T, Harrap S, Chalmers J, Macmahon S, Fox K, Ferrari R, Simoons ML, Danser AJ (2011) A pharmacogenetic analysis of determinants of hypertension and blood pressure response to angiotensin-converting enzyme inhibitor therapy in patients with vascular disease and healthy individuals. J Hypertens 29:509-519

[43] He J, Gu D, Kelly TN, Hixson JE, Rao DC, Jaquish CE, Chen J, Zhao Q, Gu C, Huang J, Shimmin LC, Chen JC, Mu J, Ji X, Liu DP, Whelton PK (2011) Genetic variants in the renin-angiotensin-aldosterone system and blood pressure responses to potassium intake. J Hypertens 29:1719-1730

[44] Katsuya T, Iwashima Y, Sugimoto K, Motone M, Asai T, Fukuda M, Fu Y, Hatanaka Y, Ohishi M, Rakugi H, Higaki J, Ogihara T (2001) Effects of antihypertensive drugs and gene variants in the renin-angiotensin system. Hypertens Res 24:463-467

[45] Konoshita T (2011) Do genetic variants of the Renin-Angiotensin system predict blood pressure response to Renin-Angiotensin system-blocking drugs?: a systematic review of pharmacogenomics in the Renin-Angiotensin system. Curr Hypertens Rep 13:356-361

[46] Kraja AT, Hunt SC, Rao DC, Davila-Roman VG, Arnett DK, Province MA (2011) Genetics of hypertension and cardiovascular disease and their interconnected pathways: lessons from large studies. Curr Hypertens Rep 13:46-54

[47] Ceyhan K, Kadi H, Celik A, Burucu T, Koc F, Sogut E, Sahin S, Onalan O (2012) Angiotensin-converting enzyme DD polymorphism is associated with poor coronary collateral circulation in patients with coronary artery disease. J Investig Med 60:49-55

[48] Prasad A, Narayanan S, Husain S, Padder F, Waclawiw M, Epstein N, Quyyumi AA (2000) Insertion-deletion polymorphism of the ACE gene modulates reversibility of endothelial dysfunction with ACE inhibition. Circulation 102:35-41

[49] Stavroulakis GA, Makris TK, Krespi PG, Hatzizacharias AN, Gialeraki AE, Anastasiadis G, Triposkiadis P, Kyriakidis M (2000) Predicting response to chronic antihypertensive treatment with fosinopril: the role of angiotensin-converting enzyme gene polymorphism. Cardiovasc Drugs Ther 14:427-432

[50] Ohmichi N, Iwai N, Uchida Y, Shichiri G, Nakamura Y, Kinoshita M (1997) Relationship between the response to the angiotensin converting enzyme inhibitor imidapril and the angiotensin converting enzyme genotype. Am J Hypertens 10:951-955

[51] O'Toole L, Stewart M, Padfield P, Channer K (1998) Effect of the insertion/deletion polymorphism of the angiotensin-converting enzyme gene on response to angiotensin-converting enzyme inhibitors in patients with heart failure. J Cardiovasc Pharmacol 32:988-994

[52] Takahashi T, Yamaguchi E, Furuya K, Kawakami Y (2001) The ACE gene polymorphism and cough threshold for capsaicin after cilazapril usage. Respir Med 95:130-135

[53] Schunkert H, Hense HW, Gimenez-Roqueplo AP, Stieber J, Keil U, Riegger GA, Jeunemaitre X (1997) The angiotensinogen T235 variant and the use of antihypertensive drugs in a population-based cohort. Hypertension 29:628-633

[54] van Geel PP, Pinto YM, Zwinderman AH, Henning RH, van Boven AJ, Jukema JW, Bruschke AV, Kastelein JJ, van Gilst WH (2001) Increased risk for ischaemic events is related to combined RAS polymorphism. Heart 85:458-462

[55] Benetos A, Topouchian J, Ricard S, Gautier S, Bonnardeaux A, Asmar R, Poirier O, Soubrier F, Safar M, Cambien F (1995) Influence of angiotensin II type 1 receptor polymorphism on aortic stiffness in never-treated hypertensive patients. Hypertension 26:44-47

[56] Benetos A, Cambien F, Gautier S, Ricard S, Safar M, Laurent S, Lacolley P, Poirier O, Topouchian J, Asmar R (1996) Influence of the angiotensin II type 1 receptor gene polymorphism on the effects of perindopril and nitrendipine on arterial stiffness in hypertensive individuals. Hypertension 28:1081-1084

[57] Filigheddu F, Argiolas G, Bulla E, Troffa C, Bulla P, Fadda S, Zaninello R, Degortes S, Frau F, Pitzoi S, Glorioso N (2008) Clinical variables, not RAAS polymorphisms, predict blood pressure response to ACE inhibitors in Sardinians. Pharmacogenomics 9:1419-1427

[58] Kurland L, Melhus H, Karlsson J, Kahan T, Malmqvist K, Ohman KP, Nystrom F, Hagg A, Lind L (2001) Angiotensin converting enzyme gene polymorphism predicts blood pressure response to angiotensin II receptor type 1 antagonist treatment in hypertensive patients. J Hypertens 19:1783-1787

[59] Bremer T, Man A, Kask K, Diamond C (2006) CACNA1C polymorphisms are associated with the efficacy of calcium channel blockers in the treatment of hypertension. Pharmacogenomics 7:271-279

[60] Langaee TY, Gong Y, Yarandi HN, Katz DA, Cooper-DeHoff RM, Pepine CJ, Johnson JA (2007) Association of CYP3A5 polymorphisms with hypertension and antihypertensive response to verapamil. Clin Pharmacol Ther 81:386-391

[61] Makris M, van Veen JJ, Maclean R (2010) Warfarin anticoagulation reversal: management of the asymptomatic and bleeding patient. J Thromb Thrombolysis 29:171-181

[62] Watson HG, Baglin T, Laidlaw SL, Makris M, Preston FE (2001) A comparison of the efficacy and rate of response to oral and intravenous Vitamin K in reversal of over-anticoagulation with warfarin. Br J Haematol 115:145-149

[63] Horne BD, Lenzini PA, Wadelius M, Jorgensen AL, Kimmel SE, Ridker PM, Eriksson N, Anderson JL, Pirmohamed M, Limdi NA, Pendleton RC, McMillin GA, Burmester JK, Kurnik D, Stein CM, Caldwell MD, Eby CS, Rane A, Lindh JD, Shin JG, Kim HS, Angchaisuksiri P, Glynn RJ, Kronquist KE, Carlquist JF, Grice GR, Barrack RL, Li J, Gage BF (2012) Pharmacogenetic warfarin dose refinements remain significantly influenced by genetic factors after one week of therapy. Thromb Haemost 107:232-240

[64] Johnson JA, Gong L, Whirl-Carrillo M, Gage BF, Scott SA, Stein CM, Anderson JL, Kimmel SE, Lee MT, Pirmohamed M, Wadelius M, Klein TE, Altman RB (2011) Clinical Pharmacogenetics Implementation Consortium Guidelines for CYP2C9 and VKORC1 genotypes and warfarin dosing. Clinical pharmacology and therapeutics 90:625-629

[65] Limdi NA, Wadelius M, Cavallari L, Eriksson N, Crawford DC, Lee MT, Chen CH, Motsinger-Reif A, Sagreiya H, Liu N, Wu AH, Gage BF, Jorgensen A, Pirmohamed M, Shin JG, Suarez-Kurtz G, Kimmel SE, Johnson JA, Klein TE, Wagner MJ (2010) Warfarin pharmacogenetics: a single VKORC1 polymorphism is predictive of dose across 3 racial groups. Blood 115:3827-3834

[66] Palareti G, Leali N, Coccheri S, Poggi M, Manotti C, D'Angelo A, Pengo V, Erba N, Moia M, Ciavarella N, Devoto G, Berretini M, Musolesi S (1997) [Hemorrhagic complications of oral anticoagulant therapy: results of a prospective multicenter study ISCOAT (Italian Study on Complications of Oral Anticoagulant Therapy)]. G Ital Cardiol 27:231-243

[67] Hirsh J, Bates SM (2001) Clinical trials that have influenced the treatment of venous thromboembolism: a historical perspective. Ann Intern Med 134:409-417

[68] Jones DR, Kim SY, Guderyon M, Yun CH, Moran JH, Miller GP (2010) Hydroxywarfarin metabolites potently inhibit CYP2C9 metabolism of S-warfarin. Chem Res Toxicol 23:939-945

[69] Kamali F, Wynne H (2010) Pharmacogenetics of warfarin. Annu Rev Med 61:63-75

[70] Kaminsky LS, Zhang ZY (1997) Human P450 metabolism of warfarin. Pharmacol Ther 73:67-74

[71] Adcock DM, Koftan C, Crisan D, Kiechle FL (2004) Effect of polymorphisms in the cytochrome P450 CYP2C9 gene on warfarin anticoagulation. Arch Pathol Lab Med 128:1360-1363

[72] Takahashi H, Echizen H (2001) Pharmacogenetics of warfarin elimination and its clinical implications. Clin Pharmacokinet 40:587-603

[73] Rettie AE, Wienkers LC, Gonzalez FJ, Trager WF, Korzekwa KR (1994) Impaired (S)-warfarin metabolism catalysed by the R144C allelic variant of CYP2C9. Pharmacogenetics 4:39-42

[74] Haining RL, Hunter AP, Veronese ME, Trager WF, Rettie AE (1996) Allelic variants of human cytochrome P450 2C9: baculovirus-mediated expression, purification, structural characterization, substrate stereoselectivity, and prochiral selectivity of the wild-type and I359L mutant forms. Arch Biochem Biophys 333:447-458

[75] Steward DJ, Haining RL, Henne KR, Davis G, Rushmore TH, Trager WF, Rettie AE (1997) Genetic association between sensitivity to warfarin and expression of CYP2C9*3. Pharmacogenetics 7:361-367

[76] Margaglione M, Colaizzo D, D'Andrea G, Brancaccio V, Ciampa A, Grandone E, Di Minno G (2000) Genetic modulation of oral anticoagulation with warfarin. Thromb Haemost 84:775-778

[77] Scordo MG, Pengo V, Spina E, Dahl ML, Gusella M, Padrini R (2002) Influence of CYP2C9 and CYP2C19 genetic polymorphisms on warfarin maintenance dose and metabolic clearance. Clin Pharmacol Ther 72:702-710

[78] Visser LE, van Vliet M, van Schaik RH, Kasbergen AA, De Smet PA, Vulto AG, Hofman A, van Duijn CM, Stricker BH (2004) The risk of overanticoagulation in patients with cytochrome P450 CYP2C9*2 or CYP2C9*3 alleles on acenocoumarol or phenprocoumon. Pharmacogenetics 14:27-33

[79] Furuya H, Fernandez-Salguero P, Gregory W, Taber H, Steward A, Gonzalez FJ, Idle JR (1995) Genetic polymorphism of CYP2C9 and its effect on warfarin maintenance dose requirement in patients undergoing anticoagulation therapy. Pharmacogenetics 5:389-392

[80] Aithal GP, Day CP, Kesteven PJ, Daly AK (1999) Association of polymorphisms in the cytochrome P450 CYP2C9 with warfarin dose requirement and risk of bleeding complications. Lancet 353:717-719

[81] Higashi MK, Veenstra DL, Kondo LM, Wittkowsky AK, Srinouanprachanh SL, Farin FM, Rettie AE (2002) Association between CYP2C9 genetic variants and anticoagulation-related outcomes during warfarin therapy. Jama 287:1690-1698

[82] Tabrizi AR, Zehnbauer BA, Borecki IB, McGrath SD, Buchman TG, Freeman BD (2002) The frequency and effects of cytochrome P450 (CYP) 2C9 polymorphisms in patients receiving warfarin. J Am Coll Surg 194:267-273

[83] Taube J, Halsall D, Baglin T (2000) Influence of cytochrome P-450 CYP2C9 polymorphisms on warfarin sensitivity and risk of over-anticoagulation in patients on long-term treatment. Blood 96:1816-1819

[84] Wadelius M, Sorlin K, Wallerman O, Karlsson J, Yue QY, Magnusson PK, Wadelius C, Melhus H (2004) Warfarin sensitivity related to CYP2C9, CYP3A5, ABCB1 (MDR1) and other factors. Pharmacogenomics J 4:40-48

[85] Freeman BD, Zehnbauer BA, McGrath S, Borecki I, Buchman TG (2000) Cytochrome P450 polymorphisms are associated with reduced warfarin dose. Surgery 128:281-285

[86] Takahashi H, Echizen H (2003) Pharmacogenetics of CYP2C9 and interindividual variability in anticoagulant response to warfarin. Pharmacogenomics J 3:202-214

[87] London SJ, Daly AK, Leathart JB, Navidi WC, Idle JR (1996) Lung cancer risk in relation to the CYP2C9*1/CYP2C9*2 genetic polymorphism among African-Americans and Caucasians in Los Angeles County, California. Pharmacogenetics 6:527-533

[88] Nasu K, Kubota T, Ishizaki T (1997) Genetic analysis of CYP2C9 polymorphism in a Japanese population. Pharmacogenetics 7:405-409

[89] Bhasker CR, Miners JO, Coulter S, Birkett DJ (1997) Allelic and functional variability of cytochrome P4502C9. Pharmacogenetics 7:51-58

[90] Schalekamp T, Klungel OH, Souverein PC, de Boer A (2008) Increased bleeding risk with concurrent use of selective serotonin reuptake inhibitors and coumarins. Arch Intern Med 168:180-185

[91] Dalton SO, Sorensen HT, Johansen C (2006) SSRIs and upper gastrointestinal bleeding: what is known and how should it influence prescribing? CNS Drugs 20:143-151

[92] Meijer WE, Heerdink ER, Leufkens HG, Herings RM, Egberts AC, Nolen WA (2004) Incidence and determinants of long-term use of antidepressants. Eur J Clin Pharmacol 60:57-61

[93] Greenblatt DJ, von Moltke LL, Harmatz JS, Shader RI (1998) Drug interactions with newer antidepressants: role of human cytochromes P450. J Clin Psychiatry 59 Suppl 15:19-27

[94] DeVane CL (1998) Differential pharmacology of newer antidepressants. J Clin Psychiatry 59 Suppl 20:85-93

[95] Duncan D, Sayal K, McConnell H, Taylor D (1998) Antidepressant interactions with warfarin. Int Clin Psychopharmacol 13:87-94

[96] Sayal KS, Duncan-McConnell DA, McConnell HW, Taylor DM (2000) Psychotropic interactions with warfarin. Acta Psychiatr Scand 102:250-255

[97] Hauta-Aho M, Tirkkonen T, Vahlberg T, Laine K (2009) The effect of drug interactions on bleeding risk associated with warfarin therapy in hospitalized patients. Ann Med 41:619-628

[98] Wallerstedt SM, Gleerup H, Sundstrom A, Stigendal L, Ny L (2009) Risk of clinically relevant bleeding in warfarin-treated patients--influence of SSRI treatment. Pharmacoepidemiol Drug Saf 18:412-416

[99] Wessinger S, Kaplan M, Choi L, Williams M, Lau C, Sharp L, Crowell MD, Keshavarzian A, Jones MP (2006) Increased use of selective serotonin reuptake inhibitors in

patients admitted with gastrointestinal haemorrhage: a multicentre retrospective analysis. Aliment Pharmacol Ther 23:937-944

[100] Castro TA, Heineck I (2012) Interventions to Improve Anticoagulation With Warfarin. Ther Drug Monit 34:209-216

[101] Zhang Q, Bal-dit-Sollier C, Drouet L, Simoneau G, Alvarez JC, Pruvot S, Aubourg R, Berge N, Bergmann JF, Mouly S, Mahe I (2011) Interaction between acetaminophen and warfarin in adults receiving long-term oral anticoagulants: a randomized controlled trial. Eur J Clin Pharmacol 67:309-314

[102] Burgess JK, Lindeman R, Chesterman CN, Chong BH (1995) Single amino acid mutation of Fc gamma receptor is associated with the development of heparin-induced thrombocytopenia. Br J Haematol 91:761-766

[103] Carlsson LE, Santoso S, Baurichter G, Kroll H, Papenberg S, Eichler P, Westerdaal NA, Kiefel V, van de Winkel JG, Greinacher A (1998) Heparin-induced thrombocytopenia: new insights into the impact of the FcgammaRIIa-R-H131 polymorphism. Blood 92:1526-1531

[104] Arepally G, McKenzie SE, Jiang XM, Poncz M, Cines DB (1997) Fc gamma RIIA H/R 131 polymorphism, subclass-specific IgG anti-heparin/platelet factor 4 antibodies and clinical course in patients with heparin-induced thrombocytopenia and thrombosis. Blood 89:370-375

[105] Waters DD (2001) What do the statin trials tell us? Am J Manag Care 7:S138-143

[106] Poduri A, Khullar M, Bahl A, Sehrawat BS, Sharma Y, Talwar KK (2010) Common variants of HMGCR, CETP, APOAI, ABCB1, CYP3A4, and CYP7A1 genes as predictors of lipid-lowering response to atorvastatin therapy. DNA Cell Biol 29:629-637

[107] Chasman DI, Posada D, Subrahmanyan L, Cook NR, Stanton VP, Jr., Ridker PM (2004) Pharmacogenetic study of statin therapy and cholesterol reduction. Jama 291:2821-2827

[108] Boekholdt SM, Kuivenhoven JA, Hovingh GK, Jukema JW, Kastelein JJ, van Tol A (2004) CETP gene variation: relation to lipid parameters and cardiovascular risk. Curr Opin Lipidol 15:393-398

[109] Kuivenhoven JA, Hovingh GK, van Tol A, Jauhiainen M, Ehnholm C, Fruchart JC, Brinton EA, Otvos JD, Smelt AH, Brownlee A, Zwinderman AH, Hayden MR, Kastelein JJ (2003) Heterozygosity for ABCA1 gene mutations: effects on enzymes, apolipoproteins and lipoprotein particle size. Atherosclerosis 171:311-319

[110] de Maat MP, Kastelein JJ, Jukema JW, Zwinderman AH, Jansen H, Groenemeier B, Bruschke AV, Kluft C (1998) -455G/A polymorphism of the beta-fibrinogen gene is associated with the progression of coronary atherosclerosis in symptomatic men: proposed role for an acute-phase reaction pattern of fibrinogen. REGRESS group. Arterioscler Thromb Vasc Biol 18:265-271

[111] Bray PF, Cannon CP, Goldschmidt-Clermont P, Moye LA, Pfeffer MA, Sacks FM, Braunwald E (2001) The platelet Pl(A2) and angiotensin-converting enzyme (ACE) D allele polymorphisms and the risk of recurrent events after acute myocardial infarction. Am J Cardiol 88:347-352

[112] Sacks FM, Pfeffer MA, Moye LA, Rouleau JL, Rutherford JD, Cole TG, Brown L, Warnica JW, Arnold JM, Wun CC, Davis BR, Braunwald E (1996) The effect of pravastatin on coronary events after myocardial infarction in patients with average cholesterol levels. Cholesterol and Recurrent Events Trial investigators. N Engl J Med 335:1001-1009

[113] Gerdes LU, Gerdes C, Kervinen K, Savolainen M, Klausen IC, Hansen PS, Kesaniemi YA, Faergeman O (2000) The apolipoprotein epsilon4 allele determines prognosis and the effect on prognosis of simvastatin in survivors of myocardial infarction : a substudy of the Scandinavian simvastatin survival study. Circulation 101:1366-1371

[114] Donnelly LA, Doney AS, Dannfald J, Whitley AL, Lang CC, Morris AD, Donnan PT, Palmer CN (2008) A paucimorphic variant in the HMG-CoA reductase gene is associated with lipid-lowering response to statin treatment in diabetes: a GoDARTS study. Pharmacogenet Genomics 18:1021-1026

[115] Kajinami K, Brousseau ME, Ordovas JM, Schaefer EJ (2004) CYP3A4 genotypes and plasma lipoprotein levels before and after treatment with atorvastatin in primary hypercholesterolemia. Am J Cardiol 93:104-107

[116] Wang A, Yu BN, Luo CH, Tan ZR, Zhou G, Wang LS, Zhang W, Li Z, Liu J, Zhou HH (2005) Ile118Val genetic polymorphism of CYP3A4 and its effects on lipid-lowering efficacy of simvastatin in Chinese hyperlipidemic patients. Eur J Clin Pharmacol 60:843-848

[117] Gao Y, Zhang LR, Fu Q (2008) CYP3A4*1G polymorphism is associated with lipid-lowering efficacy of atorvastatin but not of simvastatin. Eur J Clin Pharmacol 64:877-882

[118] Krauss RM, Mangravite LM, Smith JD, Medina MW, Wang D, Guo X, Rieder MJ, Simon JA, Hulley SB, Waters D, Saad M, Williams PT, Taylor KD, Yang H, Nickerson DA, Rotter JI (2008) Variation in the 3-hydroxyl-3-methylglutaryl coenzyme a reductase gene is associated with racial differences in low-density lipoprotein cholesterol response to simvastatin treatment. Circulation 117:1537-1544

[119] Mangravite LM, Wilke RA, Zhang J, Krauss RM (2008) Pharmacogenomics of statin response. Curr Opin Mol Ther 10:555-561

[120] Wilke RA, Moore JH, Burmester JK (2005) Relative impact of CYP3A genotype and concomitant medication on the severity of atorvastatin-induced muscle damage. Pharmacogenet Genomics 15:415-421

[121] Pasanen MK, Neuvonen M, Neuvonen PJ, Niemi M (2006) SLCO1B1 polymorphism markedly affects the pharmacokinetics of simvastatin acid. Pharmacogenet Genomics 16:873-879

[122] Voora D, Shah SH, Spasojevic I, Ali S, Reed CR, Salisbury BA, Ginsburg GS (2009) The SLCO1B1*5 genetic variant is associated with statin-induced side effects. J Am Coll Cardiol 54:1609-1616

[123] Donnelly LA, Doney AS, Tavendale R, Lang CC, Pearson ER, Colhoun HM, McCarthy MI, Hattersley AT, Morris AD, Palmer CN (2011) Common nonsynonymous substitutions in SLCO1B1 predispose to statin intolerance in routinely treated individuals with type 2 diabetes: a go-DARTS study. Clin Pharmacol Ther 89:210-216

[124] Li Y, Sabatine MS, Tong CH, Ford I, Kirchgessner TG, Packard CJ, Robertson M, Rowland CM, Bare LA, Shepherd J, Devlin JJ, Iakoubova OA (2011) Genetic variants in the KIF6 region and coronary event reduction from statin therapy. Hum Genet 129:17-23

[125] Catapano AL (2012) Statin-induced myotoxicity: pharmacokinetic differences among statins and the risk of rhabdomyolysis, with particular reference to pitavastatin. Curr Vasc Pharmacol 10:257-267

[126] Priori SG, Barhanin J, Hauer RN, Haverkamp W, Jongsma HJ, Kleber AG, McKenna WJ, Roden DM, Rudy Y, Schwartz K, Schwartz PJ, Towbin JA, Wilde AM (1999) Genetic and molecular basis of cardiac arrhythmias: impact on clinical management parts I and II. Circulation 99:518-528

[127] Thorn HA, Lundahl A, Schrickx JA, Dickinson PA, Lennernas H (2011) Drug metabolism of CYP3A4, CYP2C9 and CYP2D6 substrates in pigs and humans. Eur J Pharm Sci 43:89-98

[128] Ylitalo P, Ruosteenoja R, Leskinen O, Metsa-Ketela T (1983) Significance of acetylator phenotype in pharmacokinetics and adverse effects of procainamide. Eur J Clin Pharmacol 25:791-795

[129] Roden DM (2006) Long QT syndrome: reduced repolarization reserve and the genetic link. J Intern Med 259:59-69

[130] Paulussen AD, Gilissen RA, Armstrong M, Doevendans PA, Verhasselt P, Smeets HJ, Schulze-Bahr E, Haverkamp W, Breithardt G, Cohen N, Aerssens J (2004) Genetic variations of KCNQ1, KCNH2, SCN5A, KCNE1, and KCNE2 in drug-induced long QT syndrome patients. J Mol Med (Berl) 82:182-188

[131] Yang P, Kanki H, Drolet B, Yang T, Wei J, Viswanathan PC, Hohnloser SH, Shimizu W, Schwartz PJ, Stanton M, Murray KT, Norris K, George AL, Jr., Roden DM (2002) Allelic variants in long-QT disease genes in patients with drug-associated torsades de pointes. Circulation 105:1943-1948

[132] Itoh H, Sakaguchi T, Ding WG, Watanabe E, Watanabe I, Nishio Y, Makiyama T, Ohno S, Akao M, Higashi Y, Zenda N, Kubota T, Mori C, Okajima K, Haruna T, Miya-

moto A, Kawamura M, Ishida K, Nagaoka I, Oka Y, Nakazawa Y, Yao T, Jo H, Sugimoto Y, Ashihara T, Hayashi H, Ito M, Imoto K, Matsuura H, Horie M (2009) Latent genetic backgrounds and molecular pathogenesis in drug-induced long-QT syndrome. Circ Arrhythm Electrophysiol 2:511-523

[133] Becker ML, Visser LE, Newton-Cheh C, Hofman A, Uitterlinden AG, Witteman JC, Stricker BH (2009) A common NOS1AP genetic polymorphism is associated with increased cardiovascular mortality in users of dihydropyridine calcium channel blockers. Br J Clin Pharmacol 67:61-67

[134] Crotti L, Monti MC, Insolia R, Peljto A, Goosen A, Brink PA, Greenberg DA, Schwartz PJ, George AL, Jr. (2009) NOS1AP is a genetic modifier of the long-QT syndrome. Circulation 120:1657-1663

[135] Tomas M, Napolitano C, De Giuli L, Bloise R, Subirana I, Malovini A, Bellazzi R, Arking DE, Marban E, Chakravarti A, Spooner PM, Priori SG (2010) Polymorphisms in the NOS1AP gene modulate QT interval duration and risk of arrhythmias in the long QT syndrome. J Am Coll Cardiol 55:2745-2752

[136] Undas A, Sanak M, Musial J, Szczeklik A (1999) Platelet glycoprotein IIIa polymorphism, aspirin, and thrombin generation. Lancet 353:982-983

[137] Goodman T, Ferro A, Sharma P (2008) Pharmacogenetics of aspirin resistance: a comprehensive systematic review. Br J Clin Pharmacol 66:222-232

[138] Goodall AH, Curzen N, Panesar M, Hurd C, Knight CJ, Ouwehand WH, Fox KM (1999) Increased binding of fibrinogen to glycoprotein IIIa-proline33 (HPA-1b, PlA2, Zwb) positive platelets in patients with cardiovascular disease. Eur Heart J 20:742-747

[139] Walter DH, Schachinger V, Elsner M, Dimmeler S, Zeiher AM (1997) Platelet glycoprotein IIIa polymorphisms and risk of coronary stent thrombosis. Lancet 350:1217-1219

[140] Kastrati A, Koch W, Gawaz M, Mehilli J, Bottiger C, Schomig K, von Beckerath N, Schomig A (2000) PlA polymorphism of glycoprotein IIIa and risk of adverse events after coronary stent placement. J Am Coll Cardiol 36:84-89

[141] Abbate R, Marcucci R, Camacho-Vanegas O, Pepe G, Gori AM, Capanni M, Simonetti I, Prisco D, Gensini GF (1998) Role of platelet glycoprotein PL(A1/A2) polymorphism in restenosis after percutaneous transluminal coronary angioplasty. Am J Cardiol 82:524-525

[142] Savi P, Nurden P, Nurden AT, Levy-Toledano S, Herbert JM (1998) Clopidogrel: a review of its mechanism of action. Platelets 9:251-255

[143] Shuldiner AR, O'Connell JR, Bliden KP, Gandhi A, Ryan K, Horenstein RB, Damcott CM, Pakyz R, Tantry US, Gibson Q, Pollin TI, Post W, Parsa A, Mitchell BD, Faraday N, Herzog W, Gurbel PA (2009) Association of cytochrome P450 2C19 genotype with the antiplatelet effect and clinical efficacy of clopidogrel therapy. Jama 302:849-857

[144] Mega JL, Simon T, Collet JP, Anderson JL, Antman EM, Bliden K, Cannon CP, Danchin N, Giusti B, Gurbel P, Horne BD, Hulot JS, Kastrati A, Montalescot G, Neumann FJ, Shen L, Sibbing D, Steg PG, Trenk D, Wiviott SD, Sabatine MS (2010) Reduced-function CYP2C19 genotype and risk of adverse clinical outcomes among patients treated with clopidogrel predominantly for PCI: a meta-analysis. Jama 304:1821-1830

[145] Roden DM, Stein CM (2009) Clopidogrel and the concept of high-risk pharmacokinetics. Circulation 119:2127-2130

[146] Santos PC, Soares RA, Santos DB, Nascimento RM, Coelho GL, Nicolau JC, Mill JG, Krieger JE, Pereira AC (2011) CYP2C19 and ABCB1 gene polymorphisms are differently distributed according to ethnicity in the Brazilian general population. BMC Med Genet 12:13

[147] Solus JF, Arietta BJ, Harris JR, Sexton DP, Steward JQ, McMunn C, Ihrie P, Mehall JM, Edwards TL, Dawson EP (2004) Genetic variation in eleven phase I drug metabolism genes in an ethnically diverse population. Pharmacogenomics 5:895-931

[148] Jaitner J, Morath T, Byrne RA, Braun S, Gebhard D, Bernlochner I, Schulz S, Mehilli J, Schomig A, Koch W, Kastrati A, Sibbing D (2012) No association of ABCB1 C3435T genotype with clopidogrel response or risk of stent thrombosis in patients undergoing coronary stenting. Circ Cardiovasc Interv 5:82-88, S81-82

[149] Kubica A, Kozinski M, Grzesk G, Fabiszak T, Navarese EP, Goch A (2011) Genetic determinants of platelet response to clopidogrel. J Thromb Thrombolysis 32:459-466

[150] Luo M, Li J, Xu X, Sun X, Sheng W (2011) ABCB1 C3435T polymorphism and risk of adverse clinical events in clopidogrel treated patients: A meta-analysis. Thromb Res

[151] Preskorn SH (2003) Relating clinical trials to psychiatric practice: part I: the case of a 13-year old on aripiprazole and fluoxetine. J Psychiatr Pract 9:307-313

Chapter 4

Interactions with Drugs and Dietary Supplements Used For Weight Loss

Melanie A. Jordan

Additional information is available at the end of the chapter

http://dx.doi.org/10.5772/51145

1. Introduction

Obesity and overweight have increasingly become major global health issues. Data from the World Health Organization (WHO) reports a near doubling of the prevalence of obesity worldwide from 1998 to 2008 [1]. In the European Region, an average of over 50% of adults are overweight and nearly 23% obese, with the prevalence of overweight and obesity being highest in Finland (67.1%), Germany (67.2%), the United Kingdom (67.8%), Malta (73.3%), and Greece (77.5%) [2]. Similar alarming trends are seen in the United States NHANES data where 68% of adults have a body mass index (BMI) greater than 25 (overweight or obese) and nearly 37% of the population is considered obese [3-7]. A large burden of health care costs can be attributed to overweight and obesity since multiple disease states such as diabetes, cancer, heart disease can be linked overweight and obesity [8-10]. The WHO estimates that up to 6% of health care expenditures in the European Region, while estimates for the United States have been estimated at 5.7% of the National Health Expenditure [8-11]. Most major organizations, like the WHO, and governmental agencies such as the U.S. Department of Agriculture Center for Nutrition Policy and Promotion have a major focus on the treatment of the obesity epidemic through promotion of proper healthy lifestyle changes [11, 12]. Although multiple anti-obesity agents have progressed through the development process, few drug products have made it through the approval process due to safety or lack of efficacy concerns. Several products, such as amphetamine, fenfluramine and sibutramine, have had their approval removed and/or have been removed from the market following reports linking the drugs to cardiovascular side effects (e.g. hypertension and myocardial infarction), addiction, and death [13-15]. As an alternative, overweight or obese patients may turn to less regulated dietary supplements as a means to assist in weight loss. Multiple herbal products are available that are indicated, often without significant scientific basis, for the treatment of overweight and obesity. The safety and efficacy of herbal products is often unknown, especially given the presence of multiple chemical compounds, lack of known active constituents or lack of standardization of known compounds [16-19].This chapter presents a review of the chemistry and pharmacology of approved anti-obesity drug products, the proposed mechanism of action for common dietary supplements used in the management of weight loss, and potential drug-drug or herb-drug interactions.

2. Drugs used in weight LOcSS

2.1. Sympathomiometic agents

2.1.1. Diethylpropion hydrochloride (Tenuate®; Tenuate® Dospan®; Durad®)

Diethylpropion HCl (amfepramone, Figure 1a) is a sympathomimetic aminoketone agent with some similarity both chemically and pharmacologically to amphetamines and other related stimulant drugs. Similarly to amphetamine, diethylpropion stimulates release while inhibiting reuptake of dopamine, norepinephrine, and 5-hydroxytryptamine [20, 21]. The increase in norepinephrine and dopamine levels along with inhibition of their reuptake is proposed as the mechanism of diethylpropion anorectic effects [22]. Diethylpropion is indicated for short term management of obesity in patients with a body mass index (BMI) of > 30 kg/m^2 who have not responded to diet and exercise alone [23]. Because of its similarity to amphetamine, some patients become psychologically dependent on diethylpropion with an increased risk of self-medicating at higher dosages, increasing potential for drug interactions.

Diethylpropion is a monoamine and therefore can interact with monoamine oxidase inhibitors (MAOI), resulting in hypertension [23]. The manufacturer recommends avoiding use of diethylpropion during or within 14 days of discontinuation of MAOI administration. There is also one reported case of diethylpropion -induced psychosis in a 26 year old female patient taking phenelzine [24]. The authors hypothesized that chronic diethylpropion use led to an increased sensitivity to MAOI psychosis-inducing effects. Although the additive effects of diethylpropion in combination with other anorectic agents has not been studied, combined use of these agents is contraindicated due to the potential increased risk of cardiovascular issues [23]. In an early study of diethylpropion in 32 obese hypertensive patients, a drop in blood pressure was observed [25]. However, it was unclear if the drop in blood pressure in these subjects was due to weight loss or the additive effect of additional hypertensive agents that the patients were taking. The manufacturer also recommends potential modification of insulin dosing, although no strong evidence to support this statement can be found. In one study done in the rat, it was determined that anorectic drugs acting via the dopaminergic system antagonize hyperphagia induced by 2-deoxy-D-glucose, although the authors did not find any modifications to insulin-induced hypoglycemia [26]. There are no reported cases of drug-herb interactions with diethylpropion. However, theoretically herbal products with CNS stimulant properties (e.g. ephedra, caffeine, bitter orange), potential for interaction with sympathomimetic agents (e.g. Indian snakeroot), or MAOI activity (e.g. yohimbe) should be avoided due to an increased risk of hypertension, cardiovascular effects, and changes in blood pressure [27].

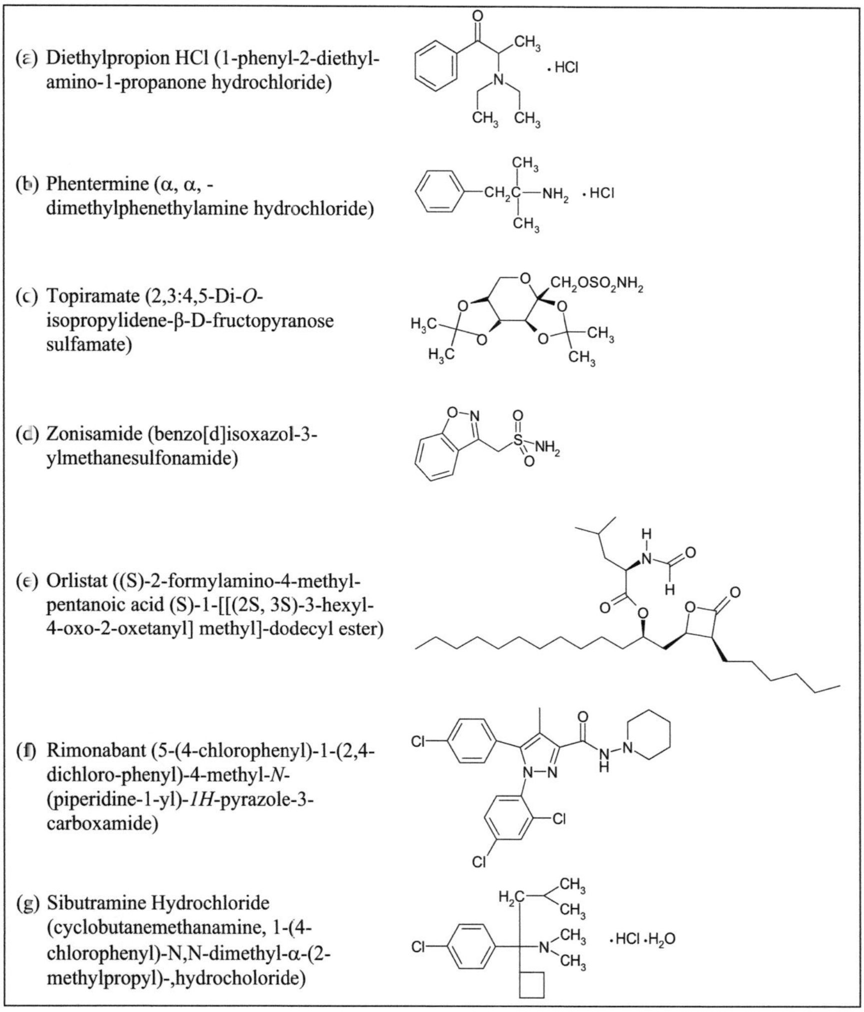

Figure 1. Molecular structures of anorectic drugs.

2.1.2. Phentermine / Phentermine hydrochloride (Fastin®, Ionamin®, Adipex-P®, Suprenza®)

Phentermine (Figure 1b), a member of the β-phenylethylamine family of compounds, exerts anorectic activity centrally through appetite suppression and is indicated in the short term treatment of obesity in patients with a BMI ≥ 30 kg/m^2 [28]. A meta-analysis of six randomized controlled trials of phentermine cumulatively show an added 3.6 kg weight loss over 2 to 24 weeks compared to control groups [29]. Phentermine acts by increasing the release of and inhibiting the reuptake of norepinephrine or dopamine [22]. Although one of the oldest approved anti-obesity drugs, the safety of monotherapy of phentermine is relatively scarce due to the long history of combination products, most notably phentermine/fenfluramine (Phen-Fen), which was removed from the market due to serious and potentially fatal cardiovascular effects [30, 31]. More recently a combination product containing phentermine and topiramate has been investigated (see *Topiramate* below) and is currently under review by the US Food and Drug Administration (FDA).

Because of the similarity in activity and mechanism of action, drug interactions with phentermine are similar to those for diethylpropion (see *Diethylpropion* above) including avoidance of alcohol, potential changes to antidiabetic agent therapy, and avoidance of coadministration of MAOIs [28]. There is one case report of a female patient experiencing two penropative hypertensive crises, which were attributed to an interaction between phentermine and anesthetic agents [32].

2.2. Antiepileptic agents

Several antiepileptic agents are known to have an effect on weight gain [33]. However, two newer antiepileptic agents, topiramate and zonisamide, have shown an associated decrease in weight in patients taking these medications [34]. Therefore, these two drugs are being looked at as potential anorectic agents.

2.2.1. Topiramate (Topamax®)

Topiramate is a carbonic anhydrase inhibitor (Figure 1c) that is typically used in the treatment of migraines and as an anticonvulsant [35]. Topiramate is proposed to exert its antiepileptic activity via gamma-aminobutyric acid (GABA)-A-mediated inhibition via a benzodiazepine insensitive pathway, although the drug also blocks voltage dependent sodium channels [35-37]. Weight loss has been a commonly reported adverse effect of topiramate; therefore, the drug has recently come into focus as a potential anorectic agent [38-42]. Topiramate has shown promise as a combination low-dose therapy with phentermine (Qsymia(R) (originally Qnexa(R), Vivus Pharmaceuticals, Mountain View, CA, USA) for long term treatment of obesity [43-46]. Despite, safety concerns related to teratogenicity and cardiovascular effects, the product has recently been approved by the U.S. Food and Drug Administration."

Drug interactions with topiramate include coadministration with other antiepileptic agents. Although no changes in carbamazepine or phenytoin levels were seen, topiramate levels decreased by 40% or 48%, respectively [35]. However, there have been two case reports of antiepileptic drug intoxications in patients initiated on topiramate who were already taking the maximum carbamazepine dose [47]. Decrease in carbamazepine dosage resolved the interaction. Hyperammonemia, hypothermia and potentially encephalopathy can result from a synergistic interaction between topiramate, valproic acid, and phenobarbital, although the exact mechanism of this interaction is unknown [35, 48-50]. Levels of ethinyl estradiol can be significantly decreased in patients taking topiramate as an adjunctive therapy with valproic acid [35]. As a carbonic anhydrase inhibitor, topiramate can cause metabolic acidosis, and therefore is contraindicated in patients taking metformin, while patients taking other carbonic anhydrase inhibitors should be monitored due to the potential additive effects when coadministered with topiramate [51-55]. High doses of topiramate (600 mg/day) can increase systemic exposure to lithium. However, since topiramate dosage proposed to anorectic effects is low, this interaction may not be a significant concern when used as anti-obesity treatment [56]. No clinical studies or case studies are available for interactions with CNS depressants (e.g alcohol), although combined use is contraindicated by the manufacturer due to combined CNS depression [35]. No data supporting herb-drug interactions are available specifically related to use of topiramate at low doses as an anorectic agent [27].

2.2.2. *Zonisamide (Zonegran®)*

Zonisamide (Figure 1d), a methanesulfonamide, is an antiepileptic agent which has broad spectrum activity and has proven to be useful in patients not responding to other antiepileptic treatments [57]. The drug blocks sustained and repetitive neuronal firing by blocking voltage sensitive sodium channels and decreasing voltage sensitive T-type calcium channels [58, 59]. Additionally, it was found that zonisamide has dopaminergic and serotonergic activity, which contributes to the anorectic effects of the drug [60, 61]. In one randomized placebo-controlled trial, 30 subjects were administered zonisamide 100 mg daily along with a low calorie diet (500 kcal/day) for a period of 16 weeks. Dosage was increased to up to 600 mg/day for patients not losing >5% of their initial body weight within the first 12 weeks. The zonisamide group lost significantly more body weight at the end of the trial compared to the placebo group (approx. 6% loss vs. 1% loss) [62].

Zonisamide is metabolized by the cytochrome P450 3A4 system and therefore can potentially interact with other drugs metabolized via this route. In one study, the half-life of zonisamide ($t_{½}$ = 60 h) was decreased in patients receiving both zonisamide and phenytoin ($t_{½}$ = 27 h), carbamazepine ($t_{½}$ = 38 h, and sodium valproate ($t_{½}$ = 46 h) [57, 63]. Another study in the dog demonstrated decreased plasma levels of zonisamide during administration of phenobarbital [64]. However, any associated decrease in levels of other antiepileptic drugs was not found to be clinically significant [65, 66]. Cigarette smoking may alter the pharmacokinetics of zonisamide. Coadministration of carbonic anhydrase inhibitors may increase risk of metabolic acidosis and kidney stone formation, therefore monitoring is recommended in this patient population [66]. One study on the effects of cigarette smoke on zonisamide concentrations in rats suggests that cigarette smoke may decrease plasma levels of the drug due to decreased oral absorption [67]. Brain, but not plasma levels of zonisamide may be affected by chronic ethanol consumption. In one study inbred EL mice were administered zonisamide 75 mg/kg for 1 – 4 weeks along with 10% ethanol *ad libidum*. In groups with 4 week coadministration, representing chronic use of alcohol, a decrease in zonisamide brain concentrations, but not serum concentration were observed [68].

2.3. Orlistat (Xenical®, Alli®)

Orlistat (Figure 1e) is a gastrointestinal lipase inhibitor approved both as a prescription (Xenical®) and over-the-counter (Alli®) weight loss aid in the long term treatment of obesity [69]. The drug exhibits antiobesity activity by inhibiting the absorption of dietary fat from the lumen of the stomach and small intestine through covalent binding with gastric and pancreatic lipase active serine residues [70]. Multiple randomized controlled trials have reported significant weight loss in patients taking orlistat compared to placebo controlled groups. One meta-analysis cites mean weight loss compared to control of -2.59 kg [95%CI, -3.46 to -1.74] or -2.9 kg [95%CI, -3.2 to -2.5] over 6 or 12 months, respectively, with a corresponding decrease in waist circumference, blood pressure, and blood glucose and lipid profiles [71-73].

A large number of preclinical and clinical studies and case reports related to potential drug interactions with orlistat have been published. There have been several cases of orlistat interaction with cyclosporine [74-79]. In all cases, significant decreases in plasma cyclosporine levels were observed following adjunct treatment with orlistat for cyclosporine-associated weight gain. Although one proposed mechanism for the reduction in plasma cyclosporine is a decrease in drug absorption, decreased levels may be due to rapid gastrointestinal transit time resulting from contraindicated high fat diets rather than a true drug-drug interaction [80]. Because orlistat is designed to inhibit gastrointestinal lipases, theoretically absorption of lipophilic molecules would also be inhibited [81-83]. In one open-label, placebo-controlled randomized two-way crossover study, orlistat (120 mg) was administered to 12 healthy subjects three times daily for 9 days followed by administration of Vitamin A (25,000 IU) or Vitamin E (400 IU) [82]. Although no effect was seen on Vitamin A levels, a significant reduction in C_{max} (approx. 43%) and AUC (approx. 60%) were observed for Vitamin E, suggesting impaired absorption of Vitamin E by orlistat. In another study, approximately a 30% reduction in beta-carotene levels was observed after administration of orlistat (120 mg) for four days followed by administration of 0 – 120 mg of beta-carotene three times a day for six days [83]. Absorption of lipophilic drugs such as the CNS agent lamotrigene can also be affected by orlistat. In one report, increased frequency of seizures was reported in an 18 year old female taking lamotrigene following initiation of an orlistat regimen [84]. One case of hypothyroidism in thyroid carcinoma was reported, presumably due to decreased absorption of thyroxine [85]. Although orlistat was not found to alter warfarin kinetics *per se*, but the drug may alter absorption of the fat soluble vitamin K which can have an effect warfarin levels and therefore these patients should be monitored for changes in coagulation parameters [86].

2.4. Rimonabant (Acomplia®, Zumulti®)

Rimonabant (Figure 1f) is a cannabanoid receptor antagonist that suppresses appetite by preventing activation of CB_1 receptors by the endogenous cannabanoids anandamide and 2-arachidonoyl-glycerol [87]. In clinical trials the drug resulted in improvement of multiple endpoints associated with obesity and metabolic syndrome compared to control groups including significant weight loss, reduction in waist circumference, decreased triglycerides, blood glucose, fasting insulin, and leptin levels with increased HDL cholesterol and adiponectin levels [88-96]. Although rimonabant proved a potentially successful drug in the treatment of obesity, especially given lack of cardiovascular risks compared to other weight loss drugs (see *Sibutramine* below), the drug has not been approved by the U.S. Food and Drug Administration (FDA). Additionally, although the drug was initially approved in 2006 by the European Medicines Agency (EMEA), later studies indicating serious neuropsychiatric

http://dx.doi.org/10.5772/51145

adverse events, especially related to increased risk of suicide, caused the Agency to rescind the approval in 2009. Although rimonabant is not available in most major markets, ongoing investigations surrounding the development of the drug continue, while the drug has been approved in other markets [97-100]. Additionally, the drug appears to be available readily via online pharmacy services and has been identified as an adulterant in dietary supplements marketed for weight loss (see *Adulteration of Dietary Supplements* below) [101-103].

Given the limited and short-lived approval status of rimonabant, there is little information regarding potential drug-drug and herb-drug interactions available. According to package insert data submitted to the EMEA, rimonabant is known to be eliminated hepatically and into the bile by amidohydrolase and CYP3A4, with a 104% increase in rimonabant AUC (95% CI 40 – 197%) upon coadministration of ketoconazole [92, 96, 104, 105]. Therefore, the manufacturer indicated potential interactions with strong CYP3A4 inhibitors (e.g. ketoconazole, itraconazole, ritonavir, telithromycin, clarithromycin, and nefazodone) and inducers (e.g. rifampicin, phenytoin, phenobarbital, carbamazepine, and St. John's Wort). Because rimonabant can decrease levels of fasting insulin and blood sugar, use of rimonabant in diabetic patients taking anti-diabetic agents is cautioned [92, 96, 104, 105].

2.5. Sibutramine (Meridia®, Reductil®)

Sibutramine hydrocholoride (Figure 1g), and its active primary (M_1) and secondary (M_2) metabolites, is a selective serotonin (5-hydroxytryptamine, 5-HT) and norepinephrine reuptake inhibitor [106-110]. Clinical data supported the efficacy of sibutramine as a weight loss agent, reporting significant weight loss compared to placebo for patients taking at least 10 mg/day for up to one year [107, 110-114]. The drug was approved as an anti-obesity agent in 1997 by the U.S. FDA and in 2002 by the EMEA, despite evidence of increased risk of hypertension and tachycardia, with a requirement that additional post-marketing safety data be collected relative to cardiotoxicity. As a result, the SCOUT (Sibutramine Cardiovascular OUTcomes) trial was implemented, which enrolled 10,000 overweight or obese patients aged 55 and older with coexisting diabetes and/or heart disease in a randomized controlled trial with a 6-month lead in period [115-118]. At the end of the six year study period, data showed a significant decrease in body weight compared to placebo but increased cardiovascular morbidity in the randomized sibutramine group [115-118]. Following publication of the SCOUT trial results in 2010, the EMEA and most other major markets pulled sibutramine while the United States and Australia required stricter labeling. By 2011 sibutramine was pulled from all major markets globally. However, as with the case of rimonabant (see above), sibutramine is of note since it is the primary contaminant found in dietary weight loss supplements (see *Adulteration of Dietary Supplements* below).

Sibutramine is known to be metabolized by CYP 3A4 into two active metabolites (M_1 and M_2). Data reported by the manufacturer in limited clinical trials (n = 12 – 27 patients) suggest potential pharmacokinetic changes in AUC and C_{max} for sibutramine when taken in combination with CYP 3A4 inhibitors such as cimetidine, ketoconazole, erythromycin, simvastatin, and omeprazole; while sibutramine does not generally have a significant impact on the levels of these drugs in return [106]. Because of the role of CYP 3A4 in sibutramine elimination, use of the drug with other CYP 3A4 substrates, including coadministration with grapefruit juice, is contraindicated [111]. One case report describes a possible interaction between sibutramine and citalopram in a 43 year old female patient who experienced hypomanic symptoms shortly after adding 10 mg sibutramine to her current citalopram and fluoxetine regimen [119]. Symptoms ceased within one day of discontinuing sibutramine. Although the exact mechanism of the interaction is unknown, the author hypothesized a possible amphetamine-like hypomania or serotonin syndrome due to increased brain serotonin levels via the combination of a serotonin reuptake inhibitor and serotonin-norepinephrine reuptake inhibitor. Another case report notes a possible interaction between sibutramine and cyclosporine in a 26 year old transplant patient resulting in significant increases in cyclosporine trough plasma levels, likely due to inhibition of CYP 3A4 metabolism [120]. Coadministration of α_2 adrenergic blockers, such as the herb yohimbine, with sibutramine has been recognized as potentially life threatening due to potential sympathetic side effects resulting in hypertension and tachycardia [121]. Due to the potential risk of bleeding caused by sibutramine, the drug should be used with caution in patients taking warfarin and other anticoagulants [106].

3. Herbs and dietary supplements used in weight loss

3.1. Açaí (*Euterpe oleracea*)

The açaí berry is harvested from the palm species *Euterpe oleracea* and is used mainly for dietary consumption as whole fruit, juice, or as a flavoring and coloring agent [27]. The fruit, widely used in Brazil, has gained in popularity as a food product and dietary supplement in the past several years, mainly due to its antioxidant and anti-inflammatory effects related to high polyphenol content [122-126]. Although there is little scientific evidence to support the berry for any of its purported health benefits, it can be found in several dietary supplements promoted for weight loss. In a pilot study investigating the effect of açaí supplementation on metabolic parameters in healthy overweight patients, the authors found a significant decrease in fasting glucose, insulin and cholesterol levels and a mild decrease in LDL-cholesterol and ratio of total cholesterol to HDL-cholesterol [127]. However, the authors did not assess weight loss in this study and therefore the activity of açaí as an anorectic agent cannot be determined. There have been no reported adverse drug interactions or interactions with others herbs and açaí [27].

3.2. Bitter orange (*Citrus aurantium, Citrus naringin, synephrine*)

Bitter orange is the fruit of *Citrus aurantium* or *Citrus naringin*, used as both a food product and the medicinal properties of the juice and peel [27]. There are multiple active constituents in bitter orange including several flavonoids (e.g. naringin) and the adrenergic agonists synephrine and octopamine [128-134]. Synephrine is structurally similar to ephedrine, therefore prompting the replacement of ephedra with bitter orange in weight loss supplements, although the fruit has been used dichotomously as both an appetite stimulant and for weight loss [27]. However, there is insufficient evidence to confirm the efficacy of bitter orange as an anti-obesity agent, especially given its inclusion in combination products [27].

Interactions with bitter orange are varied. Synephrine, like ephedrine, is known to cause adverse cardiovascular effects at high doses, the risk of which are heightened when combination products also including caffeine are ingested and therefore patients taking cardiac medications should be cautioned on its use [135, 136]. Some evidence demonstrates that bitter orange can inhibit cytochrome P450 3A4, although to a lesser extent than with grapefruit [137-140]. A 76% increase in AUC was observed following administration of 10 mg extended release felodipine administered with 240 mL Seville orange juice compared to control [139]; while a significant increase in indinavir t_{max} was observed with administration of 8 ounces of Seville orange juice compared to control [140]. Because synephrine and octopamine, both endogenous substances, can interact with monoamine oxidase there is a theoretical interaction of bitter orange with MAOIs [141, 142].

3.3. Caffeine-containing herbs

Caffeine is a methylxanthine that is commonly found in food, beverages, and dietary supplements. It is used as an additive in beverages and dietary supplements for its energy enhancing properties. Many dietary supplements marketed for weight loss contain high levels of caffeine, often from multiple sources, for increased thermogenesis and lipid metabolism [143, 144]. Most studies investigating the anti-obesity effects of caffeine have been done using combination products that include ephedra, or have looked at enhancement of athletic endurance [145-151]. Therefore, it is difficult to assess the effect of caffeine alone on weight loss. One study demonstrated an increase in thermogenic metabolic rate in subjects drinking coffee along with food, compared to ingestion of decaffeinated coffee [144].

Adverse effects associated with caffeine consumption include restlessness, jitteriness, anxiety, insomnia, and cardiovascular effects [152-156]. Most drug and herb interactions with caffeine are mild to moderate and are related to increased adverse effects resulting from decreased caffeine elimination or additive effects with other methylxanthine containing products [157]. For example, estrogen drugs (e.g. oral contraceptives and estrogen replacement therapy) have been shown to decrease clearance of caffeine up to 50 – 65% [158, 159]. The most significant caffeine interaction occurs with coadministration of *Ephedra* or ephedrine containing products (see *Ephedra* below). The ban on ephedra in the United States has resulted in marketing of "ephedra-free" dietary supplements using ephedra alternatives, including caffeine containing herbs and bitter orange (see *Bitter Orange* above). In one randomized controlled trial study, subjects were administered products containing *Citrus aurantium* standardized to either a high dose of synephrine (46.9 mg) or a product containing caffeine and a low synephrine dose (5.5 mg) [136]. A significant increase on blood pressure was observed in patients taking the product containing both caffeine and synephrine, but not high dose synephrine alone, suggesting an interaction between the two herbs.

3.3.1. Green tea (Camellia sinensis; EGCG)

Green tea has gained in popularity for the treatment of a wide variety of diseases and for promotion of general wellbeing. The addition of green tea to weight loss supplements is due in part to the caffeine content of *Camellia sinensis*. However, in addition to alkaloid content (caffeine, theobromine, theophylline) green tea also contains polyphenols, most notably the catechin epigallocatechin-3-gallate (EGCG) [160-164]. EGCG, in concert with caffeine, is proposed to elicit anti-obesity effects via inhibition of catechol O-methyl transferase and phosphodiesterase [164]. A meta-analysis of clinical trials involving green tea in weight loss concluded that weight loss is decreased, relative to placebo, in treatment involving both green tea ECGC and caffeine but not with decaffeinated green tea products [165].

As expected, the majority of drug interactions associated with green tea are related to caffeine content. However, a few interactions described in the literature are due to other constituents of green tea. Green tea may be contraindicated, especially at high doses, in patients taking anticoagulants such as warfarin due to the high Vitamin K content of the herb. There is one case report of a patient taking warfarin who experienced a significant reduction in INR following initiation of daily consumption of one-half to one gallon of green tea [166]. Once green tea consumption was stopped INR normalized. Green tea is also thought to cause decreased estrogen levels and combination products containing the herb have been used to improve fertility and relieve menopausal symptoms [167-170]. Therefore, use of high doses of green tea in patients taking oral contraceptives or estrogen replacement therapy may be cautioned.

3.3.2. Guarana (Paullinia cupana)

Guarana (*Paullinia cupana*) is a plant native to South America that is used traditionally and in anti-obesity supplements for its high caffeine content, although other minor constituents including theophylline, theobromine, catechin and epicatechin are found in these extracts [171-176]. There are no studies investigating the effects of Guarana alone on weight loss so it is difficult to determine the anti-obesity properties of the herb. In one double-blind, parallel, placebo controlled trial 47 subjects were administered three capsules containing yerba mate (*Ilex paraguayensis,* 112 mg), guarana (95 mg) and damiana (*Turnera diffusa,* 36 mg) daily for 45 days, resulting in significant weight loss (-5.1 ± 0.5 kg) compared to placebo (-0.3 ± 0.08 kg) [145]. One of the few interactions reported with guarana not related to caffeine content suggests possible interference with anticoagulants since platelet aggregation was observed *in vitro* and in animal studies [177].

3.4. Dandelion (*Taraxacum officinale*)

Dandelion is a perennial herb of multiple global varieties that has traditionally been used for liver, spleen, kidney, and gastrointestinal disorders, although there have been no clinical trials investigating the effects of dandelion in weight loss [27, 178]. It is commonly added to weight loss supplements, mainly for its diuretic properties, although the herb does possess some mild laxative properties [179-181]. There are no known drugs interactions between *Taraxacum* and other herbs or drugs, although one study in rats suggests a probable interaction with quinolone antibiotics due to the high mineral content of *Taraxacum* [182]. In the study, ciprofloxacin (20 mg/kg) C_{max} significantly decreased while V_d and $t_{½}$ significantly increased when administered with crude dandelion extract (2 g/kg) compared to control. There is one case report of hypoglycemia in a 58 year old diabetic patient following a 2-week period of dandelion consumption in salads [183].

The patient denied changes in calorie consumption, exercise, or insulin dosing. Diabetic patients taking hypoglycemic agents while consuming dandelion should be monitored.

3.5. Ephedra (*Ephedra sinica*, ma huang)

Ephedra, derived from the evergreen shrub *Ephedra sinica*, contains multiple plant alkaloids including ephedrine and pseudoephedrine that are chemically related to amphetamines. These compounds act by increasing availability and activity of endogenous neurotransmitters such as epinephrine and norepinephrine, resulting in brain and cardiovascular catecholamine receptor stimulation [184]. The herb has traditionally been used for bronchodilation in the treatment of respiratory ailments such as asthma, as an athletic performance enhancer, and for its thermogenic properties in weight loss [148, 185-189]. Ephedra as a weight loss dietary supplement is commonly found in combination products also containing caffeine or caffeine-containing herbs. In one study a product containing 90 mg and 192 mg of ephedra alkaloids and caffeine, respectively, administered daily over six months in a randomized, double-blind placebo controlled trial resulted in significant decreases in body weight, body fat and LDL-cholesterol with an increase in HDL-cholesterol [148]. The addition of aspirin to ephedrine containing products can potentiate the thermogenic properties of ephedra, improving weight loss compared to products containing ephedra alone [190-201]. Due to high risk of cardiovascular toxicities and cardiomyopathies, ephedra has been banned in the United States [202-211]. However, the herb is still available in other countries [212].

Because of the controversial nature of ephedra related to cardiac toxicity and its eventual ban via the U.S. FDA, there are a significant number of clinical studies and case reports related to toxicities and interactions with ephedra and ephedrine. Ephedra can potentially interact with anesthetics since it is known that administration of ephedrine can reverse anesthesia induced hypotension and regression of analgesia following epidural blockade [213, 214]. Ephedrine has both chrontropic and inotropic effects, and therefore interactions with cardiovascular agents may be possible [184, 211, 215, 216]. However, no effects on heart rate or blood pressure were seen in clinical trials investigating the efficacy of ephedra in weight loss [192, 217, 218]. Theoretically interactions with antiadrenergic agents and MAOIs can occur due to sympathomimetic effects of ephedrine, potentially increasing risk of hypertensive crisis. There is a case report of a patient taking a product containing caffeine, ephedrine, and theophylline who experienced multiple adverse effects including encephalopathy, hypotension, tachycardia, and hypothermia 24 hours following discontinuation of phenelzine [219]. Interactions with ephedrine and tricyclic antidepressants are also possible [220]. Some evidence from clinical trials suggests that ephedra in combination with caffeine can cause hyperglycemia, and therefore interactions with antidiabetic agents is possible [147, 148, 221]. A lowering of seizure threshold has been observed in patients taking ephedrine, and therefore use of ephedra in this patient population is cautioned [222]. A major interaction between ephedra and methylxanthines (e.g. caffeine, theophylline) is possible due to increased risk of cardiovascular, neurologic and psychiatric adverse effects due to additive sympathomimetic and CNS stimulant activity [184, 223, 224]. One case study reports a 21 year old male patient admitted to the hospital emergency room with a blood pressure of 220/110 mmHg and ventricular arrhythmia following ingestion of a caffeine/ephedra containing product ("Herbal Ecstasy") [225].

3.6. Glucomannan (*Amorphophallus konjac*)

Glucomannan is a soluble but highly viscous dietary fiber derived from the root of the *Amorphophallus konjac* (elephant yam) plant that grows native to Asia [27]. Although traditionally used as a food, the plant has gained popularity as an additive in weight loss supplements since the dietary fiber absorbs water in the gastrointestinal tract, helping to promote a sense of satiety and act as a bulk laxative [226-228]. There is also evidence that fiber content of glucomannan helps to reduce cholesterol levels [67, 229-232]. In a double blind crossover study involving 63 healthy males, 3.9 grams of glucomannan administered daily for four weeks resulted in a 10% reduction in total cholesterol, 7.2% reduction in LDL cholesterol, and a 23% decrease in triglyceride levels [67]. A meta-analysis of clinical trials involving glucomannan reported overall decreases in the above markers as well as fasting blood glucose [230].

There are relatively few reported drug interactions with glucomannan, most of which are likely due to associated decreases in cholesterol and lipid levels as well as interference with absorption of some drugs. Monitoring of patients taking antihypertensives, antilipemics, and other anti-obesity agents is warranted. Several studies note a significant decrease in fasting blood glucose levels following glucomannan administration while decreased absorption of the sulfonylurea drugs is possible [230, 231, 233-237]. Glucomannan can significantly decrease circulating levels of T3, T4, and FT3 in the treatment of thyrotoxicosis and therefore its use may be contraindicated in patients taking thyroid medications [238]. Glucomannan can potentially affect the absorption of certain drugs and supplements as demonstrated in one study in which absorption of the fat soluble Vitamin E was decreased potentially via the reduction of bile acids necessary for absorption of the vitamin [239].

3.7. *Hoodia gordonii*

Hoodia gordonii, a small succulent of the Apocynaceae family native to the Kalahari Desert, has been used traditionally by native tribes for its appetite and thirst suppressing properties [240, 241]. The active constituent of Hoodia (P57 or P57AS3) is an oxypregnane steroidal glycoside which is purported to increase ATP production in the hypothalamus, resulting in a feeling of satiety [242]. There is little known regarding potential drug or herb interactions with *Hoodia*, although *in vitro* studies suggest a potential interaction with drugs metabolized by CYP 3A4 [243].

3.8. Hydroxycitric acid (HCA, *Garcinia cambogia*)

Garcinia cambogia is a plant native to Southeast Asia which yields a small purple fruit used in weight loss products for its hydroxycitric acid (HCA) content [27, 244]. The anorectic activity of HCA is due to the inhibition of the adenosine triphosphate-citrate (pro-3S)-lyase, which catalyzes the formation of acetyl-CoA, resulting in decreased fatty acid synthesis and lipogenesis [245]. The evidence for HCA as an effective weight loss agent is contradictory. One randomized controlled trial reported a 5-6% reduction in weight and BMI following approximately a 4.5 gram daily dose of HCA, while two other studies reported no significant weight loss or effect on appetite at lower doses of 1.5 – 2.4 gram daily HCA doses [246-248]. There are a minimal number of reported interactions with *Garcinia* or HCA. Antilipemic agents such as HMG-CoA reductase inhibitors should be avoided due to an increased risk of rhabdomyolysis. In one case report a healthy 54 year old female patient reported chest pain following ingestion of an herbal product containing ephedra, guarana, chitosan, *Gymnena sylvestre, Garcinia cambogia* (50% HCA), and chromium. Lab results indicated elevated serum creatine kinase (1028 IU/mL), which declined following cessation of the supplement [249]. Although the exact interaction was not determined, cautionary use of HCA-containing products in patients at risk of rhabdomyolysis is warranted.

3.9. Herbal laxatives

Frequently laxatives and diuretics are used alone or in combination products to promote weight loss. However, there is little to no evidence supporting these supplements as anti-obesity agents, although subgroups of this patient population may abuse laxatives and diuretics for the purpose of weight loss [250].

3.9.1. Bulk laxatives

Bulk laxatives generally consist of soluble dietary fiber which expands in the gastrointestinal tract in the presence of water resulting in improved bowel function. Common sources of bulk laxatives include *Amorphophallus konjac* (glucomannan, *see above*), guar gum (*Cyamopsis tetragonoloba*), and psyllium husk (*Plantago psyllium*). Although the efficacy of bulk laxatives for weight loss is not proven, adsorption of dietary glucose and lipids to these agents in the gastrointestinal tract results in decreased absorption of lipids, cholesterol, and carbohydrates into the body, thereby promoting weight loss [230, 234, 251-253]. Because of changes in carbohydrate and glucose absorption, dosing of antidiabetic agents may require modification and therefore patients in this population should be monitored when taking bulk laxatives [254-261]. Bulk laxatives appear to have some effect on the absorption of orally administered medications, which can result in changes in drug plasma levels [262-272]. For example, in one study the effect of guar gum on digoxin and phenoxymethyl penicillin absorption was studied in 10 healthy volunteers, with significant reductions in both peak penicillin plasma concentrations and AUC, but little effect on overall digoxin levels [269]. In one case report of a patient with adrenal insufficiency treated with fludrocortisone and prednisolone, the patient experienced symptoms of acute adrenal crisis including fatigue, nausea, abdominal pain, and weakness approximately 3 – 4 days after initiation of psyllium [262]. The authors postulated that psyllium inhibited absorption of fludrocortisone and/or prednisolone. Other evidence related to changes in absorption of ethinyl estradiol, metformin, and lithium have also been reported [264-266, 270, 272].

3.9.2. Stimulant laxatives

Stimulant laxatives act by irritating the lining of the gastrointestinal tract, resulting in increased propulsive muscle contractions that aid elimination of intestinal contents. Because of the quick and efficacious activity, stimulant laxatives are most frequently abused to promote weight loss by increasing gastrointestinal transit time [273, 274]. The most common stimulant laxative herbs are senna (*Cassia senna*), aloe latex (*Aloe vera*), and Cascara sagrada (*Frangula purshiana*). The leaves and pods from *Cassia senna* contain anthroquinone stimulant laxative compounds effective in the treatment of constipation and for bowel evacuation prior to medical procedures [27, 275-295]. The herb has been approved by the U.S. FDA as a non-prescription medication. Similarly, aloe latex, derived from the peripheral bundle sheath cells of the aloe leaf, contains anthracene compounds that are cleaved in the colon by bacterial enzymes into active anthrone compounds with stimulant laxative properties [296-299]. However, concerns over possible carcinogenic properties of certain anthraquinones in aloe latex, along with lack of safety evidence, prompted the U.S. FDA to ban aloe latex in 2002, although the herb is still used in other countries [178, 300, 301]. The bark of the deciduous buckthorn shrub Cascara sagrada is effective for the treatment of constipation due to the stimulant laxative properties of its anthraglycoside constituents [27, 302]. Like aloe latex, Cascara had previously been approved by the U.S. FDA as a non-prescription medication, but the designation was withdrawn into 2002 based on lack of safety and efficacy evidence, although the herb is still available as a supplement [300].

Stimulant laxatives share multiple common adverse effects and potential drug interactions. Because of decreased gastrointestinal transit time, absorption of some drugs, especially those with poor permeability, may be decreased [303, 304]. Experimental evidence in rats suggests absorption of carbohydrates may result in decreased blood glucose levels and therefore monitoring of patients receiving hypoglycemic agents or insulin is warranted [305-307]. Concomitant use of stimulant laxatives with diuretics, cardiac glycosides and licorice is contraindicated due to hypokalemic effects, especially with long term use of these laxatives [27, 178, 304, 308, 309]. Senna can potentially interfere with antiplatelet and anticoagulant activity by causing excessive bleeding [310]. There is one case report of a possible interaction of aloe and sevoflurane, in which a 35 year old female patient undergoing surgery for hemangioma experienced perioperative bleeding [311]. Although the size and vascularization of the hemangioma were noted as partial root causes of the bleeding episodes, the authors felt that the combination of anesthetic and aloe administration (4 tablets daily for 2 weeks prior to surgery) may have contributed to the adverse event.

3.10. Licorice (*Glycyrrhiza glabra*)

Licorice has historically been used both medicinally and as a food product and its relative safety at low doses has placed it on the U.S. FDA GRAS (generally recognized as safe) list, although at high doses licorice can cause severe adverse effects [27]. The main active components of licorice are glycyrrhizin and glycyrrhizic acid, although several other active constituents have been identified [312, 313]. One of the main adverse effects of high licorice consumption includes mineralocorticoid excess syndrome and resulting hypokalemia with associated increases in blood pressure, as well as secondary pseudohyperaldosteronism [314-338]. Licorice consumption may also alter blood glucose levels, potentially via binding to PPAR-γ [339, 340]. Although licorice is used in dietary supplements for weight loss, contradictory evidence reports weight gain with licorice consumption [341-343]. However, one study in which 3.5 grams daily licorice consumption was administered to 15 normal

http://dx.doi.org/10.5772/51145

weight subjects for two months reports a significant decrease in body fat mass but not body mass index [344, 345].

Acquisition of mineralocorticoid excess syndrome following high dose consumption of licorice results in the potential for licorice-drug interactions with multiple drug classes, including aldosterone receptor antagonists, antiarrhythmics, antihypertensives, cardiac glycosides, corticosteroids, diuretics, and potassium lowering agents [321-324, 326]. In one study, 10 healthy subjects were given 32 grams of licorice daily for two weeks along with 25 mg of hydrochlorothiazide (HCTZ); a significant reduction in potassium levels was observed, while two patients experience hypokalemia, compared to HCTZ alone [346]. Glycyrrhizin and β-glycyrrhetinic acid may also affect complement activity and decrease neutrophil generated oxides and peroxides, resulting in anti-inflammatory activity [347-350]. Therefore, licorice should be used with caution in patients taking other anti-inflammatory medications. Licorice constituents may also have an effect on hormonal agents via anti-estrogenic activity, inhibition of 17β-hydroxysteroid dehydrogenase, or associated decreases in prolactin levels [351-358]. In *in vitro* and animal studies it has been shown that constituents in licorice can promote the intestinal absorption of some drugs and therefore it is recommended that oral drugs be taken at least an hour before or two hours after licorice consumption [359]. Theoretically licorice may interact with antidepressant agents, since increases in norepinephrine and dopamine have been observed in mice while *in vitro* cell culture studies suggest potential serotonin reuptake inhibition [360, 361].

3.11. St. John's Wort (*Hypericum perforatum*)

St. John's Wort (SJW) is a perennial herb native to Europe that is commonly used to treat depression, anxiety, post-menopausal symptoms, attention deficit hyperactivity disorder (ADHD), and other mood disorders [362-367]. The active constituents of SJW are hypericin and hyperforin, which are thought to act by inhibiting the synaptic uptake of serotonin (5-HT), GABA, noradrenaline, dopamine, and L-glutamate via a novel mechanism compared to synthetic antidepressants [362, 368-373]. Although there are no official studies regarding the use of SJW for weight loss, anecdotal reports suggest a positive effect on satiety, which may be attributable to the serotonergic uptake inhibition (see *Sibutramine* above). Following the removal of fenfluramine, an anorectic agent commonly used in the combination product "Phen-Fen" (phentermine – fenfluramine), from the market in 1997, SJW was combined with *Ephedra* or *Citrus aurantium* (see above) and marketed for weight loss as "Herbal Phen-Fen". Because of the expanding popularity of SJW in the 1990s – 2000s, a great deal of research on the mechanism of action and herb-drug interactions has been reported.

Drug interactions with SJW are primarily related to binding of active constituents to the pregnane X receptor leading to induction of cytochrome P450 metabolizing or induction of p-glycoprotein efflux mechanisms via the MDR-1 drug transporter [374-388]. As a result, pharmacokinetics of many cytochrome P450 drug substrates is altered, often leading to decreased plasma concentrations and reduced efficacy [27]. There have been numerous studies that have demonstrated potential metabolism-related drug interactions with CYP 3A4, 1A2, 2C9 and 2C19 [389]. Kinetics of antiplatelet and anticoagulant agents may be altered in the presence of SJW [390, 391]. In one open-label, three-way crossover randomized study, 12 healthy male subjects were given 1 gram of SJW (standardized to hypericin 0.825 mg/g and hyperforin 12.5 mg/g) for 21 days, with administration of a single 25 mg dose of warfarin on day 14 [390]. A significant increase in warfarin (Cl/F) was observed compared to warfarin alone, with a corresponding decrease in AUC and half-life. However, there was no significant impact on INR or platelet aggregation. The interaction is likely caused not only by alteration of drug metabolism via CYP 450 induction, but also binding of warfarin to the SJW constituents hypericin and pseudohypericin, leading to decreased absorption of the drug [392]. In another study, patients not responding to clopidogrel therapy alone experienced an increase in therapeutic activity when clopidogrel and SJW were coadministered; therefore it is possible that patients responding to stand alone clopidogrel treatment may be at increased risk of bleeding [391]. There has been one case report of a possible interaction between theophylline and SJW in which theophylline levels significantly increased following discontinuation of SJW in a smoker also taking 11 other drugs [393]. However, another study in healthy subjects showed no impact of SJW on theophylline kinetics [394]. Plasma concentrations of protease inhibitors such as indinavir may be reduced in the presence of SJW due to induction of p-glycoprotein efflux in the gastrointestinal tract [395-398]. Decreased plasma levels of the "statins" simvastatin and atorvastatin have been reported in controlled, randomized, cross-over studies [399, 400]. Reports of pharmacokinetic interactions have also been reported for digoxin, gliclazide, imatinib, irinotecan, methadone, omeprazole, verapamil, and voriconazole have also been published [401-412]. In general, coadministration of SJW with drugs significantly eliminated via these enzymes should be avoided.

Several studies and case reports describe interactions between SJW and oral contraceptives, resulting in breakthrough or irregular bleeding and unplanned pregnancy [413-416]. In one case report, an unwanted pregnancy occurred in a 36-year old patient while taking an ethinyl estradiol/dinogesterol oral contraceptive (Valette®). The patient had previously been taking fluvastatin (20 mg/day) for 2 years, but had discontinued the drug and started 1700 mg SJW extract daily for 3 months prior to conception [414]. One randomized controlled trial in 18 female subjects taking low dose oral contraceptives (0.02 mg ethinyl estradiol / 0.150 mg desogestrel) in combination with 300 mg SJW twice daily reported a significant increase in breakthrough bleeding compared to subjects taking oral contraceptive alone [417]. Progestins and estrogens contained in oral contraceptives are known to be metabolized by various CYP enzymes and therefore induction of these enzymes by SJW results in decreased plasma concentrations and therapeutic failure [417-420].

Interactions between SJW and with drugs used in the prevention of organ transplant rejection such as tacrolimus and cyclosporine have been reported [421-431]. Several transplant patients have experienced transplant rejection potentially related to coadministration of SJW. In one case report a patient treated with 75 mg cyclosporine daily for several years following kidney transplant experienced a drop in cyclosporin plasma levels attributed to SJW administration [427]. Levels returned to normal when SJW was discontinued and dropped upon rechallenge with SJW extract. Similarly, tacrolimus plasma levels markedly decreased in a study involving 10 stabilized renal transplant patients administered 600 mg SJW extract for two weeks,

http://dx.doi.org/10.5772/51145

requiring dosage adjustments during and for up to two weeks following discontinuation of SJW [431].

SJW may interact with selective serotonin reuptake inhibitors (SSRIs), monoamines, and other antidepressant and psychiatric medications due to the serotonin uptake inhibitory properties of hypericin and hyperforin, although metabolic induction plays a role for some drugs [368, 370-373, 432-446]. In one case report, a patient who had been taking paroxetine 40 mg daily for treatment of depression discontinued her medication and began taking SJW 600 mg daily [434]. No adverse events were reported with the switch, but upon coadministration of a 20 mg dose of paroxetine to aid in sleep the patient experience extreme grogginess, weakness, fatigue, and incoherency. The author cited the potential for additive serotonin uptake inhibition resulting in "serotonin syndrome". One case of a male adult patient stabilized on methylphenidate for attention deficit hyperactivity disorder (ADHD) is reported in which the patient experienced increased ADHD symptoms after taking SJW 600 mg daily for four months [438]. The mechanism of the interaction is unknown. Interactions have also been reported for amitriptyline, clozapine, fexofenadine, and sertraline; therefore administration of SJW in patients taking these and similar drugs should be avoided [440, 443, 444, 446, 447].

An interaction between SJW and drugs known to cause phototoxic adverse reactions is also possible, due to the photosensitizing nature of hypericin [448-450]. In one study, 11 subjects were exposed to UVA1 radiation at baseline and following 10 days treatment with 1020 mg (3000 mcg hypericin) extract [449]. Minimum erythemal dose (MED) as measured 8, 24 and 48 hours after exposure to radiation and was found to be significantly lower at 8 and 48, but not 24 hours, after exposure compared to control. There is one case report of a patient experiencing severe phototoxicity upon exposure to laser light (532 nm) and pulsed dye laser light (585 nm), presumably due to ingestion of SJW [451]. SJW may also increase the sensitivity and skin toxicity of radiation treatment in patients undergoing radiation therapy, possibly through photosensitizing effects although the exact underlying mechanism is not known [452].

3.12. Willow bark (*Salix alba*)

Willow bark from the *Salix alba* tree is often contained in weight loss supplements, presumably due to earlier studies that noted enhanced thermogenic properties of ephedra in combination products also including aspirin (see *Ephedra* above). The active constituents of white willow are predominantly the salicylates (acetylsalicylic acid) and, therefore, the bark has traditionally been used in the treatment of pain [27, 453, 454]. The analgesic and anti-inflammatory activity of willow bark is due to inhibition of cyclooxygenase-2 (COX-2) mediated prostaglandin E2 release [455, 456]. Although there are few case reports dealing with willow bark extract specifically, drug and herb interactions seen with other salicylates are possible [455, 457]. Generally, caution should be used in concomitant administration of drugs contraindicated for aspirin, such as beta-blockers, NSAIDs, carbonic anhydrase inhibitors (e.g. acetazolamide), probenecid, alcohol, and salicylates, while the kinetics of protein bound drugs can also be modified [27]. Salicin may also have an effect on platelet aggregation, and therefore interactions with anticoagulants and antiplatelet drugs are possible [458, 459]. In one randomized double-blind study involving 16 patients administered standardized extracts of *Salicis cortex* (240 mg salicin/day), mean arachidonic induced platelet aggregation was reduced (61% compared to 78% in placebo group), but not as significantly as in the acetylsalicylic acid group (13% reduction) [458]. One randomized placebo-controlled trial investigating the efficacy of willow bark extract in osteoarthritis reported an increase in triglyceride levels, suggesting a potential interaction between willow bark and antihyperlipidemics [460]. Some patients in another randomized controlled trial, who were given 240 mg salicin daily for four weeks, suffered blood pressure instability and edema; use of willow bark in patients taking antihypertensives should be cautioned [461].

4. Adulteration of dietary supplements

A final note is necessary regarding the adulteration of weight loss supplements with drug products and other chemical substances. This adulteration is often the underlying cause for the purported activity of a dietary supplement and can result in serious toxicity. The most commonly cited contaminant in weight loss supplements is sibutramine (Meridia®; see above), a weight loss supplement removed from the market in October 2010 for significant cardiac toxicities [462-466]. One U.S. FDA report cites 72 different herbal products containing adulterants, 94.4% of which contained sibutramine as an additive [102]. Multiple products listed in the report were contaminated with phenolphthalein (11.1%) or the anti-seizure drug phenytoin (2.8%). Other reported contaminants (1.4%) included the experimental anti-obesity agent cetilistat, the recalled anti-obesity agent rimonabant (see above), the anti-obesity amphetamine stimulant drug fenproporex, the antidepressant fluoxetine, or the diuretics furosemide and bumetanide[103]. Phenophthalein was previously used as a laxative in over-the-counter products but was removed from the U.S. market in 1999 due to concerns of carcinogenicity and genotoxicity [467]. Another study investigating contamination of 20 different dietary supplements using 1H-NMR methods found contamination of 14 of the products (70%), with eight products containing sibutramine, five containing both sibutramine and phenolphthalein, and one formulation containing undeclared synephrine [468]. There have been other reports of contamination of weight loss supplements with the diuretic hydrochlorothiazide [462, 469]. Given that tainting of weight loss supplements is common, patients and health care professionals should be made aware of the risks associated with ingestion of herbal products, especially those with minimal evidence backing their claims of efficacy.

Author details

Melanie A. Jordan

Midwestern University, College of Pharmacy – Glendale, Glendale, AZ, USA

References

[1] World Health Organization, *Obesity: Facts and Figures*, 2012; Available from: http://www.euro.who.int/en/what-we-do/health-topics/noncommunicable-diseases/obesity/facts-and-figures [accessed 06/20/12].

[2] World Health Organization, *WHO Global Infobase*, 2012; Available from: https://apps.who.int/infobase/Comparisons.aspx [accessed 06/20/12]

[3] Ogden, C.L., et al., *Prevalence of overweight and obesity in the United States, 1999-2004.* JAMA, 2006. 295(13): p. 1549-55.

[4] Flegal, K.M., et al., *Prevalence of obesity and trends in the distribution of body mass index among US adults, 1999-2010.* JAMA, 2012. 307(5): p. 491-7.

[5] James, W.P., *WHO recognition of the global obesity epidemic.* Int J Obes (Lond), 2008. 32 Suppl 7: p. S120-6.

[6] Ogden, C.L., et al., *Prevalence of obesity in the United States, 2009-2010.* NCHS Data Brief, 2012(82): p. 1-8.

[7] Samaranayake, N.R., et al., *Management of obesity in the National Health and Nutrition Examination Survey (NHANES), 2007-2008.* Ann Epidemiol, 2012. 22(5): p. 349-53.

[8] Manton, K.G., *The global impact of noncommunicable diseases: estimates and projections.* World Health Stat Q, 1988. 41(3-4): p. 255-66.

[9] Wang, Y., et al., *Will all Americans become overweight or obese? estimating the progression and cost of the US obesity epidemic.* Obesity (Silver Spring), 2008. 16(10): p. 2323-30.

[10] Wolf, A.M. and G.A. Colditz, *Current estimates of the economic cost of obesity in the United States.* Obes Res, 1998. 6(2): p. 97-106.

[11] *European Charter on Counteracting Obesity*, in *WHO European Ministerial Conference on Counteracting Obesity*. 2006, World Health Organization: Istanbul, Turkey.

[12] U.S. Department of Agriculture, Cente rfor Nutrition Policy and Promotion, 2012. *ChooseMyPlate.gov*; Available from: http://www/ChooseMyPlate.gov [accessed 06/20/12].

[13] J. Steenhuysen, S.H., J. Lentz, L. Richwine, *Factbox: A troubled history for weight-loss drugs*, in *Reuters*. 2011, Thomson Reuters.

[14] Sam, A.H., V. Salem, and M.A. Ghatei, *Rimonabant: From RIO to Ban.* J Obes, 2011. 2011: p. 432607.

[15] U.S. Food and Drug Adminsitration, *FDA Drug Safety Communication: FDA Recommends Against the Continued Use of Meridia (sibutramine)*, 2010: Silver Spring, MD.

[16] Basch, E.M., J.C. Servoss, and U.B. Tedrow, *Safety assurances for dietary supplements policy issues and new research paradigms.* J Herb Pharmacother, 2005. 5(1): p. 3-15.

[17] Harris, I.M., *Regulatory and ethical issues with dietary supplements.* Pharmacotherapy, 2000. 20(11): p. 1295-302.

[18] Jordan, S.A., D.G. Cunningham, and R.J. Marles, *Assessment of herbal medicinal products: challenges, and opportunities to increase the knowledge base for safety assessment.* Toxicol Appl Pharmacol, 2010. 243(2): p. 198-216.

[19] Tsutani, K. and H. Takuma, *[Regulatory sciences in herbal medicines and dietary supplements].* Yakugaku Zasshi, 2008. 128(6): p. 867-80.

[20] Garcia-Mijares, M., A.M. Bernardes, and M.T. Silva, *Diethylpropion produces psychostimulant and reward effects.* Pharmacol Biochem Behav, 2009. 91(4): p. 621-8.

[21] Ollo, C., et al., *Lack of neurotoxic effect of diethylpropion in crack-cocaine abusers.* Clin Neuropharmacol, 1996. 19(1): p. 52-8.

[22] Samanin, R. and S. Garattini, *Neurochemical mechanism of action of anorectic drugs.* Pharmacol Toxicol, 1993. 73(2): p. 63-8.

[23] *Prescribing Information. Tenuate (diethylpropion hydrochloride).* November 2003, Aventis Pharmaceuticals, Inc.: Bridgewater, NJ.

[24] Martin, C.A. and E.T. Iwamoto, *Diethylpropion-induced psychosis reprecipitated by an MAO inhibitor: case report.* J Clin Psychiatry, 1984. 45(3): p. 130-1.

[25] Seedat, Y.K. and J. Reddy, *Diethylpropion hydrochloride (Tenuate Dospan) in combination with hypotensive agents in the treatment of obesity associated with hypertension.* Curr Ther Res Clin Exp, 1974. 16(5): p. 398-413.

[26] Carruba, M.O., et al., *Dopaminergic and serotoninergic anorectics differentially antagonize insulin- and 2-DG-induced hyperphagia.* Life Sci, 1985. 36(18): p. 1739-49.

[27] Jellin, J. et al. (Eds), *Natural Medicines Comprehensive Database.* 1995 - 2012, Therapeutic Research Faculty.

[28] *Suprenza (phentermine hydrochloride) Prescribing Information.* 2011, Akrimax Pharmaceuticals, LLC: Cranford, NJ.

[29] Haddock, C.K., et al., *Pharmacotherapy for obesity: a quantitative analysis of four decades of published randomized clinical trials.* Int J Obes Relat Metab Disord, 2002. 26(2): p. 262-73.

[30] Fleming, R.M. and L.B. Boyd, *The longitudinal effects of fenfluramine-phentermine use.* Angiology, 2007. 58(3): p. 353-9.

[31] Barasch, A. and M.M. Safford, *Diet medications and valvular heart disease: the current evidence.* Spec Care Dentist, 2002. 22(3): p. 108-14.

http://dx.doi.org/10.5772/51145

[32] Stephens, L.C. and S.G. Katz, *Phentermine and anaesthesia.* Anaesth Intensive Care, 2005. 33(4): p. 525-7.

[33] Biton, V., *Clinical pharmacology and mechanism of action of zonisamide.* Clin Neuropharmacol, 2007. 30(4): p. 230-40.

[34] Antel, J. and J. Hebebrand, *Weight-reducing side effects of the antiepileptic agents topiramate and zonisamide.* Handb Exp Pharmacol, 2012(209): p. 433-66.

[35] *Topamax (topiramate) Prescribing Information.* 2009, Janssen Pharmaceuticals, Inc.: Titusville, NJ.

[36] Czuczwar, S.J., *[GABA-ergic system and antiepileptic drugs].* Neurol Neurochir Pol, 2000. 34 Suppl 1: p. 13-20.

[37] White, H.S., et al., *Topiramate modulates GABA-evoked currents in murine cortical neurons by a nonbenzodiazepine mechanism.* Epilepsia, 2000. 41 Suppl 1: p. S17-20.

[38] Eliasson, B., et al., *Weight loss and metabolic effects of topiramate in overweight and obese type 2 diabetic patients: randomized double-blind placebo-controlled trial.* Int J Obes (Lond), 2007. 31(7): p. 1140-7.

[39] Gordon, A. and L.H. Price, *Mood stabilization and weight loss with topiramate.* Am J Psychiatry, 1999. 156(6): p. 968-9.

[40] Littrell, K.H., et al., *Weight loss with topiramate.* Ann Pharmacother, 2001. 35(9): p. 1141-2.

[41] Roy Chengappa, K.N., et al., *Long-term effects of topiramate on bipolar mood instability, weight change and glycemic control: a case-series.* Eur Psychiatry, 2001. 16(3): p. 186-90.

[42] Shapira, N.A., T.D. Goldsmith, and S.L. McElroy, *Treatment of binge-eating disorder with topiramate: a clinical case series.* J Clin Psychiatry, 2000. 61(5): p. 368-72.

[43] Allison, D.B., et al., *Controlled-release phentermine/topiramate in severely obese adults: a randomized controlled trial (EQUIP).* Obesity (Silver Spring), 2012. 20(2): p. 330-42.

[44] Bays, H.E. and K.M. Gadde, *Phentermine/topiramate for weight reduction and treatment of adverse metabolic consequences in obesity.* Drugs Today (Barc), 2011. 47(12): p. 903-14.

[45] Powell, A.G., C.M. Apovian, and L.J. Aronne, *The combination of phentermine and topiramate is an effective adjunct to diet and lifestyle modification for weight loss and measures of comorbidity in overweight or obese adults with additional metabolic risk factors.* Evid Based Med, 2012. 17(1): p. 14-5.

[46] Shah, K. and D.T. Villareal, *Combination treatment to CONQUER obesity?* Lancet, 2011. 377(9774): p. 1295-7.

[47] Mack, C.J., et al., *Interaction of topiramate with carbamazepine: two case reports and a review of clinical experience.* Seizure, 2002. 11(7): p. 464-7.

[48] Cano-Zuleta, A., et al., *Report of three cases of hyperammonaemic encephalopathy associated with valproic acid due to possible synergism with phenobarbital and topiramate.* Farm Hosp, 2012.

[49] Deutsch, S.I., J.A. Burket, and R.B. Rosse, *Valproate-induced hyperammonemic encephalopathy and normal liver functions: possible synergism with topiramate.* Clin Neuropharmacol, 2009. 32(6): p. 350-2.

[50] Gomez-Ibanez, A., E. Urrestarazu-Bolumburu, and C. Viteri-Torres, *Hyperammonemic encephalopathy related to valproate, phenobarbital, and topiramate synergism.* Epilepsy Behav, 2011. 21(4): p. 480-2.

[51] *Metabolic acidosis due to topiramate.* Prescrire Int, 2004. 13(73): p. 186.

[52] Burmeister, J.E., et al., *Topiramate and severe metabolic acidosis: case report.* Arq Neuropsiquiatr, 2005. 63(2B): p. 532-4.

[53] Fernandez-de Orueta, L., et al., *Topiramate-induced metabolic acidosis: a case study.* Nefrologia, 2012. 32(3): p. 403-404.

[54] Ko, C.H. and C.K. Kong, *Topiramate-induced metabolic acidosis: report of two cases.* Dev Med Child Neurol, 2001. 43(10): p. 701-4.

[55] Ozer, Y. and H. Altunkaya, *Topiramate induced metabolic acidosis.* Anaesthesia, 2004. 59(8): p. 830.

[56] Vivius, I., *VI-0521 (Qnexa) Advisory Committee Briefing Document*, E.a.M.D.A. Committee, Editor. 2012, Vivius, Inc.: Mountain View, CA. p. 1 - 166.

[57] Leppik, I.E., *Zonisamide: chemistry, mechanism of action, and pharmacokinetics.* Seizure, 2004. 13 Suppl 1: p. S5-9; discussion S10.

[58] Czapinski, P., B. Blaszczyk, and S.J. Czuczwar, *Mechanisms of action of antiepileptic drugs.* Curr Top Med Chem, 2005. 5(1): p. 3-14.

[59] Suzuki, S., et al., *Zonisamide blocks T-type calcium channel in cultured neurons of rat cerebral cortex.* Epilepsy Res, 1992. 12(1): p. 21-7.

[60] Okada, M., et al., *Effects of zonisamide on dopaminergic system.* Epilepsy Res, 1995. 22(3): p. 193-205.

[61] Okada, M., et al., *Biphasic effects of zonisamide on serotonergic system in rat hippocampus.* Epilepsy Res, 1999. 34(2-3): p. 187-97.

[62] Gadde, K.M., et al., *Zonisamide for weight loss in obese adults: a randomized controlled trial.* JAMA, 2003. 289(14): p. 1820-5.

[63] Ojemann, L.M., et al., *Comparative pharmacokinetics of zonisamide (CI-912) in epileptic patients on carbamazepine or phenytoin monotherapy.* Ther Drug Monit, 1986. 8(3): p. 293-6.

[64] Orito, K., et al., *Pharmacokinetics of zonisamide and drug interaction with phenobarbital in dogs.* J Vet Pharmacol Ther, 2008. 31(3): p. 259-64.

[65] Shinoda, M., et al., *The necessity of adjusting the dosage of zonisamide when coadministered with other anti-epileptic drugs.* Biol Pharm Bull, 1996. 19(8): p. 1090-2.

[66] *Zonegran (zonisamide) Package Insert.* 2006, Eisai Inc.: Teaneck, NJ.

[67] Arvill, A. and L. Bodin, *Effect of short-term ingestion of konjac glucomannan on serum cholesterol in healthy men.* Am J Clin Nutr, 1995. 61(3): p. 585-9.

[68] Nagatomo, I., et al., *Alcohol intake decreases brain Zonisamide concentration in inbred EL mice.* Neuroreport, 1997. 8(2): p. 391-4.

[69] *Xenical Prescribing Information.* 2012, Genentech USA, Inc.: South San Francisco, CA.

[70] Drent, M.L. and E.A. van der Veen, *Lipase inhibition: a novel concept in the treatment of obesity.* Int J Obes Relat Metab Disord, 1993. 17(4): p. 241-4.

[71] Li, Z., et al., *Meta-analysis: pharmacologic treatment of obesity.* Ann Intern Med, 2005. 142(7): p. 532-46.

[72] Davidson, M.H., et al., *Weight control and risk factor reduction in obese subjects treated for 2 years with orlistat: a randomized controlled trial.* JAMA, 1999. 281(3): p. 235-42.

[73] Torgerson, J.S., et al., *XENical in the prevention of diabetes in obese subjects (XENDOS) study: a randomized study of orlistat as an adjunct to lifestyle changes for the prevention of type 2 diabetes in obese patients.* Diabetes Care, 2004. 27(1): p. 155-61.

[74] Colman, E. and M. Fossler, *Reduction in blood cyclosporine concentrations by orlistat.* N Engl J Med, 2000. 342(15): p. 1141-2.

[75] Errasti, P., et al., *Reduction in blood cyclosporine concentration by orlistat in two renal transplant patients.* Transplant Proc, 2002. 34(1): p. 137-9.

[76] Evans, S., et al., *Drug interaction in a renal transplant patient: cyclosporin-Neoral and orlistat.* Am J Kidney Dis, 2003. 41(2): p. 493-6.

[77] Le Beller, C., et al., *Co-administration of orlistat and cyclosporine in a heart transplant recipient.* Transplantation, 2000. 70(10): p. 1541-2.

[78] Nagele, H., et al., *Effect of orlistat on blood cyclosporin concentration in an obese heart transplant patient.* Eur J Clin Pharmacol, 1999. 55(9): p. 667-9.

[79] Schnetzler, B., et al., *Orlistat decreases the plasma level of cyclosporine and may be responsible for the development of acute rejection episodes.* Transplantation, 2000. 70(10): p. 1540-1.

[80] Barbaro, D., et al., *Obesity in transplant patients: case report showing interference of orlistat with absorption of cyclosporine and review of literature.* Endocr Pract, 2002. 8(2): p. 124-6.

[81] McDuffie, J.R., et al., *Effects of orlistat on fat-soluble vitamins in obese adolescents.* Pharmacotherapy, 2002. 22(7): p. 814-22.

[82] Melia, A.T., S.G. Koss-Twardy, and J. Zhi, *The effect of orlistat, an inhibitor of dietary fat absorption, on the absorption of vitamins A and E in healthy volunteers.* J Clin Pharmacol, 1996. 36(7): p. 647-53.

[83] Zhi, J., et al., *The effect of orlistat, an inhibitor of dietary fat absorption, on the pharmacokinetics of beta-carotene in healthy volunteers.* J Clin Pharmacol, 1996. 36(2): p. 152-9.

[84] Bigham, S., C. McGuigan, and B.K. MacDonald, *Reduced absorption of lipophilic anti-epileptic medications when used concomitantly with the anti-obesity drug orlistat.* Epilepsia, 2006. 47(12): p. 2207.

[85] Madhava, K. and A. Hartley, *Hypothyroidism in thyroid carcinoma follow-up: orlistat may inhibit the absorption of thyroxine.* Clin Oncol (R Coll Radiol), 2005. 17(6): p. 492.

[86] Zhi, J., et al., *The effect of orlistat on the pharmacokinetics and pharmacodynamics of warfarin in healthy volunteers.* J Clin Pharmacol, 1996. 36(7): p. 659-66.

[87] Xie, S., et al., *The endocannabinoid system and rimonabant: a new drug with a novel mechanism of action involving cannabinoid CB1 receptor antagonism--or inverse agonism--as potential obesity treatment and other therapeutic use.* J Clin Pharm Ther, 2007. 32(3): p. 209-31.

[88] Banerji, M.A. and M. Tiewala, *Rimonabant--the RIO North America trial: a new strategy to sustaining weight loss and related morbidity.* Curr Diab Rep, 2006. 6(3): p. 228-9.

[89] Kintscher, U., *The cardiometabolic drug rimonabant: after 2 years of RIO-Europe and STRADIVARIUS.* Eur Heart J, 2008. 29(14): p. 1709-10.

[90] Nissen, S.E., et al., *Effect of rimonabant on progression of atherosclerosis in patients with abdominal obesity and coronary artery disease: the STRADIVARIUS randomized controlled trial.* JAMA, 2008. 299(13): p. 1547-60.

[91] Pan, C., H.J. Yoo, and L.T. Ho, *Perspectives of CB1 Antagonist in Treatment of Obesity: Experience of RIO-Asia.* J Obes, 2011. 2011: p. 957268.

[92] Pi-Sunyer, F.X., et al., *Effect of rimonabant, a cannabinoid-1 receptor blocker, on weight and cardiometabolic risk factors in overweight or obese patients: RIO-North America: a randomized controlled trial.* JAMA, 2006. 295(7): p. 761-75.

[93] Scheen, A.J., *CB1 receptor blockade and its impact on cardiometabolic risk factors: overview of the RIO programme with rimonabant.* J Neuroendocrinol, 2008. 20 Suppl 1: p. 139-46.

[94] Topol, E.J., et al., *Rimonabant for prevention of cardiovascular events (CRESCENDO): a randomised, multicentre, placebo-controlled trial.* Lancet, 2010. 376(9740): p. 517-23.

[95] Van Gaal, L.F., et al., *Long-term effect of CB1 blockade with rimonabant on cardiometabolic risk factors: two year results from the RIO-Europe Study.* Eur Heart J, 2008. 29(14): p. 1761-71.

[96] Despres, J.P., A. Golay, and L. Sjostrom, *Effects of rimonabant on metabolic risk factors in overweight patients with dyslipidemia.* N Engl J Med, 2005. 353(20): p. 2121-34.

[97] Rasmussen, E.B., et al., *Rimonabant reduces the essential value of food in the genetically obese Zucker rat: an exponential demand analysis.* Physiol Behav, 2012. 105(3): p. 734-41.

[98] Verty, A.N., et al., *Anti-obesity effects of the combined administration of CB1 receptor antagonist rimonabant and melanin-concentrating hormone antagonist SNAP-94847 in diet-inudced obese mice.* Int J Obes (Lond), 2012.

[99] Zaitone, S.A. and S. Essawy, *Addition of a low dose of rimonabant to orlistat therapy decreases weight gain and reduces adiposity in dietary obese rats.* Clin Exp Pharmacol Physiol, 2012. 39(6): p. 551-9.

[100] Taj Pharmaceuticals Limited, *Indian Pharmaceuticals Company Taj Pharmaceuticals receives FDA Approval for Generic Rimonabant.* 2010; Available from: http://www.tajpharma.com/media/media_r/Indian%20Pharmaceuticals%20Company%20Taj %20Pharmaceuticals%20receives%20FDA%20approval%20for%20Generic%20Rimonabant.pdf [accessed 06/20/12].

[101] Venhuis, B.J., et al., *The identification of rimonabant polymorphs, sibutramine and analogues of both in counterfeit Acomplia bought on the internet.* J Pharm Biomed Anal, 2011. 54(1): p. 21-6.

[102] U.S. Food and Drug Adminsitration, Department of Health and Human Services, *Questions and Answers about FDA's Initiative Against Contaminated Weight Loss Products*, 2008: Silver Spring, MD.

[103] U.S. Food and Drug Adminsitration, Department of Health and Human Services, *FDA Uncovers Additional Tainted Weight Loss Products: Agency Alerts Consumers to the Finding of New Undeclared Drug Ingredients.*, 2009: Rockville, MD.

[104] European Medicines Agency (EMEA), *Acomplia: EPAR - Product Information*, 2009.

[105] Mandhane, S., et al., *Induction of Glucose Intolerance by Acute Administration of Rimonabant.* Pharmacology, 2012. 89(5-6): p. 339-347.

[106] *Meridia (sibutramine hydrocholoride) Package Insert.* 2010, Abbott Laboratories: North Chicago, IL.

[107] Heal, D.J., et al., *Sibutramine: a novel anti-obesity drug. A review of the pharmacological evidence to differentiate it from d-amphetamine and d-fenfluramine.* Int J Obes Relat Metab Disord, 1998. 22 Suppl 1: p. S18-28; discussion S29.

[108] Liu, Y.L., D.J. Heal, and M.J. Stock, *Mechanism of the thermogenic effect of Metabolite 2 (BTS 54 505), a major pharmacologically active metabolite of the novel anti-obesity drug, sibutramine.* Int J Obes Relat Metab Disord, 2002. 26(9): p. 1245-53.

[109] McNeely, W. and K.L. Goa, *Sibutramine. A review of its contribution to the management of obesity.* Drugs, 1998. 56(6): p. 1093-124.

[110] Nisoli, E. and M.O. Carruba, *An assessment of the safety and efficacy of sibutramine, an anti-obesity drug with a novel mechanism of action.* Obes Rev, 2000. 1(2): p. 127-39.

[111] Bailey, D.G. and G.K. Dresser, *Interactions between grapefruit juice and cardiovascular drugs.* Am J Cardiovasc Drugs, 2004. 4(5): p. 281-97.

[112] Greenway, F.L. and M.K. Caruso, *Safety of obesity drugs.* Expert Opin Drug Saf, 2005. 4(6): p. 1083-95.

[113] Wellman, P.J., S.L. Jones, and D.K. Miller, *Effects of preexposure to dexfenfluramine, phentermine, dexfenfluramine-phentermine, or fluoxetine on sibutramine-induced hypophagia in the adult rat.* Pharmacol Biochem Behav, 2003. 75(1): p. 103-14.

[114] Yalcin, A.A., et al., *Elevation of QT dispersion after obesity drug sibutramine.* J Cardiovasc Med (Hagerstown), 2010. 11(11): p. 832-5.

[115] Caterson, I.D., et al., *Maintained intentional weight loss reduces cardiovascular outcomes: results from the Sibutramine Cardiovascular OUTcomes (SCOUT) trial.* Diabetes Obes Metab, 2012. 14(6): p. 523-30.

[116] Coutinho, W.F., *The obese older female patient: CV risk and the SCOUT study.* Int J Obes (Lond), 2007. 31 Suppl 2: p. S26-30; discussion S31-2.

[117] Maggioni, A.P., *SCOUT trial reports on the safety profile of sibutramine in patients with cardiovascular diseases.* Phys Sportsmed, 2009. 37(3): p. 95-7.

[118] Torp-Pedersen, C., et al., *Cardiovascular responses to weight management and sibutramine in high-risk subjects: an analysis from the SCOUT trial.* Eur Heart J, 2007. 28(23): p. 2915-23.

[119] Benazzi, F., *Organic hypomania secondary to sibutramine-citalopram interaction.* J Clin Psychiatry, 2002. 63(2): p. 165.

[120] Clerbaux, G., E. Goffin, and Y. Pirson, *Interaction between sibutramine and cyclosporine.* Am J Transplant, 2003. 3(7): p. 906.

[121] Jordan, J. and A.M. Sharma, *Potential for sibutramine-yohimbine interaction?* Lancet, 2003. 361(9371): p. 1826.

[122] Chin, Y.W., et al., *Lignans and other constituents of the fruits of Euterpe oleracea (Acai) with antioxidant and cytoprotective activities.* J Agric Food Chem, 2008. 56(17): p. 7759-64.

[123] Jensen, G.S., et al., *In vitro and in vivo antioxidant and anti-inflammatory capacities of an antioxidant-rich fruit and berry juice blend. Results of a pilot and randomized, double-blinded, placebo-controlled, crossover study.* J Agric Food Chem, 2008. 56(18): p. 8326-33.

[124] Lichtenthaler, R., et al., *Total oxidant scavenging capacities of Euterpe oleracea Mart. (Acai) fruits.* Int J Food Sci Nutr, 2005. 56(1): p. 53-64.

[125] Mertens-Talcott, S.U., et al., *Pharmacokinetics of anthocyanins and antioxidant effects after the consumption of anthocyanin-rich acai juice and pulp (Euterpe oleracea Mart.) in human healthy volunteers.* J Agric Food Chem, 2008. 56(17): p. 7796-802.

[126] Xie, C., et al., *Acai juice attenuates atherosclerosis in ApoE deficient mice through antioxidant and anti-inflammatory activities.* Atherosclerosis, 2011. 216(2): p. 327-33.

[127] Udani, J.K., et al., *Effects of Acai (Euterpe oleracea Mart.) berry preparation on metabolic parameters in a healthy overweight population: a pilot study.* Nutr J, 2011. 10: p. 45.

[128] Allison, D.B., et al., *Exactly which synephrine alkaloids does Citrus aurantium (bitter orange) contain?* Int J Obes (Lond), 2005. 29(4): p. 443-6.

[129] Dandekar, D.V., G.K. Jayaprakasha, and B.S. Patil, *Simultaneous extraction of bioactive limonoid aglycones and glucoside from Citrus aurantium L. using hydrotropy.* Z Naturforsch C, 2008. 63(3-4): p. 176-80.

[130] Haaz, S., et al., *Citrus aurantium and synephrine alkaloids in the treatment of overweight and obesity: an update.* Obes Rev, 2006. 7(1): p. 79-88.

[131] Liu, L., et al., *Naringenin and hesperetin, two flavonoids derived from Citrus aurantium up-regulate transcription of adiponectin.* Phytother Res, 2008. 22(10): p. 1400-3.

[132] Nelson, B.C., et al., *Mass spectrometric determination of the predominant adrenergic protoalkaloids in bitter orange (Citrus aurantium).* J Agric Food Chem, 2007. 55(24): p. 9769-75.

[133] Pellati, F., et al., *Determination of adrenergic agonists from extracts and herbal products of Citrus aurantium L. var. amara by LC.* J Pharm Biomed Anal, 2002. 29(6): p. 1113-9.

[134] Penzak, S.R., et al., *Seville (sour) orange juice: synephrine content and cardiovascular effects in normotensive adults.* J Clin Pharmacol, 2001. 41(10): p. 1059-63.

[135] Bui, L.T., D.T. Nguyen, and P.J. Ambrose, *Blood pressure and heart rate effects following a single dose of bitter orange.* Ann Pharmacother, 2006. 40(1): p. 53-7.

[136] Haller, C.A., N.L. Benowitz, and P. Jacob, 3rd, *Hemodynamic effects of ephedra-free weight-loss supplements in humans.* Am J Med, 2005. 118(9): p. 998-1003.

[137] Di Marco, M.P., et al., *The effect of grapefruit juice and seville orange juice on the pharmacokinetics of dextromethorphan: the role of gut CYP3A and P-glycoprotein.* Life Sci, 2002. 71(10): p. 1149-60.

[138] Edwards, D.J., et al., *6',7'-Dihydroxybergamottin in grapefruit juice and Seville orange juice: effects on cyclosporine disposition, enterocyte CYP3A4, and P-glycoprotein.* Clin Pharmacol Ther, 1999. 65(3): p. 237-44.

[139] Malhotra, S., et al., *Seville orange juice-felodipine interaction: comparison with dilute grapefruit juice and involvement of furocoumarins.* Clin Pharmacol Ther, 2001. 69(1): p. 14-23.

[140] Penzak, S.R., et al., *Effect of Seville orange juice and grapefruit juice on indinavir pharmacokinetics.* J Clin Pharmacol, 2002. 42(10): p. 1165-70.

[141] Suzuki, O., et al., *Oxidation of synephrine by type A and type B monoamine oxidase.* Experientia, 1979. 35(10): p. 1283-4.

[142] Visentin, V., et al., *Dual action of octopamine on glucose transport into adipocytes: inhibition via beta3-adrenoceptor activation and stimulation via oxidation by amine oxidases.* J Pharmacol Exp Ther, 2001. 299(1): p. 96-104.

[143] Acheson, K.J., et al., *Metabolic effects of caffeine in humans: lipid oxidation or futile cycling?* Am J Clin Nutr, 2004. 79(1): p. 40-6.

[144] Acheson, K.J., et al., *Caffeine and coffee: their influence on metabolic rate and substrate utilization in normal weight and obese individuals.* Am J Clin Nutr, 1980. 33(5): p. 989-97.

[145] Andersen, T. and J. Fogh, *Weight loss and delayed gastric emptying following a South American herbal preparation in overweight patients.* J Hum Nutr Diet, 2001. 14(3): p. 243-50.

[146] Astrup, A., et al., *The effect of ephedrine/caffeine mixture on energy expenditure and body composition in obese women.* Metabolism, 1992. 41(7): p. 686-8.

[147] Astrup, A., et al., *Thermogenic synergism between ephedrine and caffeine in healthy volunteers: a double-blind, placebo-controlled study.* Metabolism, 1991. 40(3): p. 323-9.

[148] Boozer, C.N., et al., *Herbal ephedra/caffeine for weight loss: a 6-month randomized safety and efficacy trial.* Int J Obes Relat Metab Disord, 2002. 26(5): p. 593-604.

[149] Coffey, C.S., et al., *A randomized double-blind placebo-controlled clinical trial of a product containing ephedrine, caffeine, and other ingredients from herbal sources for treatment of overweight and obesity in the absence of lifestyle treatment.* Int J Obes Relat Metab Disord, 2004. 28(11): p. 1411-9.

[150] Dulloo, A.G., *Herbal simulation of ephedrine and caffeine in treatment of obesity.* Int J Obes Relat Metab Disord, 2002. 26(5): p. 590-2.

[151] Dulloo, A.G., J. Seydoux, and L. Girardier, *Peripheral mechanisms of thermogenesis induced by ephedrine and caffeine in brown adipose tissue.* Int J Obes, 1991. 15(5): p. 317-26.

[152] Cannon, M.E., C.T. Cooke, and J.S. McCarthy, *Caffeine-induced cardiac arrhythmia: an unrecognised danger of healthfood products.* Med J Aust, 2001. 174(10): p. 520-1.

[153] Heseltine, D., et al., *The effect of caffeine on postprandial hypotension in the elderly.* J Am Geriatr Soc, 1991. 39(2): p. 160-4.

[154] Heseltine, D., et al., *The effect of caffeine on postprandial blood pressure in the frail elderly.* Postgrad Med J, 1991. 67(788): p. 543-7.

[155] Katan, M.B. and E. Schouten, *Caffeine and arrhythmia.* Am J Clin Nutr, 2005. 81(3): p. 539-40.

[156] Nurminen, M.L., et al., *Coffee, caffeine and blood pressure: a critical review.* Eur J Clin Nutr, 1999. 53(11): p. 831-9.

[157] Upton, R.A., *Pharmacokinetic interactions between theophylline and other medication (Part I).* Clin Pharmacokinet, 1991. 20(1): p. 66-80.

[158] Del Rio, G., et al., *Increased cardiovascular response to caffeine in perimenopausal women before and during estrogen therapy.* Eur J Endocrinol, 1996. 135(5): p. 598-603.

[159] Pollock, B.G., et al., *Inhibition of caffeine metabolism by estrogen replacement therapy in postmenopausal women.* J Clin Pharmacol, 1999. 39(9): p. 936-40.

[160] Dulloo, A.G., et al., *Efficacy of a green tea extract rich in catechin polyphenols and caffeine in increasing 24-h energy expenditure and fat oxidation in humans.* Am J Clin Nutr, 1999. 70(6): p. 1040-5.

[161] Dulloo, A.G., et al., *Green tea and thermogenesis: interactions between catechin-polyphenols, caffeine and sympathetic activity.* Int J Obes Relat Metab Disord, 2000. 24(2): p. 252-8.

[162] Jagdeo, J. and N. Brody, *Complementary antioxidant function of caffeine and green tea polyphenols in normal human skin fibroblasts.* J Drugs Dermatol, 2011. 10(7): p. 753-61.

[163] Samanidou, V., A. Tsagiannidis, and I. Sarakatsianos, *Simultaneous determination of polyphenols and major purine alkaloids in Greek Sideritis species, herbal extracts, green tea, black tea, and coffee by high-performance liquid chromatography-diode array detection.* J Sep Sci, 2012. 35(4): p. 608-15.

[164] Westerterp-Plantenga, M.S., *Green tea catechins, caffeine and body-weight regulation.* Physiol Behav, 2010. 100(1): p. 42-6.

[165] Phung, O.J., et al., *Effect of green tea catechins with or without caffeine on anthropometric measures: a systematic review and meta-analysis.* Am J Clin Nutr, 2010. 91(1): p. 73-81.

[166] Taylor, J.R. and V.M. Wilt, *Probable antagonism of warfarin by green tea.* Ann Pharmacother, 1999. 33(4): p. 426-8.

[167] Sun, J., *Morning/evening menopausal formula relieves menopausal symptoms: a pilot study.* J Altern Complement Med, 2003. 9(3): p. 403-9.

[168] Westphal, L.M., M.L. Polan, and A.S. Trant, *Double-blind, placebo-controlled study of Fertilityblend: a nutritional supplement for improving fertility in women.* Clin Exp Obstet Gynecol, 2006. 33(4): p. 205-8.

[169] Westphal, L.M., et al., *A nutritional supplement for improving fertility in women: a pilot study.* J Reprod Med, 2004. 49(4): p. 289-93.

[170] Wu, A.H., et al., *Tea and circulating estrogen levels in postmenopausal Chinese women in Singapore.* Carcinogenesis, 2005. 26(5): p. 976-80.

[171] Abourashed, E.A., et al., *Two new flavone glycosides from paullinia pinnata.* J Nat Prod, 1999. 62(8): p. 1179-81.

[172] Avato, P., et al., *Seed oil composition of Paullinia cupana var. sorbilis (Mart.) Ducke.* Lipids, 2003. 38(7): p. 773-80.

[173] Belliardo, F., A. Martelli, and M.G. Valle, *HPLC determination of caffeine and theophylline in Paullinia cupana Kunth (guarana) and Cola spp. samples.* Z Lebensm Unters Forsch, 1985. 180(5): p. 398-401.

[174] Saldana, M.D., et al., *Extraction of methylxanthines from guarana seeds, mate leaves, and cocoa beans using supercritical carbon dioxide and ethanol.* J Agric Food Chem, 2002. 50(17): p. 4820-6.

[175] Weckerle, C.S., M.A. Stutz, and T.W. Baumann, *Purine alkaloids in Paullinia.* Phytochemistry, 2003. 64(3): p. 735-42.

[176] Zamble, A., et al., *Paullinia pinnata extracts rich in polyphenols promote vascular relaxation via endothelium-dependent mechanisms.* J Cardiovasc Pharmacol, 2006. 47(4): p. 599-608.

[177] Bydlowski, S.P., R.L. Yunker, and M.T. Subbiah, *A novel property of an aqueous guarana extract (Paullinia cupana): inhibition of platelet aggregation in vitro and in vivo.* Braz J Med Biol Res, 1988. 21(3): p. 535-8.

[178] Blumenthal, M., W.R. Busse, and Bundesinstitut für Arzneimittel und Medizinprodukte (Germany), *The complete German Commission E monographs, Therapeutic guide to herbal medicines*. 1998, Austin, Texas; Boston: American Botanical Council ;Integrative Medicine Communications. xxii, 685 p.

[179] Escudero, N.L., DeArellano, M.L., Fernandez, S., Albarracin, G., and Mucciarelli, S., *Taraxacum officinale as a food source.* Plant Foods for Human Nutrition, 2003. 58(3): p. 1 - 10.

[180] Tabassum, N., Qazi, M.A., and Shah, A., *Curative Activity of Ethanol Extract of Taraxacum officinale Weber. Against CCl4 Induced Hepatocellular Damage in Albino Rats.* J. Pharmacy Res., 2011. 4(3): p. 687 - 689.

http://dx.doi.org/10.5772/51145

[181] Clare, B.A., R.S. Conroy, and K. Spelman, *The diuretic effect in human subjects of an extract of Taraxacum officinale folium over a single day.* J Altern Complement Med, 2009. 15(8): p. 929-34.

[182] Zhu, M., P.Y. Wong, and R.C. Li, *Effects of taraxacum mongolicum on the bioavailability and disposition of ciprofloxacin in rats.* J Pharm Sci, 1999. 88(6): p. 632-4.

[183] Goksu, E., et al., *First report of hypoglycemia secondary to dandelion (Taraxacum officinale) ingestion.* Am J Emerg Med, 2010. 28(1): p. 111 e1-2.

[184] Kalix, P., *The pharmacology of psychoactive alkaloids from ephedra and catha.* J Ethnopharmacol, 1991. 32(1-3): p. 201-8.

[185] Greenway, F.L., et al., *Effect of a dietary herbal supplement containing caffeine and ephedra on weight, metabolic rate, and body composition.* Obes Res, 2004. 12(7): p. 1152-7.

[186] Hackman, R.M., et al., *Multinutrient supplement containing ephedra and caffeine causes weight loss and improves metabolic risk factors in obese women: a randomized controlled trial.* Int J Obes (Lond), 2006. 30(10): p. 1545-56.

[187] Magkos, F. and S.A. Kavouras, *Caffeine and ephedrine: physiological, metabolic and performance-enhancing effects.* Sports Med, 2004. 34(13): p. 871-89.

[188] Williams, A.D., et al., *The effect of ephedra and caffeine on maximal strength and power in resistance-trained athletes.* J Strength Cond Res, 2008. 22(2): p. 464-70.

[189] Willis, S.L., et al., *Hypertensive retinopathy associated with use of the ephedra-free weight-loss herbal supplement Hydroxycut.* MedGenMed, 2006. 8(3): p. 82.

[190] *Ephedrine, Xanthines, Aspirin and Other Thermogenic Drugs to Assist the Dietary Management of Obesity. Proceedings of an international symposium. Geneva, 24-26 September 1992.* Int J Obes Relat Metab Disord, 1993. 17 Suppl 1: p. S1-83.

[191] Battig, K., *Acute and chronic cardiovascular and behavioural effects of caffeine, aspirin and ephedrine.* Int J Obes Relat Metab Disord, 1993. 17 Suppl 1: p. S61-4.

[192] Daly, P.A., et al., *Ephedrine, caffeine and aspirin: safety and efficacy for treatment of human obesity.* Int J Obes Relat Metab Disord, 1993. 17 Suppl 1: p. S73-8.

[193] Dulloo, A.G., *Ephedrine, xanthines and prostaglandin-inhibitors: actions and interactions in the stimulation of thermogenesis.* Int J Obes Relat Metab Disord, 1993. 17 Suppl 1: p. S35-40.

[194] Dulloo, A.G. and D.S. Miller, *Aspirin as a promoter of ephedrine-induced thermogenesis: potential use in the treatment of obesity.* Am J Clin Nutr, 1987. 45(3): p. 564-9.

[195] Dulloo, A.G. and D.S. Miller, *Ephedrine, caffeine and aspirin: "over-the-counter" drugs that interact to stimulate thermogenesis in the obese.* Nutrition, 1989. 5(1): p. 7-9.

[196] Geissler, C.A., *Effects of weight loss, ephedrine and aspirin on energy expenditure in obese women.* Int J Obes Relat Metab Disord, 1993. 17 Suppl 1: p. S45-8.

[197] Horton, T.J. and C.A. Geissler, *Aspirin potentiates the effect of ephedrine on the thermogenic response to a meal in obese but not lean women.* Int J Obes, 1991. 15(5): p. 359-66.

[198] Horton, T.J. and C.A. Geissler, *Post-prandial thermogenesis with ephedrine, caffeine and aspirin in lean, pre-disposed obese and obese women.* Int J Obes Relat Metab Disord, 1996. 20(2): p. 91-7.

[199] Krieger, D.R., et al., *Ephedrine, caffeine and aspirin promote weight loss in obese subjects.* Trans Assoc Am Physicians, 1990. 103: p. 307-12.

[200] Loose, I. and M. Winkel, *Clinical, double-blind, placebo-controlled study investigating the combination of acetylsalicylic acid and pseudoephedrine for the symptomatic treatment of nasal congestion associated with common cold.* Arzneimittelforschung, 2004. 54(9): p. 513-21.

[201] Lucker, P.W., et al., *Pharmacokinetic interaction study of a fixed combination of 500 mg acetylsalicylic acid/30 mg pseudoephedrine versus each of the single active ingredients in healthy male volunteers.* Arzneimittelforschung, 2003. 53(4): p. 260-5.

[202] Chen, C., et al., *Ischemic stroke after using over the counter products containing ephedra.* J Neurol Sci, 2004. 217(1): p. 55-60.

[203] Clark, B.M. and R.S. Schofield, *Dilated cardiomyopathy and acute liver injury associated with combined use of ephedra, gamma-hydroxybutyrate, and anabolic steroids.* Pharmacotherapy, 2005. 25(5): p. 756-61.

[204] Dhar, R., et al., *Cardiovascular toxicities of performance-enhancing substances in sports.* Mayo Clin Proc, 2005. 80(10): p. 1307-15.

[205] Figueredo, V.M., *Chemical cardiomyopathies: the negative effects of medications and nonprescribed drugs on the heart.* Am J Med, 2011. 124(6): p. 480-8.

[206] Flanagan, C.M., et al., *Coronary artery aneurysm and thrombosis following chronic ephedra use.* Int J Cardiol, 2010. 139(1): p. e11-3.

[207] Miller, S.C., *Safety concerns regarding ephedrine-type alkaloid-containing dietary supplements.* Mil Med, 2004. 169(2): p. 87-93.

[208] Peters, C.M., et al., *Is there an association between ephedra and heart failure? a case series.* J Card Fail, 2005. 11(1): p. 9-11.

[209] Shekelle, P.G., et al., *Efficacy and safety of ephedra and ephedrine for weight loss and athletic performance: a meta-analysis.* JAMA, 2003. 289(12): p. 1537-45.

[210] Thomas, J.E., et al., *STEMI in a 24-year-old man after use of a synephrine-containing dietary supplement: a case report and review of the literature.* Tex Heart Inst J, 2009. 36(6): p. 586-90.

[211] White, L.M., et al., *Pharmacokinetics and cardiovascular effects of ma-huang (Ephedra sinica) in normotensive adults.* J Clin Pharmacol, 1997. 37(2): p. 116-22.

[212] Siegrid Keline, C.R., Robert Rister, *The Complete German Commissions E Monographs: Therapeutic Guide to Herbal Medicines*. 1998, Boston, MA: Integrative Medicine Communications. 685.

[213] Kanaya, N., et al., *Propofol anesthesia enhances the pressor response to intravenous ephedrine*. Anesth Analg, 2002. 94(5): p. 1207-11, table of contents.

[214] Ueda, W., et al., *Ephedrine-induced increases in arterial blood pressure accelerate regression of epidural block*. Anesth Analg, 1995. 81(4): p. 703-5.

[215] Lee, A., W.D. Ngan Kee, and T. Gin, *Prophylactic ephedrine prevents hypotension during spinal anesthesia for Cesarean delivery but does not improve neonatal outcome: a quantitative systematic review*. Can J Anaesth, 2002. 49(6): p. 588-99.

[216] Lee, A., W.D. Ngan Kee, and T. Gin, *A dose-response meta-analysis of prophylactic intravenous ephedrine for the prevention of hypotension during spinal anesthesia for elective cesarean delivery*. Anesth Analg, 2004. 98(2): p. 483-90, table of contents.

[217] Astrup, A., et al., *The effect and safety of an ephedrine/caffeine compound compared to ephedrine, caffeine and placebo in obese subjects on an energy restricted diet. A double blind trial*. Int J Obes Relat Metab Disord, 1992. 16(4): p. 269-77.

[218] Martinet, A., K. Hostettmann, and Y. Schutz, *Thermogenic effects of commercially available plant preparations aimed at treating human obesity*. Phytomedicine, 1999. 6(4): p. 231-8.

[219] Dawson, J.K., S.M. Earnshaw, and C.S. Graham, *Dangerous monoamine oxidase inhibitor interactions are still occurring in the 1990s*. J Accid Emerg Med, 1995. 12(1): p. 49-51.

[220] Boada, S., et al., *[Hypotension refractory to ephedrine after sympathetic blockade in a patient on long-term therapy with tricyclic antidepressants]*. Rev Esp Anestesiol Reanim, 1999. 46(8): p. 364-6.

[221] Astrup, A. and S. Toubro, *Thermogenic, metabolic, and cardiovascular responses to ephedrine and caffeine in man*. Int J Obes Relat Metab Disord, 1993. 17 Suppl 1: p. S41-3.

[222] Samenuk, D., et al., *Adverse cardiovascular events temporally associated with ma huang, an herbal source of ephedrine*. Mayo Clin Proc, 2002. 77(1): p. 12-6.

[223] Tormey, W.P. and A. Bruzzi, *Acute psychosis due to the interaction of legal compounds--ephedra alkaloids in 'vigueur fit' tablets, caffeine in 'red bull' and alcohol*. Med Sci Law, 2001. 41(4): p. 331-6.

[224] Theoharides, T.C., *Sudden death of a healthy college student related to ephedrine toxicity from a ma huang-containing drink*. J Clin Psychopharmacol, 1997. 17(5): p. 437-9.

[225] Zahn, K.A., R.L. Li, and R.A. Purssell, *Cardiovascular toxicity after ingestion of "herbal ecstacy"*. J Emerg Med, 1999. 17(2): p. 289-91.

[226] Cairella, M. and G. Marchini, *[Evaluation of the action of glucomannan on metabolic parameters and on the sensation of satiation in overweight and obese patients].* Clin Ter, 1995. 146(4): p. 269-74.

[227] Chen, H.L., et al., *Konjac acts as a natural laxative by increasing stool bulk and improving colonic ecology in healthy adults.* Nutrition, 2006. 22(11-12): p. 1112-9.

[228] Chen, H.L., et al., *Supplementation of konjac glucomannan into a low-fiber Chinese diet promoted bowel movement and improved colonic ecology in constipated adults: a placebo-controlled, diet-controlled trial.* J Am Coll Nutr, 2008. 27(1): p. 102-8.

[229] Chen, H.L., et al., *Konjac supplement alleviated hypercholesterolemia and hyperglycemia in type 2 diabetic subjects--a randomized double-blind trial.* J Am Coll Nutr, 2003. 22(1): p. 36-42.

[230] Sood, N., W.L. Baker, and C.I. Coleman, *Effect of glucomannan on plasma lipid and glucose concentrations, body weight, and blood pressure: systematic review and meta-analysis.* Am J Clin Nutr, 2008. 88(4): p. 1167-75.

[231] Vuksan, V., et al., *Beneficial effects of viscous dietary fiber from Konjac-mannan in subjects with the insulin resistance syndrome: results of a controlled metabolic trial.* Diabetes Care, 2000. 23(1): p. 9-14.

[232] Yoshida, M., et al., *Effect of plant sterols and glucomannan on lipids in individuals with and without type II diabetes.* Eur J Clin Nutr, 2006. 60(4): p. 529-37.

[233] Shima, K., et al., *Effect of dietary fiber, glucomannan, on absorption of sulfonylurea in man.* Horm Metab Res, 1983. 15(1): p. 1-3.

[234] Doi, K., *Effect of konjac fibre (glucomannan) on glucose and lipids.* Eur J Clin Nutr, 1995. 49 Suppl 3: p. S190-7.

[235] Doi, K., et al., *Treatment of diabetes with glucomannan (konjac mannan).* Lancet, 1979. 1(8123): p. 987-8.

[236] Huang, C.Y., et al., *Effect of Konjac food on blood glucose level in patients with diabetes.* Biomed Environ Sci, 1990. 3(2): p. 123-31.

[237] Vuksan, V., et al., *Konjac-Mannan and American ginsing: emerging alternative therapies for type 2 diabetes mellitus.* J Am Coll Nutr, 2001. 20(5 Suppl): p. 370S-380S; discussion 381S-383S.

[238] Azezli, A.D., T. Bayraktaroglu, and Y. Orhan, *The use of konjac glucomannan to lower serum thyroid hormones in hyperthyroidism.* J Am Coll Nutr, 2007. 26(6): p. 663-8.

[239] Doi, K., et al., *Influence of dietary fiber (konjac mannan) on absorption of vitamin B12 and vitamin E.* Tohoku J Exp Med, 1983. 141 Suppl: p. 677-81.

[240] van Heerden, F.R., *Hoodia gordonii: a natural appetite suppressant.* J Ethnopharmacol, 2008. 119(3): p. 434-7.

[241] Vermaak, I., J.H. Hamman, and A.M. Viljoen, *Hoodia gordonii: an up-to-date review of a commercially important anti-obesity plant.* Planta Med, 2011. 77(11): p. 1149-60.

[242] MacLean, D.B. and L.G. Luo, *Increased ATP content/production in the hypothalamus may be a signal for energy-sensing of satiety: studies of the anorectic mechanism of a plant steroidal glycoside.* Brain Res, 2004. 1020(1-2): p. 1-11.

[243] Madgula, V.L., et al., *In vitro metabolic stability and intestinal transport of P57AS3 (P57) from Hoodia gordonii and its interaction with drug metabolizing enzymes.* Planta Med, 2008. 74(10): p. 1269-75.

[244] Jena, B.S., et al., *Chemistry and biochemistry of (-)-hydroxycitric acid from Garcinia.* J Agric Food Chem, 2002. 50(1): p. 10-22.

[245] Soni, M.G., et al., *Safety assessment of (-)-hydroxycitric acid and Super CitriMax, a novel calcium/potassium salt.* Food Chem Toxicol, 2004. 42(9): p. 1513-29.

[246] Heymsfield, S.B., et al., *Garcinia cambogia (hydroxycitric acid) as a potential antiobesity agent: a randomized controlled trial.* JAMA, 1998. 280(18): p. 1596-600.

[247] Preuss, H.G., et al., *Effects of a natural extract of (-)-hydroxycitric acid (HCA-SX) and a combination of HCA-SX plus niacin-bound chromium and Gymnema sylvestre extract on weight loss.* Diabetes Obes Metab, 2004. 6(3): p. 171-80.

[248] Mattes, R.D. and L. Bormann, *Effects of (-)-hydroxycitric acid on appetitive variables.* Physiol Behav, 2000. 71(1-2): p. 87-94.

[249] Mansi, I.A. and J. Huang, *Rhabdomyolysis in response to weight-loss herbal medicine.* Am J Med Sci, 2004. 327(6): p. 356-7.

[250] Levy, A.S. and A.W. Heaton, *Weight control practices of U.S. adults trying to lose weight.* Ann Intern Med, 1993. 119(7 Pt 2): p. 661-6.

[251] Boban, P.T., B. Nambisan, and P.R. Sudhakaran, *Hypolipidaemic effect of chemically different mucilages in rats: a comparative study.* Br J Nutr, 2006. 96(6): p. 1021-9.

[252] Pittler, M.H. and E. Ernst, *Guar gum for body weight reduction: meta-analysis of randomized trials.* Am J Med, 2001. 110(9): p. 724-30.

[253] Salas-Salvadó, J., et al., *Effect of two doses of a mixture of soluble fibres on body weight and metabolic variables in overweight or obese patients: a randomised trial.* Br J Nutr, 2008. 99(6): p. 1380-7.

[254] Blackburn, N.A., et al., *The mechanism of action of guar gum in improving glucose tolerance in man.* Clin Sci (Lond), 1984. 66(3): p. 329-36.

[255] Frati-Munari, A.C., et al., *Effect of Plantago psyllium mucilage on the glucose tolerance test.* Arch Invest Med (Mex), 1985. 16(2): p. 191-7.

[256] Jenkins, D.J. and A.L. Jenkins, *Dietary fiber and the glycemic response.* Proc Soc Exp Biol Med, 1985. 180(3): p. 422-31.

[257] Leclere, C.J., et al., *Role of viscous guar gums in lowering the glycemic response after a solid meal.* Am J Clin Nutr, 1994. 59(4): p. 914-21.

[258] McCarty, M.F., *Glucomannan minimizes the postprandial insulin surge: a potential adjuvant for hepatothermic therapy.* Med Hypotheses, 2002. 58(6): p. 487-90.

[259] Ou, S., et al., *In vitro study of possible role of dietary fiber in lowering postprandial serum glucose.* J Agric Food Chem, 2001. 49(2): p. 1026-9.

[260] Russo, A., et al., *Guar attenuates fall in postprandial blood pressure and slows gastric emptying of oral glucose in type 2 diabetes.* Dig Dis Sci, 2003. 48(7): p. 1221-9.

[261] Torsdottir, I., et al., *Dietary guar gum effects on postprandial blood glucose, insulin and hydroxyproline in humans.* J Nutr, 1989. 119(12): p. 1925-31.

[262] Ahi, S., et al., *A bulking agent may lead to adrenal insufficiency crisis: a case report.* Acta Med Iran, 2011. 49(10): p. 688-9.

[263] Chiu, A.C. and S.I. Sherman, *Effects of pharmacological fiber supplements on levothyroxine absorption.* Thyroid, 1998. 8(8): p. 667-71.

[264] Garcia, J.J., et al., *Influence of two dietary fibers in the oral bioavailability and other pharmacokinetic parameters of ethinyloestradiol.* Contraception, 2000. 62(5): p. 253-7.

[265] Gin, H., M.B. Orgerie, and J. Aubertin, *The influence of Guar gum on absorption of metformin from the gut in healthy volunteers.* Horm Metab Res, 1989. 21(2): p. 81-3.

[266] González, A., et al., *Effect of glucomannan and the dosage form on ethinylestradiol oral absorption in rabbits.* Contraception, 2004. 70(5): p. 423-7.

[267] Heaney, R.P. and C.M. Weaver, *Effect of psyllium on absorption of co-ingested calcium.* J Am Geriatr Soc, 1995. 43(3): p. 261-3.

[268] Holt, S., et al., *Effect of gel fibre on gastric emptying and absorption of glucose and paracetamol.* Lancet, 1979. 1(8117): p. 636-9.

[269] Huupponen, R., P. Seppala, and E. Iisalo, *Effect of guar gum, a fibre preparation, on digoxin and penicillin absorption in man.* Eur J Clin Pharmacol, 1984. 26(2): p. 279-81.

[270] Perlman, B.B., *Interaction between lithium salts and ispaghula husk.* Lancet, 1990. 335(8686): p. 416.

[271] Reissell, P. and V. Manninen, *Effect of administration of activated charcoal and fibre on absorption, excretion and steady state blood levels of digoxin and digitoxin. Evidence for intestinal secretion of the glycosides.* Acta Med Scand Suppl, 1982. 668: p. 88-90.

[272] Toutoungi, M., et al., *[Probable interaction of psyllium and lithium].* Therapie, 1990. 45(4): p. 358-60.

[273] Roerig, J.L., et al., *Laxative abuse: epidemiology, diagnosis and management.* Drugs, 2010. 70(12): p. 1487-503.

http://dx.doi.org/10.5772/51145

[274] Tozzi, F., et al., *Features associated with laxative abuse in individuals with eating disorders.* Psychosom Med, 2006. 68(3): p. 470-7.

[275] Amato, A., et al., *Half doses of PEG-ES and senna vs. high-dose senna for bowel cleansing before colonoscopy: a randomized, investigator-blinded trial.* Am J Gastroenterol, 2010. 105(3): p. 675-81.

[276] Branco, A., et al., *Anthraquinones from the bark of Senna macranthera.* An Acad Bras Cienc, 2011. 83(4): p. 1159-64.

[277] Brouwers, J.R., et al., *A controlled trial of senna preparations and other laxatives used for bowel cleansing prior to radiological examination.* Pharmacology, 1980. 20 Suppl 1: p. 58-64.

[278] El-Gengaihi, S., A.H. Agiza, and A. El-Hamidi, *Distribution of anthraquinones in Senna plants.* Planta Med, 1975. 27(4): p. 349-53.

[279] Franz, G., *The senna drug and its chemistry.* Pharmacology, 1993. 47 Suppl 1: p. 2-6.

[280] Godding, E.W., *Laxatives and the special role of senna.* Pharmacology, 1988. 36 Suppl 1: p. 230-6.

[281] Gould, S.R. and C.B. Williams, *Castor oil or senna preparation before colonoscopy for inactive chronic ulcerative colitis.* Gastrointest Endosc, 1982. 28(1): p. 6-8.

[282] Hietala, P., et al., *Laxative potency and acute toxicity of some anthraquinone derivatives, senna extracts and fractions of senna extracts.* Pharmacol Toxicol, 1987. 61(2): p. 153-6.

[283] Izard, M.W. and F.S. Ellison, *Treatment of drug-induced constipation with a purified senna derivative.* Conn Med, 1962. 26: p. 589-92.

[284] Khafagy, S.M., et al., *Estimation of sennosides A, B, C and D in Senna leaves, pods and formulations.* Planta Med, 1972. 21(3): p. 304-9.

[285] Kinnunen, O., et al., *Safety and efficacy of a bulk laxative containing senna versus lactulose in the treatment of chronic constipation in geriatric patients.* Pharmacology, 1993. 47 Suppl 1: p. 253-5.

[286] Kositchaiwat, S., et al., *Comparative study of two bowel preparation regimens for colonoscopy: senna tablets vs sodium phosphate solution.* World J Gastroenterol, 2006. 12(34): p. 5536-9.

[287] Krumbiegel, G. and H.U. Schulz, *Rhein and aloe-emodin kinetics from senna laxatives in man.* Pharmacology, 1993. 47 Suppl 1: p. 120-4.

[288] Lamphier, T.A. and R. Ehrlich, *Evaluation of standardized senna in the management of constipation.* Am J Gastroenterol, 1957. 27(4): p. 381-4.

[289] Lemli, J., *The Estimation of Anthracene Derivatives in Senna and Rhubarb.* J Pharm Pharmacol, 1965. 17: p. 227-32.

[290] Marlett, J.A., et al., *Comparative laxation of psyllium with and without senna in an ambulatory constipated population.* Am J Gastroenterol, 1987. 82(4): p. 333-7.

[291] Mc, N.G., *The effect of a standardised senna preparation on the human bowel.* J Pharm Pharmacol, 1958. 10(8): p. 499-506.

[292] Monias, M.B., *Standardized senna concentrate in postpartum bowel rehabilitation.* Md State Med J, 1966. 15(2): p. 32-3.

[293] Putalun, W., et al., *Sennosides A and B production by hairy roots of Senna alata (L.) Roxb.* Z Naturforsch C, 2006. 61(5-6): p. 367-71.

[294] Radaelli, F., et al., *High-dose senna compared with conventional PEG-ES lavage as bowel preparation for elective colonoscopy: a prospective, randomized, investigator-blinded trial.* Am J Gastroenterol, 2005. 100(12): p. 2674-80.

[295] Valverde, A., et al., *Senna vs polyethylene glycol for mechanical preparation the evening before elective colonic or rectal resection: a multicenter controlled trial. French Association for Surgical Research.* Arch Surg, 1999. 134(5): p. 514-9.

[296] Ishii, Y., H. Tanizawa, and Y. Takino, *[Studies of aloe. II. Mechanism of cathartic effect].* Yakugaku Zasshi, 1988. 108(9): p. 904-10.

[297] Ishii, Y., H. Tanizawa, and Y. Takino, *Studies of aloe. III. Mechanism of cathartic effect. (2).* Chem Pharm Bull (Tokyo), 1990. 38(1): p. 197-200.

[298] Ishii, Y., H. Tanizawa, and Y. Takino, *Studies of aloe. V. Mechanism of cathartic effect. (4).* Biol Pharm Bull, 1994. 17(5): p. 651-3.

[299] Ishii, Y., H. Tanizawa, and Y. Takino, *Studies of aloe. IV. Mechanism of cathartic effect. (3).* Biol Pharm Bull, 1994. 17(4): p. 495-7.

[300] *Status of certain additional over-the-counter drug category II and III active ingredients. Final rule.* Fed Regist, 2002. 67(90): p. 31125-7.

[301] *Final report on the safety assessment of AloeAndongensis Extract, Aloe Andongensis Leaf Juice,aloe Arborescens Leaf Extract, Aloe Arborescens Leaf Juice, Aloe Arborescens Leaf Protoplasts, Aloe Barbadensis Flower Extract, Aloe Barbadensis Leaf, Aloe Barbadensis Leaf Extract, Aloe Barbadensis Leaf Juice,aloe Barbadensis Leaf Polysaccharides, Aloe Barbadensis Leaf Water, Aloe Ferox Leaf Extract, Aloe Ferox Leaf Juice, and Aloe Ferox Leaf Juice Extract.* Int J Toxicol, 2007. 26 Suppl 2: p. 1-50.

[302] Quercia, V., *[Separation of anthraquinone compounds of Cascara sagrada by means of high-pressure liquid chromatography].* Boll Chim Farm, 1976. 115(4): p. 309-16.

[303] Fugh-Berman, A., *Herb-drug interactions.* Lancet, 2000. 355(9198): p. 134-8.

[304] Laitinen, L., et al., *Anthranoid laxatives influence the absorption of poorly permeable drugs in human intestinal cell culture model (Caco-2).* Eur J Pharm Biopharm, 2007. 66(1): p. 135-45.

[305] Huseini, H.F., et al., *Anti-hyperglycemic and anti-hypercholesterolemic effects of Aloe vera leaf gel in hyperlipidemic type 2 diabetic patients: a randomized double-blind placebo-controlled clinical trial.* Planta Med, 2012. 78(4): p. 311-6.

[306] Musabayane, C.T., P.T. Bwititi, and J.A. Ojewole, *Effects of oral administration of some herbal extracts on food consumption and blood glucose levels in normal and streptozotocin-treated diabetic rats.* Methods Find Exp Clin Pharmacol, 2006. 28(4): p. 223-8.

[307] Rajasekaran, S., et al., *Hypoglycemic effect of Aloe vera gel on streptozotocin-induced diabetes in experimental rats.* J Med Food, 2004. 7(1): p. 61-6.

[308] Lewis, S.J., et al., *Lower serum oestrogen concentrations associated with faster intestinal transit.* Br J Cancer, 1997. 76(3): p. 395-400.

[309] Lewis, S.J., R.E. Oakey, and K.W. Heaton, *Intestinal absorption of oestrogen: the effect of altering transit-time.* Eur J Gastroenterol Hepatol, 1998. 10(1): p. 33-9.

[310] Kittisupamongkol, W., V. Nilaratanakul, and W. Kulwichit, *Near-fatal bleeding, senna, and the opposite of lettuce.* Lancet, 2008. 371(9614): p. 784.

[311] Lee, A., et al., *Possible interaction between sevoflurane and Aloe vera.* Ann Pharmacother, 2004. 38(10): p. 1651-4.

[312] Kitagawa, I., et al., *Chemical studies of Chinese licorice-roots. I. Elucidation of five new flavonoid constituents from the roots of Glycyrrhiza glabra L. collected in Xinjiang.* Chem Pharm Bull (Tokyo), 1994. 42(5): p. 1056-62.

[313] Mitscher, L.A., et al., *Antimicrobial agents from higher plants. Antimicrobial isoflavanoids and related substances from Glycyrrhiza glabra L. var. typica.* J Nat Prod, 1980. 43(2): p. 259-69.

[314] Grossman, E. and F.H. Messerli, *Drug-induced hypertension: an unappreciated cause of secondary hypertension.* Am J Med, 2012. 125(1): p. 14-22.

[315] Kaleel, M., et al., *Licorice: a patient's shocking presentation.* Del Med J, 2011. 83(7): p. 211-5.

[316] Knobel, U., et al., *Gitelman's syndrome with persistent hypokalemia - don't forget licorice, alcohol, lemon juice, iced tea and salt depletion: a case report.* J Med Case Rep, 2011. 5: p. 312.

[317] Brayley, J. and J. Jones, *Life-threatening hypokalemia associated with excessive licorice ingestion.* Am J Psychiatry, 1994. 151(4): p. 617-8.

[318] Famularo, G., F.M. Corsi, and M. Giacanelli, *Iatrogenic worsening of hypokalemia and neuromuscular paralysis associated with the use of glucose solutions for potassium replacement in a young woman with licorice intoxication and furosemide abuse.* Acad Emerg Med, 1999. 6(9): p. 960-4.

[319] Joseph, R. and J. Kelemen, *Paraparesis due to licorice-induced hypokalemia.* N Y State J Med, 1984. 84(6): p. 296.

[320] Mumoli, N. and M. Cei, *Licorice-induced hypokalemia.* Int J Cardiol, 2008. 124(3): p. e42-4.

[321] Pelner, L., *Licorice induced hypokalemia.* N Y State J Med, 1984. 84(12): p. 591.

[322] Yasue, H., et al., *Severe hypokalemia, rhabdomyolysis, muscle paralysis, and respiratory impairment in a hypertensive patient taking herbal medicines containing licorice.* Intern Med, 2007. 46(9): p. 575-8.

[323] Yoshida, S. and Y. Takayama, *Licorice-induced hypokalemia as a treatable cause of dropped head syndrome.* Clin Neurol Neurosurg, 2003. 105(4): p. 286-7.

[324] Armanini, D., et al., *Further studies on the mechanism of the mineralocorticoid action of licorice in humans.* J Endocrinol Invest, 1996. 19(9): p. 624-9.

[325] Stoving, R.K., et al., *Is glycyrrhizin sensitivity increased in anorexia nervosa and should licorice be avoided? Case report and review of the literature.* Nutrition, 2011. 27(7-8): p. 855-8.

[326] Wynn, G.J., G.K. Davis, and B. Maher, *Trick or treat? Pseudohyperaldosteronism due to episodic licorice consumption.* J Clin Hypertens (Greenwich), 2011. 13(3): p. E3-4.

[327] Armanini, D., M. Wehling, and P.C. Weber, *Mineralocorticoid effector mechanism of liquorice derivatives in human mononuclear leukocytes.* J Endocrinol Invest, 1989. 12(5): p. 303-6.

[328] Berlango Jimenez, A., et al., *[Acute rhabdomyolysis and tetraparesis secondary to hypokalemia due to ingested licorice].* An Med Interna, 1995. 12(1): p. 33-5.

[329] Brasseur, A. and J. Ducobu, *[Severe hypokalemia after holidays return].* Rev Med Brux, 2008. 29(5): p. 490-3.

[330] Carretta, R. and S. Muiesan, *[Pseudohyperaldosteronism caused by the abuse of licorice].* G Clin Med, 1986. 67(1): p. 55-6.

[331] Cataldo, F., et al., *[Pseudohyperaldosteronism secondary to licorice poisoning associated with hemorrhagic gastritis].* Pediatr Med Chir, 1997. 19(3): p. 219-21.

[332] Ferrari, P. and B.N. Trost, *[A case from practice (169). Liquorice-induced pseudohyperaldosteronism in a previously alcoholic woman caused by the drinking of an alcohol-free Pastis substitute beverage].* Schweiz Rundsch Med Prax, 1990. 79(12): p. 377-8.

[333] Ghielmini, C. and A. Hoffmann, *[A case from practice (171). Pseudohyperaldosteronism in licorice abuse].* Schweiz Rundsch Med Prax, 1990. 79(15): p. 472-3.

[334] Gomez Fernandez, P., et al., *[Primary pseudohyperaldosteronism produced by chronic licorice consumption].* Rev Clin Esp, 1981. 163(4): p. 277-8.

[335] Holmes, A.M., et al., *Pseudohyperaldosteronism induced by habitual ingestion of liquorice.* Postgrad Med J, 1970. 46(540): p. 625-9.

[336] Russo, S., et al., *Low doses of liquorice can induce hypertension encephalopathy.* Am J Nephrol, 2000. 20(2): p. 145-8.

[337] Scali, M., et al., *Pseudohyperaldosteronism from liquorice-containing laxatives.* J Endocrinol Invest, 1990. 13(10): p. 847-8.

[338] Sontia, B., et al., *Pseudohyperaldosteronism, liquorice, and hypertension.* J Clin Hypertens (Greenwich), 2008. 10(2): p. 153-7.

[339] Kimura, I., et al., *The antihyperglycaemic blend effect of traditional chinese medicine byakko-ka-ninjin-to on alloxan and diabetic KK-CA(y) mice.* Phytother Res, 1999. 13(6): p. 484-8.

[340] Kuroda, M., et al., *Phenolics with PPAR-gamma ligand-binding activity obtained from licorice (Glycyrrhiza uralensis roots) and ameliorative effects of glycyrin on genetically diabetic KK-A(y) mice.* Bioorg Med Chem Lett, 2003. 13(24): p. 4267-72.

[341] Bardhan, K.D., et al., *Clinical trial of deglycyrrhizinised liquorice in gastric ulcer.* Gut, 1978. 19(9): p. 779-82.

[342] Engqvist, A., et al., *Double-blind trial of deglycyrrhizinated liquorice in gastric ulcer.* Gut, 1973. 14(9): p. 711-5.

[343] MacKenzie, M.A., et al., *The influence of glycyrrhetinic acid on plasma cortisol and cortisone in healthy young volunteers.* J Clin Endocrinol Metab, 1990. 70(6): p. 1637-43.

[344] Armanini, D., et al., *Effect of licorice on the reduction of body fat mass in healthy subjects.* J Endocrinol Invest, 2003. 26(7): p. 646-50.

[345] Armanini, D., et al., *Glycyrrhetinic acid, the active principle of licorice, can reduce the thickness of subcutaneous thigh fat through topical application.* Steroids, 2005. 70(8): p. 538-42.

[346] Hukkanen, J., O. Ukkola, and M.J. Savolainen, *Effects of low-dose liquorice alone or in combination with hydrochlorothiazide on the plasma potassium in healthy volunteers.* Blood Press, 2009. 18(4): p. 192-5.

[347] Kawakami, F., Y. Shimoyama, and K. Ohtsuki, *Characterization of complement C3 as a glycyrrhizin (GL)-binding protein and the phosphorylation of C3alpha by CK-2, which is potently inhibited by GL and glycyrrhetinic acid in vitro.* J Biochem, 2003. 133(2): p. 231-7.

[348] Kroes, B.H., et al., *Inhibition of human complement by beta-glycyrrhetinic acid.* Immunology, 1997. 90(1): p. 115-20.

[349] Akamatsu, H., et al., *Mechanism of anti-inflammatory action of glycyrrhizin: effect on neutrophil functions including reactive oxygen species generation.* Planta Med, 1991. 57(2): p. 119-21.

[350] Rackova, L., et al., *Mechanism of anti-inflammatory action of liquorice extract and glycyrrhizin.* Nat Prod Res, 2007. 21(14): p. 1234-41.

[351] Armanini, D., et al., *Licorice consumption and serum testosterone in healthy man.* Exp Clin Endocrinol Diabetes, 2003. 111(6): p. 341-3.

[352] Armanini, D., G. Bonanni, and M. Palermo, *Reduction of serum testosterone in men by licorice.* N Engl J Med, 1999. 341(15): p. 1158.

[353] Armanini, D., et al., *History of the endocrine effects of licorice.* Exp Clin Endocrinol Diabetes, 2002. 110(6): p. 257-61.

[354] Armanini, D., et al., *Licorice reduces serum testosterone in healthy women.* Steroids, 2004. 69(11-12): p. 763-6.

[355] Kraus, S.D., *Glycyrrhetinic acid--a triterpene with antioestrogenic and anti-inflammatory activity.* J Pharm Pharmacol, 1960. 12: p. 300-6.

[356] Kraus, S.D. and A. Kaminskis, *The anti-estrogenic action of beta-glycyrrhetinic acid.* Exp Med Surg, 1969. 27(4): p. 411-20.

[357] Yamada, K., et al., *Effectiveness of shakuyaku-kanzo-to in neuroleptic-induced hyperprolactinemia: a preliminary report.* Psychiatry Clin Neurosci, 1996. 50(6): p. 341-2.

[358] Yamada, K., et al., *Effectiveness of herbal medicine (shakuyaku-kanzo-to) for neuroleptic-induced hyperprolactinemia.* J Clin Psychopharmacol, 1997. 17(3): p. 234-5.

[359] Imai, T., et al., *In vitro and in vivo evaluation of the enhancing activity of glycyrrhizin on the intestinal absorption of drugs.* Pharm Res, 1999. 16(1): p. 80-6.

[360] Ofir, R., et al., *Inhibition of serotonin re-uptake by licorice constituents.* J Mol Neurosci, 2003. 20(2): p. 135-40.

[361] Dhingra, D. and A. Sharma, *Antidepressant-like activity of Glycyrrhiza glabra L. in mouse models of immobility tests.* Prog Neuropsychopharmacol Biol Psychiatry, 2006. 30(3): p. 449-54.

[362] Tadros, M.G., et al., *Involvement of serotoninergic 5-HT1A/2A, alpha-adrenergic and dopaminergic D1 receptors in St. John's wort-induced prepulse inhibition deficit: a possible role of hyperforin.* Behav Brain Res, 2009. 199(2): p. 334-9.

[363] Shelton, R.C., et al., *Effectiveness of St John's wort in major depression: a randomized controlled trial.* JAMA, 2001. 285(15): p. 1978-86.

[364] Kasper, S., et al., *Better tolerability of St. John's wort extract WS 5570 compared to treatment with SSRIs: a reanalysis of data from controlled clinical trials in acute major depression.* Int Clin Psychopharmacol, 2010. 25(4): p. 204-13.

[365] Niederhofer, H., *St. John's wort may improve some symptoms of attention-deficit hyperactivity disorder.* Nat Prod Res, 2010. 24(3): p. 203-5.

[366] Canning, S., et al., *The efficacy of Hypericum perforatum (St John's wort) for the treatment of premenstrual syndrome: a randomized, double-blind, placebo-controlled trial.* CNS Drugs, 2010. 24(3): p. 207-25.

[367] Balk, J., *The effects of St. John's wort on hot flashes.* Menopause, 2010. 17(5): p. 1089-90.

[368] Chatterjee, S.S., A. Biber, and C. Weibezahn, *Stimulation of glutamate, aspartate and gamma-aminobutyric acid release from synaptosomes by hyperforin.* Pharmacopsychiatry, 2001. 34 Suppl 1: p. S11-9.

[369] Gobbi, M., et al., *In vitro binding studies with two hypericum perforatum extracts--hyperforin, hypericin and biapigenin--on 5-HT6, 5-HT7, GABA(A)/benzodiazepine, sigma, NPY-Y1/Y2 receptors and dopamine transporters.* Pharmacopsychiatry, 2001. 34 Suppl 1: p. S45-8.

[370] Muller, W.E., A. Singer, and M. Wonnemann, *Hyperforin--antidepressant activity by a novel mechanism of action.* Pharmacopsychiatry, 2001. 34 Suppl 1: p. S98-102.

[371] Muller, W.E., et al., *Hyperforin represents the neurotransmitter reuptake inhibiting constituent of hypericum extract.* Pharmacopsychiatry, 1998. 31 Suppl 1: p. 16-21.

[372] Roz, N., et al., *Inhibition of vesicular uptake of monoamines by hyperforin.* Life Sci, 2002. 71(19): p. 2227-37.

[373] Singer, A., M. Wonnemann, and W.E. Muller, *Hyperforin, a major antidepressant constituent of St. John's Wort, inhibits serotonin uptake by elevating free intracellular Na+1.* J Pharmacol Exp Ther, 1999. 290(3): p. 1363-8.

[374] Wentworth, J.M., et al., *St John's wort, a herbal antidepressant, activates the steroid X receptor.* J Endocrinol, 2000. 166(3): p. R11-6.

[375] Weber, C.C., et al., *Modulation of P-glycoprotein function by St John's wort extract and its major constituents.* Pharmacopsychiatry, 2004. 37(6): p. 292-8.

[376] Wang, Z., et al., *The effects of St John's wort (Hypericum perforatum) on human cytochrome P450 activity.* Clin Pharmacol Ther, 2001. 70(4): p. 317-26.

[377] Wang, L.S., et al., *St John's wort induces both cytochrome P450 3A4-catalyzed sulfoxidation and 2C19-dependent hydroxylation of omeprazole.* Clin Pharmacol Ther, 2004. 75(3): p. 191-7.

[378] Wang, E.J., M. Barecki-Roach, and W.W. Johnson, *Quantitative characterization of direct P-glycoprotein inhibition by St John's wort constituents hypericin and hyperforin.* J Pharm Pharmacol, 2004. 56(1): p. 123-8.

[379] Ott, M., et al., *St. John's Wort constituents modulate P-glycoprotein transport activity at the blood-brain barrier.* Pharm Res, 2010. 27(5): p. 811-22.

[380] Obach, R.S., *Inhibition of human cytochrome P450 enzymes by constituents of St. John's Wort, an herbal preparation used in the treatment of depression.* J Pharmacol Exp Ther, 2000. 294(1): p. 88-95.

[381] Noldner, M. and S. Chatterjee, *Effects of two different extracts of St. John's wort and some of their constituents on cytochrome P450 activities in rat liver microsomes.* Pharmacopsychiatry, 2001. 34 Suppl 1: p. S108-10.

[382] Markowitz, J.S., et al., *Effect of St John's wort on drug metabolism by induction of cytochrome P450 3A4 enzyme.* JAMA, 2003. 290(11): p. 1500-4.

[383] Markowitz, J.S., et al., *Effect of St. John's wort (Hypericum perforatum) on cytochrome P-450 2D6 and 3A4 activity in healthy volunteers.* Life Sci, 2000. 66(9): p. PL133-9.

[384] Karyekar, C.S., N.D. Eddington, and T.C. Dowling, *Effect of St. John's Wort extract on intestinal expression of cytochrome P4501A2: studies in LS180 cells.* J Postgrad Med, 2002. 48(2): p. 97-100.

[385] Dresser, G.K., et al., *Coordinate induction of both cytochrome P4503A and MDR1 by St John's wort in healthy subjects.* Clin Pharmacol Ther, 2003. 73(1): p. 41-50.

[386] Dostalek, M., et al., *Effect of St John's wort (Hypericum perforatum) on cytochrome P-450 activity in perfused rat liver.* Life Sci, 2005. 78(3): p. 239-44.

[387] Chaudhary, A. and K.L. Willett, *Inhibition of human cytochrome CYP 1 enzymes by flavonoids of St. John's wort.* Toxicology, 2006. 217(2-3): p. 194-205.

[388] Durr, D., et al., *St John's Wort induces intestinal P-glycoprotein/MDR1 and intestinal and hepatic CYP3A4.* Clin Pharmacol Ther, 2000. 68(6): p. 598-604.

[389] Zhou, S.F. and X. Lai, *An update on clinical drug interactions with the herbal antidepressant St. John's wort.* Curr Drug Metab, 2008. 9(5): p. 394-409.

[390] Jiang, X., et al., *Effect of St John's wort and ginseng on the pharmacokinetics and pharmacodynamics of warfarin in healthy subjects.* Br J Clin Pharmacol, 2004. 57(5): p. 592-9.

[391] Lau, W.C., et al., *The effect of St John's Wort on the pharmacodynamic response of clopidogrel in hyporesponsive volunteers and patients: increased platelet inhibition by enhancement of CYP3A4 metabolic activity.* J Cardiovasc Pharmacol, 2011. 57(1): p. 86-93.

[392] Groning, R., J. Breitkreutz, and R.S. Muller, *Physico-chemical interactions between extracts of Hypericum perforatum L. and drugs.* Eur J Pharm Biopharm, 2003. 56(2): p. 231-6.

[393] Nebel, A., et al., *Potential metabolic interaction between St. John's wort and theophylline.* Ann Pharmacother, 1999. 33(4): p. 502.

[394] Morimoto, T., et al., *Effect of St. John's wort on the pharmacokinetics of theophylline in healthy volunteers.* J Clin Pharmacol, 2004. 44(1): p. 95-101.

[395] *Toxicity. St. John's wort--interactions with indinavir and other drugs.* TreatmentUpdate, 2000. 12(2): p. 9-11.

[396] Hu, Y.F., et al., *Effects of St. John's wort extract on indinavir pharmacokinetics in rats: differentiation of intestinal and hepatic impacts.* Life Sci, 2009. 85(7-8): p. 296-302.

[397] Miller, J.L., *Interaction between indinavir and St. John's wort reported.* Am J Health Syst Pharm, 2000. 57(7): p. 625-6.

[398] Piscitelli, S.C., et al., *Indinavir concentrations and St John's wort.* Lancet, 2000. 355(9203): p. 547-8.

[399] Andren, L., A. Andreasson, and R. Eggertsen, *Interaction between a commercially available St. John's wort product (Movina) and atorvastatin in patients with hypercholesterolemia.* Eur J Clin Pharmacol, 2007. 63(10): p. 913-6.

[400] Eggertsen, R., A. Andreasson, and L. Andren, *Effects of treatment with a commercially available St John's Wort product (Movina) on cholesterol levels in patients with hypercholesterolemia treated with simvastatin.* Scand J Prim Health Care, 2007. 25(3): p. 154-9.

[401] Andelic, S., *[Bigeminy--the result of interaction between digoxin and St. John's wort].* Vojnosanit Pregl, 2003. 60(3): p. 361-4.

[402] Birdsall, T.C., *St. John's wort and irinotecan-induced diarrhea.* Toxicol Appl Pharmacol, 2007. 220(1): p. 108; author reply 109-10.

[403] Dasgupta, A., *Herbal supplements and therapeutic drug monitoring: focus on digoxin immunoassays and interactions with St. John's wort.* Ther Drug Monit, 2008. 30(2): p. 212-7.

[404] Frye, R.F., et al., *Effect of St John's wort on imatinib mesylate pharmacokinetics.* Clin Pharmacol Ther, 2004. 76(4): p. 323-9.

[405] Hu, Z., et al., *St. John's Wort modulates the toxicities and pharmacokinetics of CPT-11 (irinotecan) in rats.* Pharm Res, 2005. 22(6): p. 902-14.

[406] Hu, Z.P., et al., *A mechanistic study on altered pharmacokinetics of irinotecan by St. John's wort.* Curr Drug Metab, 2007. 8(2): p. 157-71.

[407] Mathijssen, R.H., et al., *Effects of St. John's wort on irinotecan metabolism.* J Natl Cancer Inst, 2002. 94(16): p. 1247-9.

[408] Mueller, S.C., et al., *Effect of St John's wort dose and preparations on the pharmacokinetics of digoxin.* Clin Pharmacol Ther, 2004. 75(6): p. 546-57.

[409] Rengelshausen, J., et al., *Opposite effects of short-term and long-term St John's wort intake on voriconazole pharmacokinetics.* Clin Pharmacol Ther, 2005. 78(1): p. 25-33.

[410] Tannergren, C., et al., *St John's wort decreases the bioavailability of R- and S-verapamil through induction of the first-pass metabolism.* Clin Pharmacol Ther, 2004. 75(4): p. 298-309.

[411] Xie, H.G., *Additional discussions regarding the altered metabolism and transport of omeprazole after long-term use of St John's wort.* Clin Pharmacol Ther, 2005. 78(4): p. 440-1.

[412] Eich-Hochli, D., et al., *Methadone maintenance treatment and St. John's Wort - a case report.* Pharmacopsychiatry, 2003. 36(1): p. 35-7.

[413] Sarino, L.V., et al., *Drug interaction between oral contraceptives and St. John's Wort: appropriateness of advice received from community pharmacists and health food store clerks.* J Am Pharm Assoc (2003), 2007. 47(1): p. 42-7.

[414] Schwarz, U.I., B. Buschel, and W. Kirch, *Unwanted pregnancy on self-medication with St John's wort despite hormonal contraception.* Br J Clin Pharmacol, 2003. 55(1): p. 112-3.

[415] Will-Shahab, L., et al., *St John's wort extract (Ze 117) does not alter the pharmacokinetics of a low-dose oral contraceptive.* Eur J Clin Pharmacol, 2009. 65(3): p. 287-94.

[416] Hall, S.D., et al., *The interaction between St John's wort and an oral contraceptive.* Clin Pharmacol Ther, 2003. 74(6): p. 525-35.

[417] Pfrunder, A., et al., *Interaction of St John's wort with low-dose oral contraceptive therapy: a randomized controlled trial.* Br J Clin Pharmacol, 2003. 56(6): p. 683-90.

[418] Bhavnani, B.R., *Pharmacokinetics and pharmacodynamics of conjugated equine estrogens: chemistry and metabolism.* Proc Soc Exp Biol Med, 1998. 217(1): p. 6-16.

[419] Tsuchiya, Y., M. Nakajima, and T. Yokoi, *Cytochrome P450-mediated metabolism of estrogens and its regulation in human.* Cancer Lett, 2005. 227(2): p. 115-24.

[420] Ranney, R.E., *Comparative Metabolism of 17alpha-Ethynyl Steroids Used in Oral-Contraceptives.* Journal of Toxicology and Environmental Health, 1977. 3(1-2): p. 139-166.

[421] Alscher, D.M. and U. Klotz, *Drug interaction of herbal tea containing St. John's wort with cyclosporine.* Transpl Int, 2003. 16(7): p. 543-4.

[422] Barone, G.W., et al., *Drug interaction between St. John's wort and cyclosporine.* Ann Pharmacother, 2000. 34(9): p. 1013-6.

[423] Bauer, S., et al., *Alterations in cyclosporin A pharmacokinetics and metabolism during treatment with St John's wort in renal transplant patients.* Br J Clin Pharmacol, 2003. 55(2): p. 203-11.

[424] Breidenbach, T., et al., *Profound drop of cyclosporin A whole blood trough levels caused by St. John's wort (Hypericum perforatum).* Transplantation, 2000. 69(10): p. 2229-30.

[425] Karliova, M., et al., *Interaction of Hypericum perforatum (St. John's wort) with cyclosporin A metabolism in a patient after liver transplantation.* J Hepatol, 2000. 33(5): p. 853-5.

[426] Mai, I., et al., *Hyperforin content determines the magnitude of the St John's wort-cyclosporine drug interaction.* Clin Pharmacol Ther, 2004. 76(4): p. 330-40.

[427] Mai, I., et al., *Hazardous pharmacokinetic interaction of Saint John's wort (Hypericum perforatum) with the immunosuppressant cyclosporin.* Int J Clin Pharmacol Ther, 2000. 38(10): p. 500-2.

[428] Moschella, C. and B.L. Jaber, *Interaction between cyclosporine and Hypericum perforatum (St. John's wort) after organ transplantation.* Am J Kidney Dis, 2001. 38(5): p. 1105-7.

[429] Bolley, R., et al., *Tacrolimus-induced nephrotoxicity unmasked by induction of the CYP3A4 system with St John's wort.* Transplantation, 2002. 73(6): p. 1009.

[430] Hebert, M.F., et al., *Effects of St. John's wort (Hypericum perforatum) on tacrolimus pharmacokinetics in healthy volunteers.* J Clin Pharmacol, 2004. 44(1): p. 89-94.

[431] Mai, I., et al., *Impact of St John's wort treatment on the pharmacokinetics of tacrolimus and mycophenolic acid in renal transplant patients.* Nephrol Dial Transplant, 2003. 18(4): p. 819-22.

[432] Buchholzer, M.L., et al., *Dual modulation of striatal acetylcholine release by hyperforin, a constituent of St. John's wort.* J Pharmacol Exp Ther, 2002. 301(2): p. 714-9.

[433] Chatterjee, S.S., et al., *Hyperforin as a possible antidepressant component of hypericum extracts.* Life Sci, 1998. 63(6): p. 499-510.

[434] Gordon, J.B., *SSRIs and St.John's Wort: possible toxicity?* Am Fam Physician, 1998. 57(5): p. 950,953.

[435] Hirano, K., et al., *Effects of oral administration of extracts of Hypericum perforatum (St John's wort) on brain serotonin transporter, serotonin uptake and behaviour in mice.* J Pharm Pharmacol, 2004. 56(12): p. 1589-95.

[436] Kiewert, C., et al., *Stimulation of hippocampal acetylcholine release by hyperforin, a constituent of St. John's Wort.* Neurosci Lett, 2004. 364(3): p. 195-8.

[437] Kobak, K.A., et al., *St. John's wort in generalized anxiety disorder: three more case reports.* J Clin Psychopharmacol, 2003. 23(5): p. 531-2.

[438] Niederhofer, H., *St. John's wort may diminish methylphenidate's efficacy in treating patients suffering from attention deficit hyperactivity disorder.* Med Hypotheses, 2007. 68(5): p. 1189.

[439] Saraga, M. and D.F. Zullino, *[St. John's Wort, corticosteroids, cocaine, alcohol... and a first manic episode].* Praxis (Bern 1994), 2005. 94(23): p. 987-9.

[440] Schneck, C., *St. John's wort and hypomania.* J Clin Psychiatry, 1998. 59(12): p. 689.

[441] Turkanovic, J., S.N. Ngo, and R.W. Milne, *Effect of St John's wort on the disposition of fexofenadine in the isolated perfused rat liver.* J Pharm Pharmacol, 2009. 61(8): p. 1037-42.

[442] Uebelhack, R. and L. Franke, *In vitro effects of St. John's wort extract and hyperforin on 5 HT uptake and efflux in human blood platelets.* Pharmacopsychiatry, 2001. 34 Suppl 1: p. S146-7.

[443] Van Strater, A.C. and J.P. Bogers, *Interaction of St John's wort (Hypericum perforatum) with clozapine.* Int Clin Psychopharmacol, 2012. 27(2): p. 121-4.

[444] Wang, Z., et al., *Effect of St John's wort on the pharmacokinetics of fexofenadine.* Clin Pharmacol Ther, 2002. 71(6): p. 414-20.

[445] Wonnemann, M., A. Singer, and W.E. Muller, *Inhibition of synaptosomal uptake of 3H-L-glutamate and 3H-GABA by hyperforin, a major constituent of St. John's Wort: the role of amiloride sensitive sodium conductive pathways.* Neuropsychopharmacology, 2000. 23(2): p. 188-97.

[446] Johne, A., et al., *Decreased plasma levels of amitriptyline and its metabolites on comedication with an extract from St. John's wort (Hypericum perforatum).* J Clin Psychopharmacol, 2002. 22(1): p. 46-54.

[447] Barbenel, D.M., et al., *Mania in a patient receiving testosterone replacement postorchidectomy taking St John's wort and sertraline.* J Psychopharmacol, 2000. 14(1): p. 84-6.

[448] *Final report on the safety assessment of Hypericum perforatum extract and Hypericum perforatum oil.* Int J Toxicol, 2001. 20 Suppl 2: p. 31-9.

[449] Beattie, P.E., et al., *Can St John's wort (hypericin) ingestion enhance the erythemal response during high-dose ultraviolet A1 therapy?* Br J Dermatol, 2005. 153(6): p. 1187-91.

[450] Traynor, N.J., et al., *Photogenotoxicity of hypericin in HaCaT keratinocytes: implications for St. John's Wort supplements and high dose UVA-1 therapy.* Toxicol Lett, 2005. 158(3): p. 220-4.

[451] Cotterill, J.A., *Severe phototoxic reaction to laser treatment in a patient taking St John's Wort.* J Cosmet Laser Ther, 2001. 3(3): p. 159-60.

[452] Putnik, K., et al., *Enhanced radiation sensitivity and radiation recall dermatitis (RRD) after hypericin therapy -- case report and review of literature.* Radiat Oncol, 2006. 1: p. 32.

[453] Kammerer, B., et al., *HPLC-MS/MS analysis of willow bark extracts contained in pharmaceutical preparations.* Phytochem Anal, 2005. 16(6): p. 470-8.

[454] Li, L.S., et al., *[Determination of salicin in extract of willow bark by high performance liquid chromatography].* Se Pu, 2001. 19(5): p. 446-8.

[455] Fiebich, B.L. and K. Appel, *Anti-inflammatory effects of willow bark extract.* Clin Pharmacol Ther, 2003. 74(1): p. 96; author reply 96-7.

[456] Wagner, I., et al., *Influence of willow bark extract on cyclooxygenase activity and on tumor necrosis factor alpha or interleukin 1 beta release in vitro and ex vivo.* Clin Pharmacol Ther, 2003. 73(3): p. 272-4.

[457] Khayyal, M.T., et al., *Mechanisms involved in the anti-inflammatory effect of a standardized willow bark extract.* Arzneimittelforschung, 2005. 55(11): p. 677-87.

[458] Krivoy, N., Pavltzky, F., Eisenberg, E., et al., *Salix coretex (willow bark dry extract) effect on platelet aggregation.*. Drug Monitor, 1999. 21: p. 202.

[459] Krivoy, N., Pavlotzky, E., Chrubasik, S., Eisenberg, E., and Brook, G., *Effect of salicis cortex extract on human platelet aggregation.* Planta Med., 2001. 67(3): p. 209-212.

[460] Schmid, B., et al., *Efficacy and tolerability of a standardized willow bark extract in patients with osteoarthritis: randomized placebo-controlled, double blind clinical trial.* Phytother Res, 2001. 15(4): p. 344-50.

[461] Chrubasik, S., et al., *Treatment of low back pain exacerbations with willow bark extract: a randomized double-blind study.* Am J Med, 2000. 109(1): p. 9-14.

[462] U.S. Food and Drug Adminsitration, *Tainted Products Marketed as Dietary Supplements Potnetially Dangerous.* Available from: http://www.fda.gov/NewsEvents/Newsroom/PressAnnouncements/2010/ucm236967.htm [accessed 06/20/12].

[463] Deitel, M., *Sibutramine warning: hypertension and cardiac arrhythmias reported.* Obes Surg, 2002. 12(3): p. 422.

[464] Ernest, D., et al., *Sibutramine-associated QT interval prolongation and cardiac arrest.* Ann Pharmacother, 2008. 42(10): p. 1514-7.

[465] Geyer, H., et al., *Nutritional supplements cross-contaminated and faked with doping substances.* J Mass Spectrom, 2008. 43(7): p. 892-902.

[466] Wooltorton, E., *Obesity drug sibutramine (Meridia): hypertension and cardiac arrhythmias.* CMAJ, 2002. 166(10): p. 1307-8.

[467] Coogan, P.F., et al., *Phenolphthalein laxatives and risk of cancer.* J Natl Cancer Inst, 2000. 92(23): p. 1943-4.

[468] Vaysse, J., et al., *Analysis of adulterated herbal medicines and dietary supplements marketed for weight loss by DOSY 1H-NMR.* Food Addit Contam Part A Chem Anal Control Expo Risk Assess, 2010. 27(7): p. 903-16.

[469] Halbsguth, U., et al., *Necrotising vasculitis of the skin associated with an herbal medicine containing amfepramone.* Eur J Clin Pharmacol, 2009. 65(6): p. 647-8.

Chapter 5

Small Molecule Screens to Identify Inhibitors of Infectious Disease

Elizabeth Hong-Geller and Sofiya Micheva-Viteva

Additional information is available at the end of the chapter

http://dx.doi.org/10.5772/52502

1. Introduction

In the 1940's, the development of penicillin as a potent broad-range antibiotic revolutionized the treatment of infectious disease and ushered in a prolific discovery period of natural small molecules produced by microorganisms that were antagonistic towards the growth of other bacteria. Antibiotics have generally been classified by their mechanism of action. For example, the β-lactam compounds, penicillin and cephalosporins, disrupt the synthesis of the peptidoglycan layer of the bacterial cell wall, whereas protein synthesis inhibitors, such as tetracycline and some aminoglycosides, bind to the 30S ribosomal subunit and block addition of amino acids to the growing peptide chain. By the 1960's, the majority of all antibiotics in use today had been isolated and developed for public consumption, leading the U.S. Surgeon General to declare in 1968 that the war on infectious disease had been won.

Unfortunately, nature has found a way to thwart mankind's effort to contain infectious disease. Under the selective pressure of antibiotics that target different cell processes, bacteria have evolved to become resistant to the lethal effects of many classes of antibiotics. One stark example that has emerged as a major public health threat is methicillin-resistant *Staphylococcus aureus* (MRSA), which is estimated to cause ~19,000 deaths in the US annually [1]. MRSA has become resistant to β-lactam antibiotics by acquiring the resistance gene *mecA*, which encodes for a unique penicillin binding protein PBP2A that can function as a surrogate for native staphylococcal PBPs normally inactivated by β-lactam antibiotics. In the last decades of the 20th century, MRSA has continued to evolve in response to a continually changing human environment, from a primary agent of hospital-acquired infections to a multi-drug resistant strain that has also acquired Tn1546 transposon-based vancomycin resistance. Furthermore, the appearance of MRSA strains in a community setting may be a stepping stone to the evolution of a completely drug-resistant strain.

There is no question that new strategies that target different aspects of pathogen function are urgently needed to combat multi-drug resistant bacteria. However, very few new scaffolds for drug discovery developed after the 1960s have been found to be effective [2]. To date, only four new classes of antibiotics, including mutilins and lipopeptides, have been introduced, but none of these have proven to be as effective as the panel of classic antibiotics. Instead, established scaffolds have been modified or re-purposed to develop successive generations of effective antibiotics. For example, the core structure of cephalosporins have been left intact to preserve activity, but the peripheral chemical groups have been modified to impart the molecule with the ability to penetrate the bacterial membrane more efficiently or be more resistant to β-lactamase [3]. Modifications of four classic antibiotics, cephalosporin, penicillin, quinolone, and macrolide, account for ~73% of the "new" antibiotics filed between 1981 and 2005 [4]. It is also important to note that small compounds need to exhibit not only anti-microbial activity, but also minimized cytotoxic properties to widen their therapeutic window.

Although advances in organic synthesis have extended the lifetime of classic antibiotics through synthetic modifications, new scaffolds are also needed. Recent efforts to search for new modalities amongst previously-overlooked natural sources, such as unmined bacterial taxa and ecological niches, have started to bear fruit. The increasingly rapid data acquisition and low cost of ultra high-throughput sequencing has provided rich coverage of bacterial genomes and transcriptomes. For example, genomic analyses of a vancomycin-resistant strain of *Amycolatopsis orientalis* revealed the presence of genetic loci that encode for at least 10 other secondary metabolites. One compound, ECO-0501, exhibited strong anti-bacterial properties against Gram-positive pathogens, including several strains of MRSA [5]. Mass spectroscopy (MS) is another primary methodology used to identify small molecule metabolites with potential anti-microbial properties. The polycyclic small molecule, abyssomicin C, from the marine actinomycete *Verrucosispora* was characterized as an inhibitor of *p*-aminobenzoate biosynthesis by MS and also exhibited antimicrobial properties against MRSA strains [6].

2. Methodology for high-throughput screens (HTS) using small molecule libraries

The workhorse platform for anti-bacterial drug discovery is a chemical genetics HTS approach using small molecule compound libraries to identify candidates that inhibit bacterial growth or the function of key bacterial enzymes. Small molecules, generally <500 molecular weight, have the potential to enter cells and selectively perturb specific protein activity, thus functioning as therapeutic agents against disease. In general, the precise mechanism of inhibitor activity remains unknown in the initial screen. Subsequent identification of the molecular targets of small molecules will have to be performed to implicate the specific bacterial functions that were inactivated in the screen. Thus, HTS can sample a large unbiased collection of structurally diverse molecules to select compounds that perturb the defined cell phenotype of interest. (Fig. 1)

http://dx.doi.org/10.5772/52502

Various chemical compound libraries are now available through commercial and public resources that include FDA-approved bioactive compounds, therapeutic agents, and natural products. To maximize the structural complexity and diversity of small molecule libraries, scientists have also employed diversity-oriented synthesis,

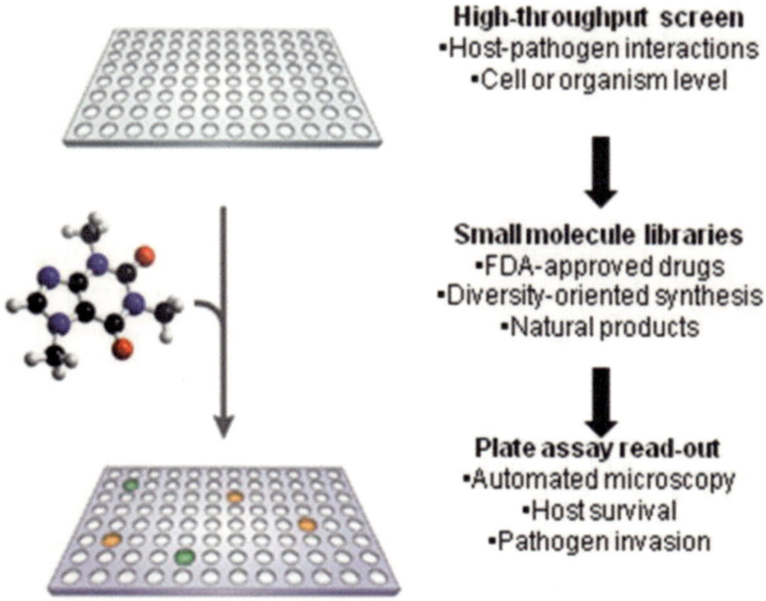

Figure 1. General flowchart of high-throughput methodology to screen small molecule libraries for inhibitors of host-pathogen interactions

in which different scaffolds are modified with highly diverse functional groups. [7, 8]. To bolster academic research in chemical biology efforts for HTS-driven identification of bioactive compounds, the NIH launched the Molecular Libraries Program in 2005 to offer access to ten large-scale automated HTS centers in the Molecular Libraries Probe Production Centers Network, including diverse compound libraries through the Small Molecule Repository and information on biological activities of small molecules in the PubChem BioAssay public database.

A variety of different molecular and cellular methods have been developed for HTS using small molecule libraries. Automated microscopy has been utilized for high-content, image-based screens of cells exposed to small molecules. Acquired cell images can be analyzed by automated image analysis software to quantitate physiological changes at the single-cell level, including phenotypes such as morphology and cell toxicity. Small molecule microarrays, in which ~10,000 small molecules are covalently bound to a glass slide, has been generated to detect high affinity binding to a protein of interest, as a potential inhibitor of function. Binding of the protein of interest to specific compounds on the microarray was then detected with fluorescent antibodies [9].

3. Disruption of host-pathogen interactions for novel drug discovery

Given the innovation gap in the discovery of novel antibiotics post-1960, strategies to inhibit novel targets are greatly needed to combat infectious disease. Multiple studies have identified small molecule inhibitors that target gene expression of pathogen TTSS components in *P. aeruginosa*, enteropathogenic *E. coli*, and *Y. pestis* [10, 11, 12]. The small molecule virstatin, 4-[N1,8-naphthalimide)]-n-butyric acid, was identified as an inhibitor of the transcriptional regulator ToxT in *Vibrio cholerae* [13]. The small molecule, 2-imino-5-arylidene thiazolidinone, which blocks TTSS-dependent functions in *S. typhimurium*, was also found to inhibit virulence in *Yersinia, Pseudomonas,* and *Francisella* strains, indicating that compounds can be identified that target common processes in multiple pathogens [14].

Research efforts have recently begun to focus on disruption of host-pathogen interactions as a new approach to identify potential targets for drug discovery, rather than solely on specific pathogen targets or processes. In particular, the screening of small molecule libraries to identify inhibitors that block pathogen infection of the host, using such phenotypes as pathogen invasion, host morphology, and pathogen replication in the host, is a powerful approach for therapeutic development that may uncover fundamental mechanisms of pathogenesis and potentially lead to discovery of new classes of anti-infective agents. Here, we describe case studies of the use of small molecules in host infection screens to identify novel inhibitors against infectious disease, including bacterial, viral, parasitic, and fungal infections. We will discuss these studies in the context of re-purposing known drugs, inhibitor specificity, and discovery of basic mechanisms of host-pathogen interactions. The screen results are summarized in Table 1.

Screening for inhibitors of intracellular infection

Intracellular pathogens, including viruses, parasites, and some bacteria, manipulate specific host factors in order to downregulate the host immune response or modulate host actin cytoskeleton rearrangements to induce phagocytic uptake of the pathogen. *L. monocytogenes,* an intracellular Gram-positive bacteria, infects the human host primarily through ingestion of contaminated foods and causes gastrointestinal infection. In 2011, *Listeria* contamination of cantaloupes led to at least 30 deaths and ~150 illnesses in 28 states. Following internalization of *L. monocytogenes* in host membrane-bound vacuoles, the pore-forming cytolysin, listeriolysin O (LLO) and a phosphatidylinositol-specific phospholipase C (PI-PLC) mediates lysis of the vacuoles to release the pathogen into the host cell cytosol. *L. monocytogenes* then polymerizes host actin to propel itself into adjacent host cells to continue the infection process. To identify compounds that inhibited *L. monocytogenes* intracellular infection, a screen of 480 small molecules from the Biomol ICCB Known Bioactives library was performed using automated microscopy and image analysis [15]. Murine bone marrow-derived macrophages were infected with a GFP-expressing *L. monocytogenes* strain to assess efficiency of invasion, survival, and replication in the host. Twenty-one compounds, affecting cell functions such as actin polymerization, calcium signaling, and apoptosis, were identified that markedly decreased *Listeria monocytogenes* infection efficiency. In particular, the FDA-approved anti-psychotic drug pimozide, used to treat Tourette's syndrome and schizophrenia, was shown to

http://dx.doi.org/10.5772/52502

decrease internalization of not just *L. monocytogenes*, but other bacterial species as well, including *Bacillus subtilis, Salmonella typhimurium,* and *E. coli.* Furthermore, pimozide decreased vacuole escape and cell-to-cell spread of *L. monocytogenes* in the host. Thus, pimozide is an example of a small molecule that can be re-purposed to treat infectious disease with potential for broad spectrum anti-microbial applications.

Parasites also employ a life cycle of host cell invasion, replication, and host cell lysis during onset of infection. *Taxoplasma gondii* is the protozoan intracellular human parasite of the phylum Apicomplexa and is related to *Plasmodium* and *Cryptosporidium*, the causative agents of malaria and diarrheal disease, respectively. To discover inhibitors of *T. gondii* invasion, a high-throughput

Pathogen	#Compounds	#Hits	Assay and methods	Ref
Bacteria				
L. monocytogenes	480	21	Host cell invasion, automated microscopy	15
P. aeruginosa	50,000	88	ExoU-,edoated host cytotoxicity	18
	56,280	6	Cytotoxicity in yeast model	19
Y. pseudotuberculosis	100,000	45	Translocation of Yops into the host	20
B. anthracis	70,094	30	Lethal factor entry into host	21
	10,000	24	Interaction between edema factor and CaM	22
P. syringae	~200	3	Bleaching of *Arabidopsis* seedlings	23
	80	1	Bleaching of *Arabidopsis* seedlings	24
Parasite				
T. gondii	12,160	24	Host cell invasion, motility, adhesins	16
Virus				
HIV	~200,000	27	Induction of viral latency	49

Table 1 Small molecule screens using host-pathogen systems

microscopy assay was developed to distinguish between extracellular and intracellular parasites in a BS-C-1 epithelial cell model, using differential labeling with fluorescent dyes [16]. Out of a 12,160 structurally-diverse small molecule library, 24 non-cytotoxic inhibitors were identified that reduced parasite invasion to <20% compared to control wells. These molecules inhibited different aspects of the infection process, including gliding motility and secretion of host cell adhesins. One of these inhibitors, tachypleginA, was found to post-translationally modify TgMLC1, a myosin light chain component of the *T. gondii* myosin motor complex, which drives host cell penetration and parasite mobility [17]. TgMLC1 exposed to the small molecule exhibited a rapid and irreversible change in electrophoretic mobility on SDS-PAGE gels. Although the exact nature of the modification remains unclear, the modification has been mapped to amino acids V46-R59 by mass spectroscopy. These studies provide key mechanistic information on the importance of *T. gondii* motility in pathogenesis and illustrate the potential for small molecules to form covalent interactions with target proteins.

Targeting virulence toxin mechanisms of infection

Many Gram-negative bacteria, including *Pseudomonas* and *Yersinia*, utilize the TTSS as a primary mechanism of virulence to inject effector proteins into the host cytosol to downregulate the host immune response. A host cytotoxicity assay was designed to screen for small molecule inhibitors of *Pseudomonas aeruginosa,* a leading cause of hospital-acquired infections in cystic fibrosis patients. *P. aeruginosa* ExoU, a TTSS effector protein, is a member of the patatin family of phospholipase A_2 (PLA_2) that can lyse host cell membranes during infection. A high-throughput screen of 50,000 compounds from the Chembridge Microformat Library E was performed using a colorimetric live/dead assay to identify small molecules that protected Chinese hamster ovary (CHO) cells from cytotoxicity mediated by *P. aeruginosa* expressing ExoU as the sole TTSS effector [18]. A primary list of 88 compounds exhibited rescue of CHO cells from ExoU-mediated cytotoxicity. The most effective compound, pseudolipasin A, inhibited ExoU function downstream of TTSS delivery into the host. In addition to inhibition of CHO cytotoxicity, pseudolipasin A also protected the amoeba *Dictyolstelium discoideum* from ExoU-mediated killing by *P. aeruginosa* and inhibited cytotoxicity in the yeast *Saccharomyces cerevisiae* expressing ExoU. Interestingly, pseudolipasin A did not affect eukaryotic PLA_2, suggesting that this small molecule may specifically target bacterial PLA_2. Pseudolipasin A is representative of small molecules that do not kill or inhibit the growth of pathogens, but instead attenuate their virulence.

Inhibitors of *P. aeruginosa* virulence have also been identified using a cell-based yeast phenotypic assay in combination with a large-scale small molecule screen. A total of 505 *P. aeruginosa* virulence factors and essential genes were individually overexpressed in *S. cerevisae* to downselect genes that inhibited yeast growth [19]. Nine genes strongly or partially impaired yeast growth, including three TTSS effectors, ExoS, ExoT, and ExoY. ExoS has been previously shown to ADP-ribosylate multiple downstream targets, including vimentin, the Ras family of small GTP-binding proteins, and cyclophilin A. Given that ExoS is a critical mediator of *P. aeruginosa* chronic infections, a library of 56,280 compounds was screened to find inhibitors of ExoS ADP-ribosylation activity that rescued cytotoxicity in yeast. Six compounds were identified that restored yeast growth. The most promising compound, exosin, was found to modulate ExoS enzymatic activity *in vitro* and exhibited a protective effect against *P. aeruginosa* infection in mammalian CHO cells. This study demonstrates the effective use of a simple eukaryotic host, baker's yeast, as a tool for drug screening for applications in controlling infectious disease in humans.

Another pathogen family that employs the TTSS is *Yersinia,* which secrete Yop effectors into the host cell. There are three *Yersinia* human pathogens, *Y. pestis,* the etiological agent of plague via intradermal fleabites or inhalation, and *Y. pseudotuberculosis* and *Y. enterocolitica,* which cause mild and self-limiting enteric disease by the oral route. HTS strategies have been developed to identify small molecules that inhibit translocation of the Yops into host cells. A recombinant *Y. pseudotuberculosis* strain was constructed to express a chimeric protein containing the first 100 amino acids of YopE, which contains the proper translocation signals to inject into the host, fused to a fragment of β-lactamase. [20]. This bacterial strain was used to infect HEp-2 host cells treated with a non-membrane-permeating, non-fluorescent dye CCF2-AM, which fluoresces green at 520nm, as a result of intramolecular FRET between the 7-hydroxycoumarin and fluorescein molecules, conjugated by a lactam ring. Upon cellular uptake, CCF2-AM is modified by cytoplasmic esterases and is trapped in the host cell. If the YopE-β-lactamase fusion is introduced into the host, the β-lactamase will cleave the lactam ring in CCF2-AM and liberate the fluorescein, leaving the coumarin to fluoresce blue at 447nm. Using this differential fluorescence assay, 100,000 compounds from a number of sources, including the ChemDiv 2, ChemDiv 3, ChemDiv 4, Maybridge 3, Maybridge 4, and Biomol ICCB libraries, were screened for low ratios of blue-to-green fluorescence. In total, 200 compounds were deemed potential hits, and 45 were assessed further using secondary assays, including rounded host morphology in response to *Yersinia* infection. Finally, 6 compounds were found that inhibited translocation of effectors into the host without affecting expression and function of TTSS components. Several of these compounds also inhibited host cell rounding when induced by *Pseudomonas* effectors, suggesting that these compounds may have a broad-spectrum anti-infective effect.

A screen to identify small molecule inhibitors of *B. anthracis* also employed the CCF2-AM FRET assay. *B. anthracis*, the Gram-positive causative agent of anthrax, secretes three major toxins during infection, lethal factor (LF), protective antigen (PA), and edema factor (EF). A fusion protein between LF and β-lactamase was introduced into host cells by PA-directed endocytosis to hydrolyze the CCF2-AM fluorogenic substrate [21]. Out of 70,094 compounds tested, 1170 initial hits exhibited concentration-dependent inhibition of β-lactamase activity. Thirty compounds with known biological activities and/or were high confidence hits were selected for further analysis. Three compounds, NCGC00084148-01, diphyllin, and niclosamide, exhibited protective effects from anthrax LF, a LF fusion to *Pseudomonas* exotoxin, and diphtheria toxin in RAW264.7 murine macrophages and CHO cells, and are thought to interfere with toxin internalization in the host.

The interaction between *B. anthracis* EF and its cellular activator, calmodulin (CaM), became the basis of a two-step tandem screen to identify small molecule inhibitors of anthrax infection. A library of 10,000 compounds (Chembridge, Library # ET350-1) in pools of 8 was screened to identify small molecules that blocked an EF-induced flat to round morphology change in Y1 murine adrenocortical cells [22]. Twenty-four initial hits were then individually tested using surface plasmon resonance (SPR) to identify molecules that block interactions between EF and immobilized CaM. One compound, (4-[4-(3,4-cichlorophenyl)-thiazolylamino]-benzenesulfonamide) 10506-2A, efficiently inhibited EF-CaM binding in a dose-dependent manner, and was found to specifically target the CaM binding region of EF by fluorescence spectroscopy. Since this compound was found to be toxic in cultured mammalian cells, a series of structurally-related compounds was synthesized, and a new inhibitory compound with reduced toxicity was subsequently identified.

Small molecule discovery in plant-pathogen interactions

Discovery of small molecule inhibitors has also been extended to plant pathogen systems as an approach to develop commercially-relevant chemicals to protect crops assets from disease. The Gram-negative pathogen *Pseudomonas syringae* expresses a TTSS, enters plant tissues through the stomata or wounds, and infects a wide range of plant species. A major challenge in the application of small molecule screens to plant-pathogen interactions is the development of high-throughput methodology with a plant model system. A high-throughput liquid assay was developed based on *P. syringae*-induced bleaching of *Arabidopsis thali-*

ana cotyledon seedlings, which signifies a loss of chlorophyll from plant tissues and is indicative of bacterial pathogenesis [23]. A screen of ~200 small molecules active in *Arabidopsis* (LATCA, Library of Active Compounds in Arabidopsis) identified several sulfanilamide compounds, including sulfamethoxazole, sulfadiazine, and sulfapyridine, that prevented cotyledon bleaching upon *P. syringae* infection. The most potent compound, sulfamethoxazole, also inhibited *P. syringae* growth in mature soil-grown plants. A similar assay was used to implicate the same compound, sulfamethoxazole, and the indole alkaloid gramine as inhibitors of *Fusarium graminearum* fungal infection in *Arabidopsis* and wheat, indicating that this strategy represents a relevant surrogate system for identification of compounds that can prevent agriculturally-important infectious disease [24].

Combinational antiviral therapies for HIV

Given that viral pathogens are absolutely dependent on the host for propagation, even more so than bacterial pathogens, research in host-directed anti-virals has advanced at a faster pace than that for anti-bacterial agents. Human Immunodeficiency virus type 1 (HIV-1), a lentivirus of the retroviral family and the causative agent of AIDS, is the most-widely studied viral pathogen to date. HIV-1 infection causes a dramatic decline in host CD4+ T cell numbers and a progressive failure of the immune response, which makes the host susceptible to opportunistic infections and cancer. The highly glycosylated HIV-1 envelope, in combination with the extreme diversity of circulating viral strains, have presented daunting challenges for development of an effective vaccine. Furthermore, the virus establishes chronic infection that resists the highly active antiretroviral therapy (HAART). Conventional HAART for HIV-1 infection combines three main classes of anti-viral drugs:

1. nucleoside reverse transcriptase inhibitors (NRTIs),
2. non-nucleoside RT inhibitors (NNRTIs), which target the non-catalytic domain of RT, and
3. protease inhibitors (PIs).

HAART is usually patient-specific, and its formulation is determined by the viral load and drug resistance. A traditional HAART consists of two NRTIs and a NNRTI or a PI [25]. More advanced combination therapies include a fourth class of antiretroviral drugs, HIV entry inhibitors. HIV-1 entry into human cells is dependent on several sequential steps that include binding of viral envelope protein gp120 to the CD4 receptor, and conformational change in gp120 that increases its affinity to the chemokine co-receptors (CCR5 or CXCR4) and exposes gp41, an HIV envelope protein that executes the fusion of HIV and host cell membranes.

Currently, there are two approved inhibitors of HIV-1 entry:

1. enfuvirtide, a peptide fusion inhibitor that binds to gp41 and
2. maraviroc, a small molecule entry inhibitor that prevents interaction between gp120 and CCR5.

The β-chemokine receptor CCR5 was found to act as a major co-receptor for the macrophage-tropic HIV-1 R5 strains, predominant in the early asymptomatic stages of virus infec-

http://dx.doi.org/10.5772/52502

tion, whereas the T-cell-tropic strains (using the CXCR4 co-receptor) become prevalent in the symptomatic stages concomitant with the decline of CD4+ T-cells [26]. CCR5 is an attractive target for development of HIV-1 entry inhibitors, given the discovery that HIV-1 non-progressors, individuals homozygous for a 32-bp deletion in the coding region of CCR5 gene (CCR5Δ32) were naturally resistant to infection with R5 HIV-1 [27]. Natural and synthetic CCR5 ligands such as RANTES, AOP-RANTES, Mip-1α, Mip-1β,and Met-RANTES were found to efficiently protect against R5 HIV-1 infection [28, 29]. Thus, the first published high throughput screen (HTS) for discovery of non- peptide inhibitors of HIV-1 entry was performed in a virus-free cell-based system using [^{125}I]-labeled RANTES. A strong inhibitor of RANTES binding to CCR5 stably expressed on the surface of CHO cells was identified from the library of Takeda Chemical Industries. Further chemical modifications of the lead compound designated TAK-779 produced a potent (IC50 1.4 nM in CHO/CCR cells) and selective CCR5 antagonist capable of blocking R5 HIV-1 infection *in vitro* [30].

The number of CCR5 inhibitors has significantly grown since the discovery of TAK-779, but very few compounds have entered clinical trials, and only maraviroc has been approved for clinical use [31]. A radiolabeled-chemokine binding assay similar to one applied for the identification of TAK-779 was used in a HTS of a small molecule library at Pfizer for the discovery of UK-107,543, which had become a scaffold for intensive medicinal chemistry, producing ~1,000 analog compounds, from which maraviroc (UK-427,857) was selected for its excellent preclinical pharmacokinetics (90% inhibitory concentration of 2 nM in pool of PBMCs from various donors) [32]. Despite its proven efficacy against HIV-1 R5 infection, maraviroc is vulnerable to gp120 escape mutations [33]. Site-directed mutagenesis and molecular modeling studies have identified a common binding pocket on CCR5 that is shared by various small-molecule CCR5 inhibitors [34, 35, 36]. Emerging details on gp120 and CCR5 points of interaction and binding thermodynamics provide valuable information that can be applied in developing tools for rational design of novel HIV-1 entry inhibitors [37, 38]. Efficient block of HIV entry into host cells is essential to curtail virus dissemination and is a key step towards eradication of HIV infection. The current HAART regiment can reduce HIV replication to very low levels (below 50 copies/ml plasma) and can lead to recovery of CD4$^+$ T-cell counts but not cure the infection. Patients that have been successfully treated with HAART for years have experienced a rapid virus rebound upon termination of the therapeutic regiment [39, 40]. Such clinical cases present evidence that HIV establishes a chronic infection that resists current HAART designed to target actively replicating virus. A deliberate and controllable induction of HIV-1 replication from its latent reservoirs in combination with HAART is a novel and actively pursued approach that aims to eliminate both active and latent viral pools [41].

Researchers often seek new anti-infective agents amongst small molecules that have previously been approved for the treatment of cancer and neurological diseases, since they have well-established pharmacokinetics and in most cases, known molecular mechanisms of action. One example of this is the histone deacetylase (HDAC) inhibitor, valproic acid (VA), which had previously been approved for treatment of neurological and psychiatric disorders. HIV-1 has been shown to enter dormancy using epigenetic silencing via deaceylation of histones in the vicinity of the integrated viral genome [42]. Thus, VA was tested as a potential agent to disrupt HIV-1 latent infection. However, years of VA treatment in combination with HAART showed no clearance of the latent HIV reservoir [43]. A more potent HDAC inhibitor, suberoylanilide hydroxamic acid (SAHA), approved for treatment of cutaneous T-cell lymphoma, was subsequently tested as a potential agent that could 'flush out' HIV-1 from latently infected cells, based on its superior effect to VA in cell culture models [44, 45]. A substantial effort has also been invested in the design and synthesis of bryostatin chemical analogs, small molecules that activate protein kinase C (PKC) with single nanomolar concentration [46]. PKC activation leads to phosphorylation of nuclear factor κB (NFκB), a key transcription factor regulator of HIV-1 gene expression [47]. However, modulation of NFκB activity requires great caution, since abnormal NFκB signaling has been related to the pathophysiology of inflammatory diseases and neurodegenerative disorders [48].

A HTS of a small molecule library recently identified novel HIV latency activators [49]. The screen was performed using a lymphoma $CD4^+$ T-cell line (SupT1) harboring latent recombinant HIV-1 and two reporters that reflect early and late virus gene expression incorporated in the HIV-1 genome [50]. A luminescent assay based on secreted alkaline phosphatase (SEAP) activity, incorporated in the late virus gene transcripts, was applied to screen a chemical library of ~200,000 compounds. Validation of 27 hits with diverse chemical structures demonstrated induction of latent virus from various cell models. Compounds with a selective index (CC_{50}/EC_{50}) above 25 were chosen for downstream medicinal chemistry modifications. Moreover, the lead compounds were shown to reactivate latent HIV from primary resting $CD4^+$ T-cells with no induction of cell proliferation. Small molecule activators of latent HIV that act in concert using different mechanisms have a better chance of purging the virus out of infected cells [49]. Such pre-clinical data strongly suggests that successful treatment of HIV infection can be achieved only through combinational therapy consisting of diverse class of antiviral drugs.

4. Whole animal small molecule screens using *C. elegans*

In vitro high-throughput screens have several limitations for the discovery of therapeutic inhibitors with high efficacy. Synthetic compound libraries often contain toxic compounds with poor pharmacokinetic properties, and many *in vitro* assays are not physiologically-relevant in the context of which a specific drug is expected to function. In a previous section, we had described the use of a HTS whole organism-based assay based on *Arabidopsis* seedlings as the host system. Here, we detail the use of a whole animal model, the nematode worm *C. elegans*, in chemical screens that permit simultaneous assessment of the immunomodulatory effects, potential toxicity of compounds, and drug efficacy in a host with a functioning immune system. The results of these screens are summarized in Table 2. Whole animal screens have the distinct advantage of being able to directly discard compounds that induce organismal toxicity and can identify compounds that target host-pathogen interactions in a relevant physiological context.

C. elegans, a hermaphroditic nematode normally found in soil, is a versatile, more ethically-acceptable whole animal system for high-throughput analysis of host response to pathogen infection. *C. elegans* contains a fully sequenced genome that facilitates both genetic and genomic analysis, offering an ideal compromise between organismal complexity and experimental tractability. *C. elegans* offers other experimental advantages, including a rapid 2-3 week life span, simple growth conditions, target-selected gene inactivation, and a relatively low cost of maintenance compared to other whole animal systems. A wealth of experimental data has demonstrated that many developmental, neurological, and biochemical processes have been highly conserved between *C. elegans* and mammals. For example, cellular functions as diverse as innate immunity, the first line of defense against pathogen infection, and RNA interference to downregulate gene expression via double-stranded RNA, are found in both *C. elegans* and higher eukaryotes, suggesting the existence of a common ancestor of these diverse species. Thus, anti-infective compounds identified using a *C. elegans* infection model may also be translatable in humans.

C. elegans as a model host system has been well-studied for numerous bacterial pathogens, including the Gram-positive *S. aureus*, *S. pneumoniae*, and *B. thuringiensis*, and the Gram-negative *B. pseudomallei*, *P. aeruginosa*, and *S. marcescens*. In general, different types of bacteria are fed to *C. elegans* in place of their normal *E. coli* food source to provoke detectable symptoms of illness, such as locomotion dysregulation, intestinal cell lysis, and shortened life span.

Small molecule inhibitors of bacterial infection

A small manual screen of 6000 synthetic compounds and 1136 natural extracts were analyzed in an immunocompromised mutant of *C. elegans* infected with *Enterococcus faecalis* to identify compounds that promoted host survival. [51]. A total of 16 compounds and 9 extracts were identified that either modulated bacterial growth *in vitro*, impaired pathogen virulence, or boosted host innate immunity. Furthermore, 15 out the 16 compounds did not kill *C. elegans* or mammalian erythrocytes, indicating that the compounds are not toxic.

The development of automated sorting and handling of *C. elegans* rapidly enabled high-throughput screening of small chemical libraries to identify compounds that enhanced survival of *C. elegans* in response to bacterial infection. This methodology was enabled by the Complex Object Parametric Analyzer and Sorter (COPAS) BioSort worm sorter (Union Biometrica) to dispense a defined number of living worms into multi-well plates, which were then imaged using automated microscopy to quantify worm survival. A library of 37,200 compounds and natural product extracts was screened using the same *C. elegans-E. faecalis* infection system described above [52]. Twenty-eight compounds and extracts were identified that enhanced survival of infected *C. elegans*. Six structural classes of identified compounds did not affect the growth of *E. faecalis* itself, suggesting that the small molecules inhibited a specific aspect of the host-pathogen interaction. Interestingly, two structural classes are similar to compounds previously identified in a high-throughput screen to identify inhibitors of *P. aeruginosa* biofilm development, indicating the presence of common molecular targets across multiple bacterial species for drug discovery [53].

A *P. aeruginosa* infection model of *C. elegans* has also been developed to screen for novel anti-infective compounds. The high-throughput assay was based on *P. aeruginosa*-induced slow killing of *C. elegans* in the presence of 1300 bioactive extracts produced by endophytic fungi associated with medicinal plants [54]. The screen identified 36 extracts that promoted the survival of the infected worms, while 4 extracts were found to inhibit *P. aeruginosa* growth using a disc diffusion assay. Given that these extracts contain a mixture of metabolites, the specific compound against *P. aeruginosa* remains to be determined. Nevertheless, this study illustrates the rich reservoir of small molecules in natural symbiotic organisms with antibacterial activity.

Pathogen	#Compounds	#Hits	Assay and methods	Ref
E. faecalis	7136	25	Host survival	51
	37,214	28	HTS, automated microscopy of host survival	52
P. aeruginosa	1300	40	Host survival	54
C. albicans	1266	15	Host survival, inhibition of *C. albicans* filamentation	55
	3228	19	HTS, co-inoculation of worms with *C. albicans*	58

Table 2 Small molecule screens using *C. elegans* as host model for infection

Discovery of novel antifungal agents

The *C. elegans* infection model was also used to screen for compounds that prolonged host survival following infection with the human pathogenic fungus *Candida albicans*. [55]. Given that most compounds that have antifungal activity are also toxic to the human host, high-throughput methods can greatly increase the likelihood of discovering specific antifungal inhibitors. From a screen of 1266 compounds with known pharmaceutical activities, 15 small molecules were identified that increased survival of *C. albicans*-infected nematodes and inhibited *in vivo* filamentation of *C. albicans*, a mechanism of pathogenesis seen during mammalian infection. Two compounds, caffeic acid phenethyl ester (CAPE), a natural component of honeybee propolis, and the fluoroquinolone agent enoxacin, were further shown to exhibit antifungal activity in a mouse model, validating the use of a *C. elegans* model for potential targets in a mammalian system. Interestingly, CAPE is known to inhibit the mammalian transcription factor NF-κB and to induce immunomodulatory effects in mice [56, 57]. Since *C. elegans* does not express a NF-κB homolog, it may be the case that CAPE affects alternative targets to achieve antifungal activity.

An automated high-throughput screen using the COPAS Biosort was also applied to *C. albicans* infection of *C. elegans* to assess a library of 3,228 compounds consisting of 1948 bioactive compounds and 1280 small molecules derived from diversity-oriented synthesis [58]. In total, 19 compounds were identified that increased *C. elegans* survival in response to *C. albicans* infection, 7 of which are currently used antifungal agents. Several immunosuppressant agents identified in this screen, including ascomycin, cyclosporin A, and FK-506, were previously found to exhibit weak antifungal activity against *Cryptococcus* and *Aspergillus*, in addition to *C. albicans* [59, 60]. Other hits were predicted to affect an array of biological activities, such as dequalinium chloride, a potent anti-tumor and protein kinase C inhibitor, and triadimefon, an inhibitor of ergosterol biosynthesis.

5. Conclusion

Chemical library screens are a potent and valuable molecular tool for HTS identification of potential inhibitors of infectious disease. The long-standing paradigm to treat pathogen infection with small molecules that specifically target pathogen growth or metabolism has led to our current dilemma of microbial drug resistance and re-emergence of once-contained infectious diseases. Thus, new approaches to target pathogen virulence or host response factors rather than essential pathogen functions have become increasingly more attractive strategies that are less likely to induce microbial resistance. Some compounds, such as the FDA-approved anti-psychotic, pimozide, exhibited inhibitory properties against infection by several pathogens, suggesting that small molecules can potentially be developed as broad-spectrum anti-infectives. Although the molecular mechanism of inhibition by small molecules remains unknown in most cases, it may be possible to make an educated guess if targeted pathogens share a common virulence strategy, such as the Type III secretion system in Gram-negative bacteria. In other cases, identification of an inhibitor can lead to a molecular understanding of the infection mechanism. For example, the small molecule, tachyplegi-nA, was found to post-translationally modify TgMLC1, a myosin light chain component, to drive host cell penetration by the parasite *T. gondii* [17].

From the various studies detailed in this review, it is apparent that the library screens represent a first step on the road of drug discovery. There has been a growing realization that fundamental discovery of biological mechanisms oftentimes reaches a 'valley of death', in which potential translation avenues into clinical therapies and diagnostics for disease treatment comes to a standstill and is lost. NIH is addressing this widening gap between basic and clinical research with the establishment of Clinical and Translational Science Centers across the country. The research community will have to remain pro-active to move promising leads from the initial screen stage into downstream validation and development modes in a timely manner. As with any drug development strategy, there still remain multiple technical challenges that need to be overcome before small molecule inhibitors can successfully transition into the clinic. Researchers will need to assess such parameters as compound toxicity, pharmacokinetics and pharmacodynamics, and validation in animal models. However, FDA-approved small molecule libraries can be applied to HTS as a cost-effective method to identify existing licensed drugs for repurposing from diseases unrelated to microbial infection. Furthermore, the development of the *C. elegans* whole organism model for small molecule screening provides a novel methodology to simultaneously assess compound toxicity and host response to pathogen infection. It would be informative to determine whether small molecules identified from conventional host cell culture studies can also inhibit pathogen infection in the *C. elegans* model. Future anti-infective treatments will most likely be comprised of combination therapies that produce additive or synergistic effects to target key processes in both the pathogen and the host. The overall promise of discovering novel anti-infective compounds has generated great hope in the biomedical community for discovery of new countermeasures against infectious disease.

Acknowledgements

The writing of this review was supported by a Los Alamos National Laboratory LDRD-DR grant to study development of novel inhibitors that block host-pathogen interactions.

Author details

Elizabeth Hong-Geller* and Sofiya Micheva-Viteva

*Address all correspondence to: ehong@lanl.gov

Bioscience Division, Los Alamos National Laboratory, Bioscience Division, Los Alamos, NM, USA

References

[1] Klevens, R. M., Morrison, M. A., Nadle, J., Petit, S., Gershman, K., Ray, S., Harrison, L. H., Lynfield, R., Dumyati, G., Townes, J. M., Craig, A. S., Zell, E. R., Fosheim, G. E., Mc Dougal, L. K., Carey, R. B., & Fridkin, S. K. (2007). Invasive methicillin-resistant Staphylococcus aureus infections in the United States. *JAMA*, 298, 1763-71.

[2] Fischbach, M. A., & Walsh, C. T. (2009). Antibiotics for emerging pathogens. *Science*, 325, 1089-93.

[3] Neu, H. C., & Fu, K. P. (1978). Cefuroxime, a beta-lactamase-resistant cephalosporin with a broad spectrum of gram-positive and-negative activity. *Antimicrob Agents Chemother*, 13, 657-64.

[4] Newman, D. J., & Cragg, G. M. (2007). Natural products as sources of new drugs over the last 25 years. *J Nat Prod*, 70, 461-77.

[5] Banskota, A. H., Mc Alpine, J. B., Sorensen, D., Ibrahim, A., Aouidate, M., Piraee, M., Alarco, A. M., Farnet, C. M., & Zazopoulos, E. (2006). Genomic analyses lead to novel secondary metabolites. *Part 3. ECO-0501, a novel antibacterial of a new class. J Antibiot (Tokyo)*, 59, 533-42.

[6] Bister, B., Bischoff, D., Strobele, M., Riedlinger, J., Reicke, A., Wolter, F., Bull, A. T., Zahner, H., Fiedler, H. P., & Sussmuth, R. D. (2004). Abyssomicin C-A polycyclic antibiotic from a marine Verrucosispora strain as an inhibitor of the p-aminobenzoic acid/tetrahydrofolate biosynthesis pathway. *Angew Chem Int Ed Engl*, 43, 2574-6.

[7] Schreiber, S. L. (2000). Target-oriented and diversity-oriented organic synthesis in drug discovery. *Science*, 287, 1964-9.

[8] Tan, D. S. (2005). Diversity-oriented synthesis: exploring the intersections between chemistry and biology. *Nat Chem Biol*, 1, 74-84.

[9] Kuruvilla, F. G., Shamji, A. F., Sternson, S. M., Hergenrother, P. J., & Schreiber, S. L. (2002). Dissecting glucose signalling with diversity-oriented synthesis and small-molecule microarrays. *Nature*, 416, 653-7.

[10] Aiello, D., Williams, J. D., Majgier-Baranowska, H., Patel, I., Peet, N. P., Huang, J., Lory, S., Bowlin, T. L., & Moir, D. T. (2010). Discovery and characterization of inhibitors of Pseudomonas aeruginosa type III secretion. *Antimicrob Agents Chemother*, 54, 1988-99.

[11] Gauthier, A., Robertson, M. L., Lowden, M., Ibarra, J. A., Puente, J. L., & Finlay, B. B. (2005). Transcriptional inhibitor of virulence factors in enteropathogenic Escherichia coli. Antimicrob Agents Chemother , 49, 4101-9.

[12] Pan, N. J., Brady, M. J., Leong, J. M., & Goguen, J. D. (2009). Targeting type III secretion in Yersinia pestis. *Antimicrob Agents Chemother*, 53, 385-92.

[13] Hung, D. T., Shakhnovich, E. A., Pierson, E., & Mekalanos, J. J. (2005). Small-molecule inhibitor of Vibrio cholerae virulence and intestinal colonization. *Science*, 310, 670-4.

[14] Felise, H. B., Nguyen, H. V., Pfuetzner, R. A., Barry, K. C., Jackson, S. R., Blanc, M. P., Bronstein, P. A., Kline, T., & Miller, S. I. (2008). An inhibitor of gram-negative bacterial virulence protein secretion. *Cell Host Microbe*, 4, 325-36.

[15] Lieberman, L. A., & Higgins, D. E. (2009). A small-molecule screen identifies the antipsychotic drug pimozide as an inhibitor of Listeria monocytogenes infection. *Antimicrob Agents Chemother*, 53, 756-64.

[16] Carey, K. L., Westwood, N. J., Mitchison, T. J., & Ward, G. E. (2004). A small-molecule approach to studying invasive mechanisms of Toxoplasma gondii. *Proc Natl Acad Sci U S A*, 101, 7433-8.

[17] Heaslip, A. T., Leung, J. M., Carey, K. L., Catti, F., Warshaw, D. M., Westwood, N. J., Ballif, BA, & Ward, G. E. (2010). A small-molecule inhibitor of T. gondii motility induces the posttranslational modification of myosin light chain-1 and inhibits myosin motor activity. *PLoS Pathog*, 6, e1000720.

[18] Lee, V. T., Pukatzki, S., Sato, H., Kikawada, E., Kazimirova, AA, Huang, J., Li, X., Arm, J. P., Frank, D. W., & Lory, S. (2007). Pseudolipasin A is a specific inhibitor for phospholipase A2 activity of Pseudomonas aeruginosa cytotoxin ExoU. *Infect Immun*, 75, 1089-98.

[19] Arnoldo, A., Curak, J., Kittanakom, S., Chevelev, I., Lee, V. T., Sahebol-Amri, M., Koscik, B., Ljuma, L., Roy, P. J., Bedalov, A., Giaever, G., Nislow, C., Merrill, A. R., Lory,

S., & Stagljar, I. (2008). Identification of small molecule inhibitors of Pseudomonas aeruginosa exoenzyme S using a yeast phenotypic screen. *PLoS Genet*, 4, e1000005.

[20] Harmon, D. E., Davis, A. J., Castillo, C., & Mecsas, J. (2010). Identification and characterization of small-molecule inhibitors of Yop translocation in Yersinia pseudotuberculosis. Antimicrob Agents Chemother , 54, 3241-54.

[21] Zhu, P. J., Hobson, J. P., Southall, N., Qiu, C., Thomas, C. J., Lu, J., Inglese, J., Zheng, W., Leppla, S. H., Bugge, T. H., Austin, CP, & Liu, S. (2009). Quantitative high-throughput screening identifies inhibitors of anthrax-induced cell death. *Bioorg Med Chem*, 17, 5139-45.

[22] Lee, Y. S., Bergson, P., He, W. S., Mrksich, M., & Tang, W. J. (2004). Discovery of a small molecule that inhibits the interaction of anthrax edema factor with its cellular activator, calmodulin. *Chem Biol*, 11, 1139-46.

[23] Schreiber, K., Ckurshumova, W., Peek, J., & Desveaux, D. (2008). A high-throughput chemical screen for resistance to Pseudomonas syringae in Arabidopsis. Plant J , 54, 522-31.

[24] Schreiber, K. J., Nasmith, C. G., Allard, G., Singh, J., Subramaniam, R., & Desveaux, D. (2011). Found in translation: high-throughput chemical screening in Arabidopsis thaliana identifies small molecules that reduce Fusarium head blight disease in wheat. *Mol Plant Microbe Interact*, 24, 640-8.

[25] Hammer, S. M., Eron, J. J. Jr, Reiss, P., Schooley, R. T., Thompson, M. A., Walmsley, S., Cahn, P., Fischl, M. A., Gatell, J. M., Hirsch, M. S., Jacobsen, D. M., Montaner, J. S., Richman, D. D., Yeni, P. G., & Volberding, P. A. (2008). Antiretroviral treatment of adult HIV infection: 2008 recommendations of the International AIDS Society-USA panel. *JAMA*, 300, 555-70.

[26] Berger, E. A., Murphy, P. M., & Farber, J. M. (1999). Chemokine receptors as HIV-1 coreceptors: roles in viral entry, tropism, and disease. *Annu Rev Immunol*, 17, 657-700.

[27] Liu, R., Paxton, W. A., Choe, S., Ceradini, D., Martin, S. R., Horuk, R., Mac Donald., ME, Stuhlmann, H., Koup, R. A., & Landau, N. R. (1996). Homozygous defect in HIV-1 coreceptor accounts for resistance of some multiply-exposed individuals to HIV-1 infection. *Cell*, 86, 367-77.

[28] Alkhatib, G., Combadiere, C., Broder, C. C., Feng, Y., Kennedy, P. E., Murphy, P. M., & Berger, E. A. (1996). CC CKR5: a RANTES, MIP-1alpha, MIP-1beta receptor as a fusion cofactor for macrophage-tropic HIV-1. *Science*, 272, 1955-8.

[29] Simmons, G., Clapham, P. R., Picard, L., Offord, R. E., Rosenkilde, MM, Schwartz, T. W., Buser, R., Wells, T. N., & Proudfoot, A. E. (1997). Potent inhibition of HIV-1 infectivity in macrophages and lymphocytes by a novel CCR5 antagonist. *Science*, 276, 276-9.

[30] Baba, M., Nishimura, O., Kanzaki, N., Okamoto, M., Sawada, H., Iizawa, Y., Shiraishi, M., Aramaki, Y., Okonogi, K., Ogawa, Y., Meguro, K., & Fujino, M. (1999). A

small-molecule, nonpeptide CCR5 antagonist with highly potent and selective anti-HIV-1 activity. *Proc Natl Acad Sci U S A*, 96, 5698-703.

[31] Kuhmann, S. E., & Hartley, O. (2008). Targeting chemokine receptors in HIV: a status report. *Annu Rev Pharmacol Toxicol*, 48, 425-61.

[32] Dorr, P., Westby, M., Dobbs, S., Griffin, P., Irvine, B., Macartney, M., Mori, J., Rickett, G., Smith-Burchnell, C., Napier, C., Webster, R., Armour, D., Price, D., Stammen, B., Wood, A., & Perros, M. (2005). Maraviroc (UK-427,857), a potent, orally bioavailable, and selective small-molecule inhibitor of chemokine receptor CCR5 with broad-spectrum anti-human immunodeficiency virus type 1 activity. *Antimicrob Agents Chemother*, 49, 4721-32.

[33] Roche, M., Jakobsen, M. R., Sterjovski, J., Ellett, A., Posta, F., Lee, B., Jubb, B., Westby, M., Lewin, S. R., Ramsland, P. A., Churchill, MJ, & Gorry, P. R. (2011). HIV-1 escape from the CCR5 antagonist maraviroc associated with an altered and less-efficient mechanism of gp120-CCR5 engagement that attenuates macrophage tropism. *J Virol*, 85, 4330-42.

[34] Dragic, T., Trkola, A., Thompson, D. A., Cormier, E. G., Kajumo, F. A., Maxwell, E., Lin, S. W., Ying, W., Smith, S. O., Sakmar, T. P., & Moore, J. P. (2000). A binding pocket for a small molecule inhibitor of HIV-1 entry within the transmembrane helices of CCR5. *Proc Natl Acad Sci U S A*, 97, 5639-44.

[35] Nishikawa, M., Takashima, K., Nishi, T., Furuta, R. A., Kanzaki, N., Yamamoto, Y., & Fujisawa, J. (2005). Analysis of binding sites for the new small-molecule CCR5 antagonist TAK-220 on human CCR5. *Antimicrob Agents Chemother*, 49, 4708-15.

[36] Maeda, K., Das, D., Ogata-Aoki, H., Nakata, H., Miyakawa, T., Tojo, Y., Norman, R., Takaoka, Y., Ding, J., Arnold, G. F., Arnold, E., & Mitsuya, H. (2006). Structural and molecular interactions of CCR5 inhibitors with CCR5. *J Biol Chem*, 281, 12688-98.

[37] Huang, C. C., Lam, S. N., Acharya, P., Tang, M., Xiang, S. H., Hussan, S. S., Stanfield, R. L., Robinson, J., Sodroski, J., Wilson, I. A., Wyatt, R., Bewley, C. A., & Kwong, P. D. (2007). Structures of the CCR5 N terminus and of a tyrosine-sulfated antibody with HIV-1 gp120 and CD4. *Science*, 317, 1930-4.

[38] Brower, E. T., Schon, A., Klein, J. C., & Freire, E. (2009). Binding thermodynamics of the N-terminal peptide of the CCR5 coreceptor to HIV-1 envelope glycoprotein gp120. *Biochemistry*, 48, 779-85.

[39] Chun, T. W., Davey, R. T. Jr, Ostrowski, M., Shawn, Justement. J., Engel, D., Mullins, J. L, & Fauci, AS. (2000). Relationship between pre-existing viral reservoirs and the re-emergence of plasma viremia after discontinuation of highly active anti-retroviral therapy. *Nat Med*, 6, 757-61.

[40] Brooks, D. G., Hamer, D. H., Arlen, P. A., Gao, L., Bristol, G., Kitchen, C. M., Berger, E. A., & Zack, J. A. (2003). Molecular characterization, reactivation, and depletion of latent HIV. *Immunity*, 19, 413-23.

[41] Richman, D. D., Margolis, D. M., Delaney, M., Greene, W. C., Hazuda, D., & Pomerantz, R. J. (2009). The challenge of finding a cure for HIV infection. *Science, 323,* 1304-7.

[42] Lehrman, G., Hogue, I. B., Palmer, S., Jennings, C., Spina, CA, Wiegand, A., Landay, A. L., Coombs, R. W., Richman, D. D., Mellors, J. W., Coffin, J. M., Bosch, R. J., & Margolis, D. M. (2005). Depletion of latent HIV-1 infection in vivo: a proof-of-concept study. *Lancet,* 366, 549-55.

[43] Siliciano, J. D., Lai, J., Callender, M., Pitt, E., Zhang, H., Margolick, J. B., Gallant, J. E., Cofrancesco, J. Jr, Moore, R. D., Gange, S. J., & Siliciano, R. F. (2007). Stability of the latent reservoir for HIV-1 in patients receiving valproic acid. *J Infect Dis,* 195, 833-6.

[44] Edelstein, L. C., Micheva-Viteva, S., Phelan, B. D., & Dougherty, J. P. (2009). Short communication: activation of latent HIV type 1 gene expression by suberoylanilide hydroxamic acid (SAHA), an HDAC inhibitor approved for use to treat cutaneous T cell lymphoma. *AIDS Res Hum Retroviruses,* 25, 883-7.

[45] Archin, N. M., Espeseth, A., Parker, D., Cheema, M., Hazuda, D., & Margolis, D. M. (2009). Expression of latent HIV induced by the potent HDAC inhibitor suberoylanilide hydroxamic acid. *AIDS Res Hum Retroviruses,* 25, 207-12.

[46] De Christopher, B. A., Loy, B., Marsden, M., Schrier, A. J., Zack, J. A., & Wender, P. A. (2012). Designed, synthetically accessible bryostatin analogues potently induce activation of latent HIV reservoirs in vitro. *Nat Chem; In Press.*

[47] Williams, S. A., Chen, L. F., Kwon, H., Fenard, D., Bisgrove, D., Verdin, E., & Greene, W. C. (2004). Prostratin antagonizes HIV latency by activating NF-kappaB. *J Biol Chem,* 279, 42008-17.

[48] Pikarsky, E., Porat, R. M., Stein, I., Abramovitch, R., Amit, S., Kasem, S., Gutkovich-Pyest, E., Urieli-Shoval, S., Galun, E., & Ben-Neriah, Y. (2004). NF-kappaB functions as a tumour promoter in inflammation-associated cancer. *Nature,* 431, 461-6.

[49] Micheva-Viteva, S., Kobayashi, Y., Edelstein, L. C., Pacchia, A. L., Lee, H. L., Graci, J. D., Breslin, J., Phelan, B. D., Miller, L. K., Colacino, J. M., Gu, Z., Ron, Y., Peltz, S. W., & Dougherty, J. P. (2011). High-throughput screening uncovers a compound that activates latent HIV-1 and acts cooperatively with a histone deacetylase (HDAC) inhibitor. *J Biol Chem,* 286, 21083-91.

[50] Micheva-Viteva, S., Pacchia, A. L., Ron, Y., Peltz, S. W., & Dougherty, J. P. (2005). Human immunodeficiency virus type 1 latency model for high-throughput screening. *Antimicrob Agents Chemother,* 49, 5185-8.

[51] Moy, T. I., Ball, A. R., Anklesaria, Z., Casadei, G., Lewis, K., & Ausubel, F. M. (2006). Identification of novel antimicrobials using a live-animal infection model. *Proc Natl Acad Sci U S A,* 103, 10414-9.

[52] Moy, T. I., Conery, A. L., Larkins-Ford, J., Wu, G., Mazitschek, R., Casadei, G., Lewis, K., Carpenter, A. E., & Ausubel, F. M. (2009). High-throughput screen for novel antimicrobials using a whole animal infection model. *ACS Chem Biol*, 4, 527-33.

[53] Junker, L. M., & Clardy, J. (2007). High-throughput screens for small-molecule inhibitors of Pseudomonas aeruginosa biofilm development. *Antimicrob Agents Chemother*, 51, 3582-90.

[54] Zhou, Y. M., Shao, L., Li, J. A., Han, L. Z., Cai, W. J., Zhu, C. B., & Chen, D. J. (2011). An efficient and novel screening model for assessing the bioactivity of extracts against multidrug-resistant Pseudomonas aeruginosa using Caenorhabditis elegans. Biosci Biotechnol Biochem , 75, 1746-51.

[55] Breger, J., Fuchs, B. B., Aperis, G., Moy, T. I., Ausubel, F. M., & Mylonakis, E. (2007). Antifungal chemical compounds identified using a C. elegans pathogenicity assay. *PLoS Pathog*, 3, e18.

[56] Watabe, M., Hishikawa, K., Takayanagi, A., Shimizu, N., & Nakaki, T. (2004). Caffeic acid phenethyl ester induces apoptosis by inhibition of NFkappaB and activation of Fas in human breast cancer MCF-7 cells. *J Biol Chem*, 279, 6017-26.

[57] Park, J. H., Lee, J. K., Kim, H. S., Chung, S. T., Eom, J. H., Kim, K. A., Chung, S. J., Paik, S. Y., & Oh, H. Y. (2004). Immunomodulatory effect of caffeic acid phenethyl ester in Balb/c mice. *Int Immunopharmacol*, 4, 429-36.

[58] Okoli, I., Coleman, J. J., Tampakakis, E., An, W. F., Holson, E., Wagner, F., Conery, A. L., Larkins-Ford, J., Wu, G., Stern, A., Ausubel, F. M., & Mylonakis, E. (2009). Identification of antifungal compounds active against Candida albicans using an improved high-throughput Caenorhabditis elegans assay. *PLoS One*, 4, e7025.

[59] Fox, D. S., Cruz, M. C., Sia, R. A., Ke, H., Cox, G. M., Cardenas, M. E., & Heitman, J. (2001). Calcineurin regulatory subunit is essential for virulence and mediates interactions with FKBP12-FK506 in Cryptococcus neoformans. *Mol Microbiol*, 39, 835-49.

[60] Steinbach, W. J., Schell, W. A., Blankenship, J. R., Onyewu, C., Heitman, J., & Perfect, J. R. (2004). In vitro interactions between antifungals and immunosuppressants against Aspergillus fumigatus. Antimicrob Agents Chemother , 48, 1664-9.

Chapter 6

Practical Considerations of Liquid Handling Devices in Drug Discovery

Sergio C. Chai, Asli N. Goktug, Jimmy Cui,
Jonathan Low and Taosheng Chen

Additional information is available at the end of the chapter

http://dx.doi.org/10.5772/52546

1. Introduction

Automated liquid handling has become an indispensable tool in drug discovery, particularly in screening campaigns ranging millions of compounds. Intense innovations of these devices go hand in hand with the progression towards assay miniaturization, accelerating dramatically the discovery of drug candidates and chemical probes for querying biological systems. The advancement in this technology is driven in large part by much impetus in cost reduction and efficiency. In addition to increased throughput, streamlining screening operations using automated fluid devices ensures consistency and reliability while avoiding human error.

In this chapter, we provide a general overview of existing liquid handlers, with emphasis on their strengths and limitations. Notably, we discuss practical considerations in the implementation of these devices, methods to discern performance quality and potential sources of error.

2. Types of liquid handling devices

A whole array of liquid handlers has been developed for every aspect of drug discovery. These instruments encompass different technologies for distinct purposes. In terms of application, they are broadly classified as bulk liquid dispensers, transfer devices and plate washers (Rudnicki and Johnston 2009).

Based on the way the reagent is being transferred, these instruments can follow two dispensing modes: contact or non-contact (Kong et al. 2012). Contact-based devices allow the fluid to be transferred to touch the surface of the destination container or solution, offering a simple and dependable alternative to sub-microliter fluid handling. Non-contact devices utilize additional force other than gravity to eject liquids, as minute volumes cannot be dispensed efficiently with gravity alone (Kong et al. 2012). The process is faster than using permanent tips or pins (Fig.1), because there is no washing step between delivery, while reducing cross-contamination and evaporation (Dunn and Feygin 2000).

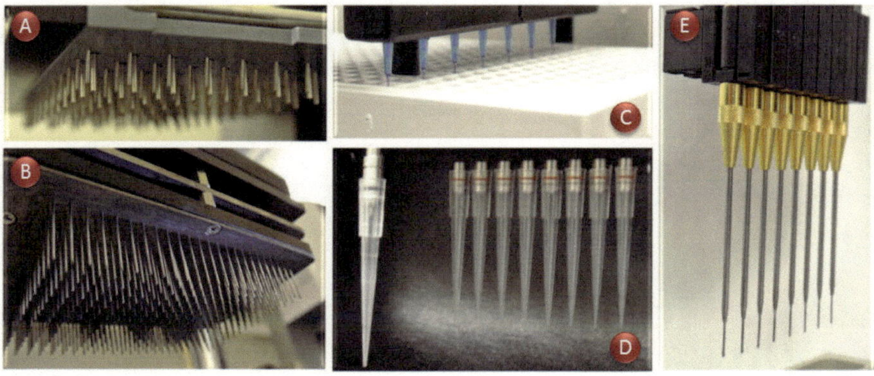

Figure 1. Various types of liquid handling tips, pins and heads from A) washer B) pintool C) peristaltic pump-based bulk dispenser D) liquid handler with single and 8-channel pipettors E) pipettor with 8-independent channels.

2.1. Peristaltic-based devices

The peristaltic pump is used for bulk reagent dispensing in conjunction with a nozzle head (Fig.1C) and a flexible tubing cartridge. The tubings stretch around a set of rollers connected to a motor. With the rotating motion of the motor, the rollers compress the tubings creating a continuous fluid motion due to positive displacement.

Typically, this type of dispenser is capable of handling volumes as low as 5 μL, offering a fast dispensing option for 96-/384-/1536-well plate formats. The disposable tubing cartridge is pre-sterilized, and the entire liquid path can be autoclaved. Additionally, these devices are normally equipped with programing capabilities that allow discrete column-wise dispensing, variable rolling speed settings and adjustable dispensing volume. The pump can roll both forward and backwards to execute priming and emptying functions, respectively. A major limitation is the lack of capabilities to dispense into individual wells.

2.2. Fixed-tip transfer devices

Fluid handlers that utilize fixed-tips (Fig.1E) are usually efficient at transferring relatively small volumes (100 μL or above) and have been largely used for compound pipetting ("cherry picking") and serial dilutions. They incorporate 2-/ 4-/ 8-channel expandable liquid handling arms in addition to 96- and 384-channel heads. This type of liquid handling device functions based on air displacement mechanism. The dilutor or syringe plunger pulls system liquid from the pipette tubing to aspirate the sample, with an air gap separating both fluids. The plunger speed, syringe size and resolution are factors that affect pipetting flow rate.

2.3. Changeable-tip transfer devices

The use of disposable tips (Fig.1D) is a simple alternative to avoid washing steps required for fixed-tip based systems, while eliminating completely the risk of cross-contamination. These instruments employ a conventional air displacement mechanism. A wide array of commercially-available tip sizes, materials and molding qualities offers the scientist great flexibility. There are even specialized tips with nanoliter-scale transfer capabilities that can be used in any conventional pipettor (Murthy et al. 2011; Ramírez et al. 2008).

2.4. Pintool transfer devices

Pintool is a contact-based dispensing method widely used for handling volumes at the nanoliter scale (Cleveland and Koutz 2005). It consists of a set of stainless steel pins (Fig. 1B) carefully crafted for consistent dimensions. The bottom end of the pins can be solid, grooved or slotted, with the option of having a hydrophobic coating to prevent non-specific binding (Dunn and Feygin 2000; Rudnicki and Johnston 2009). Solutions are transferred through a combination of capillary action and surface tension, with the volume being highly dependent on the contact surfaces and solution properties (Dunn and Feygin 2000). The pin array is normally assembled in a floating pin cassette to ensure soaking of all the pins amid uneven surfaces, which also minimizes pin damage. After liquid transfer, the pins have to cycle through washing steps to prevent cross-contamination.

2.5. Piezoelectric devices

The piezoelectric dispenser is a non-contact technology, where solutions are delivered as multiple tiny drops of defined size (Niles and Coassin 2005). This technology has been utilized in contemporary inject printers and refined to be implemented in the biological sciences. Various biochemical solutions (DNA, RNA, proteins) and bacterial suspensions have been tested with no negative effects (Schober et al. 1993). The system is composed of a capillary tube made of quartz or steel, with one end connected to the reagent reservoir and the other end ending in an orifice from which droplets are ejected (Niles and Coassin 2005). A piezoelectric crystal collar is bound to the capillary, which is filled with solution. Upon voltage application, the piezoelectric element contracts causing pressure on the capillary to generate fine drops. The ejection is at high acceleration with minimal wetting of the nozzle (Schober et al. 1993). Several thousand drops can be dispensed per second, with attainable drop sizes spanning the picoliter and nanoliter range (Schober et al. 1993). Droplet volume depends on several factors, including bore diameter, solution viscosity and the voltage pulse amplitude and frequency (James and Papen 1998; Kong et al. 2012).

2.6. Solenoid-based devices

Solenoid-based devices are non-contact dispensers that use a positive displacement mechanism (Bateman et al. 1999). The flow of pressurized liquid is occluded by a solenoid valve, which is actuated by electric current to allow for liquid to pass through the valve. The dispensed volume is regulated by the fluid pressure, duration of the valve in the open position, solution properties and orifice diameter (Bateman et al. 1999; Niles and Coassin 2005). Depending on the time the valve stays in the open position, the device can eject droplets or a continuous stream (Niles and Coassin 2005).

2.7. Acoustic devices

Acoustic droplet ejection (ADE) is a recent touch-less technology that surges in popularity in recent years. It adopts acoustic energy to propel droplets from various types of solutions with good precision (Ellson et al. 2003; Harris et al. 2008; Rudnicki and Johnston 2009; Shieh et al. 2006). The source plate remains stationary as the transducer and destination plate shuffle to allow for solution transfer from any well in the source plate to any well in the destination plate, the latter one lying in an inverted position (Olechno et al. 2006). This system does not require any additional consumable other than microplates (Olechno et al. 2006), and it speeds up the process by avoiding washing steps and having the capability to prepare assay-ready plates (Turmel et al. 2010)

2.8. Microplate washers

Microplate washers are laboratory instruments designed to automate and expedite assay applications, where a washing step is essential. They play an important role in areas such as high-content screening and enzyme-linked immunosorbent assays (ELISA). In 1990, Stobbs developed the first multiple plate washer using readily available materials as a low cost alternative to the commercially available plate washers of the era (Stobbs 1990). Over the years, fully programmable plate washers have been developed with numerous features. The development of automated plate washers has decreased the time required for laborious washing steps involved in many screening assays and improved reproducibility through standardized plate handling across multiple wash cycles (defined as a single dispense and aspirate step per cycle).

The two most critical components of a plate washer are a plate carrier and a manifold containing a number of fixed stainless steel needle probes for solution dispensing (Fig.1A). This manifold (or a separate manifold depending on the design) aspirates the liquid from the wells after an optional soaking period, leaving a pre-defined residual volume in the wells. A third component is the vacuum/pump assembly, which supplies the necessary pressure differential to drive efficient aspiration. Sunghou Lee first developed an additional vacuum filtration system integrated with a conventional plate washer to speed up the wash process for applications involving filter plates (Lee 2006). Some plate washers have a built-in magnet or a vacuum filtration module for handling bead-based assays.

Microplate washers can be categorized into two types: strip washers, which wash a single column or row of a plate at a time, and full plate washers (Rudnicki and Johnston 2009). The availability of 8-/12-/16-channel manifolds for strip washers provides both single strip washing and full-plate washing capability in the same device, but at the cost of increased wash time for full plates. On the other hand, full plate washers with either a 96- or 384-channel manifold may be preferred for time-efficient wash operations (from a few seconds to a few minutes), but lack the flexibility of the 8-/12-/16-channel units.

The combination of plate washing and bulk dispensing features within the same device may be favored for a space-efficient solution. They are designed to dispense reliably low volumes and reduce prime volume (Rudnicki and Johnston 2009). A major advantage of the washer-dispenser combination comes into play with assay protocols that require the direct addition of fluid after or between the washing steps, such as cell fixation or microplate surface coating reagents.

3. Considerations for using liquid handling devices

3.1. Determination of quality assessment descriptors

Assessment of instrument performance has become important in order to minimize false-positive and false-negative rates in high-throughput screening (Taylor et al. 2002). One of the most important figures of merit in evaluating the performance of liquid handlers is accuracy, which is commonly reported as %bias (Rose 1999):

$$\%bias = 100 \times \left(\frac{V_M - V_T}{V_T}\right) \tag{1}$$

where V_M is the measured volume and V_T is the theoretical volume (desired). %bias represents the deviation from the desired volume, with a value of 0% indicating no deviation from the true value.

The precision, a measure of reproducibility, is calculated from the mean and standard deviation (SD) of a set of measurements, and it is reported as percent coefficient of variation (%CV) or relative standard deviation (RSD), as shown in Eq. 2. For most cases, it is adequate to have a bias value below 5% and a CV below 10% (Rose 1999).

$$\%CV = 100 \times \frac{SD}{mean} \tag{2}$$

There have been several approaches for volume verification, which typically consist of gravimetric or photometric methods. Gravimetric measurements utilize the mass and the density (ϱ) of the dispensed solution to determine the volume. It has been used extensively to calibrate and verify the accuracy of liquid dispensers (Bergsdorf et al. 2006; Rhode et al. 2004; Taylor et al. 2002). Typically, the solution is dispensed across a pre-weighed microtiter plate, which is weighed immediately after dispensing to prevent evaporation. %bias can be calculated based on the total weight of the dispensed solution (W_{total}) and the number of dispensed wells (n):

$$\%\text{bias per well (gravimetric)} = 100 \times \frac{\left(\frac{W_{total}}{n \times \rho}\right) - V_T}{V_T} \quad (3)$$

Environmental conditions (e.g. temperature and humidity) have major effects on the reliability of gravimetric methods, which facilitates evaporation and water uptake for hygroscopic solvents such as dimethyl sulfoxide (DMSO). These factors of variation can be minimized by placing gasketed lids on the microtiter plates immediately following dispense (Taylor et al. 2002).

Absorbance and fluorescence are the most common photometric methods utilized to test the accuracy and precision of the transferred volumes of a liquid handling device. In a study comparing the performance of the two methods on determining the precision in 96-/384-/1536-well plates, no significant difference was observed between the 96- and 384-well plates (Petersen and Nguyen 2005). However, to achieve similar results for both fluorescence and absorbance measurements in the 1536-well plate, a centrifugation step was required because of the irregular meniscus shape enhanced by the small well geometry. In another study performed on liquid handlers with two different mechanisms, absorbance was found to be a more reliable method as long as the pH stability of the dye-buffer solution is maintained (Rhode et al. 2004).

Fluorescence signal is also known to be susceptible to photobleaching, which can be prevented by shorter excitation times, suitable buffer solutions and adequate concentration of fluorophore (Diaspro et al. 2006; Harris and Mutz 2006). To overcome the problems encountered due to signal quenching in DMSO, sulforhodamine 101 was presented as an alternative fluorescence dye (Walling 2011). Fluorescein was found to be a suitable probe to use in liquid handling performance quantification as long as the DMSO concentration in the buffer solution does not exceed 1% and the stock solutions are stored in 70-100% DMSO in a dark environment (Harris and Mutz 2006). While photobleaching is not an issue in absorbance, the method is limited by high background levels and lower sensitivity compared to fluorescence (Bradshaw et al. 2007). Based on the physical characteristics of a transferred sample and the material of the consumables, unforeseen interactions may be observed influencing the assay results. Especially, DMSO-containing samples are highly affected by the hydroscopic properties of the solvent, which inflates sample volume (Berg et al. 2001).

3.2. Considerations for using bulk reagent dispensers: Peristaltic-based devices

A single screening experiment can be costly, requiring valuable compounds and biological reagents. Routine evaluation of liquid handlers, in particularly prior to each run, is a necessary mean for preventing disastrous outcomes. Simple procedures can be integrated to identify problems in a relatively short period of time, which in many instances, can be easily corrected. Routine analysis should be performed with the actual reagents, because there are several factors that affect the dispensed volumes, including viscosity, density, and temperature (McGown and Hafeman 1998). General considerations to prevent undesirable dispensing performance and common sources of variations include:

3.2.1. *Uneven dispensing*

Tubings tend to stretch after certain period of use, affecting the intended volume to be delivered. When not in use, the cartridges should be placed in the "rest" position. In addition, autoclaving the cassettes should be minimized. Dispensing speed and the height of the tips in relation to the plate have to be optimized for the intended reagent, as viscous solutions could miss the targeted well at low dispensing speed and large spacing between the tips and microtiter plate. When working with cells, uneven dispensing can be reduced by increasing the prime volume, constant mixing/stirring the cell suspension source and minimizing cell clumps. Solutions should be dispensed in the center of the well, and plates have to be centrifuged when dispensing low volumes to force droplets at the walls to the bottom of the well. Cassettes should be calibrated regularly as recommended by the supplier and checked for tip clogging.

3.2.2. *Protein binding*

Protein binding to dispensing components is an important point to consider in the implementation of biochemical assays, particularly at low protein concentrations. In some instances, enzymes appear to be inactivated over time when dispensing multiple plates using a liquid handler, when in reality the enzymes have been depleted from the solution due to non-specific binding to plastic, silicone and other polymer-based surfaces. This effect is amplified when dispensing sizeable number of plates, as there is larger exposure time of the assay components to the surfaces of reagent reservoirs and dispensing cassette elements. In order to circumvent this problem, blocking reagents can be added to the buffer, plastic surfaces can be coated, or a combination of both. The two major types of blocking reagents are detergents and proteins. It is preferable to use non-ionic detergents such as Tween-20, Triton X-100 or Nonidet-P40. Among the most widely-used protein blockers are bovine serum albumin (BSA) and casein. Protein blockers are better suited for coating surfaces, as detergents can be easily washed away. Typical working concentrations for detergents range from 0.01 to 0.1%, while protein blockers are used between 0.1 to 3 %. The selection of the appropriate type of blocking reagent and concentration is central to a robust assay. Other less common blocking reagents include polyethylene glycol (PEG), polyvinyl alcohol (PVA) and polyvinyl pyrrolidone (PVP). Additionally, the use of glass reagent reservoirs is recommended.

3.2.3. *Clogging*

Particles can obstruct the flow of a dispensing cassette mainly by blocking the tips. Complete clogging is fairly easy to recognize, as the lack of fluid coming out of the tips can be visibly noticed. Depending on the degree of obstruction, partial clogging may not be easily perceived by the naked eye, and it is detected only by photometric or gravimetric testing. However, there are certain indications of partial clogging, such as slanted fluid spray or drop formation at the tip. To prevent clogging, the tubing should be primed with deionized water shortly after use, especially prior to priming with alcohol, as salts in the buffer may precipitate and biological reagents may clump. When working with cells, it is recommended to wet the tubing with buffer or media before dispensing cells, and if possible, not to allow the cells to settle in the tubing by emptying the contents back to the reservoir immediate after dispensing (prime/empty cycle).

3.2.4. Foaming

Solutions with high protein content can cause frothing, including media containing serum and biochemical buffers with high percentage of BSA (used as blocking protein). To minimize frothing, it is recommended not to empty the tubing between dispensing (as ordinarily performed in fully automated platforms for large screenings). If tubing emptying is unavoidable, it is advisable to empty a volume smaller than the dead volume. Other means to reduce frothing involve decreasing dispensing speed and applying grease to the cassette tips. Torn or cracked tubing can pull air generating bubbles.

3.2.5. Reservoir container

The reservoir container is an important component of a liquid dispenser that is often neglected in troubleshooting. The material of the container can have a detrimental effect on the assay robustness, such as sticking of proteins to plastic surfaces. For peristaltic pump-based dispensers, we suggest using a jacketed glass flask connected to a water chiller (waterbath with adjustable temperature). Careful monitoring of the temperature in the flask using a thermometer is recommended, as the temperature set in the chiller is not always reflected in the container. Suspensions of cells, beads or nanoparticles have to be constantly stirred to prevent settling, which could result in uneven dispensing or clogging. The stirring speed needs to be optimized, as fast stirring can create bubbles and disturb biological components (cells). When working with large reagent volumes at the start of dispensing, the stirring may have to be reduced as the volume decreases to prevent foaming or bubble formation.

3.2.6. Tubing extension

Extensions can be implemented when the dispensing tubings cannot be immersed in the reservoir container because of its large dimensions. Some commercially available extensions allow for the 8 tubings of a standard cartridge to be coupled into single elongated tubing through metallic cannulas sticking out of a joint casing. For viscous solutions, these types of elongations can introduce bubbles due to the joint design, particularly during prime/empty cycles. The metallic cannulas can easily tear the tubing during fitting, which is ameliorated by using glycerol or alcohol to smoothen the surfaces. A better alternative is to build home-made extensions by attaching each of the new tubings to separate discarded tubings through connectors, which can be made by cutting the end of a pipette tip.

http://dx.doi.org/10.5772/52546

3.2.7. Routine quality assessment

During assay development and validation, factors affecting liquid dispenser performance are identified and corrected. However, setbacks can occur randomly regardless of detailed preparations ahead of the screens. For instance, torn tubing, tip blockage or incorrect cartridge setup cannot be prevented a priori. Therefore, it is recommended to rapidly monitor dispensing variations at the start of a screen, where problems encountered at this stage can be usually corrected fairly quickly.

We normally dispense a solution of fluorescein isothiocyanate (FITC) in PBS into a couple of 384-well plates. Fluorescence intensities are analyzed for signal variations corresponding to each cassette channel, as described by %CV and %bias' (Fig.2). Determination of %CV for the entire plate is frequently performed in many laboratories, but this approach cannot distinguish issues with individual channels. In addition, a flawed channel does not necessarily change drastically the %CV of the whole plate, as illustrated by Fig. 2A. The types of problems commonly associated to high %CV include improper cassette mounting, tubing stretching and damage.

There are instances when the tip is partially obstructed, leading to reduced volume delivered. Even when a channel displays low fluorescence counts, the signal can still have small %CV values (Fig. 2B). We have adapted the concept of %bias to detect significant deviations in signal intensity for each row (S_R) compared to that of the whole plate (S_T), resulting in %bias' (Eq. 4). Values lower than 10 %CV and 10 %bias' are acceptable.

$$\% \text{ bias}' = 100 \times \left(\frac{S_R - S_T}{S_T} \right) \tag{4}$$

3.3. Considerations for using transfer devices: Pintool

The pintool has become a mature technology for transferring nanoliter to sub-microliter volumes. Even though the system is regarded as fairly simple and robust, there are a number of points to consider for a consistent and reliable performance:

3.3.1. Volume variation

The volume delivered by a pin can change due to a number of factors. To minimize volume variations, there should be consistency in immersion depth (Dunn and Feygin 2000). There is a minimum volume required in the source plate, and the destination plate should not be dry (Rudnicki and Johnston 2009). The dwell time that pins spend in the fluid and withdrawal speed from the liquid surface should be optimized for solutions of very different properties (e.g. viscosity).

The slot of a pin can be tainted by compound precipitation or formation of suspension deposits (Fig. 3B). Sufficient and robust washing and drying steps are effective in preventing deposition and being critical to avoid carry-over and cross-contamination. The pins can be physically damaged by dipping in highly uneven surfaces, particularly when using slotted pins (Fig. 3C). Coated pins should avoid harsh washing procedures, such as going through powerful sonication washes.

A

	% CV	Raw signal	% bias'		1	2	3	4	5	6	7	8	9	10	11	12	13	14	15	16	17	18	19	20	21	22	23	24
CHANNEL 1	3.4	2473	-1.9	A	2559	2618	2476	2547	2383	2532	2374	2518	2371	2497	2372	2516	2361	2517	2397	2508	2382	2520	2380	2522	2393	2561	2412	2627
	2.3	2511	-0.4	B	2630	2501	2574	2472	2555	2469	2534	2463	2543	2459	2574	2441	2527	2446	2556	2418	2561	2471	2549	2460	2569	2442	2562	2483
CHANNEL 2	1.9	2650	5.2	C	2576	2782	2712	2630	2691	2658	2583	2670	2699	2660	2647	2723	2599	2661	2594	2629	2645	2665	2570	2641	2601	2664	2610	2696
	1.6	2604	3.3	D	2639	2595	2677	2619	2694	2616	2585	2579	2621	2523	2609	2577	2627	2550	2588	2555	2598	2555	2622	2552	2643	2606	2609	2662
CHANNEL 3	2.3	2609	3.5	E	2780	2682	2664	2614	2699	2656	2603	2622	2599	2615	2589	2609	2567	2555	2553	2477	2545	2622	2586	2573	2630	2582	2589	2595
	1.6	2534	0.6	F	2559	2512	2514	2500	2566	2548	2523	2521	2586	2518	2550	2610	2516	2524	2491	2517	2515	2579	2510	2523	2501	2564	2437	2634
CHANNEL 4	4.0	2508	-0.5	G	2278	2584	2413	2573	2455	2608	2404	2587	2463	2629	2479	2624	2451	2616	2428	2574	2398	2612	2438	2550	2405	2596	2419	2620
	3.7	2503	-0.7	H	2619	2464	2601	2429	2579	2427	2565	2402	2613	2454	2617	2484	2613	2448	2602	2407	2551	2381	2547	2339	2533	2340	2581	2476
CHANNEL 5	4.1	2546	1.0	I	2523	2618	2525	2672	2488	2639	2414	2672	2468	2547	2499	2752	2533	2459	2460	2371	2472	2695	2459	2618	2463	2637	2428	2696
	4.4	2579	2.3	J	2704	2521	2716	2496	2749	2483	2662	2478	2722	2504	2714	2496	2686	2473	2669	2448	2689	2513	2669	2406	2637	2400	2562	2501
CHANNEL 6	15.0	2306	-8.5	K	2719	2090	2515	1967	2614	2040	2748	1950	2485	1946	2790	1946	2714	1929	2415	1999	2714	2084	2650	1922	2622	1928	2624	1933
	17.9	2281	-9.5	L	1979	2670	1923	2750	1703	2654	1816	2520	1720	2710	1811	2670	1905	2674	2009	2621	1983	2714	1915	2647	1954	2664	1965	2764
CHANNEL 7	4.2	2646	5.0	M	2669	2833	2792	2750	2714	2818	2689	2690	2700	2662	2661	2628	2578	2597	2714	2649	2524	2665	2602	2603	2371	2617	2574	2405
	3.4	2594	2.9	N	2755	2593	2673	2578	2683	2528	2611	2500	2647	2721	2652	2625	2597	2583	2697	2484	2592	2607	2464	2547	2460	2587	2670	2404
CHANNEL 8	5.4	2507	-0.5	O	2286	2590	2448	2730	2488	2680	2408	2626	2404	2672	2419	2616	2309	2637	2360	2595	2332	2555	2343	2555	2408	2626	2408	2662
	3.2	2468	-2.0	P	2514	2544	2534	2511	2374	2451	2518	2380	2517	2438	2382	2441	2552	2398	2479	2438	2550	2363	2441	2380	2511	2691	2459	2374
ENTIRE PLATE	7.3	2520																										

B

	% CV	Raw signal	% bias'		1	2	3	4	5	6	7	8	9	10	11	12	13	14	15	16	17	18	19	20	21	22	23	24
CHANNEL 1	3.4	2473	-0.3	A	2559	2618	2476	2547	2383	2532	2374	2518	2371	2497	2372	2516	2361	2517	2397	2508	2382	2520	2380	2522	2393	2561	2412	2627
	2.3	2511	1.2	B	2630	2501	2574	2472	2555	2469	2534	2463	2543	2459	2574	2441	2527	2446	2556	2418	2561	2471	2549	2460	2569	2442	2562	2483
CHANNEL 2	1.9	2650	6.8	C	2576	2782	2712	2630	2691	2658	2583	2670	2699	2660	2647	2723	2599	2661	2594	2629	2645	2665	2570	2641	2601	2664	2610	2696
	1.6	2604	4.9	D	2639	2595	2677	2619	2694	2616	2585	2579	2621	2523	2609	2577	2627	2550	2588	2555	2598	2555	2622	2552	2643	2606	2609	2662
CHANNEL 3	2.3	2609	5.1	E	2780	2682	2664	2614	2699	2656	2603	2622	2599	2615	2589	2609	2567	2555	2553	2477	2545	2622	2586	2573	2630	2582	2589	2595
	1.6	2534	2.1	F	2559	2512	2514	2500	2566	2548	2523	2521	2586	2518	2550	2610	2516	2524	2491	2517	2515	2579	2510	2523	2501	2564	2437	2634
CHANNEL 4	4.0	2508	1.1	G	2278	2584	2413	2573	2455	2608	2404	2587	2463	2629	2479	2624	2451	2616	2428	2574	2398	2612	2438	2550	2405	2596	2419	2620
	3.7	2503	0.9	H	2619	2464	2601	2429	2579	2427	2565	2402	2613	2454	2617	2484	2613	2448	2602	2407	2551	2381	2547	2339	2533	2340	2581	2476
CHANNEL 5	4.1	2546	2.6	I	2523	2618	2525	2672	2488	2639	2414	2672	2468	2547	2499	2752	2533	2459	2460	2371	2472	2695	2459	2618	2463	2637	2428	2696
	4.4	2579	3.9	J	2704	2521	2716	2496	2749	2483	2662	2478	2722	2504	2714	2496	2686	2473	2669	2448	2689	2513	2669	2406	2637	2400	2562	2501
CHANNEL 6	3.2	2555	3.0	K	2639	2595	2677	2619	2694	2616	2585	2579	2621	2523	2574	2441	2527	2446	2556	2418	2561	2471	2549	2460	2393	2561	2630	2582
	2.4	2593	4.5	L	2639	2595	2677	2619	2694	2555	2469	2534	2463	2543	2550	2586	2518	2550	2599	2661	2594	2629	2630	2691	2658	2583	2609	2577
CHANNEL 7	4.2	2646	6.6	M	2669	2833	2792	2750	2714	2818	2689	2690	2700	2662	2661	2628	2578	2597	2714	2649	2524	2665	2602	2603	2371	2617	2574	2405
	3.4	2594	4.5	N	2755	2593	2673	2578	2683	2528	2611	2500	2647	2721	2652	2625	2597	2583	2697	2484	2592	2607	2464	2547	2460	2587	2670	2404
CHANNEL 8	7.1	1907	-22.8	O	1686	1990	1848	2130	1888	2080	1808	2026	1804	2072	1819	2016	1709	2037	1760	1995	1732	1955	1743	1955	1808	2026	1808	2062
	4.2	1868	-24.3	P	1914	1944	1934	1911	1774	1851	1918	1780	1917	1838	1782	1841	1952	1798	1879	1838	1950	1763	1841	1780	1911	2091	1859	1774
ENTIRE PLATE	9.9	2480																										

C

		1	2	3	4	5	6	7	8	9	10	11	12
CHANNEL 1	A	5385520	5246640	4785600	4010320	3930240	3588880	3386240	3409360	2257840	1833440	1839200	1862640
	B	5159200	5311360	5430400	5021680	4097520	3672640	3787680	3306800	3129200	2183120	2146000	2101920
CHANNEL 2	C	4452480	5501120	5265600	5196480	4607280	3602240	4102480	3279440	3523280	3572560	2587040	2211120
	D	5697760	5619280	5633840	5183600	4586800	4400800	4148240	4322240	3471680	3494880	2361040	1954800
CHANNEL 3	E	5209600	5593920	4931120	4397120	4794000	4102320	3986400	4000880	4053760	4086800	3831440	2857280
	F	5838560	5811120	5694160	5386880	5198960	4600480	4711040	4998000	4393120	4330080	4025200	3537440
CHANNEL 4	G	6023680	5468960	6021200	5007680	5513280	5842160	5448960	5553440	3963200	3613520	3197920	3343920
	H	6536880	6358240	6344560	6116880	6442880	6913920	6372000	6091680	5124080	5039520	3948400	4302240
CHANNEL 5	I	5853760	5569120	4738400	5251360	5290160	3954960	3151920	3586320	3677280	2736320	2411920	1950880
	J	6194480	5629600	5933840	5863360	5771440	5247120	4340800	4513280	4100320	3046560	3047840	3140240
CHANNEL 6	K	5350880	4006320	5344080	4832880	5107360	4195840	3467840	2889680	2906960	2124560	2597840	2581680
	L	5641120	5504880	5313600	5208720	4428240	3940880	3537360	3011920	3131840	3018240	2783760	2598880
CHANNEL 7	M	5666480	5086240	5198400	4760400	4449200	3349440	3746400	2828880	2526640	2791920	2385600	2675280
	N	5707840	5489680	5657040	5331600	4843040	3897360	4529440	3117840	2447520	2352800	1849360	2253520
CHANNEL 8	O	5282160	4514800	4426640	4242320	3425360	3229760	3247600	2265360	2193360	2140000	1835040	1576000
	P	5285360	5593920	5518480	5210800	4177600	3192240	3482320	3141360	2691280	2512400	1821520	2310560

Figure 2. A-B) Delivery variation by a bulk reagent dispenser distributing a FITC solution into 384-well plates. Certain dispensing cassette channels display either higher %CV or %bias' values than the anticipated cut-off of 10%. C) Cell settling in the reagent reservoir when transferring to a microtiter plate using an automated pipetting system with an 8-channel head, with 1 min delay between transfers to each column. Cell settling is uneven due to the v-shaped bottom of the reservoir, causing the intensity pattern observed in the plate. The cells (HEK293T) were incubated with Cell-Titer-Glo® for 20 min prior to luminescence reading.

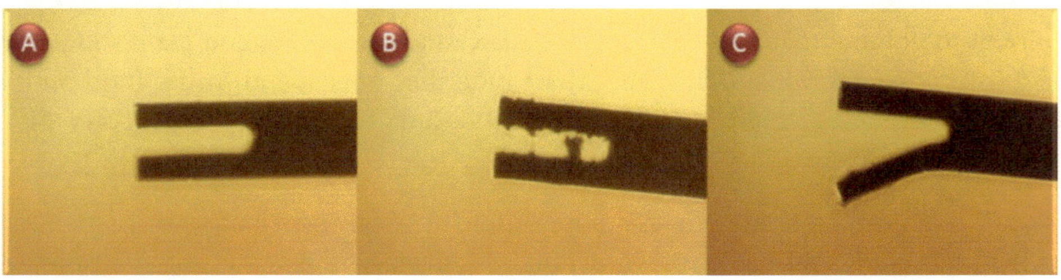

Figure 3. Magnified view of FP1NS50H pins (V&P Scientific, Inc.) with A) clean slot B) dirty slot C) damaged slot.

http://dx.doi.org/10.5772/52546

3.3.2. *Carry-over*

After transferring compounds from one plate to another, the pins are washed in DMSO, alcohol, water or a combination of these solutions. The pintool protocol involves dipping the pins in each solution bath certain number of times, at a particular speed and soaking time. The pins are then dried on lint-free blotting paper. Protocols of pintool devices used on robotic platforms are optimized for effectiveness in removing previous transfers while spending the minimum time between wash cycles. In many cases, the drugging (i.e., addition of compound to assay well) step using pintool becomes the bottleneck in a screening campaign, and the washing step accounts for most of the time consumed. However, certain assays can be very sensitive to compound carry-over, particularly if the compounds are very potent modulators and bind avidly to the pin surface. In such cases, increasing the number of dips and soaking time can improve cleanliness, albeit at the cost of increasing total transfer time.

Fig. 4 illustrates the effect of four different wash protocols in a kinase assay using staurosporine as the inhibitor. After compound transfer by pintool to the first assay plate, the pins are immersed in DMSO and isopropanol reservoirs, followed by drying on blotting paper. Subsequently, the pins are dipped in a second assay plate containing the kinase system. Residual staurosporine in the pins increases the signal variation as determined by %CV of a set of multiple wells. Protocol 1 has the least number of dips and soaking time per bath, resulting in the most dramatic signal variation due to carry-over. This general approach is recommended for detecting carry-over and selecting the appropriate pintool wash.

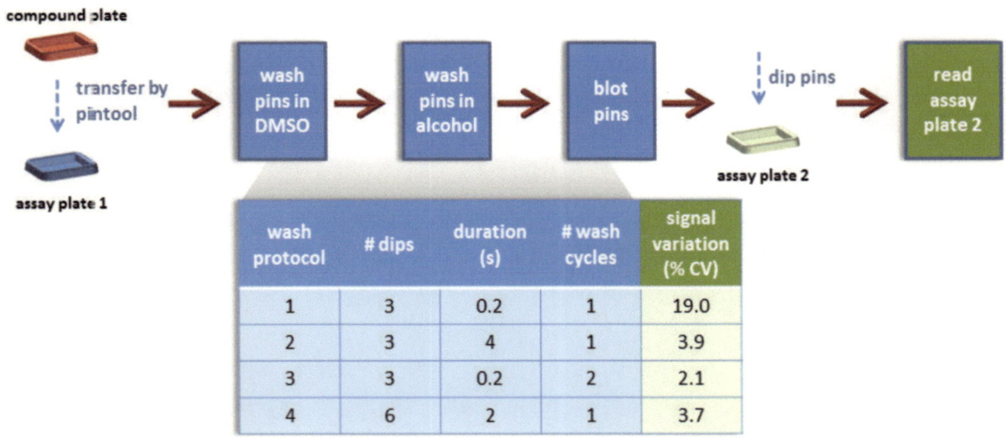

wash protocol	# dips	duration (s)	# wash cycles	signal variation (% CV)
1	3	0.2	1	19.0
2	3	4	1	3.9
3	3	0.2	2	2.1
4	6	2	1	3.7

Figure 4. General approach to detect compound carry-over and optimize pintool washing. A single wash cycle consists of dipping the pins in DMSO and isopropanol baths, followed by blotting on lint-free paper.

3.3.3. *Routine quality assessment*

Regular pintool calibration and quality assessment can considerably improve data quality. In screening runs at a single compound concentration, well-maintained pins can lead to a reduction of false negative hits, as damaged or dirty pins would usually deliver lower volumes than anticipated. In dose-response analysis, the quality of the curve fit is highly dependent on the variability of the data points.

A good quality control procedure should provide the transferred volume and the variation associated with the pin set. We implemented a relatively quick and simple procedure using a fluorescent dye (FITC). Prior to the test, the pins are washed as described above. A calibration curve is generated of fluorescence intensity as a function of FITC concentration. Using the pintool, FITC in DMSO is transferred from a source plate to several destination plates containing PBS (the use of 4 plates was shown to be sufficient). The average transferred volume per pin is calculated using the fluorescence signal of the destination plates and the calibration curve. Volume variation across the microtiter plate can be readily appreciated by plotting volume against well position (Fig. 5, top charts). The pink and green solid lines represent the upper and lower boundaries within 10% CV of the average volume, where outliers can be clearly identified. The frequency chart (Fig. 5, bottom chart) displays outliers present in 1, 2, 3 or all of the 4 destination plates, and it can be used to identify pins that consistently provide volumes outside a specified range. In the example shown in Fig. 5, pins corresponding to positions A13, B21, D8, F13, K1, N14 and P20 will have to be replaced. Depending on the need, stringency can be adjusted by changing the boundaries as specified by %CV. It is highly recommended to utilize the same freshly prepared fluorescent dye and buffer solutions in all aspects of the protocol. A template for data analysis can be easily created in conventional software such as MS-Excel.

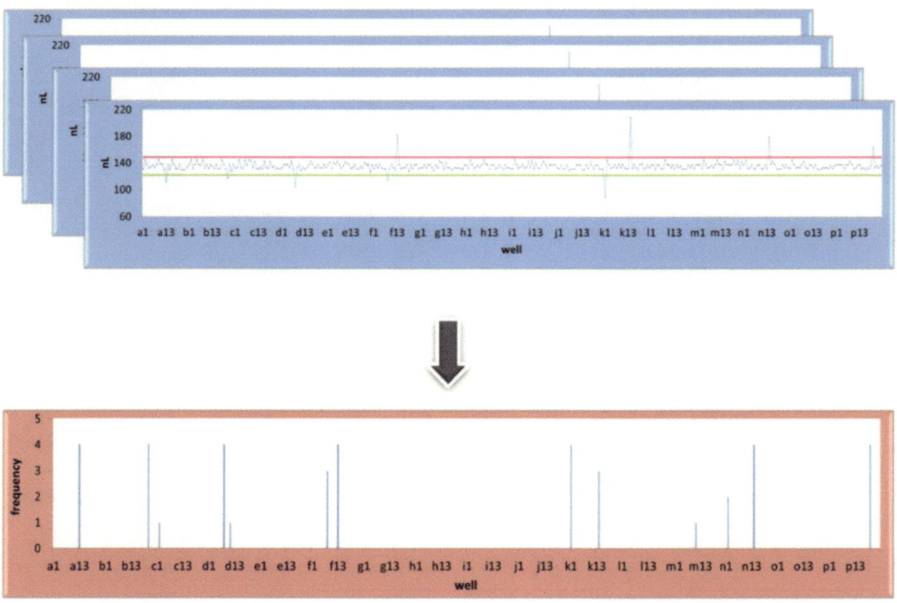

Figure 5. A simple and comprehensive approach to analyze pintool performance. Individual pins can be selected for replacement based on consistent variation across multiple transfers.

3.4. Considerations for using transfer devices: Pipettors

3.4.1. Pipette stations

The automation station is an integral part of any high throughput pipettor, regardless of the type of tips (fixed or disposable) it employs. It typically consists of ANSI/SBS standard compliant single or multiple deck positions on a stationary or moving platform to hold the labware, with a moving arm situated above the platform containing the single- or multi-channel pipette head. A major advantage of automated pipettor devices over manual or electronic multichannel hand-held pipettes is the elimination of inconsistency in the transfer process by minimizing human intervention, which also enables high throughput applications that are not otherwise feasible. The three major tasks that can be performed with suitable hardware settings are liquid transfer, cherry-picking and serial-dilution.

For plate-to-plate liquid transfers, 96- or 384-well pipette heads are preferred to work with 96-/384-/1536-well microplates to speed up the process and increase the throughput. While 4-/8-/12-/16-pipette heads can also be used for direct transfer applications, they are primarily used to perform serial-dilutions. On the other hand, a single channel pipette tip is an essential component to accomplish cherry-picking tasks.

The speed of an automated pipettor is important for time-sensitive experiments. Especially when performing small volume transfers into microplates, the amount of time spent to transfer liquids in a column-by-column or row-by-row manner may be problematic due to quick evaporation. If the speed of transfer is too slow, some evaporation in the first column or row may be observed before dispensing to the last column or row, causing inconsistent volume across the plate. To avoid evaporation issues during liquid transfers, deck size, pipettor speed, head type and the transfer volume should be considered.

3.4.2. Tip contamination

Sample carry-over is a common problem in liquid handling tasks requiring sequential dipping steps into various sample reservoirs. With fixed-tips, an adequate cleaning step is essential between two transfer operations to prevent sample carry-over. An on-deck cleaning protocol often consists of immersion in a bath (DMSO, alcohol and/or water) with optional sonication step. The tips should be allowed sufficient drying time to prevent sample dilution in the following transfer phase. Appropriate wash solutions should be selected and the optimum length of washing time should be determined during the assay development stage. Although fixed-tips may have the risk of carry-over, they enable more accurate and precise transfers in smaller volume ranges (Felton 2003).

Contamination can also be associated with disposable tips, especially when sterile and nuclease-free assay conditions are required. The speed at which the pipette tips are removed from a sample fluid was found to correlate to the amount of macroscopic droplets stuck to the outer surface of the polypropylene tips, which contributed to cross-contamination (Berg et al. 2001). It was also reported that to decrease this form of cross-contamination, which is influenced by the tip shape and the sample-polypropylene interactions, the removal speed should be slow enough to diminish droplet generation.

Impurities can also leach out of the disposable tips when in contact with solvents such as DMSO. Studies have shown that bioactive compounds released from plastic labware may interfere with assay readouts causing misleading experimental results (McDonald et al. 2008; Niles and Coassin 2008; Watson et al. 2009). Consumable materials, especially polypropylene tips, tend to adsorb certain compounds, leading to unreliable concentrations in the destination plates (Harris et al. 2010). Therefore, it is recommended to test and validate the influence of consumables on an assay during assay development and whenever there is a change in labware.

3.4.3. Foaming

Pipetting viscous and "sticky" samples is challenging due to bubble formation. Among the most important parameters to consider in avoiding these issues are the speed that the tips exit the sample fluid and the aspirate/dispense rates; they should be slow enough to avoid residuals at the inside and outside of the tips. Pre- and post-air pipetting options should be avoided.

3.4.4. Pipette behavior affecting dispensing variation

Most pipettor systems provide pre- and post-air aspiration functions to ensure accurate liquid transfers. Introduction of air into the tips before or after the aspiration of the sample liquid is recommended to improve volume accuracy by forcing all the liquid out of the tips. In a study performed to optimize the automated parameters to achieve a 10 μL transfer volume in a sequential transfer experiment, introduction of a 5 μL pre-air gap significantly reduced the relative volume inaccuracy along with the CV of the final transferred volume in a 96-well plate (Albert et al. 2007). While this method may help to achieve more precise results especially with small volume transfers, bubble formation in the destination wells may be inevitable unless proceeded by a shaking or centrifugation step. Post-air aspiration may also be applied to create an air gap between liquids, preventing unsought contamination in the source reservoirs when multiple samples are picked up sequentially into a single tip before the delivery into the destination reservoir.

When small and repetitive volume transfers into multiple destinations are needed, it is a common practice to pick up a single large volume and deliver smaller amounts in a sequential mode. However, with this method, it is hard to achieve accurate delivery in each step. In a study of multi-sequential dispense accuracy, it was shown that the first and last dispense steps led to relatively higher and lower transferred volumes, respectively, in addition to increased relative inaccuracy (Albert et al. 2007). Therefore, it is recommended to dispense the first and last steps into the source reservoir to enhance the precision in the destination plate. Delivery performance of the dry versus pre-wetted tips may also exhibit differences in variability depending on the sample characteristics.

Droplet formation at the end of the pipette tips after a dispense action remains an issue for liquids with high viscosity or low densities. Besides the selection of the optimum dispense speed, a "tip touch" function is a useful feature offered in some automated pipettors, where the tips contact the well wall at the end of a dispense step to force the release of the droplet. The path of the moving pipetting arm across the deck should be carefully determined to reduce the chance of contaminating other labware by hanging droplets.

Proper mixing of solutions in the source reservoir before aspiration and in the destination reservoir after dispensing may greatly affect the final assay quality due to the necessity of uniform sample concentrations. To avoid the formation of concentration gradient in wells, mixing can be performed by repetitive pipetting cycles. Mixing of the well contents by pipetting up and down is proven to be a quicker and more efficient method compared to free diffusion or shaking, which are not as successful due to the correlations between well size, content volume and the exerted capillary forces (Berg et al. 2001; Shieh et al. 2010; Travis et al. 2010). Mixing is necessary when dealing with suspensions (cells, beads, etc.). For instance, cell settling creates uneven cell density in the source reservoir, which would lead to aspiration of decreasing number of cells over time (Fig. 2C)

3.4.5. Routine quality assessment

Verification of transferred volumes and routine quality control (QC) are the most important and inevitable processes when working with liquid handling devices. While the verification method should be reliable enough to quantify the pipettor performance, it should also be easy and fast to be applied routinely. The performance assessment described for bulk liquid dispensers (section 3.2.7.) can also be applied to pipettors as long as the same volume is distributed throughout the plate for %CV and %bias' calculations.

As mentioned previously, liquid handlers are heavily used to perform serial dilutions, and suitable QC techniques should be employed to validate dilution performance, particularly when accurate compound potency is directly dependent on concentration accuracy. Dilution ratio, accuracy, precision and outlier distribution constitute the four major criteria that should be evaluated (Popa-Burke et al. 2009). Artel developed an approach to determine dilution and transferred volume accuracy by using dual-wavelength photometry, where two absorbance dyes with baseline resolved spectra are mixed at various ratios using a liquid handler (Albert 2007; Dong et al. 2007). This dual-dye ratiometric method can be applied by using a multichannel verification system (MVS) equipped with the necessary instrumentation and analysis (Bradshaw et al. 2005). Dual-dye photometry is also proven to be suitable to measure the efficiency of different mixing methods (Spaulding et al. 2006) and when pipetting non-aqueous solutions (Bradshaw et al. 2007).

3.5. Considerations for using microplate washers

3.5.1. General considerations

One of the major concerns with any high throughput microplate handler device is its compatibility with plates of various types and sizes. While most high throughput instruments are designed to accommodate labware with dimensions conforming to ANSI/SBS standards, an ideal plate washer is also able to support flat, v-shaped and round-bottom plates.

Both the vacuum assembly and the bottle setup are also important aspects of the plate washer. Although most washers operate through changes in vacuum pressure, pump-based vacuum-free and pressure-free systems are also offered.

Plate washers functioning by positive displacement principle are also available, enabling non-contact washing with no residual volume (Rudnicki and Johnston 2009). For assays where more than one wash buffer may need to be used, plate washers with multiple dispense channels and automatic buffer switching capability are preferred to minimize both operation time and contamination. Examples of other optional features for safe instrument operation include waste liquid level sensors and plate detection sensors to avoid unwanted overflows and jams. For BSL2 or higher level experiments, a washer with aerosol cover should be chosen to prevent spread of the contagious material.

3.5.2. *Washer performance*

Although compatibility and control properties are important, plate washers are predominantly evaluated by their wash performance. Plate washers provide a range of user-defined dispense/aspirate heights, flow rates, and needle probe positioning in reference to the well walls. By adjusting these parameters for each step of the wash cycle, optimal wash performance can be ensured. On the other hand, an adequate wash quality needs to be reached to diminish extensive background signal and high signal variations amongst wells. This can be primarily achieved by minimizing the amount of liquid left inside each well at the end of the aspiration step. Besides their effects on wash power, the above-mentioned parameters also have an impact on the residual volume and need to be fine-tuned in conjunction with the vacuum/pump settings. Some plate washers may also provide multipoint, secondary, crosswise or delayed aspiration modes aiming to deliver the best results. The number of wash cycles and the length of soaking time are other settings that can be modified to reduce background noise levels.

3.5.3. *Washer maintenance*

Since plate washers consist of tubing and needles which transport buffer solutions or waste liquid to or from the device, they require special cleaning processes as they are prone to be clogged by chemical residues such as salt and proteins from the wash liquids. Depending on the frequency of use, the fluid path may need to be rinsed daily to prevent blockage and contamination, especially if different buffers are being delivered through the same tubing. An efficient cleaning method alternates deionized water and a detergent such as Terg-a-Zyme®, which is highly recommended by plate washer manufacturers. Plate washers which provide an automatic cleaning feature or integrated ultrasonic washing technology are often easier to maintain. Models which do not contain built-in cleaning functionality are generally supplied with removable dispense/aspiration manifolds to ease the maintenance tasks.

Cleaning of the other detachable or fixed plate washer components should also be performed periodically.

3.5.4. Troubleshooting

Plate washers serve as an excellent alternative to time consuming manual wash procedures for many applications. Since all the wash parameters should be optimized for each specific application during the assay development stage, a tedious troubleshooting process may be inevitable while setting up wash protocols to meet specific assay needs. Table 1 presents a summary of wash parameters/components and their contributions to the wash performance along with various troubleshooting tips. Different assay types may require distinct considerations. With biochemical assays, minimizing the background signal and well-to-well variations are the most important tasks in the optimization process. Low background signal levels can be achieved by reducing the leftover liquid volume in each well. Decreasing the aspiration height and lowering the aspiration rate can greatly affect the residual volume leading to minimal liquid amounts in the wells. In order to prevent high standard deviations in the assay readouts, equal residual volumes should be attempted by optimizing the aspiration/dispense heights and rates. Depending on the viscosity of the wash buffer, high aspiration rates or low dispense rates may lead to unequal volumes. Inadequate priming volumes, unadjusted dispense or aspiration heights, clogged tubing, and physical misalignments between the manifolds and plate carrier should also be avoided to prevent high signal variations. The effect of the aspiration height on the final residual volume is presented in Fig. 6 for both 96- and 384-well black plates with clear bottom. The volume of the residual liquid (water) per well was measured with the gravimetric technique at several selected aspiration heights on a Biotek EL405 microplate washer, while all the other wash parameters were kept constant. A rising trend is observed in the final volume as the aspiration height is increased.

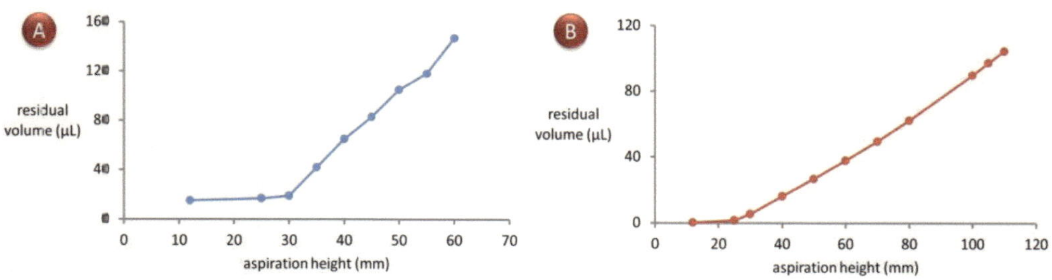

Figure 6. Effects of aspiration height on residual volume. Residual volume was measured in a) 96-well and B) 384-well plates at various aspiration heights. Residual volume was increased as the aspiration height from the bottom of the well was increased.

In cell-based assays, gentle cell washing is one of the most critical factors to produce reproducible assay results, and it can be controlled by several settings such as aspiration and dispense rates, heights and horizontal positions. For loosely-adherent cells, the cell layer attached to the bottom of the well may be easily disrupted by rigorous wash cycles, and the aspiration and dispense rates should be set low enough to prevent turbulence inside the wells. For the same purpose, wash fluid should be dispensed at a distance from the well bottom and may be even be aimed at the well walls when possible. To observe the consequences of inadequate washing and dispensing parameters on the cell layer endurance, a 3-cycle wash experiment was performed on HEK 293T cells, which are known for their low adherence and propensity to be frequently washed away in cell-based assays. The fixing solution was dispensed at medium speed, and the cells were washed before and after fixation. Representative images from wells containing an intact or damaged cell layer are presented in Fig. 7. When dealing with adherent cells, each step of the assay protocol should be optimized, including those involving other liquid handling devices such as bulk dispensers, pintools and pipettors.

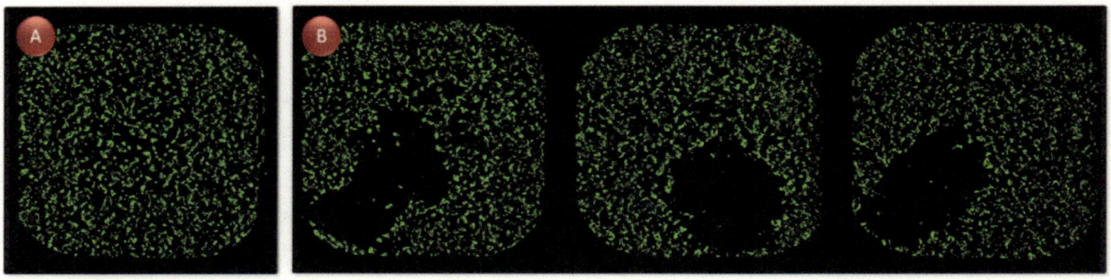

Figure 7. Effects of non-optimized dispensing and washing on low-adherent cells. HEK293T cells were fixed, stained with Hoechst 33258 and imaged with Acumen eX3 in a 384-well black clear bottom plates. The fixing solution was dispensed by a Thermo Scientific Matrix® Wellmate®. Representative images (shown here in false color green) of A) an intact cell layer and B) disrupted cell layers indicated cell loss due to harsh dispense and wash settings.

As with most high throughput instrument operations, it is a common practice to perform a periodic quality check on plate washers to assure a satisfactory wash performance at each use. It is important to perform these assessments with a wash buffer that has a similar viscosity to the buffers used in most of the applications. For evaluations on the residual volume, one can perform a mock wash with a dummy plate and measure the leftover liquid volume inside the wells with a single or multichannel manual pipettor. For more accurate results, gravimetric or colorimetric techniques can be used to calculate the average volume per well. This way, one can also test if dispensing/aspiration is consistent in all the probes, and if there is any physical failure with any of the device components.

http://dx.doi.org/10.5772/52546

parameter/component	effect	troubleshooting tips
prime	dispense performance	• prevent air bubble formation or no/uneven dispensing with adequate priming
aspiration rate	residual volume, gentle/rigorous washing	• higher residual volume if too fast • perturbed cell layer if too fast • uneven aspiration if too fast
aspiration height	residual volume, gentle/rigorous washing	• higher residual volume if too high • uneven aspiration if too low or too high • perturbed cell layer if aspiration probes touch the well bottom • undisturbed cell layer if high enough
horizontal aspirate position	gentle/rigorous washing	• prevent bead loss by offsetting the aspirate position (for magnetic bead assays)
dispense flow rate	dispense volume, gentle/rigorous washing	• uneven dispensing if too slow • fluid overflow if too slow or too fast • perturbed cell layer if too fast • air bubble formation if too slow
dispense height	dispense volume, gentle/rigorous washing	• uneven dispensing if too low or too high • fluid overflow if too high
horizontal dispense position	gentle/rigorous washing	• undisturbed cell layer if dispense position is offset to aim the well walls
assay buffer properties	residual volume, aspiration/dispense performance	• optimize for viscous/non-viscous buffer solutions • add surfactant to the buffer solution to reduce surface tension
vacuum/pump assembly	aspiration/dispense performance	• no/uneven aspiration with insufficient vacuum supply • no/uneven aspiration or leakage if tubing is defective, bent or clogged
plate carrier	aspiration/dispense performance	• uneven aspiration/dispense if plate carrier is not leveled or movement is blocked • plate is placed on the carrier with A1 in the correct position • enough plate clearance to prevent jams • higher throughput with lower plate clearance

Table 1. Wash parameters and troubleshooting advices

4. Conclusion

In order to fulfill the need for higher throughput options, the technology behind liquid handling devices is in constant progression, with systems capable of delivering smaller volumes at a faster rate with accuracy and precision. These developments should consider cost reduction by minimizing reagent and solvent expenditure, as well as reducing consumables.

The main concerns and limitations that liquid handling systems face are reproducibility and reliability. The devices should be robust to execute extensive experiments in a daily basis with minimal downtime and maintenance. However, as a single screen can generate thousands of data points, the user is required to ensure all the devices are functioning up to standards by implementing routine quality assessments. Regardless of the technological innovations and advancements, scientists are compelled to spend significant amount of time optimizing the liquid handling parameters to suit specific assay conditions. A thorough understanding of the principles, strengths and limitations of the instruments is advantageous in preventing undesirable results and facilitating troubleshooting.

Acknowledgements

This work was supported by the American Lebanese Syrian Associated Charities (ALSAC), St. Jude Children's Research Hospital, and National Cancer Institute grant P30CA027165.

Author details

Sergio C. Chai, Asli N. Goktug, Jimmy Cui, Jonathan Low and Taosheng Chen

High Throughput Screening Center, Department of Chemical Biology and Therapeutics, St. Jude Children's Research Hospital, USA

References

[1] Albert, KJ, Bradshaw, JT, Knaide, TR & Rogers, AL (2006). Verifying liquid-handler performance for complex or nonaqueous reagents: a new approach. *Journal of the Association for Laboratory Automation*, Vol. 11(4): pp. 172-80

[2] Bateman, TA, Ayers, RA & Greenway, RB (1999). An engineering evaluation of four fluid transfer devices for automated 384-well high throughput screening. *Laboratory Robotics and Automation*, Vol. 11(5): pp. 250-59

[3] Berg, M, Undisz, K, Thiericke, R, Zimmermann, P, Moore, T & Posten, C (2001). Evaluation of liquid handling conditions in microplates. *Journal of Biomolecular Screening*, Vol. 6(1): pp. 47-56

[4] Bergsdorf, C, Gewiese, N, Stolz, A, Mann, R, Parczyk, K & Bomer, U (2006). A cost-effective solution to reduce dead volume of a standard dispenser system by a factor of 5. *Journal of Biomolecular Screening*, Vol. 11(4): pp. 407-12

[5] Bradshaw, JT, Curtis, RH, Knaide, TR & Spaulding, BW (2007). Determining dilution accuracy in microtiter plate assays using a quantitative dual-wavelength absorbance method. *Journal of the Association for Laboratory Automation*, Vol. 12(5): pp. 260-66

[6] Bradshaw, JT, Knaide, T, Rogers, A & Curtis, R (2005). Multichannel Verification System (MVS): a dual-dye ratiometric photometry system for performance verification of multichannel liquid delivery devices. *Journal of the Association for Laboratory Automation*, Vol. 10(1): pp. 35-42

[7] Cleveland, PH & Koutz, PJ (2005). Nanoliter dispensing for uHTS using pin tools. *Assay and Drug Development Technologies*, Vol. 3(2): pp. 213-25

[8] Diaspro, A, Chirico, G, Usai, C, Ramoino, P & Dobrucki, J (2006). Photobleaching. In: *Handbook of Biological Confocal Microscopy*. J. B. Pawley. pp 690-702, Springer Science +Business Media, LLC, New York

[9] Dong, H, Ouyang, Z, Liu, J & Jemal, M (2006). The use of a dual dye photometric calibration method to identify possible sample dilution from an automated multichannel liquid-handling system. *Journal of the Association for Laboratory Automation*, Vol. 11(2): pp 60-64

[10] Dunn, DA & Feygin, I (2000). Challenges and solutions to ultra-high-throughput screening assay miniaturization: submicroliter fluid handling. *Drug Discovery Today*, Vol. 5(12): pp. S84-S91

[11] Ellson, R, Mutz, M, Browning, B, Lee, L, Miller, MF & Papen, R (2003). Transfer of low nanoliter volumes between microplates using focused acoustics—automation considerations. *Journal of the Association for Laboratory Automation*, Vol. 8(5): pp. 29-34

[12] Felton, MJ (2003). Liquid handling: dispensing reliability. *Analytical Chemistry*, Vol. 75(17): pp. 397a-99a

[13] Harris, D, Mutz, M, Sonntag, M, Stearns, R, Shieh, J, Pickett, S, Ellson, R & Olechno, J (2008). Low nanoliter acoustic transfer of aqueous fluids with high precision and accuracy of volume transfer and positional placement. *Journal of the Association for Laboratory Automation*, Vol. 13(2): pp. 97-102

[14] Harris, D, Olechno, J, Datwani, S & Ellson, R (2010). Gradient, contact-free volume transfers minimize compound loss in dose-response experiments. *Journal of Biomolecular Screening*, Vol. 15(1): pp. 86-94

[15] Harris, DL & Mutz, M (2006). Debunking the myth: validation of fluorescein for testing and precision of nanoliter dispensing. *Journal of the Association for Laboratory Automation*, Vol.11(4): pp. 233-39

[16] James, P & Papen, R (1998). Nanolitre dispensing - a new innovation in robotic liquid handling. *Drug Discovery Today*, Vol. 3(9): pp. 429-30

[17] Kong, F, Yuan, L, Zheng, YF & Chen, W (2012). Automatic liquid handling for life science: a critical review of the current state of the art. *Journal of Laboratory Automation*, Vol. 17(3): pp. 169-85

[18] Lee, S (2006). Development of a vacuum filtration system for the conventional microplate washer. *Journal of Pharmacologicaland Toxicololgical Methods*, Vol. 53(3): pp. 272-6

[19] McDonald, GR, Hudson, AL, Dunn, SMJ, You, HT, Baker, GB, Whittal, RM, Martin, JW, Jha, A, Edmondson, DE & Holt, A (2008). Bioactive contaminants leach from disposable laboratory plasticware. *Science*, Vol. 322(5903): pp. 917-17

[20] McGown, EL & Hafeman, DG (1998). Multichannel pipettor performance verified by measuring pathlength of reagent dispensed into a microplate. *Analytical Biochemistry*, Vol. 258(1): pp. 155-57

[21] Murthy, TV, Kroncke, D & Bonin, PD (2011). Adding precise nanoliter volume capabilities to liquid-handling automation for compound screening experimentation. *Journal of the Association for Laboratory Automation*, Vol. 16(3): pp. 221-28

[22] Niles, WD & Coassin, PJ (2005). Piezo- and solenoid valve-based liquid dispensing for miniaturized assays. *Assay and Drug Development Technologies*, Vol. 3(2): pp. 189-202

[23] Niles, WD & Coassin, PJ (2008). Cyclic olefin polymers: innovative materials for high-density multiwell plates. *Assay and Drug Development Technologies*, Vol. 6(4): pp. 577-90

[24] Olechno, J, Shieh, J & Ellson, R (2006). Improving IC50 results with acoustic droplet ejection. *Journal of the Association for Laboratory Automation*, Vol. 11: pp. 240-46

[25] Petersen, J & Nguyen, J (2005). Comparison of absorbance and fluorescence methods for determining liquid dispensing precision. *Journal of the Association for Laboratory Automation*, Vol. 10: pp. 82-87

[26] Popa-Burke, I, Lupotsky, B, Boyer, J, Gannon, W, Hughes, R, Kadwill, P, Lyerly, D, Nichols, J, Nixon, E, Rimmer, D, Saiz-Nicolas, I, Sanfiz-Pinto, B & Holland, S (2009). Establishing quality assurance criteria for serial dilution operations on liquid-handling equipment. *Journal of Biomolecular Screening*, Vol. 14(8): pp. 1017-30

[27] Ramírez, M, Tudela, C, Crespo, JB, Rubles, A, Jiménez, A, Tarazona, G, Fernández, L, Sánchez, P, Kroncke, D, Tabanera, N, Pérez, J, Sánchez, M, Tormo, JR & Peláez, F (2008). Automation of sample dispensing using pocket tips for evaluation of CYP2C9

isoenzyme reversible inhibition in an evolution precision pipetting platform. *Journal of the Association for Laboratory Automation*, Vol. 13: pp. 289-96

[28] Rhode, H, Schulze, M, Renard, S, Zimmerman, P, Moore, T, Cumme, GA & Horn, A (2004). An improved method for checking HTS/uHTS liquid-handling systems. *Journal of Biomolecular Screening*, Vol. 9(8): pp. 726-33

[29] Rose, D (1999). Microdispensing technologies in drug discovery. *Drug Discovery Today*, Vol. 4(9): pp. 411-19

[30] Rudnicki, S & Johnston, S (2009). Overview of liquid handling instrumentation for high-throughput applications. *Current Protocols in Chemical Biology*, Vol. 1(1): pp. 43-54

[31] Schober, A, Gunther, R, Schwienhorst, A, Doring, M & Lindemann, BF (1993). Accurate high-speed liquid handling of very small biological samples. *Biotechniques*, Vol. 15(2): pp. 324-29

[32] Shieh, J, Ellson, RN & Olechno, J (2006). The effects of small molecule and protein solutes on acoustic drop ejection. *Journal of the Association for Laboratory Automation*, Vol. 11(4): pp. 227-32

[33] Shieh, J, Jamieson, B & Vivek, V (2010). Evaluating five microplate mixing techniques: diffusion, centrifugation, shaking, pipetting and ultrasonic mixing. Poster presented at Society for Biomolecular Sciences, Phoenix, AZ

[34] Spaulding, BW, Bradshaw, JT & Rogers, AL (2006). A method to evaluate mixing efficiency in 384-well plates. Poster presented at Society for Biomolecular Sciences, Seattle, WA

[35] Stobbs, LW (1990). Construction of a simple, inexpensive multiple enzyme-linked immunosorbent assay microdilution plate washer. *Applied and Environmental Microbiology*, Vol. 56(6): pp. 1763-7

[36] Taylor, PB, Ashman, S, Baddeley, SM, Bartram, SL, Battle, CD, Bond, BC, Clements, YM, Gaul, NJ, McAllister, WE, Mostacero, JA, Ramon, F, Wilson, JM, Hertzberg, RP, Pope, AJ &Macarron, R (2002). A standard operating procedure for assessing liquid handler performance in high-throughput screening. *Journal of Biomolecular Screening*, Vol. 7(6): pp. 554-69

[37] Travis, M, Vivek, V, Jamieson, B, Shieh, J & Weaver, D (2010). Mixing effectiveness – amethodology and study of microplate mixing techniques including ultrasonic HENDRIX SM100. Poster presented at Association for Laboratory Automation, Palm Spring, CA

[38] Turmel, M, Itkin, Z, Liu, D & Nie, D (2010). An innovative way to create assay ready plates for concentration response testing using acoustic technology. *Journal of the Association for Laboratory Automation*, Vol. 15(4): pp. 297-305

[39] Walling, LA (2011). An inline QC method for determining serial dilution performance of DMSO-based systems. *Journal of the Association for Laboratory Automation*, Vol. 16(3): pp. 235-40

[40] Watson, J, Greenough, EB, Leet, JE, Ford, MJ, Drexler, DM, Belcastro, JV, Herbst, JJ, Chatterjee, M & Banks, M (2009). Extraction, identification, and functional characterization of a bioactive substance from automated compound-handling plastic tips. *Journal of Biomolecular Screening*, Vol. 14(5): pp. 566-72

Chapter 7

Data Analysis Approaches in High Throughput Screening

Asli N. Goktug, Sergio C. Chai and Taosheng Chen

Additional information is available at the end of the chapter

http://dx.doi.org/10.5772/52508

1. Introduction

With the advances in biotechnology, identification of new therapeutic targets, and better understanding of human diseases, pharmaceutical companies and academic institutions have accelerated their efforts in drug discovery. The pipeline to obtain therapeutics often involves target identification and validation, lead discovery and optimization, pre-clinical animal studies, and eventually clinical trials to test the safety and effectiveness of the new drugs. In most cases, screening using genome-scale RNA interference (RNAi) technology or diverse compound libraries comprises the first step of the drug discovery initiatives. Small interfering RNA (siRNA, a class of double-stranded RNA molecules 20-25 nucleotides in length capable of interfering with the expression of specific genes with complementary nucleotide sequence) screen is an effective tool to identify upstream or downstream regulators of a specific target gene, which may also potentially serve as drug targets for a more efficient and successful treatment. On the other hand, screening of diverse small molecule libraries against a known target or disease-relevant pathway facilitates the discovery of chemical tools as candidates for further development.

Conducting either genome-wide RNAi or small molecule screens has become possible with the advances in high throughput (HT) technologies, which are indispensible to carry out massive screens in a timely manner (Macarron 2006; Martis et al. 2011; Pereira and Williams 2007). In screening campaigns, large quantities of data are collected in a considerably short period of time, making rapid data analysis and subsequent data mining a challenging task (Harper and Pickett 2006). Numerous automatic instruments and operational steps participate in an HT screening process, requiring appropriate data processing tools for data quality assessment and statistical analysis. In addition to quality control (QC) and "hit" selection strategies, pre- and post-processing of the screening data are essential steps in a comprehensive HT operation for subsequent interpretation and annotation of the large data sets. In this chapter, we review statistical data analysis methods developed to meet the needs for handling large datasets generated from HT campaigns. We first discuss the influence of proper assay design on statistical outcomes of the HT screening data. We then highlight similarities and differences among various methods for data normalization, quality assessment and "hit" selection. Information presented here provides guidance to researchers on the major aspects of high throughput screening data interpretation.

2. Role of statistics in HT screening design

2.1. HT screening process

A typical HT screening campaign can be divided into five major steps regardless of the assay type and the assay read-out (Fig. 1). Once target or pathway is identified, assay development is performed to explore the optimal assay conditions, and to miniaturize the assay to a microtiter plate format. Performance of an HT assay is usually quantified with statistical parameters such as signal window, signal variability and Z-factor (see definition in section 4). To achieve acceptable assay performances, one should carefully choose the appropriate reagents, experimental controls and numerous other assay variables such as cell density or protein/substrate concentrations.

The final distribution of the activities from a screening data set depends highly on the target and pathway (for siRNA) or the diversity of the compound libraries, and efforts have been continuously made to generate more diverse libraries (Entzeroth et al. 2009; Gillet 2008; Kummel and Parker 2011; Zhao et al. 2005). Furthermore, the quality and reliability of the screening data is affected by the stability and the purity of the test samples in the screening libraries, where storage conditions should be monitored and validated in a timely manner (Baillargeon et al. 2011; Waybright et al. 2009). For small molecules, certain compounds might interfere with the detection system by emitting fluorescence or by absorbing light, and they should be avoided whenever possible to obtain reliable screening results.

Assay development is often followed by a primary screen, which is carried out at a single concentration (small molecule) or single point measurements (siRNA). As the "hits" identified in the primary screen are followed-up in a subsequent confirmatory screen, it is crucial to optimize the assay to satisfactory standards. Sensitivity - the ability to identify an siRNA or compound as a "hit" when it is a true "hit", and specificity - the ability to classify an siRNA or compound as a "non-hit" when it is not a true "hit", are two critical aspects to identify as many candidates while minimizing false discovery rates. Specificity is commonly emphasized in the confirmatory screens which follow the primary screens. For instance, the confirmatory screen for small molecules often consists of multiple measurements of each compound's activity at various concentrations using different assay formats to assess the compound's potency and selectivity. The confirmatory stage of an RNAi screen using pooled siRNA may be performed in a deconvolution mode, where each well contains a single siRNA. Pooling strategy is also applicable to primary small molecule screens, where a keen pooling design is necessary (Kainkaryam

http://dx.doi.org/10.5772/52508

and Woolf 2009). The confirmatory screens of compounds identified from small molecule libraries are followed by lead optimization efforts involving structure-activity relationship investigations and molecular scaffold clustering. Pathway and genetic clustering analysis, on the other hand, are widespread hit follow-up practices for RNAi screens. The processes encompassing hit identification from primary screens and lead optimization methods require powerful software tools with advanced statistical capabilities.

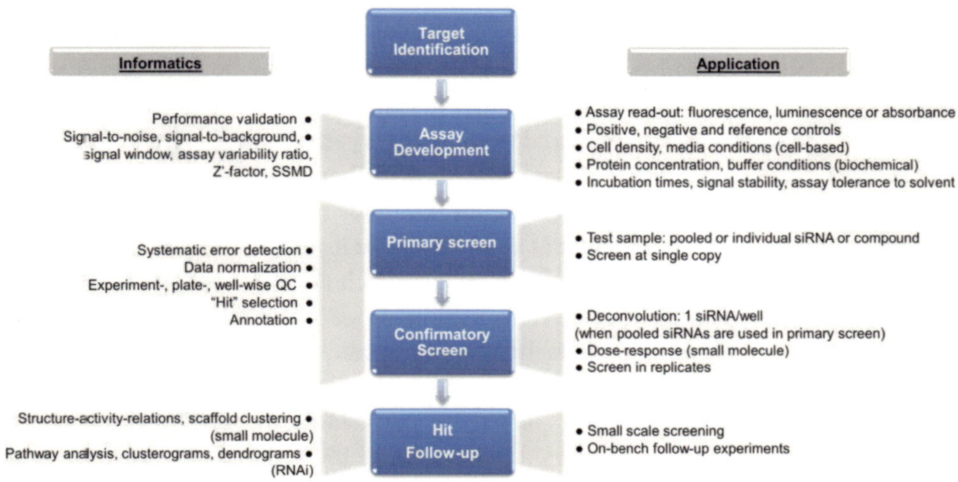

Figure 1. The HT screening process.

Accuracy and precision of an assay are also critical parameters to consider for a successful campaign. While accuracy is a measurement of how close a measured value is to its true value, precision is the proximity of the measured values to each other. Therefore, accuracy of an assay is highly dependent on the performance of the HT instruments in use. Precision, on the other hand, can be a function of sample size and control performances as well as instrument specifications, indicating that the experimental design has a significant impact on the statistical evaluation of the screening data.

2.2. Classical versus robust (resistant) statistics

One of the main assumptions when analyzing HT screening data is that the data is normally distributed, or it complies with the central limit theorem, where the mean of the distributed values converge to normal distribution unless there are systematic errors associated with the screen (Coma et al. 2009). Therefore, log transformations are often applied to the data in the pre-processing stage to achieve more symmetrically distributed data around the mean as in a normal distribution, to represent the relationship between variables in a more linear way especially for cell growth assays, and to make an efficient use of the assay quality assessment parameters (Sui and Wu 2007).

In HT screening practices, the presence of outliers - data points that do not fall within the range of the rest of the data - is generally experienced. Distortions to the normal distribution of the data caused by outliers impact the results negatively. Therefore, an HT data set with outliers needs to be analyzed carefully to avoid an unreliable and inefficient "hit" selection process. Although outliers in control wells can be easily identified, it should be clear that outliers in the test sample may be misinterpreted as real "hits" instead of random errors.

There are two approaches for statistical analysis of data sets with outliers: classical and robust. One can choose to replace or remove outliers based on the truncated mean or similar approaches, and continue the analysis process with classical methods. However, robust statistical approaches have gained popularity in HT screening data analysis in recent decades. In robust statistics, median and median absolute deviation (MAD) are utilized as statistical parameters as opposed to mean and standard deviation (std), respectively, to diminish the effect of outliers on the final analysis results. Although there are numerous approaches to detect and abolish/replace outliers with statistical methods (Hund et al. 2002; Iglewicz and Hoaglin 1993; Singh 1996), robust statistics is preferred for its insensitivity to outliers (Huber 1981). In statistics, while the robustness of an analysis technique can be determined by two main approaches, i.e. influence functions (Hampel et al. 1986) and breakdown point (Hampel 1971), the latter is a more intuitive technique in the concept of HT screening, where the breakdown point of a sample series is defined as the amount of outlier data points that can be tolerated by the statistical parameters before the parameters take on drastically different values that are not representing anymore distribution of the original dataset. In a demonstrated example on a five sample data set, robust parameters were shown to perform superior to the classical parameters after the data set was contaminated with outliers (Rousseeuw 1991). It was also emphasized that median and MAD have a breakdown point of 50%, while mean and std have 0%, indicating that sample sets with 50% outlier density can still be successfully handled with robust statistics.

2.3. False discovery rates

As mentioned previously, depending on the specificity and sensitivity of an HT assay, erroneous assessment of "hits" and "non-hits" is likely. Especially in genome-wide siRNA screens, false positive and negative results may mislead the scientists in the confirmatory studies. While the cause of false discovery results may be due to indirect biological regulations of the gene of interest through other pathways that are not in the scope of the experiment, it may also be due to random errors experienced in the screening process. Although the latter can be easily resolved in the follow-up screens, the former may require a better assay design (Stone et al. 2007). Lower false discovery rates can also be achieved by careful selection of assay reagents to avoid inconsistent measurements (outliers) during screening. The biological interference effects of the reagents in RNAi screens can be considered in two categories: sequence-dependent and sequence-independent (Echeverri et al. 2006; Mohr and Perrimon 2012). Therefore, off-target effects and low transfection efficiencies are the main challenges to be overcome in these screens. Moreover, selection of the appropriate controls for either small molecule or RNAi screens is very crucial for screen quality assessment as

http://dx.doi.org/10.5772/52508

well as for "hit" selection, so that the false discovery rates can be inherently reduced. Positive controls are often chosen from small-molecule compounds or gene silencing agents that are known to have the desired effect on the target of interest; however, this may be a difficult task if very little is known about the biological process (Zhang et al. 2008a). On the other hand, selection of negative controls from non-targeting reagents is more challenging due to higher potential of biological off-target effects in RNAi screens compared to the negative controls used in small-molecule screens (Birmingham et al. 2009). Another factor that might interfere with the biological process in an HT screening assay is the bioactive contaminants that may be released from the consumables used in the screening campaign, such as plastic tips and microplates (McDonald et al. 2008; Watson et al. 2009). Unreliable and misleading screening results may be obtained from altered assay conditions caused by leached materials, and boosted false discovery rates may be unavoidable. Hence, the effects of laboratory consumables on the assay readout should be carefully examined during assay development.

The false discovery rates are also highly dependent on the analysis methods used for "hit" selection, and they can be statistically controlled. False discovery rate is defined as the ratio of false discoveries to the total number of discoveries. A *t*-test and the associated *p* value are often used for hypothesis testing in a single experiment and can be interpreted as the false positive discovery rate (Chen et al. 2010). However, the challenge arises when multiple hypothesis testing is needed or when the comparison of results across multiple experiments is required. For HT applications, a Bayesian approach was developed to enable plate-wise and experiment-wise comparison of results in a single process, while the false discovery rates can still be controlled (Zhang et al. 2008b). Another method utilizing the strictly standardized mean difference (SSMD) parameter was proven to control the false discovery and non-discovery rates in RNAi screens (Zhang 2007a; Zhang 2010 b; Zhang et al. 2010). By taking the data variability into account, SSMD method is capable of determining "hits" with higher assurance compared to the Z-score and *t*-test methods.

3. Normalization and systematic error corrections

3.1. Normalization for assay variability

Despite meticulous assay optimization efforts considering all the factors mentioned previously, it is expected to observe variances in the raw data across plates even within the same experiment. Here, we consider these variances as "random" assay variability, which is separate from the systematic errors that can be linked to a known reason, such as failure of an instrument. Uneven assay performances may unpredictably occur at any given time during screening. Hence, normalization of data within each plate is necessary to enable comparable results across plates or experiments allowing a single cut-off for the selection of "hits".

When normalizing the HT screening data, two main approaches can be followed: controls-based and non-controls-based. In controls-based approaches, the assay-specific in-plate positive and negative controls are used as the upper (100%) and lower (0%) bounds of the assay activity, and the activities of the test samples are calculated with respect to these values. Although, it is an intuitive and easily interpretable method, there are several concerns with the use of controls for normalization purposes. With controls-based methods, too high or too low variability in the control wells does not necessarily represent the variability in the sample wells, and the outliers and biases within the control wells might impair the upper and lower activity bounds (Brideau et al. 2003; Coma et al. 2009). Therefore, non-control-based normalizations are favored for better understanding of the overall activity distribution based on the sample activities per se. In this method, most of the samples are assumed to be inactive in order to serve as their own "negative controls". However, this approach may be misleading when the majority of the wells in a plate consist of true "hits" (such as screening a library of bioactive molecules) or siRNAs (e.g., focused library). Since the basal activity level would shift upwards under these conditions, non-controls-based method would result in erroneous decision making.

Plate-wise versus experiment-wise normalization and "hit" picking is another critical point to consider when choosing the best fitting analysis technique for a screen. Experiment-wise normalizations are advantageous in screens where active samples are clustered within certain plates. In this case, each plate is processed in the context of all plates in the experiment. On the other hand, plate-wise normalizations can effectively correct systematic errors occurring in a plate-specific manner without disrupting the results in other plates (Zhang et al. 2006). Therefore, the normalization method that fits best with one's experimental results should be carefully chosen to perform efficient "hit" selection with low false discovery rates.

The calculation used in the most common controls-based normalization methods are as follows:

- Percent of control (PC): Activity of the ith sample (S_i) is divided by the mean of either the positive or negative control wells (C).

$$PC= \frac{S_i}{mean(C)} x100 \quad (1)$$

- Normalized percent inhibition (NPI): Activity of the ith sample is normalized to the activity of positive and negative controls. The sample activity is subtracted from the high control (C_{high}) which is then divided by the difference between mean of the low control (C_{low}) and the mean of the high control. This parameter may be termed normalized percent activity if the final result is subtracted from 100. Additionally, control means may be preferably substituted with the medians.

$$NPI= \frac{mean(C_{high})-S_i}{mean(C_{high})-mean(C_{low})} x100 \quad (2)$$

The calculation used in the most common non-controls-based normalization methods are as follows.

- Percent of samples (PS): The mean of the control wells in the PC parameter (only when negative control is the control of interest) is replaced with the mean of all samples (S_{all}).

$$PS=\frac{S_i}{mean(S_{all})}x100 \tag{3}$$

- Robust percent of samples (RPS): In order to desensitize the PS calculation to the outliers, robust statistics approach is preferred, where mean of S_{all} in PS calculation is replaced with the median of S_{all}.

$$RPS=\frac{S_i}{median(S_{all})}x100 \tag{4}$$

Assay Variability Normalization				
Controls-based	Percent of control $PC=\frac{S_i}{mean(C)}x100$	Non-controls-based	Percent of samples $PS=\frac{S_i}{mean(S_{all})}x100$	Z-score $Z\text{-score}=\frac{S_i-mean(S_{all})}{std(S_{all})}$
Controls-based	Normalized percent inhibition $NPI=\frac{mean(C_{high})-S_i}{mean(C_{high})-mean(C_{low})}x100$	Non-controls-based	Robust percent of samples $RPS=\frac{S_i}{median(S_{all})}x100$	Robust Z-score $Robust\ Z\text{-score}=\frac{S_i-median(S_{all})}{MAD(S_{all})}$ $MAD(S_{all})=1.4826xmedian(\lvert S_i-median(S_{all})\rvert)$

Systematic Error Corrections			
Non-controls-based	Median polish $r_{ijp}=S_{ijp}-\hat{\mu}_p-\hat{row}_i-\hat{col}_j$	BZ-score $BZ\text{-score}=\frac{r_{ijp}-mean((r_{ijp})_{all})}{std((r_{ijp})_{all})}$	Well-correction
Non-controls-based	B-score $B\text{-score}=\frac{r_{ijp}}{MAD_p}$	Background correction $z_{ij}=\frac{1}{N}\sum_{p=1}^{N}S'_{ijp}$	Diffusion state model (can be controls-based too)

Table 1. Summary of HT screening data normalization methods.

- Z-score: Unlike the above parameters, this method accounts for the signal variability in the sample wells by dividing the difference of S_i and the mean of S_{all} by the std of S_{all}. Z-score is a widely used measure to successfully correct for additive and multiplicative offsets between plates in a plate-wise approach (Brideau et al. 2003).

$$Z\text{-score}=\frac{S_i-mean(S_{all})}{std(S_{all})} \tag{5}$$

- Robust Z-score: Since Z-score calculation is highly affected by outliers, robust version of Z-score is available for calculations insensitive to outliers. In this parameter, the mean and std are replaced with median and MAD, respectively.

$$Robust\ Z\text{-score}=\frac{S_i-median(S_{all})}{MAD(S_{all})} \tag{6}$$

$$MAD(S_{all})=1.4826 \text{ x median}(|S_i\text{-median}(S_{all})|) \quad (7)$$

3.2. Normalization for systematic errors

Besides the data variability between plates due to random fluctuations in assay performance, systematic errors are one of the major concerns in HT screening. For instance plate-wise spatial patterns play a crucial role in cell-based assay failures. As an example, incubation conditions might be adjusted to the exact desired temperature and humidity settings, but the perturbed air circulations inside the incubator unit might cause an uneven temperature gradient, resulting in different cell-growth rates in each well due to evaporation issues. Therefore, depending on the positions of the plates inside the incubator, column-wise, row-wise or bowl-shape edge effects may be observed within plates (Zhang 2008b; Zhang 2011b). On the other hand, instrumental failures such as inaccurate dispensing of reagents from individual dispenser channels might cause evident temporal patterns in the final readout. Therefore, experiment-wise patterns should be carefully examined via proper visual tools. Although some of these issues might be fixed at the validation stage such as performing routine checks to test the instrument performances, there are numerous algorithms developed to diminish these patterns during data analysis, and the most common ones are listed as follows and summarized in Table 1.

- Median polish: Tukey's two-way median polish (Tukey 1977) is utilized to calculate the row and column effects within plates using a non-controls-based approach. In this method, the row and column medians are iteratively subtracted from all wells until the maximum tolerance value is reached for the row and column medians as wells as for the row and column effects. The residuals in p^{th} plate (r_{ijp}) are then calculated by subtracting the estimated plate average ($\hat{\mu}_p$), i^{th} row effect ($\widehat{row}_i$) and j^{th} column effect ($\widehat{col}_j$) from the true sample value (S_{ijp}). Since median parameter is used in the calculations, this method is relatively insensitive to outliers.

$$r_{ijp}=S_{ijp}-\hat{\mu}_p-\widehat{row}_i-\widehat{col}_j \quad (8)$$

- B-score: This is a normalization parameter which involves the residual values calculated from median polish and the sample MAD to account for data variability. The details of median polish technique and an advanced B-score method, which accounts for plate-to-plate variances by smoothing are provided in (Brideau et al. 2003).

$$\text{B-score}=\frac{r_{ijp}}{MAD_p} \quad (9)$$

$$MAD_p= 1.4826 \text{ x median}(|(r_{ijp})_{all}\text{- median}((r_{ijp})_{all})|) \quad (10)$$

- BZ-score: This is a modified version of the B-score method, where the median polish is followed by Z-score calculations. While BZ-score is more advantageous to Z-score because of its capability to correct for row and column effects, it is less powerful than B-score and does not fit very well with the normal distribution model (Wu et al. 2008).

$$\text{BZ-score}=\frac{r_{ijp}-\text{mean}((r_{ijp})_{all})}{\text{std}((r_{ijp})_{all})} \tag{11}$$

- Background correction: In this correction method, the background signal corresponding to each well is calculated by averaging the activities within each well (S'_{ijp} representing the normalized signal of a well in i^{th} row and j^{th} column in p^{th} plate) across all plates. Then, a polynomial fitting is performed to generate an experiment-wise background surface for a single screening run. The offset of the background surface from a zero plane is considered to be the consequence of present systematic errors, and the correction is performed by subtracting the background surface from each plate data in the screen. The background correction performed on pre-normalized data was found to be more efficient, and exclusion of the control wells was recommended in the background surface calculations. The detailed description of the algorithm is found in (Kevorkov and Makarenkov 2005).

$$z_{ij}=\frac{1}{N}\sum_{p=1}^{N} S'_{ijp} \tag{12}$$

- Well-correction: This method follows an analogous strategy to the background correction method; however, a least-squares approximation or polynomial fitting is performed independently for each well across all plates. The fitted values are then subtracted from each data point to obtain the corrected data set. In a study comparing the systematic error correction methods discussed so far, well-correction method was found to be the most effective for successful "hit" selection (Makarenkov et al. 2007).
- Diffusion-state model: As mentioned previously, the majority of the spatial effects are caused by uneven temperature gradients across assay plates due to inefficient incubation conditions. To predict the amount of evaporation in each well in a time and space dependent manner, and its effect on the resulting data set, a diffusion-state model was developed by (Carralot et al. 2012). As opposed to the above mentioned correction methods, the diffusion model can be generated based on the data from a single control column instead of sample wells. The edge effect correction is then applied to each plate in the screening run based on the generated model.

Before automatically applying a systematic error correction algorithm on the raw data set, it should be carefully considered whether there is a real need for such data manipulation. To detect the presence of systematic errors, several statistical methods were developed (Coma et al. 2009; Root et al. 2003). In a demonstrated study, the assessment of row and column effects was performed based on a robust linear model, so called R score, and it was shown that performing a positional correction using R score on the data that has no or very small spatial effects results in lower specificity. However, correcting a data set with large spatial effects decreases the false discovery rates considerably (Wu et al. 2008). In the same study, receiver operating characteristics (ROC) curves were generated to compare the performance of several positional correction algorithms based on sensitivity and "1-specificity" values, and R-score was found to be the most superior. On the other hand, application of well-correction or diffusion model on data sets with no spatial effects was shown to have no adverse effect on the final "hit" selection (Carralot et al. 2012; Makarenkov et al. 2007). Additionally, reduction of thermal gradients and associated edge effects in cell-based assays was shown to be possible by easy adjustments to the assay workflow, such as incubating the plates at room temperature for 1 hour immediately after dispensing the cells into the wells (Lundholt et al. 2003).

4. QC methods

There are various environmental, instrumental and biological factors that contribute to assay performance in an HT setting. Therefore, one of the key steps in the analysis of HT screening data is the examination of the assay quality. To determine if the data collected from each plate meet the minimum quality requirements, and if any patterns exist before and after data normalization, the distribution of control and test sample data should be examined at experiment-, plate- and well-level. While there are numerous graphical methods and tools available for the visualization of the screening data in various formats (Gribbon et al. 2005; Gunter et al. 2003; Wu and Wu 2010), such as scatter plots, heat maps and frequency plots, there are also many statistical parameters for the quantitative assessment of assay quality. Same as for the normalization techniques, both controls-based and non-controls-based approaches exist for data QC methods. The most commonly-used QC parameters in HT screening are listed as follows and summarized in Table 2.

- Signal-to-background (S/B): This is a simple measure of the ratio of the positive control mean to the background signal mean (i.e. negative control).

$$S/B=\frac{\mathrm{mean}(C_{pos})}{\mathrm{mean}(C_{neg})} \tag{13}$$

- Signal-to-noise (S/N): This is a similar measure to S/B with the inclusion of signal variability in the formulation. Two alternative versions of S/N are presented below. Both S/B and S/N are considered week parameters to represent dynamic signal range for an HT screen and are rarely used.

$$\begin{aligned} S/N&=\frac{\mathrm{mean}(C_{pos})-\mathrm{mean}(C_{neg})}{\mathrm{std}(C_{neg})} \quad (a) \\ S/N&=\frac{\mathrm{mean}(C_{pos})-\mathrm{mean}(C_{neg})}{\sqrt{\mathrm{std}(C_{pos})^2+\mathrm{std}(C_{neg})^2}} \quad (b) \end{aligned} \tag{14}$$

- Signal window (SW): This is a more indicative measure of the data range in an HT assay than the above parameters. Two alternative versions of the SW are presented below, which only differ by denominator.

$$SW=\frac{\left|mean\left(C_{pos}\right)-mean\left(C_{neg}\right)\right|-3x\left(std\left(C_{pos}\right)+std\left(C_{neg}\right)\right)}{std\left(C_{pos}\right)}(a)$$
$$SW=\frac{\left|mean\left(C_{pos}\right)-mean\left(C_{neg}\right)\right|-3x\left(std\left(C_{pos}\right)+std\left(C_{neg}\right)\right)}{std\left(C_{neg}\right)}(b) \quad (15)$$

- Assay variability ratio (AVR): This parameter captures the data variability in both controls as opposed to SW, and can be defined as (1-Z′-factor) as presented below.

$$AVR=\frac{3 \times std(C_{pos}) + 3 \times std(C_{neg})}{\left|mean(C_{pos}) - mean(C_{neg})\right|} \quad (16)$$

- Z′-factor: Despite of the fact that AVR and Z′-factor has similar statistical properties, the latter is the most widely used QC criterion, where the separation between positive (C_{pos}) and negative (C_{neg}) controls is calculated as a measure of the signal range of a particular assay in a single plate. Z′-factor has its basis on normality assumption, and the use of 3 std's of the mean of the group comes from the 99.73% confidence limit (Zhang et al. 1999). While Z′-factor accounts for the variability in the control wells, positional effects or any other variability in the sample wells are not captured. Although Z′-factor is an intuitive method to determine the assay quality, several concerns were raised about the reliability of this parameter as an assay quality measure. Major issues associated with the Z′-factor method are that the magnitude of the Z′-factor does not necessarily correlate with the hit confirmation rates, and that Z′-factor is not an appropriate measure to compare the assay quality across different screens and assay types (Coma et al. 2009; Gribbon et al. 2005).

$$Z'\text{-factor}=1 - \frac{3 \times std(C_{pos}) + 3 \times std(C_{neg})}{\left|mean(C_{pos}) - mean(C_{neg})\right|} \quad (17)$$

- Z-factor: This is the modified version of the Z′-factor, where the mean and std of the negative control are substituted with the ones for the test samples. Although Z-factor is more advantageous than Z′-factor due to its ability to incorporate sample variability in the calculations, other issues associated with Z′-factor (as discussed above) still apply. Additionally, in a focused library in which many possible "hits" are clustered in certain plates, Z-factor would not be an appropriate QC parameter. While assays with Z′- or Z-factor values above 0.5 are considered to be excellent, one may want to include additional measures, such as visual inspection or more advanced formulations in the decision process, especially for cell-based assays with inherently high signal variability. The power of the above mentioned parameters were discussed in multiple studies (Gribbon et al. 2005; Iversen et al. 2006; Macarron and Hertzberg 2009; Stevens et al. 1998).

$$\text{Z-factor}=1 - \frac{3 \times std(C_{pos}) + 3 \times std(S_{all})}{|mean(C_{pos}) - mean(S_{all})|} \tag{18}$$

- SSMD: It is an alternative quality metric to Z′- and Z-factor, which was recently developed to assess the assay quality in HT screens (Zhang 2007a; Zhang 2007b). Due to its basis on probabilistic and statistical theories, SSMD was shown to be a more meaningful parameter than previously mentioned methods for QC purposes. SSMD differs from Z′- and Z-factor by its ability to handle controls with different effects, which enables the selection of multiple QC criteria for assays (Zhang et al. 2008a). The application of SSMD-based QC criterion was demonstrated in multiple studies in comparison to other commonly-used methods (Zhang 2008b; Zhang 2011b; Zhang et al. 2008a). Although SSMD was developed primarily for RNAi screens, it can also be used for small molecule screens.

$$\text{SSMD}= \frac{mean(C_{pos}) + mean(C_{neg})}{\sqrt{std(C_{pos})^2 + std(C_{neg})^2}} \tag{19}$$

Signal-to-background (S/B)	$\frac{mean(C_{pos})}{mean(C_{neg})}$
Signal-to-noise (S/N)	$\frac{mean(C_{pos}) - mean(C_{neg})}{std(C_{neg})}$ or $\frac{mean(C_{pos}) - mean(C_{neg})}{\sqrt{std(C_{pos})^2 + std(C_{neg})^2}}$
Signal window (SW)	$\frac{\lvert mean(C_{pos}) - mean(C_{neg})\rvert - 3 \times (std(C_{pos}) + std(C_{neg}))}{std(C_{pos})}$ or $\frac{\lvert mean(C_{pos}) - mean(C_{neg})\rvert - 3 \times (std(C_{pos}) + std(C_{neg}))}{std(C_{neg})}$
Assay variability ratio (AVR)	$\frac{3 \times std(C_{pos}) + 3 \times std(C_{neg})}{\lvert mean(C_{pos}) - mean(C_{neg})\rvert} = 1 - \text{Z'-factor}$
Z′-factor	$1 - \frac{3 \times std(C_{pos}) + 3 \times std(C_{neg})}{\lvert mean(C_{pos}) - mean(C_{neg})\rvert}$
Z-factor	$1 - \frac{3 \times std(C_{pos}) + 3 \times std(S_{all})}{\lvert mean(C_{pos}) - mean(S_{all})\rvert}$
SSMD	$\frac{mean(C_{pos}) - mean(C_{neg})}{\sqrt{std(C_{pos})^2 + std(C_{neg})^2}}$

Table 2. Summary of HT screening data QC methods.

http://dx.doi.org/10.5772/52508

5. "Hit" selection methods

The main purpose of HT screens is to obtain a list of compounds or siRNAs with desirable activity for further confirmation. Therefore, the ultimate goal of an HT screening campaign is to narrow down a big and comprehensive compound or siRNA library to a manageable number of "hits" with low false discovery rates. While the initial library of test samples undergoes multiple phases of elimination, the most critical factor is to select as many true "hits" as possible. After data normalization is applied as necessary, "hit" selection is performed on the plates that pass the QC criterion. As stated previously in Section 2.1, HT processes in primary and confirmatory screens differ in design. The "hit" selection process following a primary screen is similar for RNAi and small-molecule screens, where the screening run is often performed in single copy, and a single data point (obtained from either endpoint or kinetic reading) is collected for each sample. On the other hand, a confirmatory RNAi screen is typically performed in replicates using pooled or individual siRNA, while the confirmatory small-molecule screens are executed in dose-response mode. Here, we classify the "hit" selection methodologies in two major categories: primary and confirmatory screen analysis.

5.1. "Hit" selection in primary screen

Although RNAi and small molecule assays differ in many ways, a common aim is to classify the test samples with relatively higher or lower activities than the reference wells as "hits". Hence, it is required to select an activity cut-off, where test samples with values above or below the cut-off are identified as "hits". It is very crucial to select a sensible cut-off value with enough difference from the noise level in order to reduce false positive rates. Depending on the specific goals of the projects, the cut-off might need to be a reasonable value that leads to a manageable quantity of "hits" for follow-up studies. To guide scientists in the process, numerous "hit" selection methods have been developed for HT screens as presented below.

- Percent inhibition cut-off: The "hits" from HT screening data that is normalized for percent inhibition (NPI method in Section 3.1) can be selected based on a percent cut-off value that is arbitrarily assigned relative to an assay's signal window. As this method does not have much statistical basis to it, it is primarily preferred for small molecule screens with strong controls.

- Mean +/- k std: In this method, cut-off is set to the value that is k std's above or below the sample mean. While the cut-off can be applied to the normalized data, a k value of 3 is typically used, which is associated with the false positive error rate of 0.00135 (Zhang et al. 2006). As this cut-off calculation method is primarily based on normality assumption, it is also equivalent to a Z-score of 3. Since the use of mean and std make this method sensitive to outliers, a more robust version is presented next.

- Median +/- k MAD: To desensitize the "hit" selection to outliers, a cut-off that is k MADs above or below the sample median was developed, and a study comparing the std- and MAD-based "hit" selection methods showed lower false non-discovery rates with the latter (Chung et al. 2008).

- Quartile-based method: Similar to the previous approaches, the quartile-based "hit" selection method is based on the idea of treating the true "hits" as outliers and identifying them by setting upper and lower cut-off boundaries based on the quartiles and interquartiles of the data. The major advantage of the quartile-based method over median +/- k MAD is its more effective cut-off calculation formulation for non-symmetrical data, where upper and lower cut-offs can be determined independently. In the comparison of the three "hit" selection criteria presented so far, the quartile-based method outperformed the other two methods to detect true "hits" with moderate effects (Zhang et al. 2006).
- SSMD and Robust SSMD: This parameter has become a widely-used method for RNAi screening data analysis mainly due to its ability to quantify RNAi effects with a statistical basis, and its better control on false negative and false positive rates (Zhang 2007a; Zhang 2007b; Zhang 2009; Zhang 2010a; Zhang 2010 b; Zhang 2011b; Zhang et al. 2010). SSMD is a robust parameter to capture the magnitude of the RNAi effects with various sample sizes. This scoring method also provides comparison of values across screens. Mean and std in the standard SSMD formula is substituted with median and MAD in the robust version. The SSMD parameter used for the primary screens without replicates holds a linear relationship with the Z-score method.
- Bayesian method: This method is used to combine both plate-wise and experiment-wise information within single "hit" selection calculation based on Bayesian hypothesis testing (Zhang et al. 2008b). Bayesian statistics incorporates a prior data distribution and a likelihood function to generate a posterior distribution function. In HT screening data analysis using this method, the experiment- and plate-wise information is incorporated into the prior and likelihood functions, respectively. With the availability of various prior distribution models, the Bayesian method can be applied either with positive and negative controls or with test sample wells. As this method enables the control of false discovery rates, it is a more powerful "hit" selection measure than the median +/- k MAD when the sample data is used to generate the prior distribution.

5.2. "Hit" selection in confirmatory screen

Different strategies are pursued for the confirmation of "hits" from RNAi and small molecule primary screens. While dose response screens are very common to test the compound activities in a dose-dependent manner in small molecule screens, this is not applicable to RNAi screens. Here, we will present the "hit" selection methods for screens with replicates in two categories: dose-response analysis and others.

5.2.1. Dose-response analysis

After running a primary screen, in which a single concentration of compound is used, a subset of compounds is selected for a more quantitative assessment. These molecules are tested at various concentrations and plotted against the corresponding assay response. These types of curves are commonly referred to as "dose-response" or "concentration-response" curves, and they are generally defined by four parameters: top asymptote (maximal response), bottom asymptote (baseline response), slope (Hill slope or Hill coefficient), and the EC_{50} value.

http://dx.doi.org/10.5772/52508

A plot of signal as a function of concentration results in a rectangular hyperbola when the hill coefficient is 1 (Fig. 2A). Because the concentration range covers several orders of magnitude, the x-axis is normally displayed in the logarithm scale, resulting in a sigmoidal curve (Fig. 2B), which is generally fitted with the Hill equation:

$$\text{signal}=B+\frac{T-B}{1+\left(\frac{EC_{50}}{x}\right)^{h}} \tag{20}$$

The most accepted benchmark for drug potency is the EC_{50} value, which corresponds to the concentration of compound (x) that generates a signal midway between the top (T) and bottom (B) asymptotes (Fig. 2B). The steepness is indicated by the Hill slope (h), also known as the Hill coefficient or the slope factor (Fig. 2C).

It is preferable to apply the Hill equation to concentrations on a logarithmic scale, because the error associated with the EC_{50} (log form) follows a Gaussian distribution (Motulsky and Neubig 2010), as indicated in Eq. 21. The x values represent log[compound].

$$\text{signal}=B+\frac{T-B}{1+\left(\frac{10^{\text{Log } EC_{50}}}{10^{x}}\right)^{h}} \tag{21}$$

In biochemical experiments, a Hill coefficient of 1 is indicative of a 1:1 stoichiometry of enzyme-inhibitor or protein-ligand complexes. Under such condition, an increase from 10% to 90% response requires 81-fold change in compound concentration. Hill coefficient values that deviate from unity could reflect mechanistic implications (such as cooperativity or multiple binding sites) or non-ideal behavior of the compound (acting as protein denaturant or causing micelle formation) (Copeland 2005).

For symmetrical curves, the inflection point corresponds to the relative EC_{50} value, which lies halfway between the asymptotes. This relative EC_{50} may be different from the actual EC_{50} if the top and bottom plateaus do not accurately represent 0% and 100% response. For instance, in Fig. 2D, the midpoint in the black curve dictates a value of 60% based on the positive and negative controls. When using the relative EC_{50}, careful analysis of data fitting is necessary to avoid deceptive results, as exemplified by the green curve in Fig. 2D. Curve fitting would provide a relative EC_{50} value of 1 for both the green and black curves, but based on controls, the compound associated with the green curve would inhibit the assay only by 20%. Therefore, it is argued that the best approach is to use a two-parameter curve fit, where only two parameters are allowed to float (EC_{50} and Hill coefficient values), while fixing the top and bottom boundaries as presented in Fig. 2E. (Copeland 2005).

Although EC_{50} is normally the main criterion to categorize compounds for downstream analysis, the value is highly dependent on assay conditions, such as cell number and enzyme/substrate amount (Copeland 2003). For enzymatic assays, a more attractive approach is to consider relative affinities. Cheng and Prusoff formulated a way to convert EC_{50} values to dissociation constants, thus reducing the overload of performing multiple titrations associated with standard enzyme kinetics (Cheng and Prusoff 1973). Nevertheless, the caveat of using this convenient alternative is to recognize the inhibitory modality of the compounds (Copeland 2005): competitive (Eq. 22), non-competitive (Eq. 23) and uncompetitive (Eq. 24).

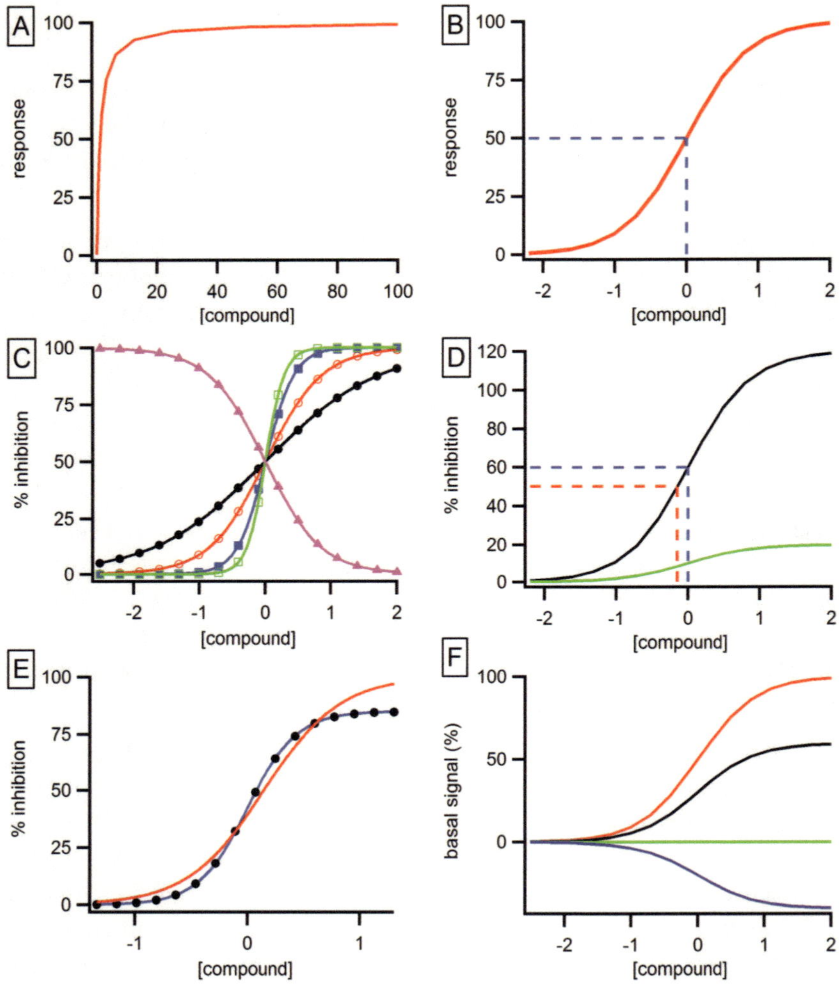

Figure 2. Dose-response curves. A) Response vs. compound concentration resulting in a rectangular hyperbola curve. B) Response vs. logarithm of compound concentration resulting in a sigmoidal curve. The dashed lines indicate the concentration corresponding to half-maximal signal. C) Curves at different Hill slopes: 0.5 (black, closed circles), 1 (red, open circles), 2 (blue, closed squares), 3 (green, open squares) and -1 (pink, closed triangles). D) Relative (blue dash lines) and actual (red dash lines) EC_{50} values for a curve with different top boundary from that of the control (black curve). The green and black curves have the same relative EC_{50}. E) The red curve fits the data points (black circles) allowing 2 parameters (EC_{50}, hill coefficient) to float, while the blue curve fits the data refining all 4 parameters (EC_{50}, hill coefficient, top and bottom asymptotes). F) Curves corresponding to a full agonist (red), partial agonist (black), antagonist (green) and inverse agonist (blue).

http://dx.doi.org/10.5772/52508

$$EC_{50}=K_i\left(1+\frac{S}{K_M}\right) \tag{22}$$

$$EC_{50}=\frac{S+K_M}{\frac{K_M}{K_i}+\frac{S}{\alpha \times K_i}} \tag{23}$$

$$EC_{50}=\alpha \times K_i\left(1+\frac{K_M}{S}\right) \tag{24}$$

The dissociation constant of a reversible compound (K_i) can be calculated based on a single substrate concentration (S) and the Michaelis constant (K_M). The constant α delineates the effect of inhibitor binding on the affinity of the substrate for the enzyme. It becomes evident that EC_{50} and K_i are roughly the same at much lower substrate concentration relative to K_M (Eq. 22) or when α=1 (Eq. 23).

Dose-response curves can follow various patterns, depending on the biological system to be investigated. For assays with certain basal level, increasing concentrations of a full agonist triggers a maximal response for the system (Fig. 2F, red curve). A partial agonist displays a reduced response (efficacy) relative to a full agonist (Fig. 2F, black curve), even though they both exhibit the same potency (i.e. same EC_{50} values). An antagonist might have certain affinity or potency, but it would not show any change in basal activity as the efficacy has a value of zero (Fig. 2F, green curve). However, an antagonist reverses the actions of an agonist. In pharmacological terms, the effects of a competitive antagonist can be overcome by augmenting the amount of agonist, but such agonist increment has no effect on the effects of non-competitive antagonists. Inverse agonists reduce the basal response of systems with constitutive activity (Fig. 2F, blue curve).

5.2.2. Other methods

In "hit" selection for confirmatory screens with single concentration of compound or siRNA, hypothesis testing is a commonly-used method to incorporate sample variability of each sample from its replicates. Therefore, confirmatory screens (or some primary screens) are chosen to be performed in replicates to statistically calculate the significance of the sample activity in relation to a negative reference group. Since previously listed Z- and robust Z-score methods assume that the variability of the test samples and the negative controls or references is equal, it is not a reliable measure for confirmatory screens with replicates, where the sample variability can be individually calculated. The most common methods to analyze screening data with replicates are listed below.

- *t*-test: For "hit" selection in confirmatory screens, *t* statistics and the associated *p* value is used to calculate if a sample compound or siRNA is behaving significantly different than the majority of the test samples or controls. A *t*-test determines whether the null hypothesis, which is the mean of a test sample being equal to the mean of the negative reference group, is accepted or not. Paired *t*-test (first pairing of the test sample and reference value within each plate, then calculating *t* statistic on the paired values) is often preferred to avoid the distortion of results due to inter-plate variability, whereas unpaired *t*-test is used for global comparison of the sample replicates with all reference values in the experiment (Zhang 2011a). The *p* value calculated from *t* statistic is then used to determine the significance of the sample activity compared to the reference. An alternative to standard *t*-test, namely randomized variance model (RVM) *t*-test (Wright and Simon 2003), was found to be more advantageous for screens with few replicates to detect relatively less strong "hits" (Malo et al. 2010).

- SSMD: While *t*-test is a useful method to calculate the significance of the sample activity by incorporating its variability across replicates, it lacks the ability to rank the samples by their effect sizes. As an alternative to *t*-test, SSMD-based "hit" selection method for replicates was proposed to enable the calculation of RNAi effects as previously illustrated in (Zhang 2011a). While SSMD-based method is more robust with small sample sizes as opposed to *t*-test (Zhang 2008a), at least 4 replicates is recommended in confirmatory screens to identify samples with moderate or higher effects (Zhang and Heyse 2009).
- Various other *p* value calculation methods (e.g., redundant siRNA activity, or RSA) (Konig et al. 2007) and rank products method (Breitling et al. 2004)) are available, which can be adapted to detect "hits" in RNAi screens (Birmingham et al. 2009).

6. Conclusion

HT screening is a comprehensive process to discover new drug targets using siRNA and drug candidates from small molecule libraries. Statistical evaluation of the assay performance is a very critical step in HT screening data analysis. A number of data analysis methods have been developed to correct for plate-to-plate assay variability and systematic errors, and assess assay quality. Statistical analysis is also pivotal in the "hit" selection process from primary screens and in the evaluation during confirmatory screens. While some of these methods may be intuitively applied using spreadsheet programs (e.g., Microsoft Excel), others may require the development of computer programs using more advanced programming environments (e.g., R, Perl, C++, Java, MATLAB). Besides commercially available comprehensive analysis tools, there are also numerous open-access software packages designed for HT screening data management and analysis for scientist with little or no programming knowledge. A short compilation of freely available analysis tools is listed in Table 3. The growing number of statistical methods will accelerate the discovery of drug candidates with higher confidence.

	Features	Programming Language
Screensaver	Web-based laboratory information management system for management of library and screen information (Tolopko et al. 2010)	Java
MScreen	Web-based compound library and siRNA plate management, QC and dose-response fitting tools (Jacob et al. 2012)	PHP, Oracle/MySQL
NEXT-RNAi	Library design and evaluation tools for RNAi screens (Horn et al. 2010)	Perl
K-Screen	Analysis, visualization, management and mining of HT screening data including dose-response curve fitting (Tai et al. 2011)	R, PHP, MySQL
HTS-Corrector	Statistical analysis, visualization and correction of systematic errors for all HT screens (Makarenkov et al. 2006)	C#
web cellHTS2	Web-based analysis toolbox for normalization, QC, "hit" selection and annotation for RNAi screens (Boutros et al. 2006; Pelz et al. 2010)	R/Bioconductor project
RNAither	Automated pipeline for normalization, QC, "hit" selection and pathway generation for RNAi screens (Rieber et al. 2009)	R/Bioconductor project
HTSanalyzeR	Gene set enrichment, network and gene set comparison analysis for post-processing of RNAi screening data (Wang et al. 2011)	R/Bioconductor project

Table 3. Examples of open-access software packages for library management and statistical analysis of HT screening data.

Acknowledgements

This work was supported by the American Lebanese Syrian Associated Charities (ALSAC), St. Jude Children's Research Hospital, and National Cancer Institute grant P30CA027165.

Author details

Asli N. Goktug, Sergio C. Chai and Taosheng Chen

High Throughput Screening Center, Department of Chemical Biology and Therapeutics, St. Jude Children's Research Hospital, USA

References

[1] Ang, K. L., Feroze, F., Ganji, G.,& Li, Y. (2004). Cell-based RNAi assay development for HTS. In: *Assay Guidance Manual*. Sittampalam, G. S., Gal-Edd, N., Arkin, M., Auld, D., Austin, C., Bejcek, B., Glicksman, M., Inglese, J., Lemmon, V., Li, Z., McGee, J., McManus, O., Minor, L., Napper, A., Riss, T., Trask, J., &Weidner J., pp. 1-20, Eli Lilly & Company, Retrieved from http://www.ncbi.nlm.nih.gov/books/NBK91998/

[2] Baillargeon, P., Scampavia, L., Einsteder, R., & Hodder, P. (2011). Monitoring of HTS compound library quality via a high-resolution image acquisition and processing instrument. *Journal of Laboratory Automation*, Vol. 16, No. 3, pp. 197-203.

[3] Birmingham, A., Selfors, L. M., Forster, T., Wrobel, D., Kennedy, C. J., Shanks, E., Santoyo-Lopez, J., Dunican, D. J., Long, A., Kelleher, D., Smith, Q., Beijersbergen, R. L., Ghazal, P., & Shamu, C. E. (2009). Statistical methods for analysis of high-throughput RNA interference screens. *Nature Methods*, Vol. 6, No. 8, pp. 569-75.

[4] Boutros, M., Bras, L. P., & Huber, W. (2006). Analysis of cell-based RNAi screens. *Genome Biology*, Vol. 7, No. 7, pp. R66.1-11.

[5] Breitling, R., Armengaud, P., Amtmann, A., & Herzyk, P. (2004). Rank products: a simple, yet powerful, new method to detect differentially regulated genes in replicated microarray experiments. *FEBS Letters*, Vol. 573, No. 1-3, pp. 83-92.

[6] Brideau, C., Gunter, B., Pikounis, B., & Liaw, A. (2003). Improved statistical methods for hit selection in high-throughput screening. *Journal of Biomolecular Screening*, Vol. 8, No. 6, pp. 634-47.

[7] Carralot, J. P., Ogier, A., Boese, A., Genovesio, A., Brodin, P., Sommer, P.,& Dorval, T. (2012). A novel specific edge effect correction method for RNA interference screenings. *Bioinformatics*,Vol. 28, No. 2, pp. 261-68.

[8] Chen, J. J., Roberson, P. K., & Schell, M. J. (2010). The false discovery rate: a key concept in large-scale genetic studies. *Cancer Control*, Vol. 17, No. 1, pp. 58-62.

[9] Cheng, Y., & Prusoff, W. H. (1973). Relationship between the inhibition constant (K1) and the concentration of inhibitor which causes 50 per cent inhibition (I50) of an enzymatic reaction. *Biochemical Pharmacology*, Vol. 22, No. 23, pp. 3099-108.

[10] Chung, N., Zhang, X. D., Kreamer, A., Locco, L., Kuan, P., Bartz, S., Linsley, P. S., Ferrer, M., & Strulovici, B. (2008). Median absolute deviation to improve hit selection

for genome-scale RNAi screens. *Journal of Biomolecular Screening,* Vol. 13, No. 2, pp. 149-58.

[11] Coma, I., Herranz, J., & Martin, J. (2009). Statistics and decision making in high-throughput screening. In: *High Throughput Screening, Methods in Molecular Biology, Methods and Protocols,* Janzen, W. P. & Bernasconi, P., pp. 69-106, Humana Press, ISBN 9781603272575, New York.

[12] Copeland, R. A. (2003). Mechanistic considerations in high-throughput screening. *Analytical Biochemistry,* Vol. 320, No. 1, pp. 1-12.

[13] Copeland, R. A. (2005). *Evaluation of Enzyme Inhibitors in Drug Discovery: A Guide for Medicinal Chemists and Pharmacologists,* John Wiley & Sons, ISBN 978-0-471-68696-5, Hoboken, New Jersey.

[14] Echeverri, C. J., Beachy, P. A., Baum, B., Boutros, M., Buchholz, F., Chanda, S. K., Downward, J., Ellenberg, J., Fraser, A. G., Hacohen, N., Hahn, W. C., Jackson, A. L.,Kiger, A., Linsley, P. S., Lum, L., Ma, Y., Mathey-Prevot, B., Root, D. E., Sabatini, D. M., Taipale, J., Perrimon, N.,& Bernards, R. (2006). Minimizing the risk of reporting false positives in large-scale RNAi screens. *Nature Methods,* Vol. 3, No. 10, pp. 777-79.

[15] Entzeroth, M., Flotow, H.,& Condron, P.(2009). Overview of high-throughput screening. In: *Current Protocols in Pharmacology,* pp. 9.4.1-27, John Wiley & Sons, Retrieved from http://onlinelibrary.wiley.com/doi/10.1002/0471141755.ph0904s44/abstract

[16] Gillet, V. J. (2008). New directions in library design and analysis. *Current Opinion in Chemical Biology,* Vol. 12, No. 3, pp. 372-78.

[17] Gribbon, P., Lyons, R., Laflin, P., Bradley, J., Chambers, C., Williams, B. S., Keighley, W., & Sewing, A. (2005). Evaluating real-life high-throughput screening data. *Journal of Biomolecular Screening,* Vol. 10, No. 2, pp. 99-107.

[18] Gunter, B., Brideau, C., Pikounis, B., &Liaw, A. (2003). Statistical and graphical methods for quality control determination of high-throughput screening data. *Journal of Biomolecular Screening,* Vol. 8, No. 6, pp. 624-33.

[19] Hampel, F. R. (1971). A General qualitative definition of robustness. *The Annals ofMathematical Statistics,* Vol. 42, No. 6, pp. 1887-96.

[20] Hampel, F. R., Ronchetti, E. M., Rousseeuw, P. J.,& Stahel, W. A. (1986). *Robust Statistics: The Approach Based on Influence Functions.* John Wiley & Sons, ISBN 9780471829218, New York.

[21] Harper, G., & Pickett, S. D. (2006). Methods for mining HTS data. *Drug Discovery Today,* Vol. 11, No. 16-16, pp. 694-99.

[22] Horn, T., Sandmann, T.,& Boutros, M. (2010). Design and evaluation of genome-wide libraries for RNA interference screens. *Genome Biology,* Vol. 11, No. 6, pp. R61.1-12.

[23] Huber, P. J. (1981). *Robust Statistics.* John Wiley& Sons, ISBN 9780471418054, New York.

[24] Hund, E., Massart, D. L., & Smeyers-Verbeke, J. (2002). Robust regression and outlier detection in the evaluation of robustness tests with different experimental designs. *AnalyticaChimica Acta,* Vol. 463, No. 1,pp. 53-73.

[25] Iglewicz, B., & Hoaglin, D. C. (1993). *How to detect and handle outliers.*ASQC Quality Press. ISBN 9780873892476, Wisconsin.

[26] Iversen, P. W., Eastwood, B. J., Sittampalam, G. S., &Cox, K. L. (2006). A comparison of assay performance measures in screening assays: Signal window, Z ' factor, andassay variability ratio. *Journal of Biomolecular Screening,* Vol. 11, No. 3, pp. 247-52.

[27] Jacob, R. T., Larsen, M. J., Scott, S. D., Kirchhoff, P. D., Sherman, D. H., & Neubig, R. R.(2012). MScreen: An Integrated Compound Management and High-Throughput Screening Data Storage and Analysis System. *Journal of Biomolecular Screening,* Vol. 20, No. 10, pp. 1-8.

[28] Kainkaryam, R. M.& Woolf, P. J. (2009). Pooling in high-throughput drug screening. Current Opinion in Drug Discovery &Development, Vo. 12, No. 3, pp. 339-50.

[29] Kevorkov, D. & Makarenkov, V. (2005). Statistical analysis of systematic errors in high-throughput screening. *Journal of Biomolecular Screening,* Vol. 10, No. 6, pp. 557-67.

[30] Konig, R., Chiang, C., Tu, B. P., Yan, S. F., DeJesus, P. D., Romero, A., Bergauer, T., Orth, A., Krueger, U., Zhou, Y., & Chanda, S. K. (2007). A probability-based approach for the analysis of large-scale RNAi screens. *Nature Methods,* Vol. 4, No. 10, pp. 847-49.

[31] Kummel, A., & Parker, C. N. (2011). The Interweaving of Cheminformatics and HTS. In: *Cheminformatics and Computational Chemical Biology, Methods in Molecular Biology,* Bajorath, J., pp. 435-457, Springer Science+Business Media, ISBN 9781607618393, New York.

[32] Lundholt, B. K., Scudder, K. M.,& Pagliaro, L. (2003). A simple techniquefor reducing edge effect in cell-based assays. *Journal of Biomolecular Screening,* Vol. 8, No. 5, pp. 566-70.

[33] Macarron, R. (2006). Critical review of the role of HTS in drug discovery. *Drug Discovery Today,* Vol. 11, No. 7-8, pp. 277-279.

[34] Macarron, R., &Hertzberg, R. P.(2009). Design and implementation of high throughput screening assays. In: *High Throughput Screening, Methods in Molecular Biology,* Janzen, W. P. & Bernasconi, P., pp. 1-32, Springer Science+Business Media, ISBN 9781603272582, New York.

[35] Makarenkov, V., Kevorkov, D., Zentilli, P., Gagarin, A., Malo, N., & Nadon, R. (2006). HTS-Corrector: software for the statistical analysis and correction of experimental high-throughput screening data. *Bioinformatics*, Vol. 22, No. 11, pp. 1408-09.

[36] Makarenkov, V., Zentilli, P., Kevorkov, D., Gagarin, A., Malo, N., &Nadon, R. (2007).An efficient method for the detection and elimination of systematic error in high-throughput screening. *Bioinformatics*, Vol. 23, No. 13, pp. 1648-57.

[37] Malo, N., Hanley, J. A., Carlile, G., Liu, J., Pelletier, J., Thomas, D. &Nadon, R. (2010). Experimental design and statistical methods for improved hit detection in high-throughput screening. *Journal of Biomolecular Screening*, Vol. 15, No. 8, pp. 990-1000.

[38] Martis, E. A., Radhakrishnan, R., & Badve, R. R. (2011). High-Throughput Screening: The Hits and Leads of Drug Discovery- An Overview. *Journal of Applied Pharmaceutical Science*, Vol. 1, No. 1, pp. 2-10.

[39] McDonald, G. R., Hudson, A. L., Dunn, S. M., You, H., Baker, G. B., Whittal, R. M., Martin, J. W., Jha, A., Edmondson, D. E., & Holt, A. (2008). Bioactive contaminants leach from disposable laboratory plasticware. *Science*, Vol. 322, No. 5903,pp. 917.

[40] Mohr, S., Bakal, C., & Perrimon, N. (2010). Genomic screening with RNAi: results and challenges. *Annual Review of Biochemistry*, Vol. 79, pp. 37-64.

[41] Mohr, S. E.,& Perrimon, N. (2012). RNAi screening: new approaches, understandings, and organisms. *Wiley Interdisciplinary Reviews*. RNA. Vol. 3, No. 2, pp. 145-158.

[42] Motulsky, H. J.,&Neubig, R. R. (2010). Analyzing binding data. In: *Currrent Protocols in Neuroscience*, pp. 7.5.1-65, John Wiley and Sons, Retrieved from http://onlinelibrary.wiley.com/doi/10.1002/0471142301.ns0705s52/full

[43] Pelz, O., Gilsdorf, M., & Boutros, M. (2010). web cellHTS2: a web-application for the analysis of high-throughput screening data. *BMC Bioinformatics*, Vol. 11, pp. 185-90.

[44] Pereira, D. A.,& Williams, J. A. (2007). Origin and evolution of high throughput screening. *British Journal of Pharmacology*, Vol. 152, No. 1, pp. 53-61.

[45] Rieber, N., Knapp, B., Eils, R.,& Kaderali, L. (2009). RNAither, an automated pipeline for the statistical analysis of high-throughput RNAi screens. *Bioinformatics*, Vol. 25, No. 5, pp. 678-679.

[46] Root, D. E., Kelley, B. P., & Stockwell, B. R. (2003). Detecting spatial patterns in biological array experiments. *Journal of Biomolecular Screening*, Vol. 8, No. 4, pp. 393-398.

[47] Rousseeuw, P. J. (1991). Tutorial to Robust Statistics. *Journal of Chemometrics*, Vol. 5, No. 1, pp. 1-20.

[48] Singh, A. (1996). Outliers and robust procedures in some chemometric applications. *Chemometrics and Intelligent Laboratory Systems*, Vol. 33, No. 2, pp. 75-100.

[49] Stevens, M. E., Bouchard. P. J., Kariv, I., Chung, T. D. Y., &Oldenburg, K. R. (1998). Comparison of automation equipment in high throughput screening. *Journal of Biomolecular Screening*, Vol. 3, No. 4, pp. 305-11.

[50] Stone, D. J., Marine, S., Majercak, J., Ray, W. J., Espeseth, A., Simon, A., & Ferrer, M. (2007). High-throughput screening by RNA interference: control of two distinct types of variance. *Cell Cycle*, Vol. 6, No. 8, pp. 898-901.

[51] Sui, Y., & Wu, Z. (2007). Alternative statistical parameter for high-throughput screening assay quality assessment. *Journal of Biomolecular Screening*, Vol. 12, No. 2, pp. 229-34.

[52] Tai, D., Chaguturu, R., & Fang, J. (2011). K-Screen: a free application for high throughput screening data analysis, visualization, and laboratory information management. *Combinatorial Chemistry & High Throughput Screening*, Vol. 14, No. 9, pp. 757-65.

[53] Tolopko, A. N., Sullivan, J. P., Erickson, S. D., Wrobel, D., Chiang, S. L., Rudnicki, K., Rudnicki, S., Nale, J., Selfors, L. M., Greenhouse, D., Muhlich, J. L., & Shamu, C. E. (2010). Screensaver: an open source lab information management system (LIMS) for high throughput screening facilities. *BMC Bioinformatics*, Vol. 11, pp. 260-73.

[54] Tukey, J. W. (1977). *Exploratory data analysis*. Addison-Wesley Publishing Company, ISBN 9780201076165, Massachusetts.

[55] Wang, X., Terfve, C., Rose, J. C., & Markowetz, F. (2011).HTSanalyzeR: an R/Bioconductor package for integrated network analysis of high-throughput screens. *Bioinformatics*, Vol. 27, No. 6, pp. 879-80.

[56] Watson, J., Greenough, E. B., Leet, J. E., Ford, M. J., Drexler. D. M., Belcastro, J. V., Herbst, J. J., Chatterjee, M., & Banks, M. (2009). Extraction, identification, and functional characterization of a bioactive substance from automated compound-handling plastic tips. *Journal of Biomolecular Screening*, Vol. 14, No. 5, pp. 566-72.

[57] Waybright, T. J., Britt, J. R., & McCloud, T. G. (2009). Overcoming problems of compound storage in DMSO: solvent and process alternatives. *Journal of Biomolecular Screening*, Vol. 14, No. 6, pp. 708-15.

[58] Wright, G. W.,& Simon, R. M. (2003). A random variance model for detection of differential gene expression in small microarray experiments. *Bioinformatics*, Vol. 19, No. 18, pp. 2448-55.

[59] Wu, Z., Liu, D.,&Sui, Y. (2008). Quantitative assessment of hit detection and confirmation in single and duplicate high-throughput screenings.*Journal of Biomolecular Screening*, Vol. 13, No. 2, pp. 159-167.

[60] Wu, Z., & Wu, Z., (2010). Exploration, visualization, and preprocessing of high-dimensional data. *Statistical Methods in Molecular Biology*, Vol. 620, pp. 267-84.

[61] Xin, H., Bernal, A., Amato, F. A., Pinhasov, A., Kauffman, J., Brenneman, D. E., Derian, C. K., Andrade-Gordon, P., Plata-Salaman, C. R., &Ilyin, S. E. (2004).High-

throughput siRNA-based functional target validation. *Journal of Biomolecular Screening*, Vol. 9, No. 4, pp. 286-93.

[62] Zhang, J., Chung, T. D. Y., & Oldenburg, K. R. (1999). A simple statistical parameter for use in evaluation and validation of high throughput screening assays. *Journal of Biomolecular Screening*, Vol. 4, No. 2, pp. 67-73.

[63] Zhang, X. D. (2007a). A new method with flexible and balanced control of false negatives and false positives for hit selection in RNA interference high-throughput screening assays. *Journal of Biomolecular Screening*, Vol. 12, No. 5, pp. 645-55.

[64] Zhang, X. D. (2007b). A pair of new statistical parameters for quality control in RNA interference high-throughput screening assays. *Genomics*, Vol. 89, No. 4, pp. 552-61.

[65] Zhang, X. D. (2008a). Genome-wide screens for effective siRNAs through assessing the size of siRNA effects. *BMC Research Notes*, Vol. 1, pp. 33-39.

[66] Zhang, X. D. (2008b). Novel analytic criteria and effective plate designs for quality control in genome-scale RNAi screens. *Journal of Biomolecular Screening*, Vol. 13, No. 5, pp. 363-77.

[67] Zhang, X. D. (2009). A method for effectively comparing gene effects in multiple conditions in RNAi and expression-profiling research. *Pharmacogenomics*, Vol. 10, No. 3, pp. 345-58.

[68] Zhang, X. D. (2010a). Assessing the size of gene or RNAi effects in multifactor high-throughput experiments. *Pharmacogenomics*, Vol. 11, No. 2, pp. 199-213.

[69] Zhang, X. D. (2010b). An effective method for controlling false discovery and false nondiscovery rates in genome-scale RNAi screens. *Journal of Biomolecular Screening*, Vol. 15, No. 9, pp. 1116-22.

[70] Zhang, X. D. (2011a). Illustration of SSMD, z score, SSMD*, z* score, and t statistic for hit selection in RNAi high-throughput screens. *Journal of Biomolecular Screening*, Vol. 16, No. 7, pp. 775-85.

[71] Zhang, X. D. (2011b). *Optimal high-throughput screening: practical experimental design and data analysis for genome-scale RNAi research.* Cambridge University Press, ISBN 9780521734448, New York.

[72] Zhang, X. D., Espeseth, Johnson. E. N., Chin, J., Gates, A., Mitnaul, L. J., Marine, S. D., Tian, J., Stec, E. M., Kunapuli, P., Holder, D. J., Heyse, J. F., Strulovici, B.,& Ferrer, M. (2008a). Integrating experimental and analytic approaches to improve data quality in genome-wide RNAi screens. *Journal of Biomolecular Screening*, Vol.13, No. 5, pp. 378-89.

[73] Zhang, X. D.,& Heyse, J. F. (2009). Determination of sample size in genome-scale RNAi screens. *Bioinformatics*, Vol. 25, No. 7, pp. 841-44.

[74] Zhang, X. D., Kuan, P. F., Ferrer, M., Shu, X., Liu, Y. C., Gates, A. T., Kunapuli, P., Stec, E. M., Xu, M., Marine, S. D., Holder, D. J., Strulovici, B., Heyse, J. F., & Espeseth,

A. S. (2008b). Hit selection with false discovery rate control in genome-scale RNAi screens. *Nucleic Acids Research,* Vol. 36, No. 14, pp. 4667-79.

[75] Zhang, X. D., Lacson, R., Yang, R., Marine, S. D., McCampbell, A., Toolan, D. M., Hare, T. R., Kajdas, J., Berger, J. P., Holder, D. J., Heyse, J. F., & Ferrer, M.(2010). The use of SSMD-based false discovery and false nondiscovery rates in genome-scale RNAi screens. *Journal of Biomolecular Screening,* Vol. 15, No. 9, pp. 1123-231.

[76] Zhang, X. D., Yang, X. C., Chung, N., Gates, A., Stec, E., Kunapuli, P., Holder, D. J., Ferrer, M., & Espeseth, A. S. (2006). Robust statistical methods for hit selection in RNA interference high-throughput screening experiments. *Pharmacogenomics,* Vol. 7, No. 3, pp. 299-309.

[77] Zhao, L., Li, T., Pan, Y., Ning, H., Liu, Z.,& Fan, D. (2005). Application of siRNA library in high-throughput genetic screens of mammalian cells. *Journal of Cancer Molecules,* Vol. 1, No. 1, pp. 19-25.

Chapter 8

Oxidative Stress in Human Infectious Diseases – Present and Current Knowledge About Its Druggability

Carsten Wrenger, Isolmar Schettert and Eva Liebau

Additional information is available at the end of the chapter

http://dx.doi.org/10.5772/53758

1. Introduction

Infectious diseases caused by parasites are a major threat for entire mankind, especially in the tropics. These infections are not only restricted to humans, they are also predominant in animal health. Just a few years ago infectious diseases caused by parasites were classified as an issue of the past. Due to the elevating level of drug resistance of these pathogens against the current chemotherapeutics, the need for new drugs became even more important. In particular parasitic diseases such as malaria, leishmaniasis, trypanosomiasis, amoebiasis, trichomoniasis, soil-transmitted helminthiasis, filariasis and schistosomiasis are major health problems, especially in "developing" areas (Renslo and McKerrow, 2006; Pal and Bandyopadhyay, 2012). A variety of these parasitic diseases, which comprises the so called neglected diseases Chagas disease, leishmaniasis, sleeping sickness, schistosomiasis, lymphatic filariasis, onchocerciasis and of course malaria (Chatelain and Ioset, 2011), are transmitted by vectors and therefore attempts to combat transmission became prominent. In contrast to the treatment of bacterial infections with antibiotics there are no "general" antiparasitic drugs. The use of a specific drug is dependent on the parasitic organism and therefore has to be individually chosen (Khaw et al., 1995).

Reactive oxygen species (ROS) and oxidative stress are the inevitable consequences of aerobic metabolism, with partially reduced and highly reactive metabolites of O_2 being formed in the mitochondria (Andreyev et al., 2005) or as by-products of other cellular sources such as the cytoplasm, the endoplasmatic reticulum, the plasma membrane and peroxisomes. Furthermore, environmental agents such as ionizing and UV radiation or xenobiotic exposure can generate intracellular ROS. O_2 metabolites include superoxide anion (O^{2-}) and hydrogen peroxide (H_2O_2), formed by one- and two electron reductions of O_2 or the highly reactive hydroxyl radical ($^{\cdot}OH$) which is formed in the presence of metal ions via Fenton and/or Haber-Weiss reactions (Massimine et al., 2006). At physiologically low levels, ROS can function as second messenger in redox signaling, with H_2O_2 best providing the specificity in its interaction with effectors in signaling processes (Forman et al., 2010). Balancing the generation and elimination of ROS maintains the proper function of redox-sensitive signalling proteins. However, severe increases of ROS induce oxidative modifications in the cellular macromolecules DNA, proteins and lipids, this leading to a disruption of redox homeostasis and irreversible oxidative damage (Trachootham et al., 2008). Depending on the cellular context, the levels of ROS and the redox state of the cells, alterations of the delicate redox balance can promote cell proliferation and survival or induce cell death.

To maintain redox homeostasis and eliminate ROS, aerobes are equipped with enzymatic/ nonenzymatic antioxidants and metal sequestering proteins to either prevent or intercept the formation of pro-oxidants. Furthermore, protective mechanisms are put in place to repair and replace damaged macromolecules. Two central thiol/disulfide couples are involved in controlling the redox state of the cell: glutathione/glutathione disulfide (GSH/GSSG) is the major redox couple that determines the antioxidative capacity of cells, other redox couples include the active site dithiol/disulfide of thioredoxins (Trx_{red}/Trx_{ox}) interacting with a different subset of proteins and thus forming a distinct but complementary redox system (Jones and Go, 2010).

Enzymatic antioxidants can be categorized into primary or secondary antioxidants, the first reacting directly with pro-oxidants (e.g. catalase, superoxide dismutase), the latter are involved in the regeneration of low molecular weight antioxidant species (Halliwell, 1999). Here, the reduced state of GSSG and Trx-enzymes is restored by the glutathione reductase (GSR) and the Trx reductase using electrons obtained from NADPH. Additionally glutaredoxins (Glrx) utilize GSH for the reduction of intracellular disulfides (Fernandes and Holmgren, 2004). While Trx, Trx reductase and Trx peroxidase (peroxiredoxin, Prx) constitute the Trx-system, the versatile GSH-system includes enzymes required for GSH synthesis and recycling, for its use in metabolism, in defense against ROS-induced damage and in a multitude of detoxification processes. Furthermore, for normal GSH turnover and disposition of GSH-conjugated metabolites and xenobiotics, export from the cell is required that is carried out by GSH efflux transporters and pumps (Sies, 1999) (Fig. 1).

In spite of the diversity of parasites, all are faced with similar biological problems that are related to their lifestyle. Besides coping with ROS levels generated from intrinsic sources, all have to deal with the oxidative stress imposed by the host's immune response. Furthermore, parasites are faced with ROS that are produced during the epithelial innate immune response of their vector, by vector-resident gut bacteria (Cirimotich et al., 2011) or during melanotic encapsulation processes (Kumar et al., 2003).

Since the redox system plays such a fundamental and indispensable role for parasite survival within their host (Massimine et al., 2006), drugs that either promote ROS generation or inhibit cellular antioxidant systems will lead to redox imbalance by pushing ROS levels above a certain threshold level that will ultimately lead to parasite death (Müller et al., 2003). In general, drugs that target vital redox reactions or promote oxidative stress are named redox-active antiparasitic drugs (Seeber et al., 2005) on which we will mainly focus within this chapter.

2. The role of the antioxidant system in *Leishmania*

Leishmaniasis is caused by the protozoan flagellate *Leishmania* which is transmitted by sandflies of the genus *Phlebotomus* (Sharma and Singh, 2008). There are several species of the genus *Leishmania* which are known to cause this infectious disease. Leishmaniasis shows a broad spectrum of clinical manifestations and includes visceral, cutaneous and mucocutaneous leishmaniasis. Whereas the two latter ones are not considered to be lethal (Herwaldt, 1999), infection with *Leishmania donovani/infantum* – resulting in kala azar or visceral leishmaniasis - can be lethal without treatment. Although treatment of leishmaniasis with chemotherapeutics is the only current option, drug resistance to first-line drugs is increasing which is accompanied by frequently occurring toxic side effects and by the high cost of treatment (Van Assche et al., 2011). Additionally, the small number of novel drugs combined with the low number of identified and subsequently validated number of *Leishmania* drug targets in clinical use, reveals an alarming situation for the current status in chemotherapy. The predominant target for the application of chemotherapy is the amastigote stage which proliferates intracellularly in tissue macrophages (Dedet et al., 2009), thereby hindering the accessibility of antileishmanial drugs to the pathogen.

3. Antimonials

Despite the fact that antimonials were already identified in 1921, they still remain the first-line treatment, although the precise mode of action is not known. But it is generally accepted that pentavalent antimonials (Sb^{V}) represent a pro-drug which is converted to trivalent antimonials (Sb^{III}) for antileishmanial activity. Recently it has been indicated that thiols act as reducing agents in this conversion. Furthermore, the participation of a unique parasite-specific trimeric glutathione transferase TDR1 in the activation of antimonial prodrugs has been suggested (Fyfe et al., 2012).

Treatment with antimonials requires parenteral administration and is accompanied by toxic side effects such as cardiac arrhythmia and acute pancreatitis (Sundar and Rai, 2002). Some studies have been carried out to investigate the activity mechanism of antimonials which correlates with an interference with the antioxidant defence system of the parasite: Trivalent antimonials decrease the thiol-reducing capacity of *Leishmania* by inducing an efflux of trypanothione. In contrast to *Leishmania*, mammalian cells depend on GSH to control their intracellular thiol-redox status. Here, ROS and oxidized cell components are efficiently reduced by GSH, thereby generating GSSG. The glutathione disulfide form can then be regenerated by the GSR (Monostori et al., 2009). In contrast, the redox metabolism of *Leishmania* relies on a modified GSH-system, *N*1,*N*8-bis(l-γ-glutamyl-l-hemicystinylglycyl) spermidine, also known as trypanothione (Fairlamb et al., 1985). The oxidised form, trypanothione disulfide, is generated when trypanothione reduces ROS and its reconversion is catalysed by the trypanothione reductase. Antimonials inhibit this enzyme, leading to an accumulation of trypanothione disulfide, which subsequently is not accessible for the reduction of ROS (Krauth-Siegel and Comini, 2008). The influence of antimonials on the parasite's redox biology has been verified on cellular level by the fact that trivalent antimonials-resistant parasites display an increased IC_{50}-value for nitric oxide donors such as $NaNO_2$, SNAP, and DETA NONOate compared to antimonial-sensitive strains (Souza et al., 2010; Holzmüller et al., 2005; Vanaerschot et al., 2010). Whether nitric oxide resistance is due to elevated trypanothione levels or due to another antioxidant mode of action is not yet clear.

4. Amphotericin B

Amphotericin B (Fig. 2), a polyene macrolide, has been employed in the treatment of *Leishmania* since 1960, but just as a second-line drug. This drug exhibits an excellent antileishmania activity with more than 90% cure rates. Because the pure compound creates severe side effects and requires long-term treatment and extensive monitoring, liposomal application of amphotericin B is used at the moment which results in cure rates of 3–5 days (up to 100%), is convenient for the patient and is less expensive (Gradoni et al., 2008; Manandhar et al., 2008; Sundar et al., 2002; Thakur et al., 1996). The mode of action can be explained based on its chemical structure, polyene macrolide has been shown to bind to ergosterol, one of the main sterols within *Leishmania* membranes. Interference with this molecule results in an increasing permeability of the cell membrane which leads to the parasite's death (Balana-Fouce et al., 1998; Amato et al., 2008). Additionally there is some evidence that amphotericin B has an effect on the oxidative response of macrophages (Mukherjee et al., 2010), however further experiments are required to verify this effect.

5. Miltefosine

Miltefosine (hexadecylphosphocholine) is the first and currently the only, orally administered antileishmanial drug (Fig. 2). However, despite cure rates of up to 98% (Roberts, 2006), the drug reveals serious side effects such as vomiting, diarrhea and can cause abnormal physiological development of the foetus. Furthermore, the drug has a relatively long half-life of about 150 hours (Seifert et al., 2007; Maltezou, 2010) which could lead to the development of rapid resistance. Related to its structure, the drug possibly interferes with membranes and membrane-linked enzymes. Currently no verified implications of the drug within the redox biology of the parasite have been found (Rakotomanga et al., 2004; Saint-Pierre-Chazalet et al., 2009).

http://dx.doi.org/10.5772/53758

6. Oxidative chemotherapeutic intervention of Trypanosoma infections

Trypanosoma infections, caused by the flagellate protozoan *Trypanosoma* are responsible for a high degree of health problems in endemic countries. They can be divided into two types of pathogens: *Trypanosoma cruzi*, the causative agent of Chagas disease, also known as American trypanosomiasis, since it occurs in Latin America and *Trypanosoma brucei ssp.*, the causative agent of sleeping sickness, or human African trypanosomiasis, since it is endemic to sub-Saharan Africa. The current medication is known for its toxicity, poor activity in immune-suppressed patients and long-term treatment combined with high costs. Moreover, vaccines are not foreseeable in the near future. The *T. cruzi* life cycle includes three fundamental forms characterized by the relative positions of the flagellum, kinetoplast and nucleus: Trypomastigotes, epimastigotes and amastigotes, the latter one characterized by their proliferation in any nucleated cell (Prata, 2001). On the one hand Chagas' disease is controlled through elimination of its vectors by using insecticides and on the other side by chemotherapy. Currently, the drugs used are nifurtimox (4[(5-nitrofurfurylidene)amino]-3-methylthiomorpholine-1,1-dioxide), derived from nitrofuran, and benznidazole (*N*-benzyl-2-nitroimidazole-1-acetamide), a nitroimidazole derivative. Nifurtimox and benznidazole (Fig. 2) are trypanocidal to all forms of the parasite (Rodriques Coura and de Castro, 2002). However, severe side effects and toxicity have been observed (Kirchhoff, 2000). In addition, there are also reports of mutagenesis resulting in DNA damage (Zahoor et al., 1987). An additional aspect that complicates treatment is the different susceptibility of different parasite strains to the applied chemotherapeutics (Filardi and Brener, 1987). The mode of action of nifurtimox and benznidazole (Fig. 2) is via the formation of free radicals and/or charged metabolites. The nitro group of both drugs is reduced to an amino group by the catalysis of nitro-reductases, leading to the formation of various free radical intermediates. Cytochrome P450-related nitro-reductases initiate this process by producing a nitro anion radical (Moreno et al., 1982). Subsequently, the radical reacts with oxygen, which regenerates the drug (Mason and Holtzman, 1975). For example, nifurtimox-derived free radicals may undergo redox cycling with O_2, thereby producing H_2O_2 in a reaction catalysed by the SOD (Temperton et al., 1998). Furthermore, in the presence of Fe^{3+} the highly reactive $^{\cdot}OH$ is also being formed according to the Haber-Weiss reaction. These free radicals can subsequently bind to cellular macromolecules such as lipids, proteins and DNA, resulting in severe damage of parasitic cells (Díaz de Toranzo et al., 1988). In contrast, the trypanocidal effect of benznidazole does not depend on ROS but it is likely that reduced metabolites of benznidazole are covalently binding to cellular macromolecules, thereby revealing their trypanocidal effect (Díaz de Toranzo et al., 1988; Maya et al., 2004). Additionally, it has been demonstrated that benznidazole inhibits the *T. cruzi* NADH-fumarate reductase (Turrens et al., 1996).

7. Approaches to increase oxidative stress within the malaria parasite

Malaria is a devastating and quite often a deadly parasitic disease, which causes important public health problems in the tropics. The population in more than 90 countries, with more than 2000 million citizens, is exposed to the infection. Malaria infection is responsible for an estimated 500 million clinical cases per annum, causing more than one million deaths; most of these are children in Africa. The malaria parasite *Plasmodium falciparum*, the causative agent of Malaria tropica, is proliferating within human red blood cells, thereby exploiting host's nutrient sources and hiding from the human immune response. A vaccine is not available and the control of the disease depends solely on the administration of a small number of drugs. Due to mutational modification of the genome of the malaria parasite, an ongoing rapid adaptation to environmental changes and drug resistance is occurring (Greenwood et al., 2008). At the moment – which is just a question of time - solely artemesinin is still effective against the malaria parasite. However, first reports already demonstrated drug resistance against artemisinin (Wangroongsarb et al., 2011). Therefore, continuous discovery and development of new drugs are urgently needed. A variety of the current anti-malaria drugs are targeting the redox balance of the parasite. As outlined above, redox systems are essential for the intracellular proliferation of the plasmodial pathogen.

In general, *P. falciparum* uses the two interacting systems, GSH- and TRX-system, to protect against reactive ROS (Kanzok et al., 2002; Kanzok et at., 2000; Kawazu et al., 2001; Kehr et al., 2011; Krnajski et al., 2001; Krnajski et al., 2002; Kumar et al., 2008; Liebau et al., 2002). Both systems can be link by the redox protein plasmoredoxin (Becker et al., 2003). Active interference by employing redox-active antiparasitic drugs, however, harms the parasite and results in its death. Compounds which disturb the redox balance can be categorised into three different groups: (i) molecules that are responsible for the *de novo* synthesis of ROS and thus lead to parasite death, (ii) molecules which inhibit the activities of redox balancing enzymes and (iii) molecules that interfere in the scavenging of pro-oxidant metabolic products like hemozoin.

8. Molecules which inhibit the activities of redox balancing enzymes

The GSH-system plays an important role in the maintenance of the redox status in *Plasmodium* (Kehr et al., 2011). It is involved in detoxifying free heme (ferriprotoporphyrin IX) (Atamna et al., 1995; Müller, 2003) and in the termination of radical-based chain reactions (Frey, 1997). Therefore, enzymatic reactions within this system are highly druggable. The GSR is one of the key enzymes of the GSH-system and consequently several compounds have been synthesized to successfully interfere with its catalysis *in vitro* and *in vivo* (Biot et al., 2004; Gallo et al., 2009; Grellier et al., 2010; Muller et al., 2011). Inhibitory compounds comprise for example isoalloxazines, quinacrines, tertiary amides that reveal antimalarial activity at low doses against the chloroquine sensitive *P. falciparum* strain 3D7 (Sarma et al., 2003; Friebolin et al., 2008; Chibale et al., 2001). Methylene blue (Fig. 2), a noncompetitive inhibitor of the *P. falciparum* GR, shows antiplasmodial activity against all blood stage forms, whereas only a marginal cytotoxic effect against mammalian cells has been reported (Biot et al., 2004; Buchholz et al., 2008; Atamna et al., 1996; Akoachere et al., 2005; Badyopadhyay et al., 2004; Krauth-Siegel et al., 2005; Garavito et al., 2007).

The GST is one of the most abundant proteins expressed in *P. falciparum*. Additionally to its detoxifying role, it efficiently binds parasitotoxic heme not only in the presence of GSH, but also when GSSG is present, thereby protecting the parasite from hemin even under severe oxidative stress conditions. Here, a peculiar loop region, that is both crucial for the glutathione-dependent tetramerization/inactivation process and for hemin-binding, represents an ideal drug target (Liebau et al., 2005; 2009). Recently chemical synthesis to design effective compounds to target GST has been performed which show some promising antiplasmodial activity (Ahmad et al., 2007; Sturm et al., 2009). Furthermore, the development of drugs that overcome resistance to available antimalarial drugs also are of great interest. The action of multidrug resistance protein (MRP)-like transporters is associated with the efflux of xenobiotics in both unaltered and GSH-conjugated form and it is conceivable that they are involved in the development of drug resistance in malarial parasites (Koenderink et al., 2010). Since coordinated expression and synergistic interactions between GST and efflux pumps have been observed (Sau et al., 2010), a promising new intervening strategy might be the inhibition of GST and/or the development of GST-activated pro-drugs that overcome drug resistance by blocking the drug binding sites of the transporters.

Another promising antimalarial drug target is the *P. falciparum* TrxR (Banerjee et al., 2009). Chalcone derivatives and Eosin B exhibit antiplasmodial activity by inhibiting the plasmodial TrxR (Li et al., 1995; Massimine et al., 2006).

For many years it was thought that the malaria parasite had no need for an endogenous SOD and simply adopted the host's enzyme for its purpose. However, in 2002, an iron-dependent SOD was described in *P. falciparum* (Boucher et al., 2006). Being quite distinct from the human tetrameric Mn and Cu/Zn SOD, it is exploited as anti-malaria drug target (Soulere et al., 2003).

9. Drugs inhibiting hemozoin formation and thereby inducing oxidative stress

Besides the attacks of the immune systems of the respective host, where ROS are deployed to kill invading pathogens, the parasite faces another even bigger challenge: *Plasmodium* relies also on the digestion of human haemoglobin to obtain amino acids for its metabolism (Sherman, 1977). Haemoglobin is the major protein inside the erythrocyte and the parasite has evolved a unique pathway to utilise this molecule (Muller et al., 2011). Heme is the degradation product of haemoglobin, which has to be detoxified and stored as hemozoin within the food vacuole of the parasite – the place where the haemoglobin degradation occurs. Non-detoxified heme is extremely toxic (Papalexis et al., 2001) and leads not only to the generation of H_2O_2, $^{\cdot}OH$ and $O^{2-\cdot}$ (Francis et al., 1997), but also to the highly reactive, non-radical molecule, singlet oxygen ($^1O_2$)

(Freinbicherler et al., 2011). Moreover, one $^1O_2$ molecule can be either synthesised by the reaction of $^{\cdot}OH$ and $O^{2-\cdot}$ or two $O^{2-\cdot}$ with two hydrogen ions (Khan and Kasha, 1994). In order to detoxify these ROS, *Plasmodium* has developed – as outlined above - multiple antioxidant defence systems. However - excluding the membrane located lipophilic tocopherol (vitamin E) (Wang and Quinn, 1999) - none of the above mentioned defense systems are capable to detoxify $^1O_2$. The fact that vitamin B6 is linked to the defense against $^1O_2$ in plants and fungi (Tambasco-Studart et al., 2005; Ehrenshaft et al., 1999), suggests that the vitamin B6 biosynthesis might also play a yet unrecognized role in combating $^1O_2$ in the malaria parasite *P. falciparum*. Very recently this role of $^1O_2$ detoxification has been verified in the malaria parasite (Wrenger et al., 2005; Knöckel et al., 2012; Butzloff et al., 2012).

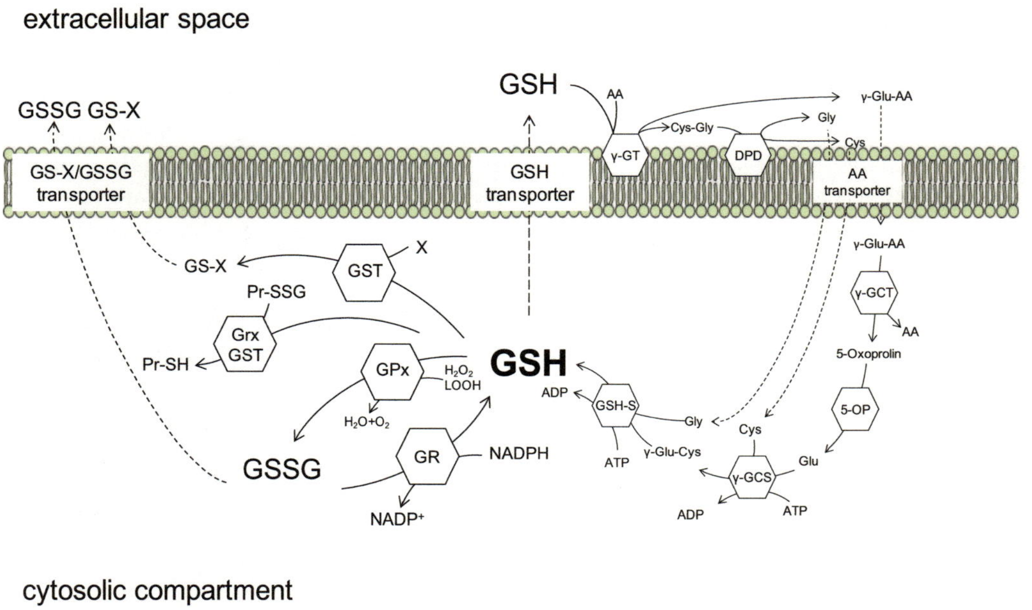

Figure 1. Schematic illustration of the glutathione (GSH) system. GSH homeostasis involves intra- and extracellular mechanisms. GSH is synthesized from amino acids (AA) by the action of γ-glutamylcysteine synthetase (γ-GCS) and glutathione synthase (GSH-S), both requiring ATP. As antioxidant, GSH participates in the reduction of peroxides, catalysed by glutathione peroxidase (GPx), in the reduction of protein-disulfides, catalysed by glutaredoxins (Grx) and in conjugation reactions with electrophils (eg. xenobiotics, X), catalysed by glutathione transferases (GSTs). The glutathione conjugates (GS-X) and GSSG are transported out of the cell via GS-X/GSSG pumps. The NADPH-dependent GSH reductase (GR) is responsible for the intracellular recycling of GSH, while extracellular GSH gets sequentially hydrolysed by γ-glutamyl transpeptidase (γ-GT) and dipeptidase (DPD), with glutamate, cysteine and glycine being recycled for GSH synthesis (γ-glutamyl cycle).

A number of drugs have been identified that act as inhibitors of the hemozoin formation by binding to heme. This leads to an accumulation of free heme, causes high levels of oxidative stress and ends in the death of the parasite (Meunier et al., 2010). Quinoline-containing derivatives such as amopyroquine, amodiaquine, tebuquine, halofantrine, pyronaridine, quinine, mepacrine, epiquinine, quinidine, bisquinoline chloroquine (see figure 2) are highly potent antimalarials that inhibit hemozoin formation at EC_{50}-values in the low nano-molar range (Egan et al., 2000; Kotecka et al., 1997; O'Neill et al., 2003; Vennerstrom et al., 1992). Azole derivatives are also inhibitors of the hemozoin formation and reveal efficacy against chloroquine sensitive as well as resistant plasmodial strains (Banerjee et al., 2009; Rodrigues et al., 2011). Another novel class, which has been identified to interact with heme and thereby prevent the hemozoin formation, are xanthones (Docampo et al., 1990; Ignatushchenko et al., 1997; Xu Kelly et al., 2001). Moreover, a variety of isonitrile derivatives gain their antimalarial activity from inhibition of the hemozoin synthesis (Kumar et al., 2007; Wright et al., 2001) resulting in EC_{50}-values in the low nano-molar range (Badyopadhyay et al., 2001; Singh et al., 2002; Kumar et al., 2007). Benzylmenadione derivatives do not show any cytotoxicity against two human cell lines while they are effective against the chloroquine resistant *P. falciparum* strain Dd2 (Muller et al., 2011). The precise mode of action of benzylmenadione remains for elucidation, but it has been suggested that the molecule is initially oxidized to a naphthoquinone derivative within the food vacuole of the parasite which leads subsequently to the inhibition of the hemozoin formation (Davioud-Charvet et al., 2003).

10. Druggability of oxidative stress systems in helminths

Helminths are parasitic worms that encompass nematodes (roundworms), cestodes and trematodes (flatworms) and affect humans in all areas of the world, with more than one-third of humans harbouring these parasites that cause chronic, debilitating morbidity. Furthermore, co-endemicity and polyparasitism increase the burden of millions (Hotez et al., 2008). In the absence of vaccines, control relies on pharmacotherapy and pharmacoprophylaxis to easy symptoms and reduce transmission. Helminthosis are treated with a limited number of anthelmintics by chemotherapy of symptomatic individuals or, more general, by control programmes that rely on mass drug administration (MDA) and require annual or bi-annual treatment of at-risk populations over prolonged period of time (Prichard et al., 2012). A major problem, however, is the development of resistance or tolerance by the parasites to these common antiparasitic drugs (Vercruysse et al., 2011). It is therefore essential to understand the underlying mechanisms of drug resistance and find new drugs to circumvent it.

Praziquantel has been used for over 20 years to treat a variety of human trematode infections. Its precise mechanism of action has not been fully elucidated, however, there is experimental evidence that praziquantel acts by increasing the permeability of cell membranes towards calcium ions and/or by interfering with adenosine uptake (Jeziorski and Greenberg, 2006; Angelucci et al., 2007). Furthermore, it has been suggested that praziquantel reduces GSH concentrations, making the parasite more susceptible to the host immune response (Ribeiro et al., 1998). Interestingly, exposure to sub-lethal concentrations of praziquantel shows that schistosomes undergo a transcriptomic response similar to that observed during oxidative stress (Aragon et al., 2009).

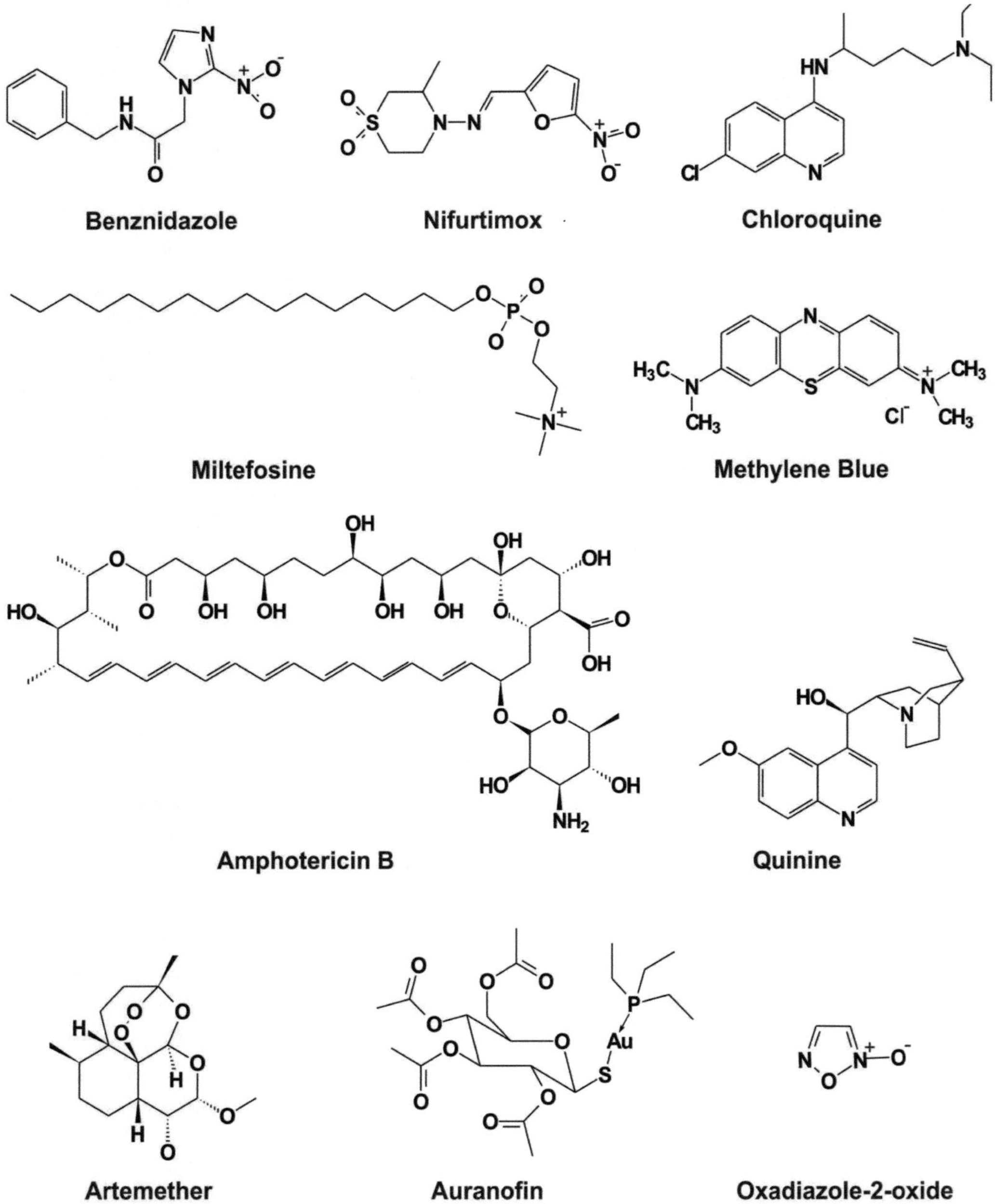

Figure 2. Molecular structures of chemotherapeutics which are used to treat infectious disease by generating directly or indirectly high levels reactive oxygen species.

Reliance on a single drug for mass treatment is risky. Therefore, anti-schistosomiasis drug development is on the way to identify new compounds with different modes of action. Recently it was demonstrated that artemisinin-based compounds (e.g. artemether, figure 2) are active against immature stages of schistosomes. Although a number of potential drug targets have been proposed, the mode of action remains ambiguous (O'Neill et al., 2010). It is thought that the primary activator of the drug is an iron source. Therefore, interaction with heme in the worm gut has been suggested, leading to the formation of an unstable species that generates ROS and thus kills the worm (Utzinger et al., 2001). Since artemisinins are critically important for malaria chemotherapy, they are not available for MDA.

Schistosomes seem to be poorly adapted to cope with oxidative stress. This is surprising, since they have to deal with host-immune and self-generated ROS and, furthermore, with ROS generated during the consumption of host haemoglobin (Huang et al., 2012).The highly restricted antioxidant network has been widely accepted as an excellent drug target for schistosomes and other platyhelminths, since it is unique and differs significantly from the human host. Interestingly, the parasites have merged the Trx- and GSH-system using a hybrid enzyme, the thioredoxin-glutathione reductase (TGR) (Salinas et al., 2004, Huang et al., 2012). Using RNA interference, the TGR was found to be essential for parasite survival (Kuntz et al., 2007). TGR was indicated to be the main target of schistosomicidal drugs used in the past (antimonyl potassium tartrate and oltipraz) and of the anti-arthritic drug auranofin (Fig. 2), with a significant worm reduction observed in infected mice (Kuntz et al., 2007; Angelucci et al., 2009). A quantitative high-throughput screen identified highly potent lead compounds against the Schistosoma TGR (Simeonov et al., 2008), with low inhibitory constants being found with derivatives of phosphinic amides, isoxazolones and the oxadiazole-2-oxide chemotype (Furoxan) (Fig. 2) (Huang et al., 2012).

Preventive chemotherapy is the mainstay in the control of human soil-transmitted helminthiasis (STH). STH is primarily caused by the nematodes *Ancylostoma duodenale* and *Necator americanus* (hookworms), *Ascaris lumbricoides* (roundworm) and *Trichuris trichiura* (whipworm) that parasitize the human gastrointestinal tract. Four anthelminthics that exhibit a broad spectrum of activity are currently recommended by the World Health Organization: The benzimidazoles albendazole and mebendazole, the synthetic phenylimidazolthiazole levamisole and the pyrimidine derivative pyrantel pamoate. While benzimidazoles bind to free β-tubulin, leading to tubule capping and degradation (Beech et al., 2011), the cholinergic agonist levamisole activates ligand-gated acetylcholine receptors (Lewis et al., 1980) and the pyrimidine derivative pyrantel pamoate induces persistent activation of nicotinic acetylcholine receptors (Utzinger and Keiser, 2004). The GABA agonist piperazine, the nicotinic acetylcholine receptor agonist tribendimidine are further drugs used in STH. Currently neither drug class used to control or treat STH, has been implicated as influencing the redox biology of parasites. Instead, most of the currently used or proposed drugs (Olliaro et al., 2011) of gastro-intestinal nematodes affect ion channel function of the neuromuscular synapses. These neuroactive drugs cause paralysis of the worm and result in its rapid expulsion or killing.

Filarial parasites are classified according to the habitat of the adult worms in the vertebral host, with the cutaneous (*Loa loa* and *Onchocerca volvulus*) and lymphatic (*Wuchereria bancrofti, Brugia malayi* and *Brugia timori*) groups being the most clinically significant. Chemotherapeutic approaches to control parasite transmission and to treat onchocerciasis rely on the macrocyclic lactone ivermectin, an effective and safe microfilaricide (Basáñez et al., 2008). Ivermectin is an agonist of ligand-gated Cl^- channels, with particular activity against glutamate-gated Cl^- channels of invertebrates (Martin et al., 1997). While ivermectin is less effective against adult worms, it causes reproductive quiescence and disappearance of microfilaria from skin or blood. Interestingly, cultured microfilariae are unaffected by ivermectin at concentrations found in treated patients (Bennett et al., 1993), making interference of the drug with protective mechanisms employed against the human immune response feasible (Geary et al., 2010). The development of ivermectin-resistant strains of *Caenorhabditis elegans* has shown that resistance to low levels of ivermectin is associated with an increased expression of drug efflux pumps and an increase in GSH-synthesis and -conjugation is observed. Since the overall levels of glutathione decrease, increased drug conjugation and removal from the cells is suggested (James and Davey, 2009). In a recent study, ivermectin has been identified as a cytotoxic agent to leukemia cells and a previously unknown indirect influence of ivermectin on the intracellular redox balance was demonstrated. Mechanistically, ivermectin induced chloride influx, membrane hyperpolarization, and generated ROS, the latter being functionally important for ivermectin-induced cell death (Shrameen et al., 2010).

Diethylcarbamazine (DEC) is still the mainstay for the treatment of lymphatic filariasis and first choice of therapy of loiasis. Surprisingly, its molecular mechanism of action is still not completely understood. Since pharmacologically relevant concentrations of DEC do not have an effect on microfilariae in culture, its mode of action must involve both the worm and its host. A possible involvement of host arachidonate- and NO-dependent pathways was observed (McGarry et al., 2005). Currently no verification of an influence on the redox biology of helminths is available.

It has been postulated that antioxidant enzymes, that defend against host-generated ROS, are of particular importance for long-lived tissue-dwelling parasites that are involved in chronic infections. Here, surface or secreted antioxidant enzymes are of great importance since they can directly neutralize ROS that pose real danger, thereby protecting surface membranes against peroxides. Secreted filarial antioxidant enzymes include SOD, GPx and Prx (Henkle-Dührsen and Kampkötter, 2001). Additionally to their antioxidant role, the Prx have recently been shown to contribute to the development of Th2-responses by altering the function of macrophages (Donnelly et al., 2008). Interestingly, GSH-dependent proteins have been observed that are capable of modifying the local environment via modulation of the immune response. Here the secretory GSTs from *O. volvulus* combine several features that make them excellent drug target: they are accessible since they are located directly at the parasite–host interface, they detoxify and/or transport various electrophilic compounds and secondary products of lipid peroxidation and they are involved in the synthesis of potential immunmodulators. Significant structural differences to the host homologues are observed in the xenobiotic binding site; this may support the structure-based design of specific inhibitors (Sommer et al., 2003; Perbandt et al., 2008; Liebau et al., 2008).

As outlined above, GSH-dependent detoxification pathways defend against current drugs and also play a role in mediating resistance to anthelmintics. The antioxidant pathways also provide the parasite with a means to protect against ROS-attack by its host and/or vector. In the model nematode *C. elegans*, GSH-synthesis and a large variety of primary and secondary antioxidant enzymes and GSH-dependent detoxification enzymes are tightly regulated by the sole NF-E2-related (Nrf) transcription factor SKN-1 (An and Blackwell, 2003). Inhibiton of SKN-1 would thus target the expression of a multitude of enzymatic antioxidants and detoxification enzymes rather than affecting only one single protein or protein class, resulting in the downregulation of xenobiotic detoxification and in an enormous increase of oxidative stress. Since SKN-1 is also essential for embryonic development, this would be an additional bonus. Nematode-specific structural differences are observed that make SKN-1 an excellent candidate for the development of specific nematocidal drugs (Choe et al., 2012).

11. Conclusion

The current bottle-neck for the treatment of parasitic diseases with chemotherapeutics is the increasing drug resistance which forces the continuous discovery and development of new antiparasitic drugs. There is an urgent need for novel chemotherapeutic targets. New drugs should be generated to specifically target the parasite with minimal (or no) toxicity to the human host. Therefore, good drug targets should be distinctly different from processes in the host, or ideally be absent in the latter. Targeting the peculiarities - which are absent in the host - is proposed as such a strategy. In this sense, the parasite-specific biosyntheses represent ideal drug targets; similar to the already exploited antifolate interference with the parasite's dihydrofolate (vitamin B9) biosynthesis. There are a variety of reports about reactive compounds that have antiparasitic activity; however, not all of these are therapeutically viable drug-like molecules due to various limitations such as toxicity, low bioavailability, rapid inactivation under *in vivo* conditions and development of resistance. Recently studies on drug synergism raised special attention, which can open new avenues to improve the efficacy of antiparasitic drugs in combination with others. Since parasites such as *Plasmodium, Trypanosoma* or helminths are highly susceptible to oxidative stress - as outlined within this chapter - the identification of new lead compounds that target the parasite's redox systems by inducing oxidative stress, will be an efficient approach to discover novel drugs.

In this chapter we have tried to give an outline of the present situation of redox-active antiparasitic molecules that target human infectious diseases. In future the mechanisms, evolutionarily developed by the parasite to circumvent the crucial presence of ROS, will open new avenues for the development of novel antiparasitic drugs that combat resistant human pathogens effectively.

Acknowledgement

The authors would like to thank FAPESP (Fundação de Amparo à Pesquisa do Estado de São Paulo) for financial support (Project No. 2009/54325-2 to CW). The support of the DFG (Deutsche Forschungsgemeinschaft, grant LI 793/5-0 to EL) is acknowledged.

Author details

Carsten Wrenger[1], Isolmar Schettert[2] and Eva Liebau[3*]

*Address all correspondence to: cwrenger@icb.usp.br or liebaue@uni-muenster.de

1 Department of Parasitology, Institute of Biomedical Science, University of São Paulo, Av. Prof. Lineu Prestes, São Paulo-SP, Brazil

2 Laboratory of Genetics and Molecular Cardiology, Heart Institute InCor, Av. Dr. Eneas de Carvalho Aguiar, São Paulo-SP, Brazil

3 Department of Molecular Physiology, University of Münster, Hindenburgplatz, Münster, Germany

References

[1] Ahmad R, Srivastava AK, Tripathi RP, Batra S, Walter RD. (2007) Synthesis and biological evaluation of potential modulators of malarial glutathione-S-transferase(s). J Enzym Inhib Med Chem. 22:327-342

[2] Akoachere M, Buchholz K, Fischer E, Burhenne J, Haefeli WE, Schirmer RH, Becker K. (2005) In vitro assessment of methylene blue on chloroquine-sensitive and -resistant *Plasmodium falciparum* strains reveals synergistic action with artemisinins. Antimicrob Agents Chemother. 49:4592-4597

[3] Amato VS, Tuon FF, Bacha HA, Neto VA, Nicodemo AC. (2008) Mucosal leishmaniasis: current scenario and prospects for treatment. Acta Trop. 105:1-9

[4] An JH, Blackwell TK. (2003) SKN-1 links C. elegans mesendodermal specification to a conserved oxidative stress response. Genes Dev. 17:1882-93

[5] Angelucci F, Basso A, Bellelli A, Brunori M, Pica Mattoccia L, Valle C. (2007) The anti-schistosomal drug praziquantel is an adenosine antagonist. Parasitology 134:1215-1221

[6] Angelucci F, Sayed AA, Williams DL, Boumis G, Brunori M, Dimastrogiovanni D, Miele AE, Pauly F, Bellelli A. (2009) Inhibition of *Schistosoma mansoni* thioredoxin-glutathione reductase by auranofin: structural and kinetic aspects. J Biol Chem. 284:28977-28985

[7] Andreyev AY, Kushnareva YE, Starkov AA. (2005) Mitochondrial metabolism of reactive oxygen species. Biochemistry (Moscow) 70:200-214

[8] Aragon AD, Imani RA, Blackburn VR, Cupit PM, Melman SD, Goronga T, Webb T, Loker ES, Cunningham C. (2009) Towards an understanding of the mechanism of action of praziquantel. Mol Biochem Parasitol. 164:57-65

[9] Atamna H, Ginsburg H. (1995) Heme degradation in the presence of glutathione. A proposed mechanism to account for the high levels of non-heme iron found in the membranes of hemoglobinopathic red blood cells. J Biol Chem. 270:24876-24883

[10] Balana-Fouce R, Reguera RM, Cubria JC, Ordonez D. (1998) The pharmacology of leishmaniasis. Gen Pharmacol. 30:435-443

[11] Bandyopadhyay U, Dey S. (2011) Antimalarial drugs and molecules inhibiting hemozoin formation. In: Apicomplexan Parasites: Molecular Approaches Toward Targeted Drug Development, edited by Becker K. Weinheim, Germany: Wiley-VCH Verlag & Co. KGaA, 205-234.

[12] Banerjee AK, Arora N, Murty US. (2009) Structural model of the *Plasmodium falciparum* thioredoxin reductase: a novel target for antimalarial drugs. J Vector Borne Dis. 46:171-183

[13] Becker K, Kanzok SM, Iozef R, Fischer M, Schirmer RH, Rahlfs S. (2003) Plasmoredoxin, a novel redox-active protein unique for malarial parasites. Eur J Biochem. 270:1057-1064

[14] Beech RN, Skuce P, Bartley DJ, Martin RJ, Prichard RK, Gilleard JS (2011) Anthelmintic resistance: markers for resistance, or susceptibility? Parasitology. 138:160–174

[15] Bennett JL, Williams JF, Dave V (1993) Pharmacology of ivermectin. Parasitol Today 4:226-228

[16] Biot C, Bauer H, Schirmer RH, Davioud-Charvet E. (2004) 5-substituted tetrazoles as bioisosteres of carboxylic acids. Bioisosterism and mechanistic studies on glutathione reductase inhibitors as antimalarials. J Med Chem. 47:5972-5983

[17] Boucher IW, Brzozowski AM, Brannigan JA, Schnick C, Smith DJ, Kyes SA, Wilkinson AJ. (2006) The crystal structure of superoxide dismutase from *Plasmodium falciparum*. BMC Struct Biol. 6:20

[18] Buchholz K, Schirmer RH, Eubel JK, Akoachere MB, Dandekar T, Becker K, Gromer S. (2008) Interactions of methylene blue with human disulfide reductases and their orthologues from *Plasmodium falciparum*. Antimicrob Agents Chemother. 52:183-191

[19] Butzloff S, Groves MR, Wrenger C, Müller IB. (2012) Cytometric quantification of singlet oxygen in the human malaria parasite *Plasmodium falciparum*. Cytometry A. 81:698-703

[20] Chatelain E, Ioset JR. (2011) Drug discovery and development for neglected diseases: the DNDi model. Drug Des Devel Ther. 5:175-181.

[21] Chibale K, Haupt H, Kendrick H, Yardley V, Saravanamuthu A, Fairlamb AH, Croft SL. (2001) Antiprotozoal and cytotoxicity evaluation of sulfonamide and urea analogues of quinacrine. Bioorg Med Chem Lett 11: 2655-2657

[22] Choe KP, Leung CK, Miyamoto MM. (2012) Unique structure and regulation of the nematode detoxification gene regulator, SKN-1: implications to understanding and controlling drug resistance. Drug Metab Rev. 44:209-23

[23] Cirimotich CM, Dong Y, Clayton AM, Sandiford SL, Souza-Neto JA, Mulenga M, Dimopoulos G (2011) Natural microbe-mediated refractoriness to Plasmodium infection in *Anopheles gambiae*. Science, 332:855-858

[24] Croft SL, Sundar S, Fairlamb AH. (2006) Drug resistance in leishmaniasis. Clin. Microbiol. Rev. 19:111-126

[25] Davioud-Charvet E, McLeish MJ, Veine DM, Giegel D, Arscott LD, Andricopulo AD, Becker K, Müller S, Schirmer RH, Williams CH, Jr., Kenyon GL. (2003) Mechanism-based inactivation of thioredoxin reductase from *Plasmodium falciparum* by Mannich bases. Implication for cytotoxicity. Biochemistry 42:13319-13330

[26] Dedet JP, Pratlong F. (2009) Protozoa infection in G. Cook, A. Zumla (Eds.), Manson's Tropical Diseases, Saunders, Philadelphia 1341-1367

[27] Díaz de Toranzo EG, Castro JA, Franke de Cazzulo BM, Cazzulo JJ. (1988) Interaction of benznidazole reactive metabolites with nuclear and kinetoplastic DNA, proteins and lipids from *Trypanosoma cruzi*. Experientia, 44:880-881

[28] Docampo R. (1990) Sensitivity of parasites to free radical damage by antiparasitic drugs. Chem Biol Interact. 73:1-27

[29] Donnelly S, Stack CM, O'Neill SM, Sayed AA, Williams DL, Dalton JP. (2008) Helminth 2-Cys peroxiredoxin drives Th2 responses through a mechanism involving alternatively activated macrophages. FASEB J 22:4022–4032

[30] Ehrenshaft M, Chung KR, Jenns AE, Daub ME. (1999) Functional characterization of SOR1, a gene required for resistance to photosensitizing toxins in the fungus *Cercospora nicotianae*. Curr Genet. 34:478-485

[31] Egan TJ, Hunter R, Kaschula CH, Marques HM, Misplon A, Walden J. (2000) Structure-function relationships in aminoquinolines: effect of amino and chloro groups on quinoline-hematin complex formation, inhibition of beta-hematin formation, and antiplasmodial activity. J Med Chem. 43:283-291

[32] Fairlamb AH, Blackburn P, Ulrich P, Chait BT, Cerami A. (1985) Trypanothione: a novel bis(glutathionyl)spermidine cofactor for glutathione reductase in trypanosomatids. Science 227:1485-1487

[33] Fernandes AP, Holmgren A (2004) Glutaredoxins: Glutathione-dependent redox enzymes with functions far beyond a simple thioredoxin backup system. Antioxid Redox Signal. 6:63-74

[34] Filardi LS, Brener Z. (1987) Susceptibility and natural resistance of *Trypanosoma cruzi* strains to drugs used clinically in Chagas disease. Trans R Soc Trop Med. Hyg. 81:755-759

[35] Forman HJ, Maiorino M, Ursini F (2010) Signaling functions of reactive oxygen species. Biochemistry 49:835-842

[36] Frey PA. (1997) Radicals in enzymatic reactions. Curr Opin Chem Biol. 1:347-356

[37] Freinbichler W, Colivicchi MA, Stefanini C, Bianchi L, Ballini C, Misini B, Weinberger P, Linert W, Varešlija D, Tipton KF, Della Corte L. (2011). Highly reactive oxygen species: detection, formation, and possible functions. Cell Mol Life Sci. 68:2067-2079

[38] Friebolin W, Jannack B, Wenzel N, Furrer J, Oeser T, Sanchez CP, Lanzer M, Yardley V, Becker K, Davioud-Charvet E. (2008) Antimalarial dual drugs based on potent inhibitors of glutathione reductase from *Plasmodium falciparum*. J Med Chem. 51:1260-1277

[39] Francis SE, Sullivan DJ, Daniel E. (1997) Hemoglobin metabolism in the malaria parasite *Plasmodium falciparum*. Annu. Rev. Microbiol. 51:97-123

[40] Fyfe PK, Westrop GD, Silva AM, Coombs GH, Hunter WN. (2012) Leishmania TDR1 structure, a unique trimeric glutathione transferase capable of deglutathionylation and antimonial prodrug activation. Proc Natl Acad Sci U S A. 109:11693-11698

[41] Geary TG, Woo K, McCarthy JS, Mackenzie CD, Horton J, Prichard RK, de Silva NR, Olliaro PL, Lazdins-Helds JK, Engels DA, Bundy DA. (2010) Unresolved issues in anthelmintic pharmacology for helminthiases of humans. Int J Parasitol. 40:1-13

[42] Gallo V, Schwarzer E, Rahlfs S, Schirmer RH, van Zwieten R, Roos D, Arese P, Becker K. (2009) Inherited glutathione reductase deficiency and *Plasmodium falciparum* malaria—a case study. PLoS One 4:e7303

[43] Garavito G, Bertani S, Rincon J, Maurel S, Monje MC, Landau I, Valentin A, Deharo E. (2007) Blood schizontocidal activity of methylene blue in combination with antimalarials against *Plasmodium falciparum*. Parasite. 14:135-140

[44] Gradoni L, Soteriadou K, Louzir H, Dakkak A, Toz SO, Jaffe C et al. (2008) Drug regimens for visceral leishmaniasis in Mediterranean countries. Trop Med Int Health 13:1272-1276

[45] Gratepanche S, Menage S, Touati D, Wintjens R, Delplace P, Fontecave M, Masset A, Camus D, Dive D. (2002) Biochemical and electron paramagnetic resonance study of the iron superoxide dismutase from *Plasmodium falciparum*. Mol Biochem Parasitol. 120:237-246

[46] Grellier P, Maroziene A, Nivinskas H, Sarlauskas J, Aliverti A, Cenas N. (2010) Antiplasmodial activity of quinones: roles of aziridinyl substituents and the inhibition of *Plasmodium falciparum* glutathione reductase. Arch Biochem Biophys. 494:32-39

[47] Halliwell B (1999) Antioxidant defense mechanisms: from the beginning to the end (of the beginning) Free Radic Res. 31:261-272.

[48] Henkle-Dührsen K, Kampkötter A (2001) Antioxidant enzyme families in parasitic nematodes. Mol Biochem Parasitol. 114:129-142.

[49] Herwaldt, BL (1999). "Leishmaniasis." Lancet 354 (9185): 1191-1199

[50] Holzmuller P, Sereno D, Lemesre JL. (2005) Lower nitric oxide susceptibility of trivalent antimony-resistant amastigotes of *Leishmania infantum*. Antimicrob Agents Chemother. 49:4406-4409

[51] Hotez PJ, Brindley PJ, Bethony JM, King CH, Pearce EJ, Jacobson J (2008) Helminth infections: the great neglected tropical diseases. J Clin Invest. 118:1311-1321

[52] Huang HH, Rigouin C, Willams DL (2012) The redox biology of schistosome parasites and application for drug development. Curr Pharm Des. 18:3595-3611

[53] Ignatushchenko MV, Winter RW, Bachinger HP, Hinrichs DJ, Riscoe MK. (1997) Xanthones as antimalarial agents; studies of a possible mode of action. FEBS Lett. 409:67-73

[54] James CE, Davey MW. (2009) Increased expression of ABC transport proteins is associated with ivermectin resistance in the model nematode *Caenorhabditis elegans*. Int J Parasitol. 39:213-20

[55] Jeziorski MC, Greenberg RM. (2006) Voltage-gated calcium channel subunits from platyhelminths: potential role in praziquantel action. Int J Parasitol 36:625–632

[56] Jones DP, Go YM. (2010) Redox compartmentalization and cellular stress. Diabetes, Obes. Metab. 12:116–125.

[57] Kanzok SM, Rahlfs S, Becker K, and Schirmer RH. (2002) Thioredoxin, thioredoxin reductase, and thioredoxin peroxidase of malaria parasite *Plasmodium falciparum*. Methods Enzymol. 347:370-381

[58] Kanzok SM, Schirmer RH, Turbachova I, Iozef R, Becker K. (2000) The thioredoxin system of the malaria parasite *Plasmodium falciparum*. Glutathione reduction revisited. J Biol Chem. 275:40180-40186

[59] Kawazu S, Komaki K, Tsuji N, Kawai S, Ikenoue N, Hatabu T, Ishikawa H, Matsumoto Y, Himeno K, Kano S. (2001) Molecular characterization of a 2-Cys peroxiredoxin from the human malaria parasite *Plasmodium falciparum*. Mol Biochem Parasitol. 116:73-79

[60] Kehr S, Jortzik E, Delahunty C, Yates JR, Rahlfs S, Becker K. (2011) Protein s-glutathionylation in malaria parasites. Antioxid Redox Signal. 15:2855-2865

[61] Khan AU, Kasha M. (1994) Singlet molecular oxygen in the Haber-Weiss reaction. Proc Natl Acad Sci USA. 91:12365-12367

[62] Khaw M, Panosian CB. (1995) Human antiprotozoal therapy: past, present, and future. Clin Microbiol Rev. 8:427-439.

[63] Kirchhoff LV. (2000) American trypanosomiasis (Chagas' disease) in R.E. Rakel (Ed.), Conn's Current Therapy, W. B. Saunders, New York: 101-102

[64] Knöckel J, Müller IB, Butzloff S, Bergmann B, Walter RD, Wrenger C. (2012) The anti-oxidative effect of *de novo* generated vitamin B6 in *Plasmodium falciparum* validated by protein interference. Biochem J. 443:397-405

[65] Koenderink JB, Kavishe RA, Rijpma SR, Russel FG. (2010) The ABCs of multidrug resistance in malaria. Trends Parasitol. 26:440-446

[66] Kotecka BM, Barlin GB, Edstein MD, Rieckmann KH. (1997) New quinoline di-Mannich base compounds with greater antimalarial activity than chloroquine, amodiaquine, or pyronaridine. Antimicrob Agents Chemother. 41:1369-1374

[67] Krauth-Siegel RL, Bauer H, Schirmer RH. (2005) Dithiol proteins as guardians of the intracellular redox milieu in parasites: old and new drug targets in trypanosomes and malaria-causing plasmodia. Angew Chem Int Ed Engl. 44:690-715

[68] Krauth-Siegel RL, Comini MA. (2008) Redox control in trypanosomatids, parasitic protozoa with trypanothione-based thiol metabolism. Biochim. Biophys. Acta 1780:1236-1248

[69] Krnajski Z, Gilberger TW, Walter RD, Cowman AF, Müller S. (2002) Thioredoxin reductase is essential for the survival of *Plasmodium falciparum* erythrocytic stages. J Biol Chem. 277:25970-25975

[70] Krnajski Z, Walter RD, Müller S. (2001) Isolation and functional analysis of two thioredoxin peroxidases (peroxiredoxins) from *Plasmodium falciparum*. Mol Biochem Parasitol. 113:303-308

[71] Kumar S, Christophides GK, Cantera R, Charles B, Han YS, Meister S, Dimopoulos G, Kafatos FC, Barillas-Mury C. (2003) The role of reactive oxygen species on Plasmodium melanotic encapsulation in *Anopheles gambiae*. Proc Natl Acad Sci USA. 100:14139-14144

[72] Kumar S, Das SK, Dey S, Maity P, Guha M, Choubey V, Panda G, Bandyopadhyay U. (2008) Antiplasmodial activity of [(aryl)arylsulfanylmethyl]Pyridine. Antimicrob Agents Chemother. 52:705-715

[73] Kuntz AN, Davioud-Charvet E, Sayed AA, Califf LL, Dessolin J, Arnér ES, Williams DL. (2007) Thioredoxin glutathione reductase from *Schistosoma mansoni:* an essential parasite enzyme and a key drug target. PLoS Med. 4:e206

[74] Lewis JA, Wu CH, Berg H, Levine JH (1980) The genetics of levamisole resistance in the nematode *Caenorhabditis elegans*. Genetics 95:905–928

[75] Li R, Kenyon GL, Cohen FE, Chen X, Gong B, Dominguez JN, Davidson E, Kurzban G, Miller RE, Nuzum EO, et al. (1995) In vitro antimalarial activity of chalcones and their derivatives. J Med Chem. 38:5031–5037

[76] Liebau E, Bergmann B, Campbell AM, Teesdale-Spittle P, Brophy PM, Luersen K, Walter RD. (2002) The glutathione S-transferase from *Plasmodium falciparum*. Mol Biochem Parasitol. 124:85-90

[77] Liebau E, De Maria F, Burmeister C, Perbandt M, Turella P, Antonini G, Federici G, Giansanti F, Stella L, Lo Bello M, Caccuri AM, Ricci G. (2005) Cooperativity and pseudo-cooperativity in the glutathione S-transferase from *Plasmodium falciparum*. J Biol Chem. 280:26121-26128.

[78] Liebau E, Höppner J, Mühlmeister M, Burmeister C, Lüersen K, Perbandt M, Schmetz C, Büttner D, Brattig N. (2008) The secretory omega-class glutathione transferase OvGST3 from the human pathogenic parasite *Onchocerca volvulus*. FEBS J. 275:3438-3453.

[79] Liebau E, Dawood KF, Fabrini R, Fischer-Riepe L, Perbandt M, Stella L, Pedersen JZ, Bocedi A, Petrarca P, Federici G, Ricci G.(2009) Tetramerization and cooperativity in *Plasmodium falciparum* glutathione S-transferase are mediated by atypic loop 113-119. J Biol Chem. 284:22133-22139.

[80] Maltezou HC. (2010) Drug resistance in visceral leishmaniasis. J. Biomed. Biotechnol. 617521

[81] Martin RJ, Robertson AP, Bjorn H (1997) Target sites of anthelmintics. Parasitology 114:111–124

[82] Massimine KM, McIntosh MT, Doan LT, Atreya CE, Gromer S, Sirawaraporn W, Elliott DA, Joiner KA, Schirmer RH, Anderson KS. (2006) Eosin B as a novel antimalarial agent for drug-resistant *Plasmodium falciparum*. Antimicrob Agents Chemother. 50:3132-3141

[83] Mason RP, Holtzman JL. (1975) The role of catalytic superoxide formation in the O2 inhibition of nitroreductase. Biochem Biophys Res Commun. 67:1267-1274

[84] Maya JD, Rodríguez A, Pino L, Pabon A, Ferreira J, Pavani M, Repetto Y, Morello A. (2004) Effects of buthionine sulfoximine nifurtimox and benznidazole upon trypanothione and metallothionein proteins in *Trypanosoma cruzi*. Biol Res. 37:61-69

[85] Maya JD, Cassels BK, Iturriaga-Vásquez P, Ferreira J, Faúndez M, Galanti N, Ferreira A, Morello A. (2007) Mode of action of natural and synthetic drugs against *Trypanosoma cruzi* and their interaction with the mammalian host. Comp Biochem Physiol A Mol Integr Physiol. 146:601-620

[86] McGarry HF, Plant LD, Taylor MJ (2005) Diethylcarbamazine activity against *Brugia malayi* microfilariae is dependent on inducible nitric-oxide synthase and the cyclooxygenase pathway. Filaria J. 4:4

[87] Monostori P, Wittmann G, Karg E, Turi S. (2009) Determination of glutathione and glutathione disulfide in biological samples: an in-depth review. J. Chromatogr. B Analyt Technol Biomed Life Sci 877:3331-3346

[88] Moreno SN, Docampo R, Mason RP, León W, Stoppani AO. (1982) Different behaviors of benznidazole as free radical generator with mammalian and *Trypanosoma cruzi* microsomal preparations. Arch Biochem Biophys. 218:585-591

[89] Mukherjee AK, Gupta G, Bhattacharjee S, Guha SK, Majumder S, Adhikari A et al. (2010) Amphotericin B regulates the host immune response in visceral leishmaniasis: reciprocal regulation of protein kinase C isoforms. J Infect. 61:173–184

[90] Meunier B, Robert A. (2010) Heme as trigger and target for trioxane-containing antimalarial drugs. Acc Chem Res 43: 1444-1451

[91] Müller S, Liebau E, Walter RD, Krauth-Siegel RL. (2003) Thiol-based redox metabolism of protozoan parasites. Trends Parasitol. 19:320-328

[92] Müller S. (2003) Thioredoxin reductase and glutathione synthesis in *Plasmodium falciparum*. Redox Rep. 8:251-255

[93] Muller T, Johann L, Jannack B, Bruckner M, Lanfranchi DA, Bauer H, Sanchez C, Yardley V, Deregnaucourt C, Schrevel J, Lanzer M, Schirmer RH, Davioud-Charvet E. (2011) A glutathione reductase-catalyzed cascade of redox reactions to bioactivate potent antimalarial 1,4-naphthoquinones-a new strategy to combat malarial parasites. J Am Chem Soc. 133:11557-11571

[94] O'Neill PM, Mukhtar A, Stocks PA, Randle LE, Hindley S, Ward SA, Storr RC, Bickley JF, O'Neil IA, Maggs JL, Hughes RH, Winstanley PA, Bray PG, Park BK. (2003) Isoquine and related amodiaquine analogues: a new generation of improved 4-aminoquinoline antimalarials. J Med Chem. 46:4933-4945

[95] O'Neill PM, Barton VE, Ward SA. (2010) The molecular mechanism of action of artemisinin--the debate continues. Molecules. 15:1705-1721

[96] Olliaro P, Seiler J, Kuesel A, Horton J, Clark JN, Don R, Keiser J. (2011) Potential drug development candidates for human soil-transmitted helminthiases. PLoS Negl Trop Dis. 5:e1138

[97] Pal C, Bandyopadhyay U. (2012) Redox-active antiparasitic drugs. Antioxid Redox Signal. 17:555-582

[98] Perbandt M, Höppner J, Burmeister C, Lüersen K, Betzel C, Liebau E. (2008) Structure of the extracellular glutathione S-transferase OvGST1 from the human pathogenic parasite *Onchocerca volvulus*. J Mol Biol. 377:501-511.

[99] Prata A. (2001) Clinical and epidemiological aspects of Chagas disease. Lancet, Infect. Dis. 1:92-100

[100] Prichard RK, Basáñez MG, Boatin BA, McCarthy JS, García HH, Yang GJ, Sripa B, Lustigman S. (2012) A research agenda for helminth diseases of humans: intervention for control and elimination. PLoS Negl Trop Dis. 6:e1549.

[101] Rakotomanga M, Loiseau PM, Saint-Pierre-Chazalet M. (2004) Hexadecylphosphocholine interaction with lipid monolayers. Biochim Biophys Acta. 1661:212-218

[102] Renslo AR, McKerrow JH. (2006) Drug discovery and development for neglected parasitic diseases. Nat Chem Biol. 2:701-710

[103] Ribeiro F, Coelho PM, Vieira LQ, Watson DG, Kusel JR. (1998) The effect of praziquantel treatment on glutathione concentration in *Schistosoma mansoni*. Parasitology. 116:229-236

[104] Roberts, MT. (2006). Current understandings on the immunology of leishmaniasis and recent developments in prevention and treatment. Br Med Bull 75-76:115-130

[105] Rodriques Coura J, de Castro SL. (2002) A critical review on Chagas disease chemotherapy. Mem. Inst. Oswaldo Cruz. 97:3-24

[106] Saint-Pierre-Chazalet M, Ben BM, Le ML, Bories C, Rakotomanga M, Loiseau PM. (2009) Membrane sterol depletion impairs miltefosine action in wild-type and miltefosine-resistant *Leishmania donovani* promastigotes. J Antimicrob Chemother. 64:993-1001

[107] Salinas G, Selkirk ME, Chalar C, Maizels RM, Fernández C. (2004) Linked thioredoxin-glutathione systems in platyhelminths. Trends Parasitol. 20:340-346

[108] Sarma GN, Savvides SN, Becker K, Schirmer M, Schirmer RH, Karplus PA. (2003) Glutathione reductase of the malarial parasite *Plasmodium falciparum*: crystal structure and inhibitor development. J Mol Biol. 328:893-907

[109] Sau A, Pellizzari Tregno F, Valentino F, Federici G, Caccuri AM. (2010) Glutathione transferases and development of new principles to overcome drug resistance. Arch Biochem Biophys. 500:116-122.

[110] Seeber F, Aliverti A, Zanetti G. (2005) The plant-type ferredoxin-NADP+reductase/ferredoxin redox system as a possible drug target against apicomplexan human parasites. Curr Pharm Des. 11:3159-3172

[111] Seifert K, Perez-Victoria FJ, Stettler M, Sanchez-Canete MP, Castanys S, Gamarro F et al. (2007) Inactivation of the miltefosine transporter, LdMT, causes miltefosine resistance that is conferred to the amastigote stage of *Leishmania donovani* and persists *in vivo*. Int J Antimicrob Agents. 30:229-235

[112] Sharma U, Singh S. (2008) Insect vectors of Leishmania: distribution, physiology and their control. J Vector Borne Dis. 45:255-272

[113] Sharmeen S, Skrtic M, Sukhai MA, Hurren R, Gronda M, Wang X, Fonseca SB, Sun H, Wood TE, Ward R, Minden MD, Batey RA, Datti A, Wrana J, Kelley SO, Schimmer AD. (2010) The antiparasitic agent ivermectin induces chloride-dependent membrane hyperpolarization and cell death in leukemia cells. Blood 116:3593-603.

[114] Sherman IW. (1977) Amino acid metabolism and protein synthesis in malarial parasites. Bull World Health Organ. 55:265-276

[115] Sies H (1999) Glutathione and its role in cellular functions. Free Radic Biol Med. 27:916-921.

[116] Simeonov A, Jadhav A, Sayed AA, Wang Y, Nelson ME, Thomas CJ, Inglese J, Williams DL, Austin CP. (2008) Quantitative high-throughput screen identifies inhibitors of the *Schistosoma mansoni* redox cascade. PLoS Negl Trop Dis. 2:e127

[117] Singh C, Srivastav NC, Puri SK. (2002) *In vivo* active antimalarial isonitriles. Bioorg Med Chem Lett. 12:2277-2279

[118] Sommer A, Rickert R, Fischer P, Steinhart H, Walter RD, Liebau E. (2003) A dominant role for extracellular glutathione S-transferase from *Onchocerca volvulus* is the production of prostaglandin D2. Infect Immun. 71:3603-3606

[119] Soulere L, Delplace P, Davioud-Charvet E, Py S, Sergheraert C, Perie J, Ricard I, Hoffmann P, Dive D. (2003) Screening of *Plasmodium falciparum* iron superoxide dismutase inhibitors and accuracy of the SOD-assays. Bioorg Med Chem. 11:4941-4944

[120] Souza AS, Giudice A, Pereira JM, Guimaraes LH, de Jesus AR, de Moura TR et al. (2010) Resistance of *Leishmania (Viannia) braziliensis* to nitric oxide: correlation with antimony therapy and TNF-alpha production. BMC Infect Dis 10:209

[121] Sturm N, Hu Y, Zimmermann H, Fritz-Wolf K, Wittlin S, Rahlfs S, Becker K. (2009) Compounds structurally related to ellagic acid show improved antiplasmodial activity. Antimicrob Agents Chemother. 53:622-630

[122] Sundar S, Rai M. (2002) Advances in the treatment of leishmaniasis. Curr Opin Infect Dis 15:593–598

[123] Tambasco-Studart M, Titiz O, Raschle T, Forster G, Amrhein N, Fitzpatrick TB. (2005) Vitamin B6 biosynthesis in higher plants. Proc Natl Acad Sci USA. 102:13687-13692

[124] Temperton NJ, Wilkinson SR, Meyer DJ, Kelly JM. (1998) Overexpression of superoxide dismutase in *Trypanosoma cruzi* results in increased sensitivity to the trypanocidal agents gentian violet and benznidazole. Mol Biochem Parasitol. 96:167-176

[125] Trachootham D, Weiqin L, Ogasawara MA, Valle NRD, Huang P. (2008) Redox Regulation of Cell Survival. Antioxid Redox Signal. 10:1343-1374

[126] Turrens JF, Watts Jr BP, Zhong L, Docampo R. (1996) Inhibition of *Trypanosoma cruzi* and *T. brucei* NADH fumarate reductase by benznidazole and anthelmintic imidazole derivatives. Mol Biochem Parasitol. 82:125-129

[127] Utzinger J, Xiao S, N'Goran EK, Bergquist R, Tanner M. (2001) The potential of artemether for the control of schistosomiasis. Int J Parasitol 31:1549-1562.

[128] Utzinger J, Keiser J. (2004) Schistosomiasis and soil-transmitted helmintiasis: common drugs for treatment and control. Expert Opin. Pharmacother. 5:263-285.

[129] Vanaerschot M, Maes I, Ouakad M, Adaui V, Maes L, De DS et al. (2010) Linking in vitro and in vivo survival of clinical *Leishmania donovani* strains. PLoS One 5:e12211

[130] Van Assche T, Deschacht M, da Luz RA, Maes L, Cos P. (2007) Leishmania-macrophage interactions: insights into the redox biology. Free Radic Biol Med. 51:337-351

[131] Vennerstrom JL, Ellis WY, Ager AL, Jr., Andersen SL, Gerena L, Milhous WK. (1992) Bisquinolines. N,N-bis(7-chloroquinolin-4-yl)alkanediamines with potential against chloroquine-resistant malaria. J Med Chem. 35:2129-2134

[132] Vercruysse J, Albonico M, Behnke J, Kotze A, Prichard R, et al.(2011) Is anthelmintic resistance a concern for the control of human soil-transmitted helminths? Int J Parasitol: Drugs Drug Res. 1:14–27

[133] Wang X, Quinn PJ. (1999). Vitamin E and its function in membranes. Prog Lipid Res. 38:309-336

[134] Wangroongsarb P, Satimai W, Khamsiriwatchara A, Thwing J, Eliades JM, Kaewkungwal J, Delacollette C. (2011) Respondent-driven sampling on the Thailand-Cambodia border. II. Knowledge, perception, practice and treatment-seeking behaviour of migrants in malaria endemic zones. Malar J. 10:117

[135] Wrenger C, Eschbach ML, Müller IB, Warnecke D, Walter RD. (2005) Analysis of the vitamin B6 biosynthesis pathway in the human malaria parasite *Plasmodium falciparum*. J Biol Chem. 280:5242-5248

[136] Wright AD, Wang H, Gurrath M, Konig GM, Kocak G, Neumann G, Loria P, Foley M, Tilley L. (2001) Inhibition of heme detoxification processes underlies the antimalarial activity of terpene isonitrile compounds from marine sponges. J Med Chem. 44:873-885

[137] Xu Kelly J, Winter R, Riscoe M, Peyton DH. (2001) A spectroscopic investigation of the binding interactions between 4,5-dihydroxyxanthone and heme. J Inorg Biochem. 86:617-625

[138] Zahoor A, Lafleur MV, Knight RC, Loman H, Edwards DI. (1987) DNA damage induced by reduced nitroimidazole drugs. Biochem Pharmacol. 36:3299–3304

Chapter 9

Discovery of Selective and Potent Inhibitors of Palmitoylation

Sonia Lobo Planey

Additional information is available at the end of the chapter

http://dx.doi.org/10.5772/52503

1. Introduction

Palmitoylation is a reversible, post-translational modification of a protein through the addition of the 16-carbon fatty acid, palmitate, to a cysteine residue. There are two types of palmitoylation, one called thio- or *S*-palmitoylation in which palmitate is added to the thiol side chain of a cysteine residue via a labile thioester bond [1]. The other type, *N*-palmitoylation, is the addition of palmitate to an N-terminal cysteine via a stable amide bond [2]. The two forms of palmitoylation are regulated by different families of palmitoyl acyltransferases (PATs)—*S*-palmitoylation via a family of multi-pass transmembrane proteins called DHHC (Asp-His-His-Cys) proteins [3] and *N*-palmitoylation via a family of multi-pass transmembrane proteins termed membrane-bound *O*-acyltransferase [4]. S-palmitoylation, the focus of this chapter, is more common and because of the labile thioester bond, can dynamically regulate protein sorting and function.

Palmitoylation increases the lipophilicity of the modified protein often changing its subcellular distribution in both dramatic and subtle ways. The larger-scale changes occur when cytoplasmic proteins relocate from the cytoplasm to membrane and when integral membrane proteins move from one membrane system to another, such as from the endoplasmic reticulum (ER) to the plasma membrane (PM). The more subtle changes, in terms of distance, occur at the nanoscale level within a membrane. The increase in lipophilicity upon palmitoylation often results in an altered affinity for a particular lipid microenvironment within that membrane [5]. For example, lipid rafts are small islands in membranes with distinct lipid compositions that selectively attract or exclude both peripheral (often exclusively by virtue of palmitoylation) and integral membrane palmitoylated proteins. Palmitoylated proteins have affinity for lipid rafts that are rich in cholesterol, while prenylated proteins have little or no affinity for these rafts [5]. Such lipophilicity-driven changes in protein distribution may alter access of a palmitoylated protein to extracellular ligands (when the protein moves from the ER to the PM), protein-protein interactions, or the engagement of the palmitoyl-protein in multi-molecular signaling complexes. The role of palmitoylation as a versatile protein sorting signal, regulating intracellular protein trafficking and targeting to membrane microdomains has been reviewed recently [6]. Palmitate may be the most common lipid species to occupy cysteine residues, but it is not the only one. Marilyn Resh and colleagues identified the lipid moieties resident on the cysteine residue of the N-terminal tail of Src family kinases [7-9]. While for these proteins the cysteine residue near the N-terminus is most frequently palmitoylated, it is also modified by palmitoleate, stearate, or oleate with a frequency that is apparently related to the abundance of palmitate in cells [10]. The physiological differences that result from proteins being modified by these other lipids has not been explored extensively; however, given their different physical properties, it seems reasonable that their impact on a protein should be subtly different than palmitate.

Unlike other forms of lipidation such as myristoylation and prenylation, palmitoylation is reversible, by virtue of the labile thioester bond. This allows for dynamic regulation of the protein's lipophilicity [11-13]. By contrast, prenyl groups are attached to cysteines by a stable thioether bond and myristate to glycines by a stable amide bond. It is now apparent that many instances of palmitoylation are enzymatically mediated by a family of palmitoyl acyltransferases (PATs), whereas the mechanisms for depalmitoylation are poorly understood. Nevertheless, it is known that palmitate cycles on and off of many proteins at variable rates ranging from minutes to days. Such dynamic regulation makes palmitoylation unique among post-translational protein lipid modifications and places it in a category similar to phosphorylation. Discovering the molecular identity of PATs was a pivotal event that dramatically accelerated the pace of discovery in the field. Likewise, there has been increased interest in palmitoylation partly because many of the genes encoding PATs have been linked to human diseases like cancer. With a greater understanding of how palmitate is enzymatically attached to proteins, some of the most interesting questions include: What are the substrate(s) of each PAT?; how does a PAT recognize and palmitoylated a substrate?; how are PATs regulated?; and how is depalmitoylation regulated? The answers to these questions are beginning to unfold due to the recent discovery of pharmacological modulators of palmitoylation as well as the development of novel assays and refinement of existing assays. Our ability to understand palmitoylation and its importance to human health and disease is only as good as the methods we use to test our hypotheses. Thus, the discovery of potent and selective inhibitors of palmitoylation as well as the continued development of assays with increased sensitivity and selectivity is critical to this venture.

2. Palmitoylation and DHHC proteins

2.1. Molecular identity of palmitoyl acyltransferases (PATs)

It has been known for many years that palmitoylation is a critical regulator of diverse and complex signaling networks, but the mechanism responsible for palmitoylation of most pro-

http://dx.doi.org/10.5772/52503

teins remained a mystery and somewhat controversial until only recently. The apparent absence of a consensus site for palmitoylation encoded by the sequence of amino acid residues surrounding palmitoyl cysteines, as well as the difficulty in purifying and identifying the enzymes capable of mediating the reaction, led many to believe that it was autocatalytic. Given these issues and the high reactivity of cysteines and palmitoyl-CoA, especially in *in vitro* protein palmitoylation assays, the possibility was not unreasonable [11, 14, 15]. Many of the arguments for and against autocatalytic palmitoylation have been reviewed recently [16].Yet, given the prevalence of palmitoylated proteins in parts of cells where signaling events are so highly concentrated, complex, and regulated, such as the neuronal synapse, it seemed somewhat unreasonable that all regulation of palmitoylation could be left to diffusion—a nagging reality that kept the search for an enzymatic mechanism alive despite the arguments to the contrary. Additionally, there was evidence over the years in support of the idea that these enzymes existed because PAT activity in detergent solubilized protein fractions had been measured using viral glycoproteins [17], p59*fyn* [18], and H-Ras [19] as substrates among others.

The experiments that conclusively provided the molecular identity of PATs were presented in a series of papers spanning almost a decade. The experimental model organism that ultimately provided the information was yeast. First, palmitoylation-dependent alleles of yeast *RAS2* were identified. A genetic screen designed to identify mutations that rendered cells non-viable if Ras2p was not palmitoylated was utilized to identify mutations in two genes- *ERF2* and *ERF4/SHR5* [20, 21]. These mutations resulted in diminished palmitoylation of Ras2p and mislocalization of GFP-Ras2p (respectively or it takes both mutations to cause both effects [20, 22]). However, it could not be decisively concluded if the mutations in *ERF2* and *ERF4* were affecting Ras2p palmitoylation directly or indirectly by altering Ras2p trafficking (which could have prevented an interaction between the palmitoyl acyltransferase and Ras2p).

In collaboration with Maurine Linder, Deschenes and colleagues used an *in vitro* palmitoylation assay to show that Erf2p and Erf4p together constituted a Ras2p PAT that used palmitoyl-CoA as a donor [23]. Erf2p is a ~42-kDa integral membrane protein that is expressed in the ER. The protein contains the DHHC-CRD (Asp-His-His-Cys-cysteine rich domain), also referred to as the NEW1 or zf-DHHC domain (PF01529), which is found in an extensive family of membrane proteins ranging from unicellular eukaryotes to humans [24, 25]. This domain is now recognized as the molecular signature for PATs that add palmitate to cysteines via a labile thioester bond.

At almost the same time that the Erf2p/Erf4p complex was identified as the Ras2p PAT, Akr1p was identified as a PAT with specificity for Yck2p [26]. An important clue leading to the relationship between these two proteins came from the fact that mutants in both Ras2p and Yck2P exhibited a reduced rate of pheromone receptor internalization [27, 28]. Akr1p contains a DHYC-CRD instead of a DHHC-CRD as well as ankyrin repeats not present in Erf2p. The DHYC motif present in three yeast proteins (Akr1p, Akr2p and Pfa5) does not appear to occur in the mammalian genome. Akr1p and Akr2p are most closely related to the mammalian HIP14 (DHHC17) and HIP14L (DHHC13) which contains the variant DQHC—the only observed mammalian deviation from DHHC [3].

2.2. The ZDHHC family of PATs

The mammalian genome contains at least 23 members of the *ZDHHC* PAT gene family identified by the presence of the signature DHHC-cysteine rich domain. Members of the family had been identified as being genes of interest (e.g., "REAM" in metastatic cancer [29]) prior to understanding their function. The genomic structure of *ZDHHC* genes varies widely, including the number and differential use of exons that are spliced together to generate the mRNA. EC gene analyses (http://genome.ewha.ac.kr/ECgene/) of the mRNAs that encode PATs suggest that all of the genes are alternatively spliced at various sites throughout the protein coding sequence as well as within untranslated regions. Many of the putative, alternatively-spliced exons are predicted to encode small peptides that change the structure of the protein in a way that may alter substrate specificity. Similarly, splicing may alter sites for other post-translational modifications, such as phosphorylation or glycosylation, all of which may regulate activity, substrate specificity, subcellular distribution, or interactions with non-substrate proteins. *ZDHHC7*, for example, alters the use of a 111 bp exon that is differentially and specifically expressed in tissues such as placenta, lung, liver, thymus, and small intestine [30]. This exon encodes a 37-residue peptide (EKSSDCRP-SACTVKTGLDPTLVGICGEGTESVQSLLL) within the intracellular loop between transmembrane domain 2 (TM2) and TM3 that contains a PKC phosphorylation site. It is conceivable that phosphorylation of this serine changes DHHC7 in such a way that substrate specificity or the rate of palmitate transfer activity is altered. In addition to alternative mRNA splicing, aberrant splicing induced by mutations or single nucleotide polymorphisms has been shown to occur in at least two ZDHHC genes. A splice-site mutation in highly conserved residues of *ZDHHC9*, a PAT that has been shown to palmitoylate H-Ras and N-Ras [31], has been described in families with X-linked mental retardation (XLMR) [32]. This mutation creates an additional, stronger splice-donor site 140 nt before (toward the 5′ end) the normal donor site. Usage of the new site results in a mRNA that is frame-shifted and that encodes a truncated protein. Single nucleotide polymorphisms that affect splicing of *ZDHHC8* have also been implicated in schizophrenia [33] (also see: [34-36]).

Hydropathy analyses predict that the PATs encoded by these genes all pass through a membrane multiple times (at least four) and are expressed predominantly in the ER and Golgi membranes [30, 37, 38]. Currently, there is little published data on the numbers of TM domains in any of the PATs with the exception of Akr1p in yeast [39]. Predictions using TopPred II 1.1 [40] as presented by Ohno and colleagues [30] show that most PATs have an even number of TM domains with the DHHC-CRD motif in the cytoplasm. However for DHHC13, -16, -11, and -22, the DHHC-CRD motif resides just C-terminal to the first or third TM domain. Assuming the N-terminus is cytoplasmic, this places the DHHC-CRD motif either in the lumen of the ER (the membrane compartment of residence reported for each by Ohno and colleagues 2006) or outside of the cell if expressed on the PM. Given that the environment in these two locations is oxidizing in nature [41, 42] and assuming this topological model is correct, it is possible that the cysteines of the DHHC-CRD motif could form inter- or intra-molecular disulfide bridges rather than being involved in the transfer of palmitate. However, while it is possible that PATs may assume duties in addition to palmitoylation, it seems somewhat unlikely they would do so in this arrangement as it represents a state in which it would be difficult to perform these functions. The highest-scoring predictions of the membrane topology using TMpred show that the human protein sequence of DHHC11 and -16 should contain four TM domains, DHHC13 eight TM domains, and DHHC22 either four or five TM domains, with each model placing the DHHC-CRD motif inside the cells. There is clear disparity among the predictions generated by the algorithms available and ultimately, any of these predictions of topology must be confirmed or disproved by experimental data. In any case, for a member of the PAT family to function as a PAT, the DHHC-CRD motif should probably reside in the cytoplasm (Figure 1A). The regions of the PAT proteins that contain the greatest diversity at the amino-acid level are the N- and C-terminal cytoplasmic tails (Figure 1B).

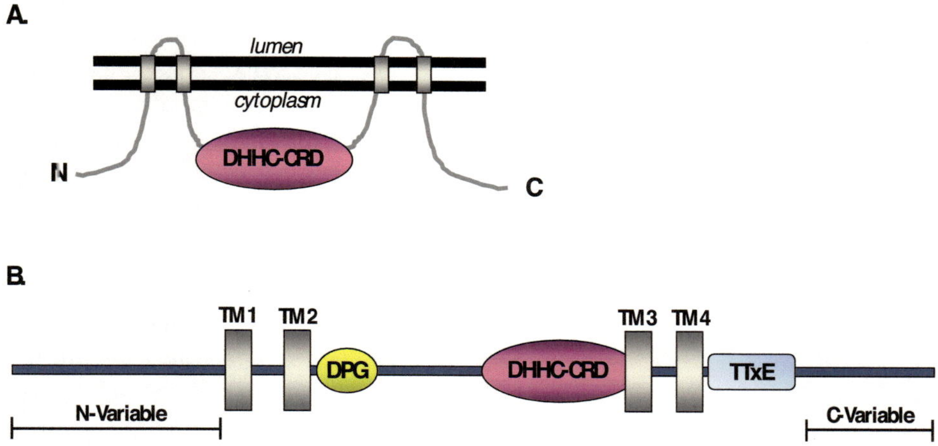

Figure 1. Predicted general structure of PATs. A) The predicted topology of PATs places the DHHC-CRD domain in the cytoplasm but such predictions must be confirmed experimentally. B) Each PAT is predicted to span the membrane four to six times; each is ~40 kDa with the greatest degree of sequence variability residing in the cytoplasmic N- and C-termini. The DHHC-CRD motif defines PATs. Palmitoylation of the cysteine in the DHHC portion is required for transfer of palmitate to a substrate. Most PATs also have a conserved DPG (aspartate-proline-glycine) motif and TTxE (threonine-threonine-asparagine-glutamate) motif, but their role in the function of PATs is not yet known.

In addition to the importance of PAT membrane topology, their membrane system of residence is likely to be an important aspect of their function. PATs have been localized to ER, Golgi, plasma membrane, endosomes, and the yeast vacuole [30, 43-48]; yet, little is known about how these proteins achieve their respective localizations. Immunolocalization of epitope-tagged DHHC proteins has been somewhat inconsistent among various cell types, between laboratories (e.g. DHHC2 [30, 37], and even in our own laboratory (unpublished observations SLP) in terms of within which membrane system a protein resides. Such inconsistencies suggest that the cell type, cell cycle, health of the cells, or even the location of the epitope tag may affect subcellular distribution. An interesting exception is DHHC2. DHHC2 has recently been shown to traffic between the PM and intracellular membranes via recycling endosomes [47]. Importantly, the C-terminal 68 amino acids of DHHC2 was shown to play an important role in defining its intracellular localization; however, a defined targeting signal present within this region of DHHC2 and in other DHHC proteins has yet to be defined.

2.3. PAT genes, palmitoylation and human disease

PATs have already been linked, in varying degrees, to human disease despite their recent discovery. At least 7 genes encoding PATs have been implicated in human disorders, including *ZDHHC8* with schizophrenia [33], *ZDHHC17* with Huntington's disease [49], *ZDHHC15* and *ZDHHC9* with X-linked mental retardation [32, 50], and *ZDHHC2*, *ZDHHC9*, *ZDHHC17*, and *ZDHHC11* with cancer [29, 51-53]; most of the demonstrated and putative connections are with cancer.

Overexpression of some PATs has also been shown to alter cancer-related signaling. DHHC17 (HIP14) is oncogenic. DHHC9 and DHHC11 display characteristics that strongly suggest they also are oncogenic. Overexpression of DHHC17 has the ability to induce colony formation and anchorage-independent growth in cell culture and tumors in mice [53]. It has been shown that these effects occur, at least in part, by DHHC17-mediated palmitoylation of H-, N-, and K2A- RAS proteins [53]. DHHC9 is strongly upregulated in some adenocarcinomas of the gastrointestinal tract at the transcript and protein levels [52] and has also been shown to palmitoylate H- and N- RAS proteins *in vitro* [31]. *ZDHHC11* has a high incidence of additional genomic copies in cases of non-small cell lung cancer and bladder cancer in which it is strongly linked to high-grade, advanced stage and disease progression [51].

Conversely to the behavior of the oncogenic PATs, a failure to express *ZDHHC2* results in an increase in metastasis in an *in vivo* model leading to the suggestion that *ZDHHC2* is a tumor/metastasis suppressor [29]. This absence of expression suggests that substrates of DHHC2 are no longer palmitoylated, and that whatever role palmitoylation had in signaling downstream from that event has been disrupted. Such is the case of DHHC2, where due to a lack of palmitoylation, one of its substrates, CKAP4, is no longer normally palmitoylated. One consequence of this is that CKAP4 no longer traffics efficiently (or at all) to the cell surface where it acts as a receptor for antiproliferative factor (APF) [37] [or presumably its other two known ligands, tissue plasminogen activator [54] and surfactant protein A [55]]. Without surface expression of CKAP4, APF is unable to initiate a wide range of downstream effects, including halting cellular proliferation and altering the expression of genes related to the progression of cancer [44].

CD9 and CD151, both tetraspanin proteins, have also been identified as substrates of DHHC2 [56]. CD9, which has been suggested to be a tumor suppressor [57, 58], is palmitoylated on multiple cysteines, but which of these are palmitoylated by DHHC2 is not known. Nonetheless, it is clear that suppression of DHHC2-mediated palmitoylation of CD9 in A431 cells affects cell behaviors that are consistent with it playing a role in tumor suppression. In particular, the cells undergo what appears to be epithelial-mesenchymal transition (EMT)—a process in which epithelial cells lose epithelial morphology and markers and gain a fibroblastic morphology during tumor progression [59-61]. It is not yet clear whether this change in cellular behavior was mediated solely by the reduction in CD9 palmitoylation or through reduced palmitoylation of this and other DHHC2 substrates such as CKAP4. It will be interesting to learn if a select subset of cysteines of CD9 is palmitoylated by DHHC2 and also how decreasing palmitoylation of specific cysteines results in the observed cellular behavior. Several other substrates of DHHC2 have been identified ranging from the neuronal adaptor/scaffold protein PSD95 [62], the SNARE proteins SNAP-23/25 [63], the non-receptor tyrosine kinase Lck [64], and the intracellular signaling proteins Gαi2 [65], GAP43 [62], R7BP [66], and eNOS [48]. Notably, there is no apparent structural similarity between the reported substrates of DHHC2, or even any sequence similarities surrounding the palmitoylated cysteine residues. Thus, DHHC2 can apparently palmitoylate cysteines located in the N-terminal regions (PSD-95, GAP-43, and Gα), internally in the protein sequence (SNAP-23/25), in the juxtamembrane region of transmembrane proteins (CD9, CD151, and CKAP4) and close to an N-terminal myristoylated glycine (Lck and eNOS).

From these examples, it is clear that upsetting the homeostatic balance of protein palmitoylation, in either direction, can have significant and deleterious effects on signaling networks. It is also clear that identification of PAT cognate substrates will provide important information concerning the molecular mechanisms underlying the oncogenic nature of the affiliated signaling systems as well as reveal important, novel targets for pharmacologic intervention. The development of specific DHHC protein inhibitors would provide vital reagents with which to study the physiological and pathophysiological importance of many palmitoylated proteins and may offer potential for therapeutic development.

2.4. PAT functions in addition to palmitoylation

It is not surprising that a disruption in the homeostatic balance of protein palmitoylation, in either direction, can have pathophysiological consequences. However, one must remain mindful that palmitoylation may not be the sole function of these proteins. Recently, two PATs—HIP14 (DHHC17) and HIP14L (DHHC13)—have been shown to mediate the transport of Mg^{2+} [67]. The first indication that these PATs were involved in Mg^{2+} regulation was that the abundance of their corresponding mRNAs was increased in cells grown in medium with reduced Mg^{2+} concentration. The authors then showed that Mg^{2+} (but not Ca^{2+}) transport was both electrogenic and voltage dependent, and that the transport required palmitoylation of the PAT. The authors concluded that these two PATs fall into a category of enzymes called "chanzymes" or ion channels that also have enzymatic activity; a type of protein previously represented only by the transient receptor potential melastatin (TRPM) family of transporters [68, 69]. The fact that GODZ (DHHC3) does not appear to mediate Mg^{2+} transport [70] but can mediate the transport of Ca^{2+} [71] suggests that this is not a general property of all PATs. The discovery that these PATs transport Mg^{2+} was astonishing especially in light of the fact that the DHHC-CRD motif appears, by sequence and predicted structure, to be a Zn^{2+}-binding protein; (a divalent cation with an atomic radius similar to Mg^{2+})—not Mg^{2+}. However, Goytain and colleagues also found that HIP14 and HIP14L transported Zn^{2+} with approximately half the efficiency as Mg^{2+}. The role of these and other PATs in binding to and/or transporting Zn^{2+} remains to be elucidated, but demonstrates the importance of not limiting ones view of PAT function (or many other proteins for that matter) only to palmitoylation.

2.5. Enzymatic mechanisms of palmitoylation

The physical and chemical mechanisms that result in enzymatic palmitoylation have yet to be defined clearly, but some progress has been made using purified proteins. It has been established that mutation of the cysteine in the DHHC motif of all PATs studied to date abolishes autoacylation of the PAT and palmitoylation of the substrate [23, 56, 62, 72]. This literature as well as discussion of potential physical mechanisms for the reaction have been reviewed recently [3, 73].

3. Palmitoyl-Cysteine prediction

Prior to the discovery of PATs, attempts were made to define stretches of amino acids that were preferred for palmitoylation. Palmitoylation near the N-terminus, following myristoylation, is among the predictable places for palmitoylation to occur provided there is one or more nearby cysteines. Navarro-Lérida et al (2002) fused a myristoylation motif (MGCTLS) to GFP with a short intervening sequence containing cysteines at various locations. These authors found a preference for cysteine palmitoylation at positions 3, 9, 15 and (to a much lesser degree) 21 residues away from the N-terminal methionine, but intervening residues were not evaluated. Commonalities in the composition of amino acid residues surrounding palmitoylated cysteines have been noted among members of the family of yeast amino acid permeases [74].

As more palmitoylated proteins and specific palmitoyl-cysteines are discovered, the task of predicting which adjacent amino acids provide a favorable environment for palmitoylation becomes easier. Algorithms trained with data from identified palmitoyl cysteines and adjacent amino acid residues are now able to provide predictions of the statistical likelihood that a cysteine of interest may be palmitoylated [75-78]. CSS-Palm 2.0, which was designed to predict potential palmitoylation sites, has been published [75]. The algorithm was trained to recognize potential palmitoyl-cysteines using a dataset of 263 experimentally determined palmitoylation sites from 109 distinct proteins. Interestingly, CSS-Palm 2.0 also successfully predicted most (~75%) of the same novel palmitoyl-cysteines in yeast proteins previously identified by Roth. et al [74] as well as palmitoyl-cysteines predicted by Roth et al., to be palmitoylated but not experimentally determined. This rate of success in both cases suggests that CSS-PALM 2.0 is more conservative at calling a site, potentially resulting in a greater rate of false negative results but is reasonably accurate nonetheless. This algorithm should prove useful when prioritizing which cysteine(s), often among multiple potential cysteines of a candidate palmitoyl protein, to analyze experimentally.

Patterns of amino acid residues surrounding palmitoyl-cysteines have emerged from these analyses. A diagram of favored residues generated by an early version of CSS-Palm 2.0 (NBA-Palm) [76] shows that leucines and additional cysteines are more commonly observed around palmitoyl-cysteines. The subsequent versions of NBA-palm used significantly improved predictive tests, but the rough sequence of preferred residues remains. An important aspect that cannot yet be considered when attempting to predict cysteine palmitoylation with these algorithms is the complexity of the PAT-substrate recognition that is encoded by residues outside of those that immediately surround the palmitoyl-cysteine; the higher order components of the recognition sites.

3.1. The physical properties of cysteines and thioester bonds

The unique physical and biochemical nature of the thioester bond that links palmitate to cysteine residues is the basis for the design of many recent assays for palmitoylation. The cysteine residue is among the most nucleophilic entities in a cell [79] and is the most common site of palmitoylation. Other residues can be modified by palmitate, but their occurrence is relatively rare and the bond chemistries are different [2, 80-83]. Palmitoylation can also occur in other ways, for example, on an amine of an N-terminal cysteine as is the case with Hedgehog [2, 83, 84], a secreted signaling protein. An example of palmitate modifying the weaker –OH nucleophile of threonine occurs on the carboxyl terminus of a spider toxin [81]. The ε-amino group of lysine can also be modified by palmitate linked by an amide bond. This occurs in several secreted proteins including a bacterial toxin [80].

The reactivity of the thiolate anion of cysteine residues makes it a key component in the structure and function of many proteins by stabilizing higher order structures via disulfide bridges and post-translational modifications like nitrosylation, prenylation, and acylation [85-87]. The high degree of reactivity has also provided a well-characterized, indispensable target for modification by synthetic, thiol-reactive ligands, allowing capture and characterization of proteins [88]. An exceptionally useful application of such thiol-specific chemistry is isotope-coded affinity tags (ICAT) for mass spectrometric determination of relative protein or peptide abundance among two or more samples [89-91]. With these probes, changes in abundance of identified proteins or peptides are determined by changes in the ratio of heavy to light-isotope-modified peptides from mixed samples. Combining ICAT technology with functional genomics methods like siRNA-mediated PAT-gene knockdown is one of several mechanisms that will allow us to identify substrates of PATs [37].

In healthy cells the cytoplasm is generally a reducing environment, meaning that solvent-exposed cysteine side chains are not typically disulfides and thus available to engage in reactions with other molecules [92]. The reactivity of a free cysteine depends on the pKa of the cysteine which is a function of the local environment surrounding the residue within the context of the whole protein. Unlike other residues with nucleophilic side chains (-OH or –NH_2), thiol side chains undergo conjugations, redox, and exchange reactions [85]. Conjugation reactions (in addition to fatty acylation) include nitric oxide (NO) or S-nitrosylation, reactive oxygen species (ROS), and reactive nitrogen species (RNS) forming bonds that are not susceptible to cleavage by hydroxylamine at neutral pH. Hydroxylamine is a reagent used to selectively remove thioester-linked palmitate [93]. Importantly, we know that hydroxylamine does not perturb disulfides [94], and that it efficiently cleaves thioesters in a quantitative manner [95].

In addition to the linkage of palmitate to cysteines, another thioester bond that occurs in cells is the transient association between ubiquitin and the E1, E2, and certain E3 ubiquitination enzymes [87, 96]. However, these thioester bonds are easily distinguished from the thioester bond that links palmitate to cysteines by their pKa; the pKa in the case of palmitoylation is near neutral pH (~7.4) whereas, for the thioester in the ubiquitin system it is pH 10.5 or greater. This wide differential allows for a high degree of selectivity when using hydroxylamine to cleave palmitate from proteins on the physical characteristics of ubiquitin-related cysteines. It is highly unlikely that they are ever in a position to be palmitoylated [97, 98].

Retinoic acid (RA) and RA-CoA have also been shown to be enzymatically attached to cysteines via a thioester bond that can be cleaved by hydroxylamine and reducing reagents such as βME at neutral pH. The reaction can be inhibited, but not fully, by myristate and palmitate suggesting that RA competes for the same cysteines as palmitate [99-107]. There is some debate in the RA field about how it binds to proteins, particularly the nuclear RA receptors, to carry out its signaling functions. RA binding to a hydrophobic cleft is the favored mechanism; however, there are many effects of RA (e.g. [108, 109]) that are independent of RA-receptor binding suggesting that cysteine modification may also have a place in the molecular mechanism of RA action.

3.2. Mass spectrometric identification of acyl groups that modify cysteines via a thioester bond

Lipid-modified thiols have been successfully identified using MALDI-TOF (matrix-assisted laser desorption ionization time-of-flight) mass spectrometry [110]. Using this method, direct information on the nature of the endogenous lipids on proteins or peptides (revealing interesting variability) can be obtained, whereas most other methods rely on surrogate markers for palmitate including thiol-reactive probes or radiolabeled palmitate. Using MALDI-TOF mass spectrometry, Marilyn Resh and colleagues found that the cysteine in the N-terminal Met-Gly-Cys of Src family kinases and two cysteines near the N-terminus of GAP43 are modified not only by palmitate but also (and to a lesser degree) by palmitoleate, stearate, or oleate [7, 8]. While palmitate appears to be the most common acyl group that forms a thioester bond to modify internal, cytoplasmic cysteines, it is clearly not the only one. The 16-carbon palmitate acyl group represents the longest chain synthesized by mammalian fatty acid synthase and is apparently the most abundant chain length present in some tissue types [111]. This relatively greater abundance may underlie the dominance of palmitate as the main acyl group to modify free thiols by S-acylation. The functional implications of incorporating lipids with shorter or longer acyl chains and especially those with different degrees of saturation may be that the proteins have different affinities for various lipid microdomains present in membranes. The specificity of PATs for chain-lengths different than 16 carbons has not been rigorously defined. However, it is known that acyl groups with differing carbon chain lengths and degrees of saturation can also be incorporated [7, 112].

3.3. PAT/Substrate recognition

Determining the nature of PAT/substrate recognition remains one of the more important tasks to be undertaken. This is especially true for PATs encoded by genes that have been linked to disease. There are two general approaches to defining PAT/substrate relationships:

http://dx.doi.org/10.5772/52503

1. identification of the PAT with specificity for a known palmitoyl protein and
2. identification of an unknown substrate of an individual PAT.

The first of these has been the most common. With this forward approach, each one of the 23 PATs is independently co-overexpressed with a known palmitoyl protein; the cells expressing the pair are metabolically labeled with ^{3}H-palmitate and the proteins analyzed by SDS-PAGE and fluorography. The incorporation of ^{3}H-palmitate onto the substrate protein in one or more of the co-overexpressions at a level significantly above background suggests that a particular PAT is responsible for palmitoylating that known substrate. Similarly, the presumptive PAT and substrate proteins can be purified and combined with ^{3}H-palmitoyl-CoA in a tube, allowed to react, and the incorporation of ^{3}H-palmitate measured as above. The current level of understanding of PAT/substrate recognition makes it unreasonable to assume that the more closely two PATs are related by sequence homology, the more likely they should palmitoylate a particular substrate. For this reason, assigning substrate status of a protein to a single PAT among a select group of tested, more closely-homologous PATs, to the exclusion of others because they are less homologous, may lead to erroneous exclusions. Similarly, we cannot yet assume that homology among residues surrounding palmitoyl cysteines of different proteins is an indication that they are palmitoylated by a particular PAT. The mechanism for molecular recognition is likely to be defined in part by the higher order structure (even quaternary as is the case with ERF2p and AKR1p) of the PATs and substrates. The reverse approach, defining unknown substrates of a single PAT can occur without these same biases as has been demonstrated in yeast and in human cells [37, 74].

4. Novel methods to discover and identify PAT/substrate specificity

The chemistry supporting novel assays to study palmitoylation and the reagents that are being incorporated into them have, for the most part, been known and available for years [88] . Most of the methods that are now being developed to study palmitoylation capitalize on many years of knowledge and development of cysteine-specific chemistries, developed mainly as methods to purify and/or specifically target proteins and peptides with various reagents. Many of the reagents that specifically label cysteines have been created as both affinity and fluorescent tags, the former for purification and structure determinations [88]and the latter as cellular reporters of protein abundance, subcellular distribution, protein conformation changes, the formation of the Golgi, and even the concentration of cellular analytes in specific subcellular domains. The following references provide a short list of some of the most clever uses of thiol chemistry [113-119]. Given the wealth of information on the unique chemistry of the palmitoyl thioester bond and the tools for capturing and characterizing cysteines in proteins, it is somewhat surprising that we are only now developing innovative assays to increase our understanding of palmitoylation. This recent increase is most likely tied to the dramatic increase in the utility of mass spectrometry as a proteomic tool. To provide a general frame of reference for the recent shift in the types of assays that are being developed, we will briefly discuss other assays that have been used successfully for a longer period of time. These assays are by no means outdated and some continue to be the most appropriate way to answer specific questions.

4.1. Chemistry and physical properties of palmitoyl cysteines: Reactions and probes

Working with palmitoylated proteins is inherently difficult due to the labile nature of the thioester bond and the increased hydrophobicity of the protein or peptide due to palmitate. On the other hand, the unique physical and chemical properties of thiols, palmitoylated thiols, and the thioester bond make them particularly amenable to modification by highly specific chemistry and a wide variety of thiol reactive probes.

Reactions of free thiols in the cytoplasm

Thiol modification occurs most commonly in cells by one of two routes: disulfide exchange or alkylation. Many of the reactive groups that undergo these two reactions are relatively stable in aqueous environments; the reactions are rapid and provide high yields of thioether and disulfide bonds [88]. Thiols will also react with many amine reactive reagents including isothiocyanates and succinimidyl esters but lack a high degree of specificity, resulting in unstable bonds that are much less useful for routine modification of thiols in proteins. Thiol-specific reagents and chemistry figure strongly into the design and development of novel assays for palmitoylation. Most investigators are limited somewhat to reagents that are available from a catalog but, fortunately, there are already many useful reagents available. Among the most useful are thio-reactive chemicals that are linked to another moiety (reactive or reporter) by a spacer arm of variable length and physical characteristics. Such hetero- and homo-bifunctional crosslinking reagents have provided much of the foundation for recent developments in palmitoylation assays and provide a fairly rich toolbox for future assay development.

Chemical moieties that react with palmitoyl-cysteines

Iodoacetamide conjugates are among the most commonly used tools for modifying cysteine thiols. These undergo nucleophilic substitution to form stable thioether bonds at physiological pH in aqueous environments. When using iodoacetamide and its conjugates, one should remember that depending on the pH of the solution, they can also react with histidine, lysine, and methionine (at pH >1.7) residues and N-terminal amines. However, when used at slightly alkaline pH in the dark and in the absence of reducing reagents, cysteine modification will be the exclusive reaction [88]. A good example of iodoacetamide-based probes are the isotope-coded affinity tags or ICAT [120]. These have proved particularly useful in determining the substrates of DHHC2 [37].

Maleimides are also common constituents of heterobifunctional crosslinking reagents and blocking reagents that target cysteines. They are ~1000 times more specific for cysteine sulfhydryls at pH 6.5-7.5, but at higher pH some cross reactivity can occur with amines. Maleimides form stable thioether bonds by adding the sulfhydryl across the double bond of the maleimide.

Phenylmercury derivatives react with thiols, including nitrosothiols, under conditions similar to iodoacetamides and maleimides to form stable mercury-thiol bonds that can be reversed in 0.1N HCl and reducing reagents like dithiothreitol (DTT) but apparently not by TCEP. Phenylmercury derivatives also react faster with thiols than do the commonly used thiol-reactive *N*-ethylmaleimide (NEM).

Compounds containing disulfide bonds are able to undergo disulfide exchange reactions with another thiol by the free thiol attacking the disulfide bond and subsequent formation of a new mixed thiol. Two examples of useful compounds in this category are Methylmethanethiosulfonate (MMTS) and pyridyl disulfide derivitives like biotin HPDP ((*N*-(6-(Biotinamido)hexyl)-3'-(2'-pyridyldithio)-propionamide). MMTS can be used in some cases to block free thiols more effectively than NEM, as it is uncharged and thus more likely to modify all free reactive cysteines. MMTS has been shown not to react with nitrosothiols or existing disulfides [121].

4.2. Metabolic labeling with radiolabeled palmitate

The most common method to identify palmitoyl proteins and to determine the residence half-life of palmitate on a specific protein or palmitate turnover (e.g. [122] for a particularly interesting example) is to metabolically label cells with radiolabled palmitate. ^{14}C-, ^{3}H- and ^{125}I-labeled palmitate have all been used, but ^{3}H-palmitate is most common because it is relatively inexpensive and widely available. However, using ^{125}I -labeled palmitate provides some advantages. In practical terms, the time required for detection is considerably shorter - hours instead of (often) weeks with ^{3}H-palmitate. The γ-irradiation from the ^{125}I is also compatible with phosphorimaging technology which is much more rapid and quantitative than densitometric measurements from films generated by autofluorography (as is used with tritium). The principle downside of using ^{125}I-labeled palmitate is that it is not commercially available, and the labeling must be done by the investigator. Reviews of the methods using radiolabeled palmitate and including technical details have been published recently [123-125].

4.3. Fluorescently-labeled peptide substrates for palmitoylation

Fluorescently-labeled peptides that mimic PAT substrates have been used to characterize PAT activity and for the discovery of inhibitors of palmitoylation [123, 126, 127]. The use of these peptides over the last several years was reviewed recently [123]. Peptide substrates for palmitoylation have also been genetically fused to fluorescent proteins and expressed in cells. This strategy has been used to determine how palmitoylation affects subcellular trafficking both between and within membranes [124]. Monomeric GFP-based reporters and fluorescence resonance energy transfer proved to be helpful in the identification of lipid rafts with an affinity for palmitate on the inner leaflet of the plasma membrane [5].

4.4. Acyl-biotin exchange: ABE

Most of the novel assays for palmitoylation utilize the same basic foundation first described for a palmitoyl protein by Schmidt and colleagues [128] and now most commonly known as acyl-exchange. First, free cysteines are blocked on proteins that have been extracted from live cells or tissue. Next, palmitates are removed from cysteines by cleavage of the thioester bond with hydroxylamine (typically 1.0M) at neutral pH. This creates a new set of free thiols unique in that they were all formerly palmitoylated; ideally, no others should exist. Finally, this new set of formerly-palmitoylated cysteines is modified by any one of the many thiol-specific reagents. The uniqueness of the individual assays that incorporate these steps lies primarily in the choice of thiol-specific reagents, and this choice depends on what questions the investigator wants to answer. There are also variations in the reagents used to block free cysteines in the first step. Both NEM and MMTS have been used in the assays described below but NEM is used most commonly.

Cysteines that are palmitoylated can also be modified by fatty acids other that palmitate [7] including stearate and oleate. The acyl-exhange method cannot yet distinguish between palmitate and the other fatty acids modifying cysteines by a thioester bond. Two additional points that relate to the specificity of this method for palmitoylation are: 1) that it will not report modification of cysteines by prenyl groups (geranylgeranyl or farnesyl) because they are attached by a thioether bond that is not susceptible to cleavage by hydroxylamine and 2) it will not report myristoylated proteins because this 14-carbon acyl group is linked to an N-terminal glutamate by an amide bond which is also insensitive to cleavage by hydroxylamine.

The recent development of novel assays using the three-step acyl exchange method to study palmitoylation in a broader sense was invigorated by two publications describing a new twist on the method that incorporated the use of radiolabeled NEM assay [129, 130]. Work described in these papers showed that labeling palmitoyl cysteines with radiolabeled NEM resulted in a remarkable 5- to 12-fold increase in sensitivity to detect several known palmitoyl proteins, including PSD-95 and SNAP-25, when compared to labeling with ^{3}H-palmitate. In addition, the authors demonstrated the utility of the biotinylated, heterobifunctional crosslinker, 4-[4′-(maleimidomethyl)cyclohexanecarboxamido] butane (Btn-BMCC), as an effective tool to capture and purify (using streptavidin-agarose) palmitoylated proteins. In doing so, they also demonstrated the general potential of using the wide variety of existing thiol-specific probes for the development of additional assays for palmitoylation that are beginning to materialize.

4.5. The palmitoyl proteome

The demonstration that one can effectively replace palmitate with a biotin group led to development of the first, large-scale, proteomic analysis of palmitoylation [74] in yeast, the model system in which the molecular identify of PATs was first determined [23, 26]. This method was dubbed "acyl biotin exchange" or ABE and used the same basic three-steps as described above. As the name implies, the proteins were labeled with a thiol-reactive, biotinylated heterobifunctional probe, [6-(Biotinamido)hexyl]-3'-(2'-pyridyldithio)propionamide (HPDP-biotin), with subsequent capture on streptavidin affinity matrix (for a detailed protocol see Wan et al. 2007 [131]). It is interesting to note the number of proteins that Roth and colleagues captured in the negative control samples (Figure 1a;[74]). The degree of overlap among proteins captured in the experimental and control samples suggests that the step in which free thiols were blocked with NEM was not quantitative and/or that the wash steps following binding of biotinylated proteins to the streptavidin matrix were not sufficiently stringent (steps 7 and 16 respectively from Wan et al, 2007 [131]) thereby resulting in the potential for a higher number of false-positive hits. However, issues of signal to noise and limits of sensitivity are by no means unique to this work (avidin-biotin affinity purification is notoriously difficult); rather they are unavoidable issues faced by all developers of novel strategies and users of nascent technologies. Incremental improvements in important assays like this always follow.

One of the key features of all proteomic methods is the system used for detection of specifically-isolated proteins or peptides. Work by Roth et al. [74] identified proteins by multi-dimensional protein identification technology (MudPIT), a high-throughput, tandem mass spectrometry (MS/MS)-based proteomic technology [132] [see also [131, 133]]. Compared to other mass spectrometric methods, MudPIT has the potential to identify less abundant proteins with a higher degree of confidence, because multiple peptides of a single protein can be used to identify a protein of interest. One downside with MudPIT in this case is that the palmitoyl cysteine(s) cannot be pinpointed, as there may be many candidates among the individual peptides of a whole protein suspected as being a palmitoyl protein. After demonstrating the usefulness of this large-scale method for purification and identification of palmitoylated proteins, the authors used mutant strains of yeast lacking one or more of the seven yeast PAT proteins to identify substrates of individual PATs. Comparison of the degree of palmitoylation of individual proteins between wild type yeast (a full set of normally palmitoylated proteins) and those not expressing one or more of the yeast PATs (each with a specific set of hypo/depalmitoylated proteins) provided the identity of the substrates of individual PATs. Together, this work represents a very significant contribution to the identification and understanding of the yeast palmitoyl proteome and provided many important clues about potential homologous PAT-substrate pairs in other systems.

The complexity of palmitoylation is greater in a vertebrate system. With at least 23 genes encoding PATs identified in humans, the diversity at the most basic level is at least three-fold greater than in yeast. When one considers the additional variants encoded by alternative splicing of PAT mRNAs, the potential diversity increases even more. The greater number of PATs suggests (but does not prove) that there are also more palmitoylated proteins in mammals. The ability to genetically manipulate mammalian cells is improving but lags behind yeast. Nevertheless, defining the palmitoyl proteome or palmitoylosome and how it is regulated in mammals (humans in particular) is a task of significant importance and interest. Now that the enzymes capable of mediating palmitoylation have been identified, one of the most important questions that we face is which substrates are palmitoylated by each PAT—a question brought sharply into focus when one considers the known connections between mutations or deletions in PAT genes and human disease, in particular cancer. DHHC2 is deleted in many types of cancer (see above). Its absence is strongly correlated with an increase in the metastatic potential of cancer cells. The simplest inverse corollary in this case is that palmitoylated substrates of DHHC2 are responsible for keeping cells from metastasizing. Identification of these substrates and their associated signaling networks using novel assays for palmitoylation has begun to provide supporting evidence for known mechanisms of cancer progression [56] as well as a novel signaling pathway for the regulation of cellular proliferation and metastasis [37].

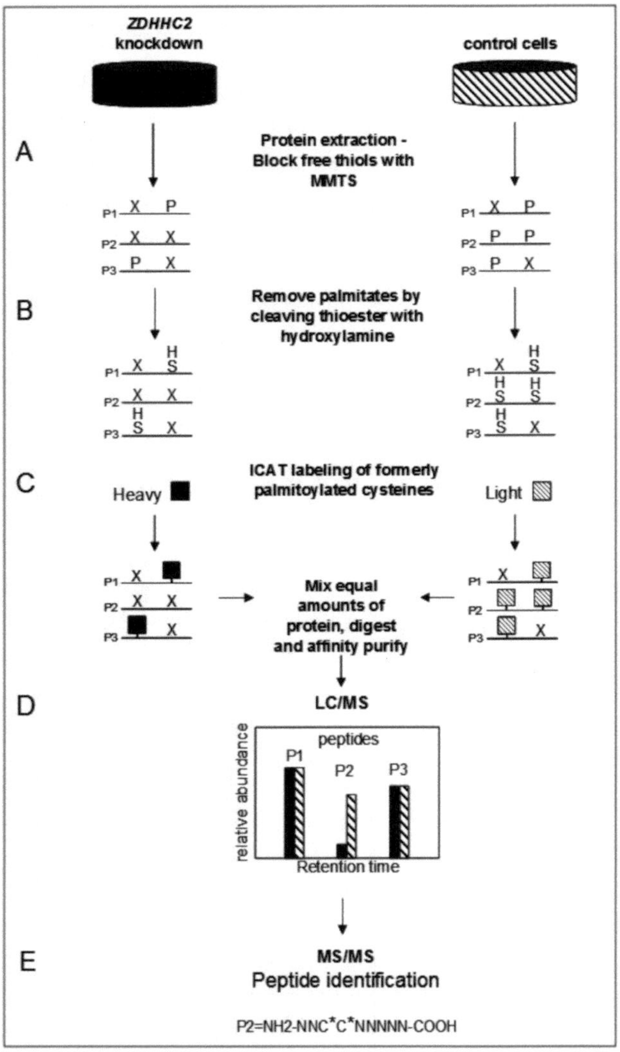

Figure 2. Palmitoyl-cysteine Identification Capture and Analysis (PICA): Determining PAT-substrate specificity by differential labeling of palmitoylated proteins with Isotope-coded Affinity Tags (ICAT) (A) In one set of cultures, *ZDHHC2* expression is knocked down by transfecting HeLa cells with *ZDHHC2*-specific siRNA (Dharmacon). Proteins are extracted from experimental and control cells and treated with the thiol-specific blocking reagent MMTS. This step chemically modifies or protects all thiols ("X" on the proteins P1-P3) that are free at physiological pH and leaves the palmitoylated cysteines (P) undisturbed as depicted on P1-P3. (B) Following the protection or blocking of free thiols, palmitates are removed by selective cleavage of the thioester bond with hydroxylamine at pH 7.4, which generates a distinctive set of free, formerly-palmitoylated, reactive thiols (C) that can be selectively labeled with ICAT reagents. Iodoacetamide at one end of the ICAT reagent binds to the thiol sidechain of cysteines; on the other end, biotin pro-

vides a mechanism for affinity purification of thiol-captured peptides on an avidin column. (D) Proteins from knockdown and control conditions are mixed in equal amounts and digested in-gel with trypsin. ICAT labeled peptides are enriched by avidin affinity and analyzed by LC/MS. A pair of ICAT-labeled peptides is chemically identical and is easily visualized, because they essentially coelute and there is a 9 Da mass difference measured in a scanning mass spectrometer. Even if equal amounts of a single protein exist in two different samples, the quantity of protein that is captured depends directly on its degree of palmitoylation; if all of a single protein is palmitoylated under one condition, then all of it will be captured; if only half of this protein is palmitoylated under another condition then the capture rate of that protein will be half as much, relative to control, making it appear half as abundant. Proteins for which there has been no change in palmitoylation (ie, equal capture rates) will yield a heavy:light (H/L) ratio of 1. The degree to which palmitoylation is diminished will register as a decrease in the H/L ratio (ie, 50% reduction in palmitoylation will correspond to a H/L ratio of 0.5). A change in the capture rate that results in a change in the post-purification abundance is measured in the LC/MS phase. (E) Finally, the peptides are further fragmented into their constituent amino acids by MS/MS, enabling identification of the proteins corresponding to the captured peptides.

4.6. Palmitoyl-cysteine Identification Capture and Analysis (PICA): Identification of PAT substrates and palmitoyl proteins in vertebrates

With the aim of defining PAT-substrate specificity in a living vertebrate system, we developed a method to identify substrates of specific PATs in mammalian cells and tissues called Palmitoyl cysteine Isolation Capture and Analysis or PICA [37]. We used this method to identify CKAP4/p63, a known palmitoyl protein [134] as one substrate of DHHC2 in HeLa cells [37]. This method is similar to ABE as described by Roth et al (2006) but was inspired [135] in part by the work of Drisdel and Green (2004) and incorporated several novel features that will be discussed below.

The ability of PICA to identify PAT substrates is based on the principle that it quantifies the differential frequency of palmitoylation of individual proteins or peptides in control conditions versus conditions in which the function of a single PAT is reduced by siRNA-mediated gene knockdown. The process to identify substrates of DHHC2 consisted of four basic steps outlined in Figure 2. In the first part we generated two distinct pools of palmitoylated proteins, one from control HeLa cells and the other from HeLa cells in which the activity of one PAT (DHHC2) was reduced. These two distinct pools of palmitoylated proteins were then captured and compared directly to identify differences in the degree of palmitoylation of individual proteins between the two pools. To do this, we reduced the expression of *ZDDHC2* mRNA (and consequently the abundance of the encoded enzyme, DHHC2) in HeLa cells using siRNA-mediated gene knockdown which resulted in a reduced level of palmitoylation of DHHC2 substrates. Total protein from knockdown and control cells was prepared by first blocking free thiols with MMTS in the presence of SDS. This was followed by selective exposure of all palmitoyl cysteines by cleavage of the palmitoyl-cysteine thioester bond with 1.0M hydroxylamine at neutral pH, thereby generating a unique population of formerly palmitoylated cysteines. Second, we selectively and differentially labeled the exposed, formerly-palmitoylated cysteines from knockdown and control cells with biotinylated, thiol-reactive heavy (H) and light (L) ICAT reagents, respectively. Third, we combined equal quantities of the ICAT-labeled protein from *ZDHHC2* knockdown and control cells and digested the mixture with trypsin. The resulting H and L ICAT-labeled tryptic peptides were captured and purified on an avidin affinity column. Finally, ICAT-labeled, putative, formerly-palmitoylated peptides were analyzed by mass spectrometry. Peptides with a reduced

H/L ratio over four independent runs were analyzed further to confirm that the identified cysteine was indeed palmitoylated by DHHC2 under physiological conditions. Details of the protocol and reagents used and outlined in Figure 2 can be found in [37].

There are several unique aspects in the PICA method. First, we used MMTS to block the free thiols in the first step. NEM is used most commonly at this step, but MMTS is more reactive and smaller than NEM or iodoacetamide, enhancing its ability to modify all free reactive cysteines. Inefficient blocking of free thiols in the first step is one factor that could easily contribute to false-positive capture of proteins in the purification step. Qualitative evaluation (silver-stained SDS-PAGE) of protein capture in experimental and control (no-hydroxylamine) conditions [Figure 2, [37]] suggests that it may be more efficient than NEM (for comparison see Figure 1A [74]). However, it may also be that we captured very few proteins under control conditions because of a more stringent wash protocol than described by Roth et al [74]. The use of ICAT reagents in PICA allowed us to combine formerly-palmitoylated peptides purified from control and experimental cells in the same pool, and subsequently, a direct, simultaneous analysis of palmitoylation in the two pools in a single analytical sample. We defined a substrate of DHHC2 as one that had a consistently reduced H/L ratio over four independent PICA runs. This approach provided us with many (the vast majority), convenient internal control peptides which are peptides that were not substrates of DHHC2 that had unchanged H/L ratios. This approach significantly reduces the potential for identification of false-positive hits because, if a protein can be falsely labeled by an ICAT, it should do so with equal efficiency in both the control and experimental cells yielding a peptide with an H/L ratio of ~1. The greater risk with this approach is the failure to identify substrates that exist in low abundance. Using tandem mass spectrometry, we analyzed a sample of significantly reduced complexity including only ICAT-tagged peptides. As is inherent in such analyses, the most abundant peptides dominate the report. However, one advantage of this approach is that when a peptide is identified, whether it is a substrate of a single PAT or not, the palmitoyl cysteine(s) is also identified. In the case of CKAP4/p63 (and the majority of other peptides) there was only a single cysteine, and it was already known to be a site for palmitoylation [134]. Spectral counting has the potential to positively identify palmitoyl proteins of lower abundance because more than a single peptide from any given protein is factored into to the identification. There is greater overall coverage (identified peptide fragments of a protein) using this method thereby increasing the confidence level of identification. However, the disadvantage inherent in analyzing a complex mixture, including non-palmitoylated peptides by spectral counting, is that identification of the palmitoyl cysteine (in the cases where there are multiple candidate cysteines) must await subsequent and tedious analyses. The tradeoff between these two complementary approaches in mass spectrometric analysis is sensitivity versus specificity. Combining these analyses will provide a much greater depth of coverage.

4.7. Forward and reverse approaches to assigning PAT-substrate pairs

The first reports that identified PAT-substrate pairings took the reverse approach: start with a known palmitoylated protein then use metabolic labeling with radiolabeled palmitate and co-overexpression of one PAT and the substrate (for a review see: [72]). Using this method, an increase in the incorporation of radiolabled palmitate on the overexpressed substrate in the presence of an overexpressed PAT is used to claim specificity. This method is an important tool for increasing our understanding of palmitoylation-related phenomena including confirmation of putative PAT-substrate pairs identified by other methods. Likewise, when starting with a known palmitoyl protein and the intention of identifying the PAT responsible for its palmitoylation, it remains a useful method. However, we should remember that just because overexpression of a PAT can increase the incorporation of palmitate onto a specific protein does not necessarily mean that it does so in a live cell. Again, problems like this are not unique to this method and simply reflect our lack of knowledge about where and when PATs and their substrates are expressed, the degree of promiscuity among PATs and, how PAT function is regulated.

The potential for specific cysteines to be modified by both palmitate and RA via a thioester bond is an issue that deserves attention from those of us interested primarily in palmitoylation for at least two reasons. One is the potential that an exchange between the two modifications is a physiologically relevant means of regulating signaling and second, the possibility that proteins identified as being palmitoylated in assays utilizing some form of ABE chemistry are RA-modified instead.

4.8. Labeling palmitoyl proteins with bioorthogonal probes

This particularly interesting approach labels cysteines with isosteric, azido-derivitives of fatty acids that are able to substitute for fatty acids that occur naturally in cells (Figure 3) [112, 136]. Once bound to cysteines, the azido group on the fatty acid is reacted, with a high degree of selectivity, via the Staudinger reaction [137] with (triaryl)phosphines that are themselves derivatized with Myc, biotin, a fluorophore, or others. Using this method Hang and colleagues [112] found that ω-azido fatty acids with 12 and 15 carbons can be efficiently metabolized by mammalian cells and accurately report myristoylation and thio-palmitoylation, respectively.

Work by Kostiuk and colleagues identified palmitoyl proteins from mitochondria using azido-palmitate [136]. To accomplish this they purified proteins from cellular mitochondrial fractions, first by differential centrifugation, then by further purification based first on charge and subsequently by size using chromatographic separation. Labeling of proteins in this study was outside of a living system presumably leaving only the possibility of autocatalytic/non-enzymatic palmitoylation. Mass spectrometric analysis of selected bands identified 21 palmitoylated proteins, 19 of which were novel. The majority of the proteins labeled were metabolic-type proteins unique to the mitochondrion. This raises the interesting possibility that the principle mechanism of palmitoylation in this organelle is autocatalytic rather than enzymatic, and that, as suggested by the authors, the key role of palmitoylation in the mitochondrion is to inhibit enzymes by palmitoylation of cysteines in the vicinity of the active site.

These so called bio-orthogonal probes have been reported to be nontoxic and very stable under physiological conditions. Importantly, this two-step reaction is rapid and more sensitive than labeling with ^{125}I-palmitoyl-CoA. These features, especially their ability to effectively substitute for endogenous fatty acids, make them ideal for labeling palmitoyl proteins in live cells, providing a significantly more direct measure of protein palmitoylation than can be achieved in any other assay format. It is easy to imagine that use of such probes will come to dominate in experimental systems for studying palmitoylation.

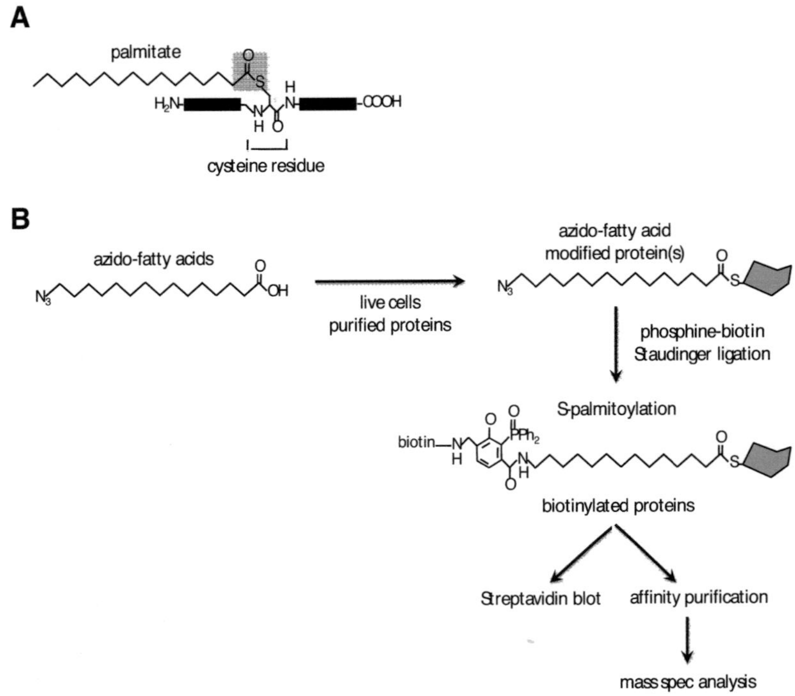

Figure 3. Using Click chemistry and bio-orthogonal probes to label palmitoyl cysteines. A) A palmitoylated protein; the shaded box indicates the thioester bond. B) Azido-palmitate is transferred to a protein forming a thioester bond with a cysteine residue. The azide moiety of the azido-palmitate reacts, via the Staudinger reaction, with the tagged (in this case biotin) phosphine, forming an amide bond. The biotin-tagged proteins can then be affinity purified and analyzed in various ways including mass spectrometry. Tags and reporters other than biotin can be added to the phosphine providing a wide array of potential methods for subsequent analyses.

5. Pharmacological modulation of Palmitoylation

5.1. Developing compounds that selectively target individual PATs

Existing chemicals used to inhibit palmitoylation are neither selective nor potent. The compounds used most commonly are 2-bromopalmitate (2BP), tunicamycin, and cerulenin. Each of these is a lipid-based molecule (Figure 4). 2BP has been used most frequently at a concentration of ~100 μM to block palmitoylation in spite of the fact that at least two studies have shown that the IC50 of 2-BP is ~10 μM [138, 139]. 2BP is not tolerated well by cultured cells and causes death even after a brief exposure to 100 μM. 2BP inhibits several enzymes involved in lipid metabolism, including carnitine palmitoyltransferase 1, fatty acid CoA ligase, glycerol-3-phosphate acyltransferase, and enzymes in the synthesis of triacylglycerol biosynthesis [140, 141]. This high degree of promiscuity as well as the toxicity of 2BP renders it nearly useless as a tool to determine anything specific about palmitoylation related signaling issues that equally plague cerulenin and tunicamycin. The uses and effects of these three inhibitors was reviewed recently [142].

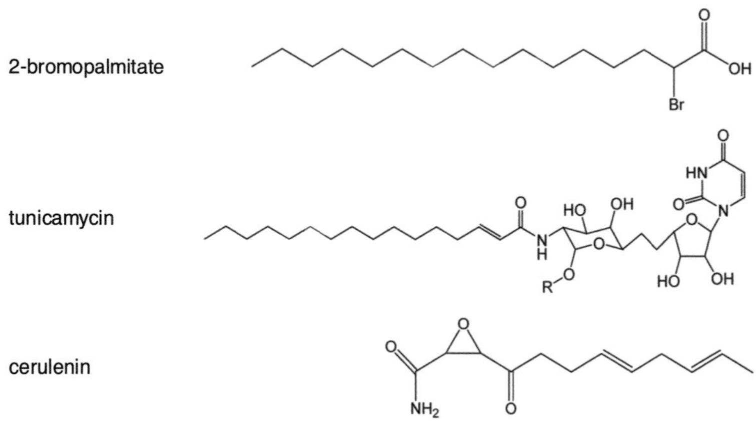

Figure 4. Lipid-based inhibitors of palmitoylation.

Smith and colleagues [126] recently screened a compound library in an attempt to identify more selective and potent inhibitors of palmitoylation, in particular inhibitors of PATs. This screen identified single compounds from five chemical classes (Compounds I-V) that inhibited cellular processes associated with palmitoylation. The assays used in the screens included: measuring the *in vivo* and *in vitro* growth rate of an NIH/3T3 cell line that overexpressed DHHC17, displacement from the plasma membrane of myristoylated or farnesylated GFP, and *in vitro* palmitoylation of small, non-complex, myristoylated or farnesylated, synthetic, fluorescent peptides intended to mimic known palmitoylation substrates [123, 126, 127]. These assays could not discriminate a direct effect of any compound on any PAT. They could only report the activity of compounds that acted at some point (not excluding direct PAT inhibition) in any pathway that leads to or affects palmitoylation; compounds like 2BP, cerulenin, and tunicamycin. This assertion was borne out in follow-up studies on the same compounds [138] (see below). Perhaps the most intriguing finding in this report was that compounds I-IV were able to suppress the oncogenic behavior of human cells that overexpressed DHHC17. However, there is no direct evidence to indicate that compounds I-IV exert these actions via inhibition of DHHC17 or through the palmitoylation of Ras proteins by DHHC17 as was speculated [53, 126]. Nevertheless, since these compounds reduced the *in vivo* growth of tumors from cells overexpressing DHHC17 [126], it would be worth determining their exact mechanism of action.

Subsequent studies by Linder, Deschenes and colleagues [138] tested four of the five compounds identified by Smith and colleagues and found that they were not selective for DHHC proteins. This report also included a wealth of information defining the mechanisms by which 2BP inhibits palmitoylation. Briefly, only one of the four compounds re-tested, compound V and 2BP, inhibited the activity of any of the four DHHC proteins tested. Neither compound V nor 2BP was selective for any of the PATs tested, and 2BP was more potent. Both compound V and 2BP blocked autoacylation of the PATs; compound V was reversible, 2BP was not. Even though compound V was able to inhibit the activity of the four PATs tested and in the same manner as 2BP, these experiments could not determine whether compound V also blocks palmitoylation indiscriminately at steps prior to the actual palmitoylation event, as is the case with 2BP, cerulenin, and tunicamycin.

There would be no compelling reason to begin a drug discovery program to identify inhibitors of just any PAT. Rather one would choose to begin with a PAT that is linked to a disease state—a situation where misregulated expression or function of that PAT was clearly linked to a pathological state. As discussed earlier, links between PAT expression (but not yet altered function) have been demonstrated for both neurological disorders and cancer; thus, candidate PATs that would be appropriate targets for drug development exist. Both overexpression and absence of PAT expression have been implicated in the development of cancer. Dampening the activity of an existing PAT is a conceptually and mechanistically simpler task than accurately restoring the specific activity of a PAT that is not expressed or absent. This review is concerned with PAT assays and PAT inhibitors, so we will address the case of PAT overexpression in ideal terms as well as the technical issues that surround the development and implementation of the assays designed to discover PAT inhibitors.

5.2. Considerations for development of high-throughput screens to discover PAT inhibitors

The DHHC motif in PATs defines the active site and is highly conserved in all mammalian PATs [3]. The regions of highest diversity are primarily in the N- and C-termini of the PAT. Mutation of the cysteine in the DHHC motif abolishes PAT autoacylation and palmitoylation of the substrate, a property of all DHHC proteins studied so far. This high degree of homology in the active site sequence among PATs could give the impression that developing highly specific, active-site inhibitors for palmitoylation will be impossible. However, this same issue exists with kinases [143, 144], and yet the development of selective and potent active-site, ATP-competitive inhibitors has been successful (eg, [145]).

The specificity of palmitoylation must be derived in part from the unique physical interactions of individual PATs with their substrates. The sequence of amino acids surrounding a substrate cysteine partially defines the potential for that cysteine to be palmitoylated. However, the physical determinants for substrate recognition will likely extend throughout the accessible portions of the PAT and substrate as was elegantly demonstrated for DHHC17 [146]. Other factors that are likely to regulate palmitoylation are the temporal and spatial aspects of PAT and substrate expression.

There are many more palmitoylated proteins than there are PATs; therefore, modulating the activity of a single PAT, even with complete compound selectivity, will likely yield a change in the palmitoylation of multiple substrates. This conundrum is common to the development of highly selective and potent pharmacological modulators of all enzymes that mediate post-translational protein modifications, again kinases being a classic example.

Another challenge is that each PAT traverses the plasma membrane multiple times. A conservative guess would suggest that the membrane environment is important for determining PAT structure and substrate recognition. However, Jennings et al.,[138] demonstrated that at least four PATs can be purified from a membrane environment and remain enzymatically active. These findings are both remarkable and encouraging evidence that enzyme activity-based and drug-binding screens for selective PAT inhibitors can be accomplished with purified proteins.

5.3. Primary screen for PAT inhibitors

The discovery and refinement of drugs to modulate PAT activity will require the use of multiple assay types. The initial success of each can only be a matter of speculation at the beginning of the project, and the success of the primary screen will influence the choice of follow up assays. However, one unique aspect of palmitoylation suggests a logical starting point. The most dramatic visible change that can occur when a protein is palmitoylated is when it moves from the cytoplasm to the plasma (or other) membrane. The technology to measure such a translocation in living cells using high-throughput microscopy has been demonstrated [139, 147] and along with many other such morphometric analyses, has become well established in drug discovery programs and the basic life sciences [148-150]. This technology is often referred to as high-content screening (HCS). To develop an assay to identify inhibitors of a single PAT using HCS, it would be ideal to have identified the most clinically relevant, cytosolic substrate of the PAT of interest and to have determined that this substrate is palmitoylated exclusively by this one PAT or, alternatively, by no other PAT expressed in the cell type that will be used for the screen. However, biological systems rarely offer ideal situations, and accommodations will inevitably need to be made. The ideal substrate would then be fused to a monomeric fluorescent protein (FP) [5, 151] to generate a fluorescent reporter of palmitoylation that localizes primarily or exclusively to the PM. Cells stably expressing this reporter would then be grown in multi-well imaging plates and exposed to a chemical compound library, and the subcellular distribution of the FP-tagged palmitoylation substrate evaluated by HCS. Compounds that cause redistribution of the fluorescent reporter from the PM to the cytoplasm are candidates (or hits) for follow up analyses that will determine if they blocked palmitoylation of the reporter by directly inhibiting the PAT of interest or indirectly by some other mechanism. Typically, compounds in a large library (tens to hundreds of thousands of compounds) are tested at a single concentration and replicated, often three times, to increase the confidence of selecting biologically active compounds. But, the relationship of replicates is solely statistical, not pharmacological. An alternative screening method for identifying hits is "titration-based screening" called qHTS [152]. This method, which has been used successfully by Jim Inglese, Doug Auld and Colleagues at the NIH Chemical Genomics Center, measures the assay system response to multiple (up to seven), different concentrations of a single compound. The increased density and accuracy of the data produced by this method can provide many benefits over screening at a single concentration (for a full description of the merits of qHTS see [152]). Among the most important benefits of screening at multiple concentrations is that it alleviates the problems of false-negatives and false-positives that plague screens run at a single concentration. The nominal, additional effort required at the front end of the process is generously compensated by a subsequent reduction in the effort required to choose which hits to pursue in follow-up assays.

Displacement or translocation of the fluorescent palmitoylation reporter from the PM to the cytoplasm in response to a compound cannot provide evidence that the compound has this effect by direct inhibition of a PAT. Secondary screens designed to determine which of the hits works by direct inhibition of PAT activity will be required. One option would be to determine the effects of each hit on the enzymatic activity of the PAT of interest. Jennings et al have demonstrated that a PAT can be purified from a membrane environment and retain its enzymatic function i.e., transfer of palmitate to a substrate. The metabolically active form of palmitate in a living system is palmitoyl-CoA. Transfer of palmitate to a substrate results in the liberation of CoA from palmitate, a chemical species that can be measured with accuracy and sensitivity in a high throughput manner (Figure 5) [153].

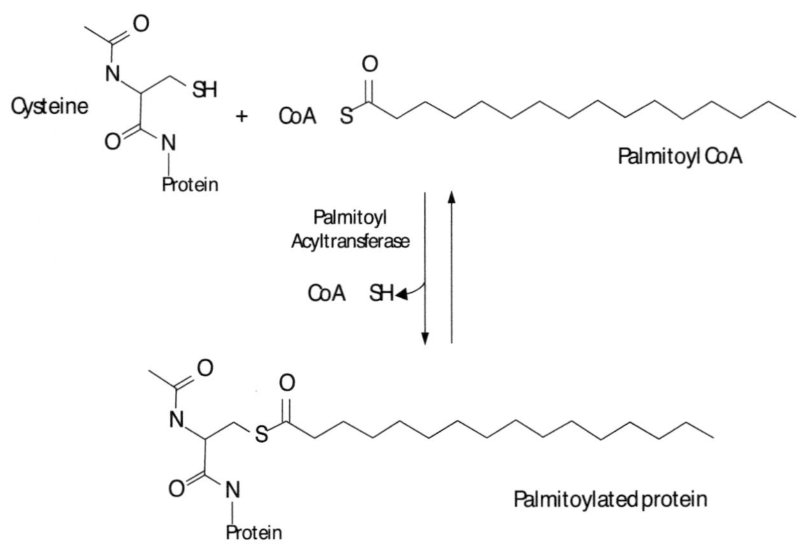

Figure 5.

http://dx.doi.org/10.5772/52503

Retesting hits from the primary screen in this secondary, enzymatic assay would determine if the compounds directly inhibited palmitoylation of the substrate in the reaction. It would also identify compounds that inhibit palmitoylation by competing with palmitoyl-CoA for access to the PAT active site, as well as allosteric inhibitors. Structural analysis of the compounds would provide information about how they inhibit palmitoylation. A binding assay in which compounds are tested for their ability to compete directly with palmitoyl-CoA for binding to the PAT would more conclusively determine the mechanism by which the compounds were inhibiting substrate palmitoylation.

It is likely that the inhibitors identified will represent multiple classes of compounds distinguished by their chemical structures. However, the chemicals identified in these screens are unlikely to represent the most potent or selective compounds that exist. Further refinement by probing and refining the chemical space of each compound in a medicinal chemistry effort will be required to achieve both objectives. Generating higher affinity analogs of the hit compounds for the PAT of interest will improve the selectivity and potency of the compounds for an individual PAT. However, the question of how selective any of these compounds is for a single PAT must be answered by determining their ability to inhibit other PATs—counterscreening. Since the family of PATs is relatively small (23 genes), it would not be unreasonable to measure the effects of the compounds on each of the other PATs in the enzymatic assay described above.

The assay development pathway proposed above is outlined only in very general and ideal terms, glossing over inevitable technical challenges that must be overcome for the project to be successful. However, even as brief as this description is, it exceeds by far the complexity of any published attempt to identify selective PAT inhibitors to date. A valuable, practical guide to choosing, developing, and validating assays including those proposed above is available at: http://ncgc.nih.gov/guidance/manual_toc.html.

6. Conclusion

The discovery of the molecular identity of PATs was a pivotal event that has fostered substantial progress in the field of lipidation, having a profoundly positive effect on many fields of biology. Many long-standing questions have been greeted with answers as well as a clearer direction in which new inquiries should proceed. While sometimes criticized as being stamp collecting, defining the palmitoyl proteome of specific cells and tissues would provide new and unforeseen insight into many cellular processes. The methods described here provide the technical foundation for defining the palmitoyl proteome. Defining the intrinsic and extrinsic mechanisms and factors that regulate PAT activity will also be crucial and challenging. Future assays to investigate such details will certainly benefit from the demonstrated usefulness of bioorthagonal probes that appear to be treated by cells as if they were palmitate. These probes may provide a more direct measure of palmitoylation than the exchange of cysteine-reactive probes for palmitate on purified proteins.

The number of signaling networks in which palmitoylation plays a pivotal role is large and growing. The relationship between PAT gene expression and cancer is perhaps the most evident as the fraction of PAT genes implicated in metastasis and tumorigenesis is notably high. There is also a remarkable confluence between our increasing understanding of palmitoylation and our increasing awareness of the importance of lipid rafts, one of the primary residences of palmitoylated proteins in cancer [154, 155]. In instances where there is a relationship between aberrant expression of PATs and cancer, the critical questions relate to the substrates of these PATs and their associated signaling networks. Identification of these signaling networks will potentially provide new therapeutic targets for the prevention or reversal of cancer progression. Given the preponderance of palmitoylated proteins resident in the neuronal synapse (which is itself a lipid raft of sorts), it is clearly another area of research that deserves (and has already received) a great deal of attention.

While there has been some progress made in identifying pharmacological modulators of palmitoylation [125, 126, 138], there is nothing yet known about how to specifically target individual PATs. From a practical standpoint, inhibiting specific PATs may be a simpler process than developing specific PAT agonists. The advent of assays with the ability to measure changes in the activity of a single PAT along with the identification of PAT-substrate associations should enable further development of new assays to identify specific pharmacological modulators of individual PATs as well as providing important information on the signaling networks associated with specific PATs.

Our ability to understand palmitoylation and its importance to human health and disease is only as good as the technological methods we use to make accurate and valid measurements. Our ability to investigate the basic mechanisms of how PATs work, of PAT/substrate relationships, and how palmitoylation affects signaling processes related to disease would be improved significantly by the development of selective and potent pharmacological tools. Until such tools are available, we should be mindful that using compounds such as 2-BP, cerulenin, and tunicamycin may lead to erroneous conclusions. Developing non-lipid, selective inhibitors that target the PAT active site is feasible. The challenges that exist are conceptually similar in some aspects to those faced during the development of selective, small-molecule inhibitors of kinases that do not resemble ATP. Based on current knowledge, the most logical PATs to target first are those for which overexpression is oncogenic. However, the motivation to initiate drug discovery programs on a large scale will probably remain below the required threshold until more conclusive data are available from more sophisticated, whole-animal experiments that link PATs to oncogenesis.

Author details

Sonia Lobo Planey

Address all correspondence to: splaney@tcmedc.org

The Commonwealth Medical College, Scranton, PA, USA

References

[1] Linder, M. E., & Deschenes, R. J. (2007). Palmitoylation: policing protein stability and traffic. *Nat Rev Mol Cell Biol. Jan*, 8(1), 74-84.

[2] Buglino, J. A., & Resh, M. D. Hhat is a palmitoylacyltransferase with specificity for N-palmitoylation of Sonic Hedgehog. *J Biol Chem*, 283(32), 22076-88.

[3] Mitchell, D. A., Vasudevan, A., Linder, M. E., & Deschenes, R. J. Protein palmitoylation by a family of DHHC protein S-acyltransferases. *J Lipid Res*, 47(6), 1118-27.

[4] Hofmann, K. A superfamily of membrane-bound O-acyltransferases with implications for wnt signaling. *Trends Biochem Sci*, 25(3), 111-2.

[5] Zacharias, D. A., Violin, J. D., Newton, A. C., & Tsien, R. Y. Partitioning of lipid-modified monomeric GFPs into membrane microdomains of live cells. *Science*, 296(5569), 913-6.

[6] Greaves, J., Prescott, G. R., Gorleku, O. A., & Chamberlain, L. H. The fat controller: roles of palmitoylation in intracellular protein trafficking and targeting to membrane microdomains (Review). *Mol Membr Biol*, 26(1), 67-79.

[7] Liang, X., Lu, Y., Neubert, T. A., & Resh, M. D. Mass spectrometric analysis of GAP-43/neuromodulin reveals the presence of a variety of fatty acylated species. *J Biol Chem*, 277(36), 33032-40.

[8] Liang, X., Lu, Y., Wilkes, M., Neubert, T. A., & Resh, M. D. The N-terminal SH4 region of the Src family kinase Fyn is modified by methylation and heterogeneous fatty acylation: role in membrane targeting, cell adhesion, and spreading. *J Biol Chem*, 279(9), 8133-9.

[9] Liang, X., Nazarian, A., Erdjument-Bromage, H., Bornmann, W., Tempst, P., & Resh, M. D. Heterogeneous fatty acylation of Src family kinases with polyunsaturated fatty acids regulates raft localization and signal transduction. *J Biol Chem*, 276(33), 30987-94.

[10] Jones, T. L., Degtyarev, M. Y., & Backlund, P. S. Jr. The stoichiometry of G alpha(s) palmitoylation in its basal and activated states. *Biochemistry*, 36(23), 7185-91.

[11] Bizzozero, O. A., Mc Garry, J. F., & Lees, M. B. Autoacylation of myelin proteolipid protein with acyl coenzyme A. *J Biol Chem*, 262(28), 13550-7.

[12] Morello, J. P., & Bouvier, M. (1996). Palmitoylation: a post-translational modification that regulates signalling from G-protein coupled receptors. *Biochem Cell Biol*, 74(4), 449-57.

[13] Wedegaertner, P. B., & Bourne, H. R. Activation and depalmitoylation of Gs alpha. *Cell*, 77(7), 1063-70.

[14] Bano, M. C., Jackson, C. S., & Magee, A. I. (1998). Pseudo-enzymatic S-acylation of a myristoylated yes protein tyrosine kinase peptide in vitro may reflect non-enzymatic S-acylation in vivo. Biochem J. Mar 1 , 330(Pt 2), 723-31.

[15] Duncan, J. A., & Gilman, A. G. (1996). Autoacylation of G protein alpha subunits. J Biol Chem. Sep 20; , 271(38), 23594-600.

[16] Dietrich, L. E., & Ungermann, C. (2004). On the mechanism of protein palmitoylation. EMBO Rep. Nov; , 5(11), 1053-7.

[17] Berger, M., & Schmidt, M. F. Cell-free fatty acid acylation of Semliki Forest viral polypeptides with microsomal membranes from eukaryotic cells. *J Biol Chem*, 259(11), 7245-52.

[18] Berthiaume, L., & Resh, M.D. Biochemical characterization of a palmitoyl acyltransferase activity that palmitoylates myristoylated proteins. *J Biol Chem*, 270(38), 22399-405.

[19] Liu, L., Dudler, T., & Gelb, M. H. Purification of a protein palmitoyltransferase that acts on H-Ras protein and on a C-terminal N-Ras peptide. *J Biol Chem*, 271(38), 23269-76.

[20] Bartels, D. J., Mitchell, D. A., Dong, X., & Deschenes, R. J. Erf2, a novel gene product that affects the localization and palmitoylation of Ras2 in Saccharomyces cerevisiae. *Mol Cell Biol*, 19(10), 6775-87.

[21] Mitchell, D. A., Farh, L., Marshall, T. K., & Deschenes, R. J. A polybasic domain allows nonprenylated Ras proteins to function in Saccharomyces cerevisiae. *J Biol Chem*, 269(34), 21540-6.

[22] Jung, V., Chen, L., Hofmann, S. L., Wigler, M., & Powers, S. Mutations in the SHR5 gene of Saccharomyces cerevisiae suppress Ras function and block membrane attachment and palmitoylation of Ras proteins. *Mol Cell Biol*, 15(3), 1333-42.

[23] Lobo, S., Greentree, W. K., Linder, M. E., & Deschenes, R. J. Identification of a Ras palmitoyltransferase in Saccharomyces cerevisiae. *J Biol Chem*, 277(43), 41268-73.

[24] Putilina, T., Wong, P., & Gentleman, S. (1999). The DHHC domain: a new highly conserved cysteine-rich motif. Mol Cell Biochem May; , 195(1-2), 219 -26 .

[25] Mesilaty-Gross, S., Reich, A., Motro, B., & Wides, R. The Drosophila STAM gene homolog is in a tight gene cluster, and its expression correlates to that of the adjacent gene ial. *Gene*, 231(1-2), 173-86.

[26] Roth, A. F., Feng, Y., Chen, L., & Davis, N. G. The yeast DHHC cysteine-rich domain protein Akr1p is a palmitoyl transferase. *J Cell Biol*, 159(1), 23-8.

[27] Feng, Y., & Davis, N. G. Akr1p and the type I casein kinases act prior to the ubiquitination step of yeast endocytosis: Akr1p is required for kinase localization to the plasma membrane. *Mol Cell Biol*, 20(14), 5350-9.

[28] Givan, S. A., & Sprague, G. F. Jr. The ankyrin repeat-containing protein Akr1p is required for the endocytosis of yeast pheromone receptors. *Mol Biol Cell*, 8(7), 1317-27.

[29] Oyama, T., Miyoshi, Y., Koyama, K., Nakagawa, H., Yamori, T., Ito, T., et al. Isolation of a novel gene on 8p21.3-22 whose expression is reduced significantly in human colorectal cancers with liver metastasis. *Genes Chromosomes Cancer*, 29(1), 9-15.

[30] Ohno, Y., Kihara, A., Sano, T., & Igarashi, Y. Intracellular localization and tissue-specific distribution of human and yeast DHHC cysteine-rich domain-containing proteins. *Biochim Biophys Acta*, 1761(4), 474-83.

[31] Swarthout, J. T., Lobo, S., Farh, L., Croke, M. R., Greentree, W. K., Deschenes, R. J., et al. DHHC9 and GCP16 constitute a human protein fatty acyltransferase with specificity for H- and N-Ras. *J Biol Chem*, 280(35), 31141-8.

[32] Raymond, F. L., Tarpey, P. S., Edkins, S., Tofts, C., O'Meara, S., Teague, J., et al. Mutations in ZDHHC9, which encodes a palmitoyltransferase of NRAS and HRAS, cause X-linked mental retardation associated with a marfanoid habitus. *Am J Hum Genet*, 80(5), 982-7.

[33] Mukai, J., Liu, H., Burt, R. A., Swor, D. E., Lai, W. S., Karayiorgou, M., et al. Evidence that the gene encoding ZDHHC8 contributes to the risk of schizophrenia. *Nat Genet*, 36(7), 725-31.

[34] Demily, C., Legallic, S., Bou, J., Houy-Durand, E., Van Amelsvoort, T., Zinkstok, J., et al. ZDHHC8 single nucleotide polymorphism rs175174 is not associated with psychiatric features of the 22q11 deletion syndrome or schizophrenia. *Psychiatr Genet*, 17(5), 311-2.

[35] Glaser, B., Schumacher, J., Williams, H. J., Jamra, R. A., Ianakiev, N., Milev, R., et al. No association between the putative functional ZDHHC8 single nucleotide polymorphism rs175174 and schizophrenia in large European samples. *Biol Psychiatry*, 58(1), 78-80.

[36] Saito, S., Ikeda, M., Iwata, N., Suzuki, T., Kitajima, T., Yamanouchi, Y., et al. No association was found between a functional SNP in ZDHHC8 and schizophrenia in a Japanese case-control population. *Neurosci Lett*, 374(1), 21-4.

[37] Zhang, J., Planey, S. L., Ceballos, C., Stevens, S. M. Jr, Keay, S. K., & Zacharias, D. A. Identification of CKAP4/63as a major substrate of the palmitoyl acyltransferase DHHC2, a putative tumor suppressor, using a novel proteomics method. *Mol Cell Proteomics*, 7(7), 1378-88.

[38] Rocks, O., Gerauer, M., Vartak, N., Koch, S., Huang, Z. P., Pechlivanis, M., et al. The palmitoylation machinery is a spatially organizing system for peripheral membrane proteins. *Cell*, 141(3), 458-71.

[39] Politis, E. G., Roth, A. F., & Davis, N. G. Transmembrane topology of the protein palmitoyl transferase Akr1. *J Biol Chem*, 280(11), 10156-63.

[40] Claros, M. G., & von, Heijne. G. TopPred II: an improved software for membrane protein structure predictions. *Comput Appl Biosci*, 10(6), 685-6.

[41] Freedman, R. B., Dunn, A. D., & Ruddock, L. W. Protein folding: a missing redox link in the endoplasmic reticulum. *Curr Biol*, 8(13), R 468-70.

[42] Huppa, J. B., & Ploegh, H. L. The eS-Sence of-SH in the ER. *Cell*, 92(2), 145-8.

[43] Hou, H., Subramanian, K., La Grassa, T. J., Markgraf, D., Dietrich, L. E., Urban, J., et al. The DHHC protein Pfa3 affects vacuole-associated palmitoylation of the fusion factor Vac8. *Proc Natl Acad Sci U S A*, 102(48), 17366-71.

[44] Planey, S. L., Keay, S. K., Zhang, C. O., & Zacharias, D. A. Palmitoylation of cytoskeleton associated protein 4 by DHHC2 regulates antiproliferative factor-mediated signaling. *Mol Biol Cell*, 20(5), 1454-63.

[45] Smotrys, J. E., & Linder, M. E. (2004). Palmitoylation of intracellular signaling proteins: regulation and function. *Annu Rev Biochem*, 73, 559-87.

[46] Lam, K. K., Davey, M., Sun, B., Roth, A. F., Davis, N. G., & Conibear, E. Palmitoylation by the DHHC protein Pfa4 regulates the ER exit of Chs3. *J Cell Biol*, 174(1), 19-25.

[47] Greaves, J., Carmichae, J. A., & Chamberlain, L. H. The palmitoyl transferase DHHC2 targets a dynamic membrane cycling pathway: regulation by a C-terminal domain. *Mol Biol Cell*, 22(11), 1887-95.

[48] Fernandez-Hernando, C., Fukata, M., Bernatchez, P. N., Fukata, Y., Lin, M. I., Bredt, D. S., et al. Identification of Golgi-localized acyl transferases that palmitoylate and regulate endothelial nitric oxide synthase. *J Cell Biol*, 174(3), 369-77.

[49] Yanai, A., Huang, K., Kang, R., Singaraja, R. R., Arstikaitis, P., Gan, L., et al. Palmitoylation of huntingtin by HIP14 is essential for its trafficking and function. *Nat Neurosci*, 9(6), 824-31.

[50] Mansouri, M. R., Marklund, L., Gustavsson, P., Davey, E., Carlsson, B., Larsson, C., et al. Loss of 5p15.33 ZDHHC15 expression in a woman with a balanced translocation t(X;15)(q13.3;cen) and severe mental retardation. *Eur J Hum Genet*, 13(8), 970-7.

[51] Yamamoto, Y., Chochi, Y., Matsuyama, H., Eguchi, S., Kawauchi, S., Furuya, T., et al. (2007). Gain of is associated with progression of bladder cancer. *Oncology*, 72(1-2), 132-8.

[52] Mansilla, F., Birkenkamp-Demtroder, K., Kruhoffer, M., Sorensen, F. B., Andersen, C. L., Laiho, P., et al. Differential expression of DHHC9 in microsatellite stable and instable human colorectal cancer subgroups. *Br J Cancer*, 96(12), 1896-903.

[53] Ducker, C. E., Stettler, E. M., French, K. J., Upson, J. J., & Smith, C. D. Huntingtin interacting protein 14 is an oncogenic human protein: palmitoyl acyltransferase. *Oncogene*, 23(57), 9230-7.

[54] Razzaq, T. M., Bass, R., Vines, D. J., Werner, F., Whawell, S. A., & Ellis, V. Functional regulation of tissue plasminogen activator on the surface of vascular smooth muscle

cells by the type-II transmembrane protein p63(CKAP4). *J Biol Chem*, 278(43), 42679-85.

[55] Gupta, N., Manevich, Y., Kazi, Tao. J. Q., Fisher, A. B., & Bates, S. R. Identification and characterization of p63 (CKAP4/ERGIC-63/CLIMP-63), a surfactant protein A binding protein, on type II pneumocytes. *Am J Physiol Lung Cell Mol Physiol*, 291(3), L 436-46.

[56] Sharma, C., Yang, X. H., & Hemler, M. E. DHHC2 Affects Palmitoylation, Stability, and Functions of Tetraspanins CD9 and CD151. *Mol Biol Cell*.

[57] Ikeyama, S., Koyama, M., Yamaoko, M., Sasada, R., & Miyake, M. Suppression of cell motility and metastasis by transfection with human motility-related protein (MRP-1/CD9) DNA. *J Exp Med*, 177(5), 1231-7.

[58] Miyake, M., Inufusa, H., Adachi, M., Ishida, H., Hashida, H., Tokuhara, T., et al. Suppression of pulmonary metastasis using adenovirally motility related protein-1 (MRP-1/CD9) gene delivery. *Oncogene*, 19(46), 5221-6.

[59] Zavadil, J., Bitzer, M., Liang, D., Yang, Y. C., Massimi, A., Kneitz, S., et al. Genetic programs of epithelial cell plasticity directed by transforming growth factor-beta. *Proc Natl Acad Sci U S A*, 98(12), 6686-91.

[60] Janda, E., Lehmann, K., Killisch, I., Jechlinger, M., Herzig, M., Downward, J., et al. Ras and TGF[beta] cooperatively regulate epithelial cell plasticity and metastasis: dissection of Ras signaling pathways. *J Cell Biol*, 156(2), 299-313.

[61] Thiery, J. P. Epithelial-mesenchymal transitions in tumour progression. *Nat Rev Cancer*, 2(6), 442-54.

[62] Fukata, M., Fukata, Y., Adesnik, H., Nicoll, R. A., & Bredt, . Identification of PSD-95 palmitoylating enzymes. *Neuron*, 44(6), 987-96.

[63] Greaves, J., Gorleku, O. A., Salaun, C., & Chamberlain, L. H. Palmitoylation of the SNAP25 protein family: specificity and regulation by DHHC palmitoyl transferases. *J Biol Chem*, 285(32), 24629-38.

[64] Zeidman, R., Buckland, G., Cebecauer, M., Eissmann, P., Davis, D. M., & Magee, A. I. DHHC2 is a protein S-acyltransferase for Lck. *Mol Membr Biol*, 28(7-8), 473-86.

[65] Tsutsumi, R., Fukata, Y., Noritake, J., Iwanaga, T., Perez, F., & Fukata, M. Identification of G protein alpha subunit-palmitoylating enzyme. *Mol Cell Biol*, 29(2), 435-47.

[66] Jia, L., Linder, M. E., & Blumer, K. J. Gi/o signaling and the palmitoyltransferase DHHC2 regulate palmitate cycling and shuttling of RGS7 family-binding protein. *J Biol Chem*, 286(15), 13695-703.

[67] Goytain, A., Hines, R. M., & Quamme, G. A. Huntingtin-interacting proteins, HIP14 and HIP14L, mediate dual functions, palmitoyl acyltransferase and Mg2+ transport. J. *Biol Chem*, 283(48), 33365-74.

[68] Schlingmann, K. P., & Gudermann, T. A critical role of TRPM channel-kinase for human magnesium transport. *J Physiol*, 566(Pt 2), 301 -8 .

[69] Schlingmann, K. P., Waldegger, S., Konrad, M., Chubanov, V., & Gudermann, T. TRPM6 and TRPM7--Gatekeepers of human magnesium metabolism. *Biochim Biophys Acta*, 1772(8), 813-21.

[70] Goytain, A., Hines, R. M., & Quamme, G. A. Huntingtin-interacting proteins, HIP14 and HIP14L, mediate dual functions:Palmitoyl acytransferase and Mg2+ transport. *J Biol Chem*.

[71] Hines, R. M., Kang, R., Goytain, A., & Quamme, G. A. Golgi-specific DHHC zinc finger protein GODZ mediates membrane Ca2+ transport. *J Biol Chem*, 285(7), 4621-8.

[72] Fukata, Y., Iwanaga, T., & Fukata, M. Systematic screening for palmitoyl transferase activity of the DHHC protein family in mammalian cells. *Methods*, 40(2), 177-82.

[73] Nadolski, M. J., & Linder, M. E. Protein lipidation. *FEBS J*, 274(20), 5202-10.

[74] Roth, A. F., Wan, J., Bailey, A. O., Sun, B., Kuchar, J. A., Green, W. N., et al. Global analysis of protein palmitoylation in yeast. *Cell*, 125(5), 1003-13.

[75] Ren, J., Wen, L., Gao, X., Jin, C., Xue, Y., & Yao, X. CSS-Palm 2.0: an updated software for palmitoylation sites prediction. *Protein Eng Des Sel*.

[76] Xue, Y., Chen, H., Jin, C., Sun, Z., & Yao, X. (2006). NBA-Palm: prediction of palmitoylation site implemented in Naive Bayes algorithm. *BMC Bioinformatics*, 7, 458 .

[77] Zhou, F., Xue, Y., Yao, X., & Xu, Y. (2006). A general user interface for prediction servers of proteins' post-translational modification sites. *Nat Protoc*, 1(3), 1318-21.

[78] Zhou, F., Xue, Y., Yao, X., & Xu, Y. CSS-Palm: palmitoylation site prediction with a clustering and scoring strategy (CSS). *Bioinformatics*, 22(7), 894-6.

[79] Bernstein, L. S., Linder, M. E., & Hepler, J. R. (2004). Analysis of RGS protein palmitoylation. *Methods Mol Biol*, 237, 195-204.

[80] Basar, T., Havlicek, V., Bezouskova, S., Halada, P., Hackett, M., & Sebo, P. The conserved lysine 860 in the additional fatty-acylation site of Bordetella pertussis adenylate cyclase is crucial for toxin function independently of its acylation status. *J Biol Chem*, 274(16), 10777-83.

[81] Branton, W. D., Rudnick, M. S., Zhou, Y., Eccleston, E. D., Fields, G. B., & Bowers, L. D. Fatty acylated toxin structure. *Nature*, 365(6446), 496-7.

[82] Kleuss, C., & Krause, E. Galpha(s) is palmitoylated at the N-terminal glycine. *Embo J*, 22(4), 826-32.

[83] Pepinsky, R. B., Zeng, C., Wen, D., Rayhorn, P., Baker, D. P., Williams, K. P., et al. Identification of a palmitic acid-modified form of human Sonic hedgehog. *J Biol Chem*, 273(22), 14037-45.

[84] Bijlsma, M. F., Spek, C. A., & Peppelenbosch, M. P. Hedgehog: an unusual signal transducer. *Bioessays*, 26(4), 387-94.

[85] Di Simplicio, P., Franconi, F., Frosali, S., & Di Giuseppe, D. Thiolation and nitrosation of cysteines in biological fluids and cells. *Amino Acids*, 25(3-4), 323 -39 .

[86] Lipton, S. A., Choi, Y. B., Takahashi, H., Zhang, D., Li, W., Godzik, A., et al. Cysteine regulation of protein function--as exemplified by NMDA-receptor modulation. *Trends Neurosci*, 25(9), 474-80.

[87] Hershko, A., & Ciechanover, A. (1998). The ubiquitin system. *Annu Rev Biochem*, 67, 425-79.

[88] Hermanson, G. T. (1996). Bioconjugate Techniques. 1st ed. *San Diego: Academic Press.*

[89] Gygi, S. P., Rist, B., Gerber, S. A., Turecek, F., Gelb, M. H., & Aebersold, R. Quantitative analysis of complex protein mixtures using isotope-coded affinity tags. *Nat Biotechnol*, 17(10), 994-9.

[90] Schrimpf, S. P., Meskenaite, V., Brunner, E., Rutishauser, D., Walther, P., Eng, J., et al. Proteomic analysis of synaptosomes using isotope-coded affinity tags and mass spectrometry. *Proteomics*, 5(10), 2531-41.

[91] Gygi, S. P., Rist, B., Griffin, T. J., Eng, J., & Aebersold, R. Proteome analysis of low-abundance proteins using multidimensional chromatography and isotope-coded affinity tags. *J Proteome Res*, 1(1), 47-54.

[92] Sitia, R., & Molteni, S. N. Stress, protein (mis)folding, and signaling: the redox connection. *Sci STKE* [239], pe27.

[93] Munro, A. P., & Williams, D. L. H. (1999). Reactivity of nitrogen nucleophiles towards S-nitrosopenicillamine. *Journal of the Chemical Society, Perkin Transactions*, 2, 1989-93.

[94] Fenton, S. S., & Fahey, R. C. Analysis of biological thiols: determination of thiol components of disulfides and thioesters. *Anal Biochem*, 154(1), 34-42.

[95] Bizzozero, O. A., & Good, L. K. Rapid metabolism of fatty acids covalently bound to myelin proteolipid protein. *J Biol Chem*, 266(26), 17092-8.

[96] Passmore, L. A., & Barford, D. Getting into position: the catalytic mechanisms of protein ubiquitylation. *Biochem J*, 379(Pt3), 513-25.

[97] Bizzozero, O. A. (1995). Chemical analysis of acylation sites and species. *Methods Enzymol*, 250, 361-79.

[98] Tolbert, B. S., Tajc, S. G., Webb, H., Snyder, J., Nielsen, J. E., Miller, B. L., et al. The active site cysteine of ubiquitin-conjugating enzymes has a significantly elevated pKa: functional implications. *Biochemistry*, 44(50), 16385-91.

[99] Cione, E., Pingitore, A., Perri, M., & Genchi, G. Influence of all-trans-retinoic acid on oxoglutarate carrier via retinoylation reaction. *Biochim Biophys Acta*, 1791(1), 3-7.

[100] Cione, E., Tucci, P., Chimento, A., Pezzi, V., & Genchi, G. Retinoylation reaction of proteins in Leydig (TM-3) cells. *J Bioenerg Biomembr*, 37(1), 43-8.

[101] Cione, E., Tucci, P., Senatore, V., Ioele, G., & Genchi, G. (2005). Binding of all-trans-retinoic acid to MLTC-1 proteins. Mol Cell Biochem Aug; , 276(1-2), 55 -60 .

[102] Kubo, Y., Wada, M., Ohba, T., & Takahashi, N. Formation of retinoylated proteins from retinoyl-CoA in rat tissues. *J Biochem*, 138(4), 493-500.

[103] Takahashi, N., & Breitman, T. R. Retinoic acid acylation (retinoylation) of a nuclear protein in the human acute myeloid leukemia cell line HL60. *J Biol Chem*, 264(9), 5159-63.

[104] Takahashi, N., & Breitman, T. R. Retinoylation of HL-60 proteins. Comparison to labeling by palmitic and myristic acids. *J Biol Chem*, 265(31), 19158-62.

[105] Takahashi, N., & Breitman, T. R. Retinoylation of proteins in leukemia, embryonal carcinoma, and normal kidney cell lines: differences associated with differential responses to retinoic acid. *Arch Biochem Biophys*, 285(1), 105-10.

[106] Takahashi, N., Liapi, C., Anderson, W. B., & Breitman, T. R. Retinoylation of the cAMP-binding regulatory subunits of type I and type II cAMP-dependent protein kinases in HL60 cells. *Arch Biochem Biophys*, 290(2), 293-302.

[107] Takahashi, N., Jetten, A. M., & Breitman, T. R. Retinoylation of cytokeratins in normal human epidermal keratinocytes. *Biochem Biophys Res Commun*, 180(1), 393-400.

[108] Djakoure, C., Guibourdenche, J., Porquet, D., Pagesy, P., Peillon, F., Li, J. Y., et al. Vitamin A and retinoic acid stimulate within minutes cAMP release and growth hormone secretion in human pituitary cells. *J Clin Endocrinol Metab*, 81(8), 3123-6.

[109] Varani, J., Burmeister, B., Perone, P., Bleavins, M., & Johnson, K. J. All-trans retinoic acid inhibits fluctuations in intracellular Ca2+ resulting from changes in extracellular Ca2+. *Am J Pathol*, 147(3), 718-27.

[110] Hensel, J., Hintz, M., Karas, M., Linder, D., Stahl, B., & Geyer, R. Localization of the palmitoylation site in the transmembrane protein p12E of Friend murine leukaemia virus. *Eur J Biochem*, 232(2), 373-80.

[111] De Mar, J. C., Jr , , & Anderson, R. E. Identification and quantitation of the fatty acids composing the CoA ester pool of bovine retina, heart, and liver. *J Biol Chem*, 272(50), 31362-8.

[112] Hang, H. C., Geutjes, E. J., Grotenbreg, G., Pollington, A. M., Bijlmakers, MJ, & Ploegh, HL. Chemical probes for the rapid detection of Fatty-acylated proteins in Mammalian cells. *J Am Chem Soc*, 129(10), 2744-5.

[113] Adams, S. R., Campbell, R. E., Gross, L. A., Martin, B. R., Walkup, G. K., Yao, Y., et al. New biarsenical ligands and tetracysteine motifs for protein labeling in vitro and in vivo: synthesis and biological applications. *J Am Chem Soc*, 124(21), 6063-76.

[114] Adams, S. R., Lev-Ram, V., & Tsien, R. Y. (1997). A new caged Ca2+, azid-1, is far more photosensitive than nitrobenzyl- based chelators. *Chem Biol*, 4(11), 867-78.

[115] Griffin, B. A., Adams, S. R., Jones, J., & Tsien, R. Y. (2000). Fluorescent labeling of recombinant proteins in living cells with FlAsH. *Methods Enzymol*, 327, 565-78.

[116] Nagai, T., Sawano, A., Park, E. S., & Miyawaki, A. (2001). Circularly permuted green fluorescent proteins engineered to sense Ca2+. *Proc Natl Acad Sci U S A*, 98(6), 3197-202.

[117] Gaietta, G. M., Giepmans, B. N., Deerinck, T. J., Smith, W. B., Ngan, L., Llopis, J., et al. Golgi twins in late mitosis revealed by genetically encoded tags for live cell imaging and correlated electron microscopy. *Proc Natl Acad Sci U S A*, 103(47), 17777-82.

[118] Martin, B. R., Giepmans, B. N., Adams, S. R., & Tsien, R. Y. Mammalian cell-based optimization of the biarsenical-binding tetracysteine motif for improved fluorescence and affinity. *Nat Biotechnol*, 23(10), 1308-14.

[119] Ju, W., Morishita, W., Tsui, J., Gaietta, G., Deerinck, T. J., Adams, S. R., et al. Activity-dependent regulation of dendritic synthesis and trafficking of AMPA receptors. *Nat Neurosci*, 7(3), 244-53.

[120] Stults, J. T., & Arnott, D. (2005). Proteomics. Methods Enzymol.; , 402, 245-89.

[121] Kenyon GL, Bruice TW. (1977). Novel sulfhydryl reagents. *Methods Enzymol*, 47, 407-30.

[122] Qanbar, R., & Bouvier, M. Determination of protein-bound palmitate turnover rates using a three-compartment model that formally incorporates [3H]palmitate recycling. *Biochemistry*, 43(38), 12275-88.

[123] Ducker, C. E., Draper, J. M., Xia, Z., & Smith, C. D. In vitro and cellular assays for palmitoyl acyltransferases using fluorescent lipidated peptides. *Methods*, 40(2), 166-70.

[124] Kenworthy, A. K. Fluorescence-based methods to image palmitoylated proteins. *Methods*, 40(2), 198-205.

[125] Resh, M. D. Use of analogs and inhibitors to study the functional significance of protein palmitoylation. *Methods*, 40(2), 191-7.

[126] Ducker, C. E., Griffel, L. K., Smith, R. A., Keller, S. N., Zhuang, Y., Xia, Z., et al. Discovery and characterization of inhibitors of human palmitoyl acyltransferases. *Mol Cancer Ther*, 5(7), 1647-59.

[127] Varner, A. S., Ducker, C. E., Xia, Z., Zhuang, Y., De Vos, M. L., & Smith, C. D. Characterization of human palmitoyl-acyl transferase activity using peptides that mimic distinct palmitoylation motifs. *Biochem J*, 373(Pt1), 91-9.

[128] Schmidt, M., Schmidt, M. F., & Rott, R. Chemical identification of cysteine as palmitoylation site in a transmembrane protein (Semliki Forest virus E1). *J Biol Chem*, 263(35), 18635-9.

[129] Drisdel, R. C., & Green, W. N. Labeling and quantifying sites of protein palmitoylation. *Biotechniques*, 36(2), 276-85.

[130] Drisdel, R. C., Manzana, E., & Green, W. N. The role of palmitoylation in functional expression of nicotinic alpha7 receptors. *J Neurosci*, 24(46), 10502-10.

[131] Wan, J., Roth, A. F., Bailey, A. O., & Davis, N. G. Palmitoylated proteins: purification and identification. 2(7), 1573-84.

[132] Liu, H., Lin, D., & Yates, J. R. 3rd. Multidimensional separations for protein/peptide analysis in the post-genomic era. *Biotechniques*, 32(4), 898 -900, 2 passim.

[133] Roth, A. F., Wan, J., Green, W. N., Yates, J. R., & Davis, N. G. Proteomic identification of palmitoylated proteins. *Methods*, 40(2), 135-42.

[134] Schweizer, A., Rohrer, J., Jeno, P., De Maio, A., Buchman, T. G., & Hauri, H. P. A reversibly palmitoylated resident protein (63 of an ER-Golgi intermediate compartment is related to a circulatory shock resuscitation protein. *J Cell Sci*, 104(Pt 3), 685-94.

[135] Zhang, J., & Zacharias, D. A. Global Analysis of the Dynamic Palmitoylosome. *Lipid Rafts and Cell Funciton*, 23-28, Steamboat Springs, Colorado: Keystone Symposia.

[136] Kostiuk, M. A., Corvi, M. M., Keller, B. O., Plummer, G., Prescher, J. A., Hangauer, M. J., et al. Identification of palmitoylated mitochondrial proteins using a bio-orthogonal azido-palmitate analogue. *FASEB J*, 22(3), 721-32.

[137] Saxon, E., & Bertozzi, C. R. (2000). Cell surface engineering by a modified Staudinger reaction. Science. Mar 17 , 287(5460), 2007-10.

[138] Jennings, B. C., Nadolski, M. J., Ling, Y., Baker, M. B., Harrison, M. L., Deschenes, R. J., et al. 2bromopalmitate and 2-(2-Hydroxy-5-nitro-benzylidene)-benzo[b]thiophen-3-one inhibit DHHC-mediated palmitoylation in vitro. *J Lipid Res*.

[139] Mikic, I., Planey, S., Zhang, J., Ceballos, C., Seron, T., Massenbach, Bv., et al. (2006). A live-cell, image based approach to understanding the enzymology and pharmacology of 2bromopalmitate and palmitoylation. *Methods in enzymology*, 414.

[140] Chase, J. F., & Tubbs, P. K. Specific inhibition of mitochondrial fatty acid oxidation by2-bromopalmitate and its coenzyme A and carnitine esters. *The Biochemical journal*, 129(1), 55-65.

[141] Coleman, R. A., Rao, P., Fogelsong, R. J., & Bardes, E. S. Bromopalmitoyl-CoA and 2-bromopalmitate: promiscuous inhibitors of membrane-bound enzymes. *Biochimica et biophysica acta*, 1125(2), 203-9.

[142] Draper, J. M., & Smith, C. D. (2009). Palmitoyl acyltransferase assays and inhibitors (Review). Mol Membr Biol. Jan , 26(1), 5-13.

[143] Fabian, M. A., Biggs, W. H. 3.r.d, Treiber, . D. K., Atteridge, C. E., Azimioara, M. D., Benedetti, M. G., et al. A small molecule-kinase interaction map for clinical kinase inhibitors. *Nature biotechnology*, 23(3), 329-36.

[144] Karaman, M. W., Herrgard, S., Treiber, D. K., Gallant, P., Atteridge, C. E., Campbell, B. T., et al. A quantitative analysis of kinase inhibitor selectivity. *Nature biotechnology*, 26(1), 127-32.

[145] Feng, Y., Yin, Y., Weiser, A., Griffin, E., Cameron, Lin. L., et al. Discovery of substituted 4-(pyrazol-4-yl)-phenylbenzodioxane-2-carboxamides as potent and highly selective Rho kinase (ROCK-II) inhibitors. *Journal of medicinal chemistry*, 51(21), 6642-5.

[146] Huang, K., Sanders, S., Singaraja, R., Orban, P., Cijsouw, T., Arstikaitis, P., et al. Neuronal palmitoyl acyl transferases exhibit distinct substrate specificity. *Faseb J*, 23(8), 2605-15.

[147] Prigozhina, N. L., Zhong, L., Hunter, E. A., Mikic, I., Callaway, S., Roop, D. R., et al. Plasma membrane assays and three-compartment image cytometry for high content screening. *Assay and drug development technologies*, 5(1), 29-48.

[148] Morelock, M. M., Hunter, E. A., Moran, T. J., Heynen, S., Laris, C., Thieleking, M., et al. Statistics of assay validation in high throughput cell imaging of nuclear factor kappaB nuclear translocation. *Assay and drug development technologies*, 3(5), 483-99.

[149] Wolff, M., Kredel, S., Wiedenmann, J., Nienhaus, G. U., & Heilker, R. Cell-based assays in practice: cell markers from autofluorescent proteins of the GFP-family. *Combinatorial chemistry & high throughput screening*, 11(8), 602-9.

[150] Collins, M. A. Generating'omic knowledge: The Role of Informatics in High Content Screening. *Combinatorial chemistry & high throughput screening*.

[151] Shaner, N. C., Campbell, R. E., Steinbach, P. A., Giepmans, B. N., Palmer, A. E., & Tsien, R. Y. Improved monomeric red, orange and yellow fluorescent proteins derived from Discosoma sp. red fluorescent protein. *Nature biotechnology*, 22(12), 1567-72.

[152] Inglese, J., Auld, Jadhav. A., Johnson, R. L., Simeonov, A., Yasgar, A., et al. Quantitative high-throughput screening: a titration-based approach that efficiently identifies biological activities in large chemical libraries. *Proceedings of the National Academy of Sciences of the United States of America*, 103(31), 11473-8.

[153] Chung, C. C., Ohwaki, K., Schneeweis, J. E., Stec, E., Varnerin, J. P., Goudreau, P. N., et al. A fluorescence-based thiol quantification assay for ultra-high-throughput screening for inhibitors of coenzyme A production. *Assay and drug development technologies*, 6(3), 361-74.

[154] Lazo, P.A. Functional implications of tetraspanin proteins in cancer biology. *Cancer Sci*; 98: 1666-77.

[155] Patra, S.K. Dissecting lipid raft facilitated cell signaling pathways in cancer. *Biochimica et biophysica acta*; 1785: 182-206.

Chapter 10

The Antibacterial Drug Discovery

Jie Yanling, Liang Xin and Li Zhiyuan

Additional information is available at the end of the chapter

http://dx.doi.org/10.5772/52510

1. Introduction

An antibacterial is a compound or substance that kills or slows down the growth of bacteria. We usually associate the beginning of the modern antibacterial era with the names of Paul Ehrlich and Alexander Fleming. Infectious diseases are the leading causes of human morbidity and mortality for most of human existence. Antibacterials are probably one of the most successful forms of chemotherapy in the history of medicine. They save countless lives and make enormous contribution to the control of infectious diseases since the beginning of antibacterial era. Perhaps most of us born since the Second World War don't know how much enthusiasm, dedication, and hardship have been put in antibacterial drug discovery, and take the success of antibacterial agents too much for granted. Therefore, let's first look back what the human did to combat the infections before antibacterial era and how the outstanding scientists discovered so many efficient antibacterial agents used clinically today and led us enter the antibacterial era.

2. The history of antibacterial discovery

2.1. Pre-antibiotic era

Before the early 20th century, treatments for infections were based primarily on medicinal folklore. Mixtures with antimicrobial properties that were used in treatments of infections were described over 2000 years ago [1]. Even the prehistoric peoples used a number of plants in wound treatment and it seems possible that many plants have the properties of antimicrobial effects [2; 3]. Tetracyclines can be incorporated into the hydroxyapatite mineral portion of bones as well as tooth enamel; once people take it, permanent markers of metabolically active areas will be left. Thus it is much conveniently to trace the exposure of these antibacterials in ancient populations. It was found than the bone sample from Sudanese Nubian (A.D. 350 to 550) was labeled by the antibiotic tetracycline and their dietary regime contained tetracycline-containing materials by X-group cemetery and other advanced technologies [4; 5]. Moreover, another study showed that, bones from the Dakhleh Oasis, Egypt, in a late Roman period, exhibit discrete fluorochromelabelling, exactly like the teeth from patients treated with tetracycline [6]. A large number of customs and anecdotes can also reveal the occurrences of other antibacterials. One popular anecdote is about the antibiotic-like properties of red soil from the Hashemite Kingdom of Jordan. Interestingly, red soil was used for treating skin infections and diaper rash in the past and is still used in some communities today as an inexpensive alternative to antibiotics [7]. In fact, recently, many pharmaceutical antibiotics, such as streptomycin, actinomycin, erythromycin, vancomycin, nystatin and amphotericin, were produced from the soil actinomycetes [8].

The traditional Chinese medicine is the summary of experience about Chinese medical treatment over millennia and may contain a lot of unknown antibiotics [9]. Many traditional Chinese medicines were tested and found effective against four common oral bacteria [10]. Discovery of active components in the ancient herbs could enrich the arsenal of antimicrobials used by the mainstream medicine.

2.2. Foundation of the antibiotic era

Bacteria were first identified in the 1670s by van Leeuwenhoek, following his invention of the microscope. The relationship between bacteria and diseases gradually set up in the nineteenth century. Since then, researchers started to try and find effective antibacterial agents.

Paul Ehrlich is the father of chemotherapy and was honored with the Nobel prize due to the molecular side-chain theory of immunity. His concept of "magic bullet" is that the chemicals selectively target only disease-causing microbes but not the host cells. In 1906, Ehrlich, together with Bertheim, developed hundreds of derivatives of Atoxyl, and finally discovered compound 606, a gold powder [9; 11]. In 1909, he found that Compound 606 could cure syphilis-infected rabbits in experiments; it could also improve terminal patients with dementia and cured early stage patients with infected sores [11]. It was publicly released as salvarsan in 1910. Despite the adverse side effects, salvarsan and it's derivative neosalvarsan kept the status of the most frequently prescribed drug until the introduction of penicillin in the 1940s [12]. Amazingly, the chemical structure of salvarsan hadn't been known until 2005 [13].

The systematic screening approach introduced by Paul Ehrlich became the cornerstone of drug search strategies in the pharmaceutical industry. Sulfonamidochrysoidine (also named prontosil), the first commercially available antibiotic, was first synthesized by Bayer chemists Josef Klarer and Fritz Mietzsch in 1930s by this approach. Then Gerhard Domagk found its effect against Streptococcus pyogenes in mice [14]. Four years later he received the Noble Prize. Eventually prontosil was recognized as a precursor for a new class of antibacterial agents— sulfonamides.

The effect of mould on bacterial colonies hadn't been investigated until 19th century, although the antibacterial properties of mold had been known since ancient times. In 1921, Alexander Fleming observed some substances called lyzosomes which could dissolve bacteria. In 1928, he discovered that a specific mould species inhibited the development of Staphylococcus bacteria. The species was known as Pencilliumnotatum and the filtrate was called penicillin [15]. In 1940, Howard Florey and Ernst Chain worked out how to purify penicillin for clinical testing [16]. All the three researchers were awarded the Nobel Prize in 1945, and since then the era of antibiotics had been initiated. Penicillin became the top therapeutic molecule because of its widespread use and the magnitude of the therapeutic outcomes, and also because of the technologies developed for production of penicillin which became the basis for production of all subsequent antibiotics and other bioproducts in use today [17].

3. Classification

Antibacterials are commonly classified based on their mechanism of action or spectrum of activity. The main classes of antibacterial drugs target only four classical bacterial functions: bacterial-cell-wall biosynthesis (e.g., penicillin and vancomycin); bacterial protein biosynthesis (e.g., aminoglycoside and macrolide); DNA and RNA replication (e.g., ciprofloxacin and rifampin); and folate coenzyme biosynthesis (e.g., sulfamethoxazole) [18]. Antibacterials that target the cell wall or cell membrane or essential bacterial enzymes are more likely to be bactericidal; but generally the bacteriostatic is the antibacterial drugs that inhibits protein synthesis [19]. Another way to distinguish the antibiotics is based on their target specificity. The broad-spectrum antibiotic affects a wide range of disease-causing bacteria, including both Gram-positive and Gram-negative bacteria, in contrast to a narrow-spectrum antibiotic, which acts against specific families of bacteria. For example, ampicillin is a widely used broad-spectrum antibiotic.

4. Antibacterial resistance and its mechanisms

Bacterial resistance to antibacterial drugs increasingly becomes a major health and economic problem, eroding the discovery of antibiotics and their application to clinical medicine. As early as 1946, Alexander Fleming predicted that "There is probably no chemotherapeutic drug to which in suitable circumstances the bacteria cannot react by in some way acquiring 'fastness' (resistance)." Today it is really the truth. Resistance to the antibiotics will emerge only a few years after it is introduced to clinic use [20]. Bacterial resistance is positively correlated with the use of antibacterial agents in clinical practice [21; 22]. Because any use of antibiotics can increase selective pressure in a population of bacteria, allowing survival of the resistant bacteria and death of the susceptible ones. We can find that pathogenic bacteria are resistant to practically all available antibacterial drugs. And many strains, which are informally called superbugs, are even resistant to several different antibiotics. Multidrug resistance has been found in Pseudomonas aeruginosa (P. aeruginosa),

Acinetobacterbaumannii (A. baumannii), E. coli, and Klebsiellapneumoniae (K. pneumoniae), producing extended-spectrum β-lactamases (ESBL), vancomycin-resistant enterococci Enterococcus faecium (E. faecium) (VRE), MRSA, vancomycin-resistant S. aureus VRSA, extensively drug-resistant (XDR) Mycobacterium tuberculosis (M. tuberculosis), Salmonella enterica (S. enterica) serovar Typhimurium, Shigelladysenteriae (S. dysenteriae), Haemophilusinfluenzae (H. influenzae), Stenotrophomonas, and Burkholderia [23; 24].

Great amount of antibiotic is used in nonhuman niches, leading to the spread of resistant bacteria too. Antibiotics have been used for improving the production of livestock and poultry for more than 50 years [25]. The Institute of Food Technologists (IFT), once convened a panel of internationally renowned experts to address the concern that, the emergence of antimicrobial resistance may result from abuse in food production, manufacturing, and elsewhere [26].

Over the past several years, people struggled to search for the mechanisms of resistance. Therefore today there is a large pool of information about how drug resistances come out. Biochemical and genetic aspects of antibiotic resistance mechanisms are shown in Fig. 1.

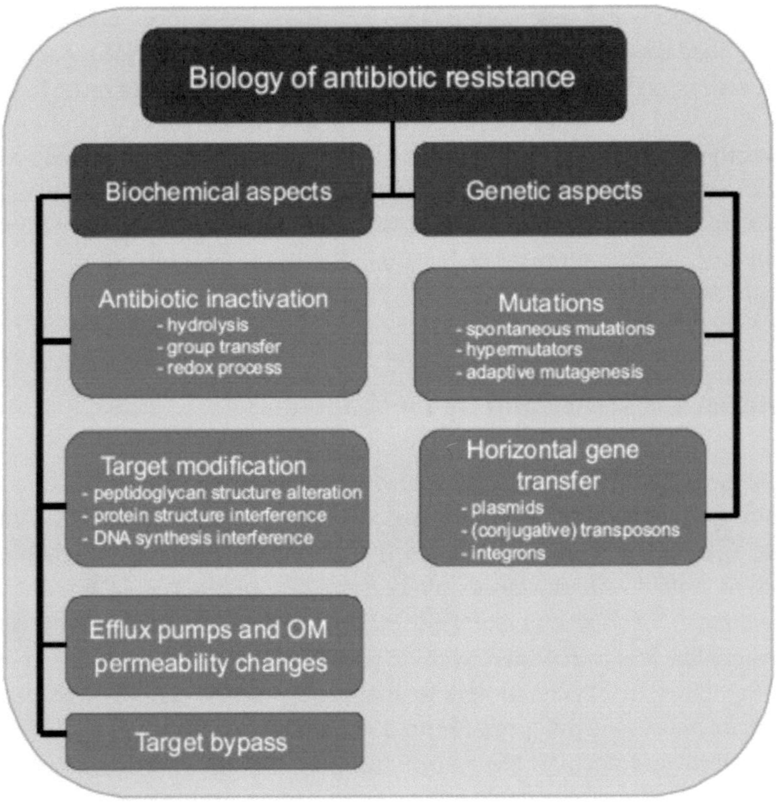

Figure 1. Kinds of antibiotic resistance mechanisms [85].

4.1. Genetics of antibiotic resistance

Resistance can be an intrinsic property of the bacteria themselves or it can be acquired. There are two main ways of acquiring antibiotic resistance: i) chromosomal mutations and ii) horizontal gene transfer. But the question is where the horizontal gene comes from? Some of these genes have an environmental origin and began their evolution before the antibiotic era; most likely, the primary genes originated and diversified within the environmental bacterial communities, then mobilized and penetrated into pathogens. [27; 28]

4.1.1. Mutations

4.1.1.1. Spontaneous mutations

These mutations occur randomly as replication errors or an incorrect repair of a damaged DNA in actively dividing cells, presenting an important mode of generating antibiotic resistance. They are also called the growth dependent mutations. Quinolone resistance in Escherichia coli resulted from the mutations in at least seven positions in the gyrA gene or three positions in the parC gene [29]. There are a large number of biochemical mechanisms of antibiotic resistance related to Spontaneous Mutations. For instance, Mutations in mexR can cause derepression of the mexAB-oprM multidrug efflux operon, causing a multidrug resistance phenotype in Pseudomonas aeruginosa [30].

4.1.1.2. Hypermutators

During a prolonged non-lethal antibiotic selective pressure a small bacterial population enters a transient state of a high mutation rate which is called hypermutable state. Hypermutators are found in many bacteria species such as E. coli, S. enterica, Neisseria meningitides (N. meningitides),H. influenzae, S. aureus, Helicobacter pylori (H. pylori), Streptococcus pneumoniae (S. pneumoniae),and P. aeruginosa [85]. Various studies suggested that hypermutations play an important role in acquisition of antibiotic resistance in pathogens [31; 32; 33].

4.1.1.3. Adaptive mutagenesis

Adaptive mutations arise in non-dividing or slowly dividing cells during the presence of a non-lethal selective pressure that favours them. A great number of antibiotic resistant mutants may come from this mutation process under bacterial natural conditions [85].

4.1.1.4. Horizontal gene transfer

Horizontal transfer of genetic material between bacteria is the most commonly used way to spread antibiotic resistance. In general, this exchange is accomplished mainly through the processes of transduction (via bacteriophages), conjugation (via plasmids and conjugative transposons), and transformation (via incorporation into the chromosome of chromosomal DNA, plasmids, and other DNAs) [34]. This type of genetic transfer not only occurred between closely related bacteria but can also occur between phylogenetically distant bacterial genera, in particular between gram-positive and gram-negative bacteria [35]. Plasmid-encoded antibiotic resistance encompasses most classes of antibiotics in practice, such as aminoglycosides, cephalosporins and fluoroquinolones [36]. Transposons spread quicker than genes in chromosomes and are transferred by conjugation, transformation, or transduction [23; 24]. Integrons acquire and exchange exogenous DNA, known as gene cassettes, by a site-specific recombination mechanism. They can integrate stably into other DNAs where they deliver multiple antibacterial resistant genes in a single exchange. Resistance gene cassettes encoding the metallo-β- lactamases IMP and VIM confer resistance to the potent carbapenem β-lactams imipenem and meropenem [36].

4.1.2. Biochemistry of antibiotic resistance

As so many scientists have been struggling to study the biochemical mechanisms of antibiotic resistance, nowadays there is a large pool of related valuable information left. Biochemical mechanisms may be varied among different bacterial species, but can be mainly classified into four categories (Fig. 2). In fact, each of these four categories also contains an amazing diversity of resistance mechanisms. Sometimes a single bacterial strain may possess several types of resistance mechanisms. Each of the four main categories will be discussed respectively below.

4.1.2.1. Antibiotic inactivation

Biochemical strategies include enzymatic modification and redox mechanisms (which is less important and will not be elaborated in this paper). Enzymes can be divided into two general classes: those such as β-lactamases that degrade antibiotics and others that perform chemical transformations. The antibiotic β-lactam has a four-atom ring known as a beta-lactamin. The β-lactamase enzyme breaks that ring open, destroying the antibacterial properties of the drugs. β-lactamase consists of enzymes with a serine residue at the active site, and metalloenzymes with zinc ion as a cofactor and with a separate heritage [37]. β-lactamase enzymes are the most common and important weapons for Gram-negative bacteria to resist the antibiotics β-lactam [38]. The group transfer approaches are the most diverse and include the modification by acyltransfer, phosphorylation, glycosylation, nucleotidylation, ribosylation, and thiol transfer. They can inactivate antibiotics (aminoglycosides, chloramphenicol, streptogramin, macrolides or rifampicin) by chemical substitution. These modifications reduce the affinity of antibiotics to a target [85]. For example, enzymatic modification is the most prevalent mechanism to destroy aminoglycosides in clinic. Aminoglycoside modifying enzymes can be divided into three classes: acetyltransferases, nucleotidyltranferases, and phosphotransferases; they mainly catalyze the modification at –OH or –NH2 groups of the 2-deoxystreptamine nucleus or the sugar moieties [39]. There are a large number of genes in the chromosomes and other mobile genetic elements coding for these enzymes which let the bacteria resist to more new antibiotics as well as horizontally spread their resistance among bacteria more easily. As a consequence, almost all pathogens are resistant to aminoglycosides through modifying enzymes [39].

4.1.2.2. Target modification

Another important resistance mechanism is the modification of antibiotic targets which makes the antibiotic unable to bind the targets properly. β-lactams target the bacterial enzymes of cell wall biosynthesis (the so-called penicillin-binding proteins, PBPs). Alterations in PBPs can reduce affinity for β-lactams, possibly causing β-lactam resistance in many bacteria strains, such as H. influenzae, N. gonorrhoeae, N. meningitidis, anaerobes, S. dysenteriae [40]. For instance, the mecA resistance gene which encodes PBP2a, a new penicillin binding protein with decreased affinity for oxacillin and most other β-lactam drugs, induces resistance to methicillin and oxacillin in S. aureus [41]. The resistance to antibiotics that interfere with protein synthesis or transcription is achieved by modification of the specific target. rRNAmethylases encoded by a number of genes modificate the 16S rRNA molecule at specific positions critical for aminoglycosides binding [42]. Modification in the 23S rRNA component of the 50S ribosomal subunit also leads to resistance to the macrolide, lincosamide and streptogramin B group of antibiotics in many pathogen strains [43; 44]. Mutations of topoisomerase IV and gyrase genes can sufficiently alter affinity of fluoroquinolones to these enzymes [45].

4.1.2.3. Efflux pumps and outer membrane (OM) permeability

Efflux pumps Membrane proteins that export antibiotics from the cell and maintain their low intracellular concentrations are called efflux pumps. Drug efflux pumps play a key role in drug resistance not just because they can produce multidrug resistance but also because they can elevate level of other resistance mechanisms [46; 47]. Bacterial drug efflux transporters are currently classified into five families: the ATP-binding cassette (ABC) superfamily, the major facilitator superfamily (MFS), the multidrug and toxic compound extrusion (MATE) family, the small multidrug resistance (SMR) family, and the resistance-nodulation-division (RND) superfamily [47]. Efflux transporters can be further classified into single or multicomponent pumps. Tetracycline and macrolide transporters are single component efflux systems that have narrow substrate profiles, while the RND family members have broader substrates and can pump out multiple structurally unrelated compounds [24; 46]. Efflux pumps exist in both Gram-positive and Gram-negative bacteria [48; 49]. MexAB-OprM efflux pumps in Pseudomonas aeruginosa, which belong to RND family, result in higher inhibitory concentration of a large number of antibiotics, such as penicillins, broad-spectrumcephalosporins, chloramphenicol, fluoroquinolones, macrolides, novobiocin, sulfonamides, tetracycline and trimethoprim, dyes and detergents [50; 51].

OM permeability The OM is an asymmetric bilayer: the phospholipid form the inner leaflet and the lipopolysaccharides (LPS) form the outer leaflet. OM of Gram-negative bacteria provides a formidable barrier that must be overcome by drugs. Drug molecules pass the OM by diffusion through porins or the bilayer, or by self-promoted uptake [85]. Small hydrophilic drugs (e.g., β-lactams), enter to the intracellular through the pore-forming porins, while macrolides and other hydrophobic drugs diffuse during their entry [52]. Some resistant clinical strains of Neisseria meningitidis, K. pneumoniae and Enterobacteraerogenes exhibit a noticeable porin variability resulting in decrease of antibacterial uptake [53]. Reduction of

LPS in the outer membrane of Polymyxin-resistant P. aeruginosa strains associates with resistance development [54].

4.1.2.4. Target bypass

This kind of resistance mechanisms is somewhat specific. Bacteria produce two kinds of targets: one is sensitive to antibiotics and the alternative one (usually an enzyme) that is resistant to inhibition of antibiotic. In ampicillin-resistant mutant Enterococcus faecium selected in vitro, bypass of the DD-transpeptidases by a novel class of peptidoglycan polymerases, the LD-transpeptidases, conveyed resistance to all β-lactams, except the carbapenems [55; 56].

5. What should we do?

5.1. Extending the lifespan of existing antibacterials

Although the emergency of antibiotic resistance seems inevitable, measures must be taken to prevent or at least delay this process. As mentioned above, many factors contribute to resistance, so we should adopt a complex approach. The most important way is to strictly control antibiotic misuse and overuse. Interestingly, the EU has implemented a comprehensive ban on the use of all antibiotics for growth promotion since 2006 [25]. And other developed countries also implement similar measures, but in many developing nations antibiotic use is relatively uncontrolled. As hospital-acquired infection is a major cause for antibiotic-resistance, strict antibiotic stewardship and policies should be adopted in the hospitals. For example, we can make some antibiotic policies to optimize the selection, dosing, route of administration, duration of the drug prescribed by the doctor, and limit the unintended consequences of antibiotic utilization [57].

5.2. New antibacterial drug discovery

As serious infectious diseases and multidrug resistance are emerging repeatedly, new antibiotics are needed badly to combat these bacterial pathogens, but the progress of discovery seems relatively slow. Most chemical scaffolds of antibiotics used now were just introduced between the mid-1930s and the early 1960s (fig 2). There are many reasons for this. The first is scientific. We have discovered the easy-to-find antibiotics. Now we have to work harder and think more cleverly to find new drugs. Another reason is commercial. Antibiotics are used much less than other drugs and the new antibiotic are just used to treat serious bacterial infections at most of the time. So antibiotics have a poor return on investment. In 2008 only five major pharmaceutical companies still kept their Enthusiasm in antibacterial discovery. It is most important to delink research and development costs from drug pricing and the return from investment on antibacterial discovery [58]. If the government could establish some subsidies and financial assistance schemes to compensate the cost, more drug companies will be attracted to this area.

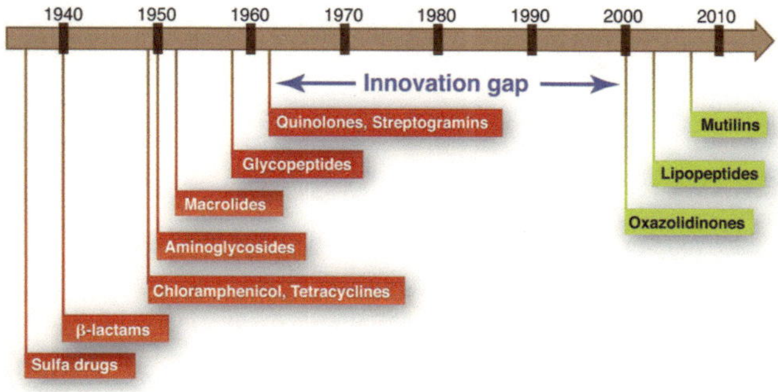

Figure 2. Innovation gap between 1962 and 2000 [59].

Despite the current grim situation in management of resistant bacteria, some new drugs have recently been approved by the FDA or are in late stages of the pipeline (Table 1, 2) [60]. The new drugs belong to the following classes of compounds: oxazolidinones, glycopeptides, ketolides, lycylcyclines, carbapenems and fluoroquinolones.

CLASS OF COMPOUND	PHASE OF DEVELO-PMENT	**ANALOGS**	MECHANISM OF ACTION	RESISTANCE MECHANISM	DRUG COMPANY
Oxazolidinones	FDA Approved 2000	Linezolid, Radezolid, Torezolid, RWJ-416457	Inhibits protein translation (initiation/ elongation)	rRNA mutations	Pfizer, Rib-X, Trius Therapeutics, Johnson & Johnson
Glycopeptides	Phase III	Oritavancin, Dalbavancin, Telavancin	Inhibit peptidoglycan biosysnthesis/ transglycosylation	unidentified	Targanta/The Medicines Co., Pfizer, Theravance
Ketolides	Phase III	Cethromycin	Inhibits protein synthesis	rRNA dimethylation, ribosomal protein mutations	Advanced Life Sciences
Glycylcyclines	FDA Approved 2005	Tigecycline, PTK0796	Inhibits protein synthesis	Efflux pumps	Wyeth, Paratek Pharmaceuticals
Carbapenems	FDA Approved 2007	Doripenem, Razupenem	Inhibits peptidoglycan biosynthesis	Carbapenemases, Efflux pumps, Porin mutations	Johnson & Johnson, Protez Pharmaceuticals
Streptogramins	Phase II	NXL103/XRP2868	Inhibits protein translation	unidentified	Novexel
Fluoroquinolones	Preclinical	JNJ-Q2, finafloxacin	Inhibit type II topoisomerase	gyrA, parC mutations	Johnson & Johnson, MerLion Pharmaceuticals

Table 1. New antibiotics of existing scaffolds

DRUG NAME	TARGET/ MECHANISM OF ACTION	SPECTRUM OF ACTIVITY	PHASE OF DEVELO-PMENT	DRUG COMPANY OR INNOVATOR
Ceftobiprole	Tight binding to PBP2a	Gram-positive, Gram-negative	Phase III	Johnson & Johnson
Ceftaroline	Tight binding to PBP2a	Gram-positive, Gram-negative	Phase III	Forrest Laboratories
Iclaprim	Increased affinity to bacterial DHFR	Gram-positive, Gram-negative	Phase III	Arpida
Sulopenem	Binding to PBPs	Gram-negative	preclinical	Pfizer
BAL30376	Monobactam/β-lactamase inhibitor combination	Multi-drug resistant Gram-negative	preclinical	Basilea
Rx100472	MethionyltRNA synthetase inhibitor	Gram-positive	preclinical	Trius Therapeutics
PC190723	Cell division protein FtsZ	S. aureus	preclinical	Prolysis
MUT7307	Enoyl-ACP FabI reductase (fatty acid biosynthesis)	Gram-positive, Gram-negative	preclinical	Mutabilis
Nitazoxanide	Inhibits vitamin cofactor of pyruvate:ferredoxin oxidoreductase (PFOR)	C. difficile	Phase II	Romark Laboratories
Fidaxomicin (OPT-80)	Inhibits RNA synthesis	C. difficile	Phase II	Optimer Pharmaceuticals
LED209	Quorum sensing	S. typhimurium F. tularensis	preclinical	University of Texas South Western Medical Center,Dallas
BPH652	Virulence factor (antioxidant)	MRSA	preclinical	University of Illinois, Chicago
Omiganan	Antimicrobial peptide; Depolarizes cytoplasmic membrane of bacteria	Gram-positive, fungi	Phase III	MIGENIX, Cadence pharmaceuticals
TMC207	ATP synthase inhibition	M. tuberculosis	Phase II	Johnson & Johnson, Tibotec
CBR2092	Dual pharmacophore	Gram-positive	Phase I	Cumbre
Amikacin	Novel drug delivery: inhaled nanoliposomes	P. aeruginosa biofilm	Phase II	Transave Inc.

Table 2. New antibiotics in development

5.2.1. Tailoring existing scaffolds

It seems that there are many ways to search for new antibacterials, but the key question is: how to search for new antibacterial drugs and where to look for them? The most convenient method is to modify the existing scaffolds to generate their derivates. All antibiotics approved between the early 1960s and 2000 were synthetic derivatives of the old scaffolds except carbapenems. Chemical modifications of old scaffolds may lead to improved bactericidal activities, better resistance profiles, safety, tolerability or superior pharmacokinetic/pharmacodynamic properties. There are four generations of β-Lactam antibiotics, all of which contains a β-lactam nucleus in their molecular structures. The second generation (e.g., cephalexin and cefaclor) and third generation (e.g., cefotaxime, ceftazidime) are not sensitive to plasmid-mediated broad-spectrum β-lactamases and have less allergic reactions, compared with the first generation (penicillins) [61]. The fourth-generation cephalosporins penetrate through the outer membrane of Gram-negative bacteria more easily and have low affinity for clinically important β-lactamases, so they have the advantage of killing many Gram-negative pathogens resistant to most third-generation [86]. Tigecycline is one of glycylcycline antibiotics derived from tetracycline and received approval from the US Food and Drug Administration for the treatment of skin, soft-tissue, and intra abdominal infections in 2005. Tigecycline can overcome the active efflux of drug from inside the bacterial cell and protection of ribosomes, which are two determinants of tetracycline resistance [62; 63]. But this approach is only a good short-term strategy to find new drugs, and but the benefit of these modified drugs will be offset quickly by the resistance to acquired through the horizontal acquisition or molecular evolution [9], which indicates that it is much more attractive to find novel chemical scaffolds.

5.2.2. *Novel scaffolds*

5.2.2.1. *Explore new places*

More than two-thirds of clinically used antibiotics come from natural products or their semi synthetic derivatives and most of them came out from soil actinomycetes. But recently researchers have shifted to underexplored ecological niches and bacterial species and found some new scaffolds. Compared to the terrestrial environment, the ocean remains an underexplored habitat with unparalleled biodiversity, leaving it the most promising place to yield new antibacterial metabolites. New antibacterial agents with novelty and/or complexity in chemical structure derived from marine bacteria have been elaborated clearly [64; 65]. Myxobacteria, a untapped bacterial strain, can produce many useful natural products which have great potential to develop into antibacterial drug [66].

5.2.2.2. *The genomics*

By the mid-1990s, pharmaceutical companies have little enthusiasm for making improvement to the existing antibacterials. Hundreds of bacterial genomes have been completely deciphered since 1995, among which are many important human pathogens, attracting large pharmaceutical companies back into antibacterial discovery [67]. Genomics influence various aspects of the antibiotic development, including new drug target identification, understanding the mechanism of antibiotic action, drug safety and efficacy assessment, bacterial resistance development, and so on [68]. Ecopia Biosciences was very skilled in using genome-scanning approach and discovered the new antibiotic scaffold ECO-0501 which is highly effective against a series of Gram-positive pathogens [59; 69]. GlaxoSmithKline also used a genomics-derived, target-based approach to screen for new drugs. They examined more than 300 genes and employed 70 high-throughput screening campaigns over a period of 7 years, but unfortunately did not create a clinical used antibacterial [70].

5.2.2.3. *New targets*

It must be admitted that target-based genomic approach has not yielded satisfactory results, nevertheless, retooled target-based strategies can still play an important role in discovery process. Most antibiotic targets are limited to peptidoglycan synthesis, ribosomal protein synthesis, folate synthesis, and nucleic acid synthesis and topoisomerization. In the future we could continue to discover new antibiotics for these old targets through improvement of the existing scaffolds or even finding new scaffolds. For instance, Lipid II is a membrane-anchored cell-wall precursor that is essential for bacterial cell-wall biosynthesis; it is not only classical target for several old antibacterial classes, but is also targeted by the new antibiotics, such as lantibiotics, mannopeptimycins and ramoplanin [71]. Grouping targets by a common inhibitor scaffold rather than by function may lead to new targets; and as mentioned above, insights from outside the antibiotic arena are also important [59].

5.2.2.4. *Forward is back*

Compared with the fruitless target-based genomic approach, traditional whole-cell assays are more effective in antibiotic discovery. Just because it is not necessary to worry about cell permeability of a novel scaffold in the development process if whole-cell assays are used. As most of the existing libraries have already been used to screen for antibacterial drugs, libraries with new chemical diversity are extremely important in this approach. Sometimes, look for libraries that don't belong to antibacterial development areas may be useful. In fact, most pharmaceutical companies of other therapeutic areas have invested considerable resources in synthesizing small molecule libraries [59]. Candidates with a strong hit in a whole-cell antibacterial assay should be tested in the right animal model early in development, because In vitro experiment results are not always reliable. For example, Antimicrobial drug target type II fatty acid synthesis (FASII) is reported to be essential for their efficacy against infections caused by multiresistant Gram-positive bacteria. But another study showed that Streptococcus agalactiae and S. aureus could take up sufficient unsaturated fatty acids from human serum to obviate the essentiality of FAS II enzymes in vivo [72].

5.2.2.5. *Focus on spectrum*

Antibacterial spectrum is a major consideration when selecting a target for lead optimization. Permeability and target distribution determine the pectrum [73]. That is to say, the drug candidates should possess two properties at the same time: one is penetrating the cell and evading efflux pump systems, another is retaining potent activity at the molecular targets. However, since almost all targets of the antibacterials in clinical use are present in all bacteria, the antibacterial drug spectra are determined largely by the ability of permeability. Therefore, some compounds are just Gram-positive organism-selective and have no effect against Gram-negative pathogens which have a second membrane acting as a permeability barrier [74; 75]. Efflux pump inhibitors (EPIs) have been explored for broadening the antibacterial spectrum and overcoming bacterial resistance. Although no clinically useful drugs have come out, extensive efforts have been made to test the effectiveness of EPIs across a range of in vitro and in vivo assays, especially the compound MC-207,110 [76].

'Broader is better' is the rule of antibacterial activity spectrum. But developing the agents with a narrower spectrum may be helpful in treating some special antibiotic resistant pathogens or the non-multiplying bacteria. One human squalene synthase inhibitor blocked staphyloxanthin biosynthesis in vitro, resulting in colorless bacteria which became more sensitive to killing by human blood and innate immune clearance [77]. Rifampicin is a standard antibiotic used for clearance of non-multiplying tuberculosis. Monoclonal antibodies (Mabs) have also become potential agents for narrow-spectrum antibacterial therapy. In clinical experiment C. difficile Mab combination MDX-066 and MDX-1388, which targets and neutralizes two main C. difficile toxins, can reduce the recurrence of C. difficile infection [78; 79]. A microbiologic diagnosis should be made before using these kinds of antibiotics for therapy. Such genus-selective agents may have the benefit of leaving more of the endogenous microfloraun unattacked compared with conventional antibiotics.

5.2.2.6. Other new methods

Bacteriophages

Bacteriophages and their fragments could kill the bacteria. They have been developed as antibacterials in humans, poultry and cattle industries, aquaculture and sewage treatment. This approach has novel mechanism of action that is completely different from current antimicrobials, but the problems are that quality control and standardization are difficult. Phage lysins, which are produced late in the viral infection cycle, can bind to cell wall peptidoglycan and rapidly induce Gram-positive bacteria lysis [80]. The sequencing of phages genomes may identify more proteins suitable for novel antibacterials [81; 82].

Other methods to find new drugs could be modulating immunity, developing monoclonal antibody for specific bacteria, designing antibacterial peptides (including antimicrobial peptides and compounds from animals and plants, the natural lipopeptides of bacteria and Fungi [83; 84]), and so on.

6. Conclusion and future issues

While the antibacterial resistance, especially multi-drug resistance continues to rise, what we should do is to investigate the potential mechanisms of drug resistance in bacteria and discover more effective antibacterials to deal with the terrible problems. Luckily there are several promising antibacterial drugs with novel mechanisms of action are in development and new types of targets have emerged. Also we need to be more precise in targeting the pathogens and limit the misuse of antimicrobials and other practices that accelerate the emergence of novel resistance mechanisms. The government must offer robust financial incentives for antibacterial R&D, and build a sustainable model for developing and using antibacterials.

Author details

Jie Yanling, Liang Xin and Li Zhiyuan

Guangzhou Institutes of Biomedicine and Health, Chinese Academy of Sciences, China

References

[1] W.J. Lindblad. Considerations for determining if a natural product is an effective wound-healing agent. Int J Low Extrem Wounds 2008;7(2):75-81.

[2] R.D. Forrest. Early history of wound treatment. J R Soc Med 1982;75(3):198-205.

[3] L.G. Nickell. Antimicrobial activity of vascular plants. Economic Botany 1959;13(4): 281-318.

[4] E.J. Bassett, M.S. Keith, G.J. Armelagos, et al. Tetracycline-labeled human bone from ancient Sudanese Nubia (A.D. 350). Science 1980;209(4464):1532-1534.

[5] M.L. Nelson, A. Dinardo, J. Hochberg, et al. Brief communication: Mass spectroscopic characterization of tetracycline in the skeletal remains of an ancient population from Sudanese Nubia 350-550 CE. Am J PhysAnthropol 2010;143(1):151-154.

[6] M. Cook, E. Molto, C. Anderson. Fluorochromelabelling in Roman period skeletons from Dakhleh Oasis, Egypt. Am J PhysAnthropol 1989;80(2):137-143.

[7] J.O. Falkinham, 3rd, T.E. Wall, J.R. Tanner, et al. Proliferation of antibiotic-producing bacteria and concomitant antibiotic production as the basis for the antibiotic activity of Jordan's red soils. Appl Environ Microbiol 2009;75(9):2735-2741.

[8] J. Clardy. Using genomics to deliver natural products from symbiotic bacteria. Genome Biol 2005;6(9):232.

[9] R.I. Aminov. A brief history of the antibiotic era: lessons learned and challenges for the future. Front Microbiol 2010;1:134.

[10] R.W. Wong, U. Hagg, L. Samaranayake, et al. Antimicrobial activity of Chinese medicine herbs against common bacteria in oral biofilm. A pilot study. Int J Oral MaxillofacSurg 2010;39(6):599-605.

[11] F. Heynick. The original 'magic bullet' is 100 years old - extra. Br J Psychiatry 2009;195(5):456.

[12] J.F. Mahoney, R.C. Arnold, A. Harris. Penicillin Treatment of Early Syphilis-A Preliminary Report. Am J Public Health Nations Health 1943;33(12):1387-1391.

[13] N.C. Lloyd, H.W. Morgan, B.K. Nicholson, et al. The composition of Ehrlich's salvarsan: resolution of a century-old debate. AngewChemInt Ed Engl 2005;44(6):941-944.

[14] J. Kimmig. [Gerhard Domagk, 1895-1964. Contribution to the chemotherapy of bacterial infections]. Internist (Berl) 1969;10(3):116-120.

[15] C. Jesman, A. Mludzik, M. Cybulska. [History of antibiotics and sulphonamides discoveries]. Pol MerkurLekarski 2011;30(179):320-322.

[16] E. Chain, H.W. Florey, A.D. Gardner, et al. THE CLASSIC: penicillin as a chemotherapeutic agent. 1940. ClinOrthopRelat Res 2005;439:23-26.

[17] N. Kardos, A.L. Demain. Penicillin: the medicine with the greatest impact on therapeutic outcomes. ApplMicrobiolBiotechnol 2011;92(4):677-687.

[18] C. Walsh. Where will new antibiotics come from? Nat Rev Microbiol 2003;1(1):65-70.

[19] R.W. Finberg, R.C. Moellering, F.P. Tally, et al. The importance of bactericidal drugs: future directions in infectious disease. Clin Infect Dis 2004;39(9):1314-1320.

[20] S.R. Palumbi. Humans as the world's greatest evolutionary force. Science 2001;293(5536):1786-1790.

[21] S.L. Bronzwaer, O. Cars, U. Buchholz, et al. A European study on the relationship between antimicrobial use and antimicrobial resistance. Emerg Infect Dis 2002;8(3): 278-282.

[22] H. Goossens, M. Ferech, R. Vander Stichele, et al. Outpatient antibiotic use in Europe and association with resistance: a cross-national database study. Lancet 2005;365(9459):579-587.

[23] A. Giedraitiene, A. Vitkauskiene, R. Naginiene, et al. Antibiotic resistance mechanisms of clinically important bacteria. Medicina (Kaunas) 2011;47(3):137-146.

[24] M.N. Alekshun, S.B. Levy. Molecular mechanisms of antibacterial multidrug resistance. Cell 2007;128(6):1037-1050.

[25] 35 years of resistance. Nat Rev Microbiol 2012;10(6):373.

[26] M.P. Doyle, F.F. Busta. Antimicrobial resistance: implications for the food system. Compr. Rev. Food Sci. Food Saf 2006;5:71-137.

[27] J.L. Martinez. Antibiotics and antibiotic resistance genes in natural environments. Science 2008;321(5887):365-367.

[28] R.I. Aminov, R.I. Mackie. Evolution and ecology of antibiotic resistance genes. FEMS MicrobiolLett 2007;271(2):147-161.

[29] D.C. Hooper. Mechanisms of fluoroquinolone resistance. Drug Resist Updat 1999;2(1):38-55.

[30] L. Adewoye, A. Sutherland, R. Srikumar, et al. The mexR repressor of the mexAB-oprM multidrug efflux operon in Pseudomonas aeruginosa: characterization of mutations compromising activity. J Bacteriol 2002;184(15):4308-4312.

[31] J. Blazquez. Hypermutation as a factor contributing to the acquisition of antimicrobial resistance. Clin Infect Dis 2003;37(9):1201-1209.

[32] A. Oliver, R. Canton, P. Campo, et al. High frequency of hypermutable Pseudomonas aeruginosa in cystic fibrosis lung infection. Science 2000;288(5469):1251-1254.

[33] I. Chopra, A.J. O'Neill, K. Miller. The role of mutators in the emergence of antibiotic-resistant bacteria. Drug Resist Updat 2003;6(3):137-145.

[34] S.B. Levy, B. Marshall. Antibacterial resistance worldwide: causes, challenges and responses. Nat Med 2004;10(12 Suppl):S122-129.

[35] P. Courvalin. Transfer of antibiotic resistance genes between gram-positive and gram-negative bacteria. Antimicrob Agents Chemother 1994;38(7):1447-1451.

[36] P. Nordmann, L. Poirel. Emerging carbapenemases in Gram-negative aerobes. Clin-Microbiol Infect 2002;8(6):321-331.

[37] G.A. Jacoby, L.S. Munoz-Price. The new beta-lactamases. N Engl J Med 2005;352(4): 380-391.

[38] S.M. Drawz, R.A. Bonomo. Three decades of beta-lactamase inhibitors. ClinMicrobiol Rev 2010;23(1):160-201.

[39] M.S. Ramirez, M.E. Tolmasky. Aminoglycoside modifying enzymes. Drug Resist Updat 2010;13(6):151-171.

[40] K. Poole. Resistance to beta-lactam antibiotics. Cell Mol Life Sci 2004;61(17): 2200-2223.

[41] F.C. Tenover. Mechanisms of antimicrobial resistance in bacteria. Am J Med 2006;119(6 Suppl 1):S3-10; discussion S62-70.

[42] S. Jana, J.K. Deb. Molecular understanding of aminoglycoside action and resistance. ApplMicrobiolBiotechnol 2006;70(2):140-150.

[43] G. Ackermann, A. Degner, S.H. Cohen, et al. Prevalence and association of macrolide-lincosamide-streptogramin B (MLS(B)) resistance with resistance to moxifloxacin in Clostridium difficile. J AntimicrobChemother 2003;51(3):599-603.

[44] B. Weisblum. Erythromycin resistance by ribosome modification. Antimicrob Agents Chemother 1995;39(3):577-585.

[45] D. Ince, X. Zhang, L.C. Silver, et al. Dual targeting of DNA gyrase and topoisomerase IV: target interactions of garenoxacin (BMS-284756, T-3811ME), a new desfluoroquinolone. Antimicrob Agents Chemother 2002;46(11):3370-3380.

[46] X.Z. Li, H. Nikaido. Efflux-mediated drug resistance in bacteria. Drugs 2004;64(2): 159-204.

[47] X.Z. Li, H. Nikaido. Efflux-mediated drug resistance in bacteria: an update. Drugs 2009;69(12):1555-1623.

[48] K.P. Langton, P.J. Henderson, R.B. Herbert. Antibiotic resistance: multidrug efflux proteins, a common transport mechanism? Nat Prod Rep 2005;22(4):439-451.

[49] M. Putman, H.W. van Veen, W.N. Konings. Molecular properties of bacterial multidrug transporters. MicrobiolMolBiol Rev 2000;64(4):672-693.

[50] J.M. Thomson, R.A. Bonomo. The threat of antibiotic resistance in Gram-negative pathogenic bacteria: beta-lactams in peril! CurrOpinMicrobiol 2005;8(5):518-524.

[51] D.M. Livermore. Multiple mechanisms of antimicrobial resistance in Pseudomonas aeruginosa: our worst nightmare? Clin Infect Dis 2002;34(5):634-640.

[52] A.H. Delcour. Outer membrane permeability and antibiotic resistance. BiochimBiophysActa 2009;1794(5):808-816.

[53] W. Achouak, T. Heulin, J.M. Pages. Multiple facets of bacterial porins. FEMS MicrobiolLett 2001;199(1):1-7.

[54] M.E. Falagas, S.K. Kasiakou. Colistin: the revival of polymyxins for the management of multidrug-resistant gram-negative bacterial infections. Clin Infect Dis 2005;40(9): 1333-1341.

[55] J.L. Mainardi, R. Legrand, M. Arthur, et al. Novel mechanism of beta-lactam resistance due to bypass of DD-transpeptidation in Enterococcus faecium. J BiolChem 2000;275(22):16490-16496.

[56] S. Triboulet, M. Arthur, J.L. Mainardi, et al. Inactivation kinetics of a new target of beta-lactam antibiotics. J BiolChem 2011;286(26):22777-22784.

[57] I.C. Gyssens. Antibiotic policy. Int J Antimicrob Ag 2011;38:11-20.

[58] T. Braine. Race against time to develop new antibiotics. Bull World Health Organ 2011;89(2):88-89.

[59] M.A. Fischbach, C.T. Walsh. Antibiotics for emerging pathogens. Science 2009;325(5944):1089-1093.

[60] G. Devasahayam, W.M. Scheld, P.S. Hoffman. Newer antibacterial drugs for a new century. Expert OpinInvestig Drugs 2010;19(2):215-234.

[61] H.C. Neu, K.P. Fu. Cefaclor: in vitro spectrum of activity and beta-lactamase stability. Antimicrob Agents Chemother 1978;13(4):584-588.

[62] G.A. Noskin. Tigecycline: a new glycylcycline for treatment of serious infections. Clin Infect Dis 2005;41Suppl 5:S303-314.

[63] P.J. Petersen, N.V. Jacobus, W.J. Weiss, et al. In vitro and in vivo antibacterial activities of a novel glycylcycline, the 9-t-butylglycylamido derivative of minocycline (GAR-936). Antimicrob Agents Chemother 1999;43(4):738-744.

[64] H. Rahman, B. Austin, W.J. Mitchell, et al. Novel anti-infective compounds from marine bacteria. Mar Drugs 2010;8(3):498-518.

[65] C.C. Hughes, W. Fenical. Antibacterials from the sea. Chemistry 2010;16(42): 12512-12525.

[66] S.C. Wenzel, R. Muller. The biosynthetic potential of myxobacteria and their impact in drug discovery. CurrOpin Drug DiscovDevel 2009;12(2):220-230.

[67] C. Freiberg, H. Brotz-Oesterhelt. Functional genomics in antibacterial drug discovery. Drug Discov Today 2005;10(13):927-935.

[68] S. Amini, S. Tavazoie. Antibiotics and the post-genome revolution. CurrOpinMicrobiol 2011;14(5):513-518.

[69] A.H. Banskota, J.B. McAlpine, D. Sorensen, et al. Genomic analyses lead to novel secondary metabolites. Part 3. ECO-0501, a novel antibacterial of a new class. J Antibiot (Tokyo) 2006;59(9):533-542.

[70] D.J. Payne, M.N. Gwynn, D.J. Holmes, et al. Drugs for bad bugs: confronting the challenges of antibacterial discovery. Nat Rev Drug Discov 2007;6(1):29-40.

[71] E. Breukink, B. de Kruijff. Lipid II as a target for antibiotics. Nat Rev Drug Discov 2006;5(4):321-332.

[72] S. Brinster, G. Lamberet, B. Staels, et al. Type II fatty acid synthesis is not a suitable antibiotic target for Gram-positive pathogens. Nature 2009;458(7234):83-86.

[73] L.L. Silver. Challenges of antibacterial discovery. ClinMicrobiol Rev 2011;24(1): 71-109.

[74] E. Andre, L. Bastide, S. Michaux-Charachon, et al. Novel synthetic molecules targeting the bacterial RNA polymerase assembly. J AntimicrobChemother 2006;57(2): 245-251.

[75] J. Wang, S. Kodali, S.H. Lee, et al. Discovery of platencin, a dual FabF and FabH inhibitor with in vivo antibiotic properties. ProcNatlAcadSci U S A 2007;104(18): 7612-7616.

[76] O. Lomovskaya, K.A. Bostian. Practical applications and feasibility of efflux pump inhibitors in the clinic--a vision for applied use. Biochemical pharmacology 2006;71(7):910-918.

[77] C.I. Liu, G.Y. Liu, Y. Song, et al. A cholesterol biosynthesis inhibitor blocks Staphylococcus aureus virulence. Science 2008;319(5868):1391-1394.

[78] I. Lowy, D.C. Molrine, B.A. Leav, et al. Treatment with monoclonal antibodies against Clostridium difficile toxins. N Engl J Med 2010;362(3):197-205.

[79] M.N. Gwynn, A. Portnoy, S.F. Rittenhouse, et al. Challenges of antibacterial discovery revisited. Ann N Y AcadSci 2010;1213:5-19.

[80] V.A. Fischetti, D. Nelson, R. Schuch. Reinventing phage therapy: are the parts greater than the sum? Nat Biotechnol 2006;24(12):1508-1511.

[81] T.D. Bugg, A.J. Lloyd, D.I. Roper. Phospho-MurNAc-pentapeptidetranslocase (MraY) as a target for antibacterial agents and antibacterial proteins. Infect Disord Drug Targets 2006;6(2):85-106.

[82] J. Liu, M. Dehbi, G. Moeck, et al. Antimicrobial drug discovery through bacteriophage genomics. Nat Biotechnol 2004;22(2):185-191.

[83] R.E. Hancock, H.G. Sahl. Antimicrobial and host-defense peptides as new anti-infective therapeutic strategies. Nat Biotechnol 2006;24(12):1551-1557.

[84] A. Makovitzki, D. Avrahami, Y. Shai. Ultrashort antibacterial and antifungal lipopeptides. ProcNatlAcadSci U S A 2006;103(43):15997-16002.

[85] S.Dzidic, J.Suskovic, B. Kos. Antibiotic resistance mechanisms in bacteria: biochemical and genetic aspects. FoodTechnolBiotechnol2008;46(1), 11-21.

[86] J.Garau, W. Wilson, M, Wood, J,Carlet. Fourth-generation cephalosporins: a review of in vitro activity, pharmacokinetics, pharmacodynamics and clinical utility.ClinMicrobiol Infect 1997;3 (Suppl 3): S87 -S101.

Chapter 11

Air, Water and Soil: Resources for Drug Discovery

Luis Jesús Villarreal-Gómez,
Irma Esthela Soria-Mercado, Ana Leticia Iglesias and
Graciela Lizeth Perez-Gonzalez

Additional information is available at the end of the chapter

http://dx.doi.org/10.5772/52659

1. Introduction

Drug discovery is the process by which new candidate drugs are discovered. The chemical compounds that are present in plants and animals have been an important source of new bioactive compounds. Also, we can found organisms that live in air, water and soil that we don`t see, but posses a great variety of chemical that we can use to create new medicines. Bioactive compounds offer an enormous diversity of chemical structures with strong biologic effect; this is one of the reasons why natural products research cannot be replaced by synthesis chemistry as a source for new bioactive compounds. Actually, more than the half of currently used medicines came from natural sources or are related to them, specifically in the situation of anticancer drugs that more than 60% belongs from nature [1].

Based on the experience in this field, it is considered that a chemical compound isolated from natural origin should be fully assessed in order to be used to combat diseases; in this manner is important to consider the type of new chemical entities potentially applicable for partial or total synthesis, as well as its use in different kind of diseases that are treatable with these compounds (2); Therefore is very important continue the search for new secondarymetabolites potentially usable as drugs by human.

2. Importance of drug discovery

The importance of look for new bioactive compounds to synthesize new drugs it's based by a main objective of saving human life that it's lose by illness. Also, it is important to recognized that the drug discovery projects, help those countries that target their efforts in this area to economically and sociality develop themselves, because when chemical compounds are discovered from microorganism that lives in natural environments, this chemical can be exploited industrially and generate more jobs.

Now, the new drugs and innovative procedures are usually able to keep people alive for a long time with better conditions that would have previously been rapidly fatal, such as cancer and end-stage heart, liver, lung, kidney, and neurologic diseases. As a result, most people in modern countries die from long-term chronic conditions that are characterized by a prolonged period of distressing symptoms and progressive loss of function.

According with World Health Organization (WHO) of *"57 million global deaths in the last report in 2008, 36 million (63%), were due to no communicable diseases (NCDs). The four main NCDs reported are cardiovascular diseases, cancers, diabetes and chronic lung diseases. The burden of these diseases is rising disproportionately among lower income countries and populations. In 2008, nearly 80% of no communicable disease deaths -- 29 million -- occurred in low- and middle-income countries with about 29% of deaths occurring before the age of 60 in these countries. The leading causes of NCD deaths in 2008 were cardiovascular diseases (17 million deaths, or 48% of all NCD deaths), cancers (7.6 million, or 21% of all NCD deaths), and respiratory diseases, including asthma and chronic obstructive pulmonary disease (4.2 million). Diabetes caused another 1.3 million deaths"* [3]. As we can see, in the WHO's statistic data, there are less number of people that die with microbial infection, it can be said to thanks to the constant development of pharmaceutical drugs.

The discovery of new bioactive compounds from microorganism present in the ambient, needs the previously determination of diversity, because by knowing the kind of microbes that live in a certain site, we can be able to design strategies and culture methods adapted for the different types of microorganism present in nature [4]. We can be able to screen chemical bioactivity only if we can culture the microorganism, because we need the microbial biomass to obtain the compounds. To culture microorganism from natural sources is not an easy topics, because, when we try to cultivate bacteria or fungi from substrates and conditions that are in constant change, and incubate them in a static temperature and nutrients; many microbes don't resist this transformation of circumstances and die.

3. Drug resistance bacteria

Some Bacteria can innately be resistant to one or more types of antimicrobial compounds and other can be capable of acquired. In actuality, it is well know the factors that provoke mutations in bacteria that create stronger species that are able to survive to the effects of currents drugs. Examples of these factors are the unnecessary use of antibiotics by humans, the use in animal feeds in low doses, availability over-the-counter in many countries, misuse by health professionals, patient failure to follow prescribed treatment, antibiotic use in agriculture, aquaria and family pets, eating raw or undercooked foods.

It can be describe several strategies of antibiotics resistance in different bacterial genera. Pathogens bacteria that have become resistant to the current antibiotic drug are an increasing public health problem. Some examples of diseases that have become very hard to treat with the current drugs are wound infections, septicemia, tuberculosis, pneumonia, and gonorrhea, to name a few. One part of the problem is that bacteria and other microbes that cause infections are remarkably adaptable and have developed several mechanisms to be immune to antibiotics and other antimicrobial drugs.

Also, it`s been reported that over-prescription and the improper use of antibiotics has led to the generation of antibiotic resistance bacteria that use to be susceptible at those antibiotics [5].

4. Mechanisms of bacteria to become antibiotics resistant

a. **Avoiding entrance of antibiotic into the bacteria cell:** Bacteria and other microbes can actually change the properties of its membrane by changing its grade of permeability by reducing the number of ion channels which are the entrance of some drugs to diffuse into the cells. Another way to get rid of antibiotics in some bacteria is use adenosine triphosphate (ATP) to obtain energy to activate this ion channels and pump it out of the cells.

b. **Editing transmembrane protein expression**: The mechanism of several antibiotics it`s to interact specifically with molecules in the membrane of the microbes and preventing it from interacting with other molecules (usually proteins) inside the cell. Some bacteria respond by changing the chemical structure or the expression of the molecule (replacing it with another molecule) so that the antibiotic can no longer recognize it or bind to it.

c. **Bacterial enzymes that destroy antibiotics:** Some bacteria can be resistant to antibiotics by neutralizing them directly. For example, some organisms may obtain new genes that encode proteins like enzymes that neutralize antibiotics agents before they get to their targets. An example of this enzymes can be found in the β–lactamases like penicillinases, cephalosporinases, carbenicillinase, cloxacilanase, carbapenamase, metalloenzyme that destroy the β-lactamics (penicillins, monobactams, carbapenems, and cephalosporins). The β–lactamases can be isolated from Gram Negative Bacteria: *Escherichia coli, Enterobacter cloacae, Citrobacter freundii, Serrati amarcescens*, and *Pseudomona aeruginosa*. The mechanism of action of β–lactamases is the breaking of β-lactam ring of the antibiotic, thus destroying the drug [6]. Other example of this is *Pseudomona sp.* erithromycinesterases that degrade erythromycin by hydrolysis of the lactone ring of erithromycin [7].

5. Cancer

Cancer is an illness that comprises more than hundred types. This disease appears when old cells are not replaced by new cells and are accumulated in a mass of tissue known as tumor" [4]. To cite some statistics data; cancer is responsible for one of every four deaths in the United States.

It's second only after heart disease as a cause of death in this country. About 1.2 million Americans were diagnosed with cancer in 1998. Of that number, more than 500,000 are expected to die of this disease. Cancer can attack anyone, but the chances of getting the disease increase with age. The most common forms of cancer are skin, lung, colon, breast and prostate cancer. Cancer is a disorder that affects the genes. There were an estimated 12.7 million cancer cases around the world in 2008, of these 6.6 million cases were in men and 6.0 million in women. This number is expected to increase to 21 million by 2030. Lung cancer is the most common cancer worldwide contributing nearly 13% of the total number of new cases diagnosed in 2008. Breast cancer (women only) is the second most common cancer with nearly 1.4 million new cases in 2008 and colorectal cancer (Figure 1) is the third most common cancer with over 1.2 million new cases in 2008 [8].

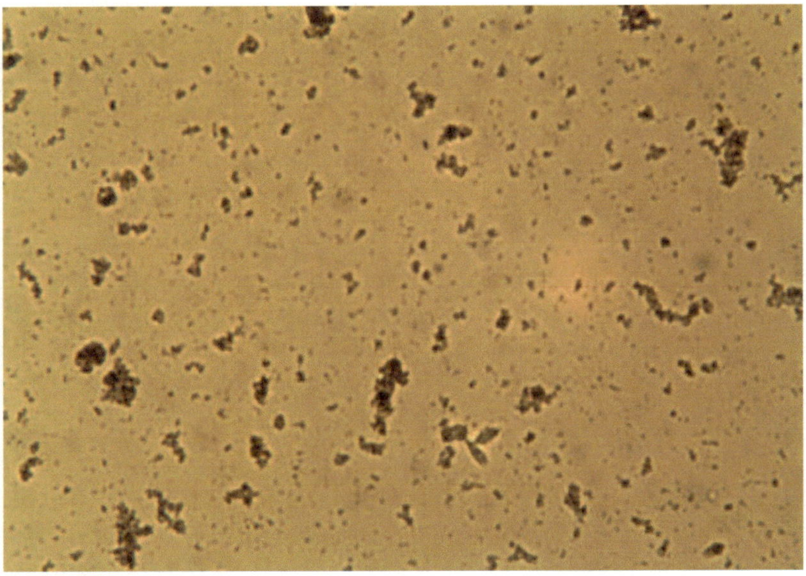

Figure 1. Cancer Colorectal HCT-116 cell culture in McCoy medium at 40 X amplification

6. Natural source for drug discovery

6.1. Drug discovery from air microorganisms

The atmosphere its well characterized for possess a good light intensity, extreme temperature variations, low concentration of organic matter and water, hence become a very hostile place for microorganism. However, there are a numerous quantity of microbes founded in the atmosphere, most of them introduced by human activity.

Bioaerosols are airborne particles that are biological in foundation. Bioaerosols can be formed from nearly any process that involves biological materials and generates enough energy to separate small particles from the larger substance, such as wind, water, air, or me-

http://dx.doi.org/10.5772/52659

chanical movement. Plants, soil, water, and animals (including humans) all serve as sources of bioaerosols and are present in most places where any of these sources live.

Microorganisms are frequently considered passive habitants of the air, dispersing via airborne dust particles (Figure 2). However, latest studies suggest that many airborne microorganisms are metabolically active, even up to altitudes of 20,000 m. Also, it has been suggested, that some airborne microbes may modify atmospheric conditions [9].

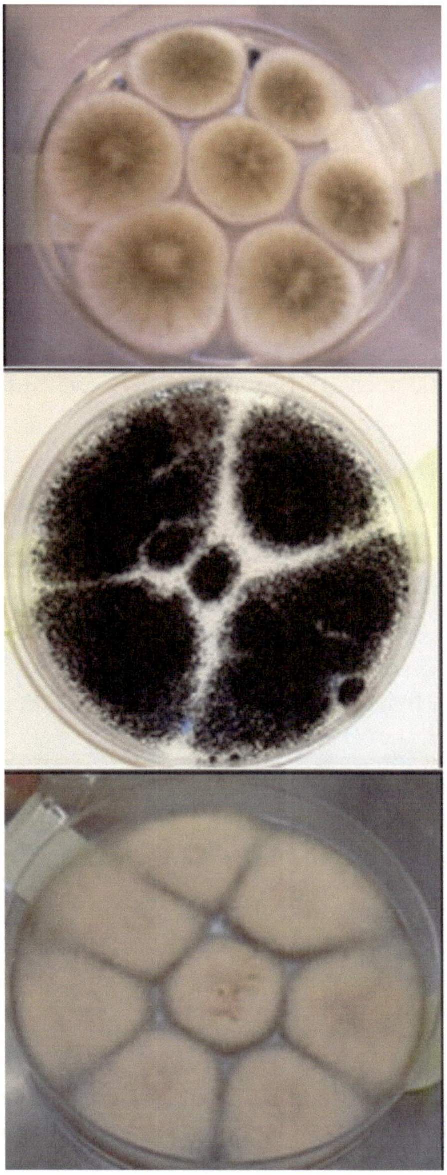

Figure 2. Fungal strains from air samples in Valle de las Palmas, Mexico.

Several studies reported a great variety of microorganism present in air samples, for example, a study realized in Mexico, in 2007, showed 21 species of bacteria founded in air samples from landfill, some of them are pathogenic and opportunistic bacteria, the most abundant are *Pasteurella haemolytica, Serratia plymuthica, Escherichia coli* y *Klebsiella pneumonia* and 19 fungal species, 7 of them allergenic, *Cladosporium herbarum, Aspergillus* sp y *Penicillium* sp. [10]. Despite this, *Serratia plymuthica*it's well known to possess 2-amino-3-(oxirane-2,3-dicarboxamido)-propanoyl-valine has been shown to inhibit the growth of the human pathogen *Candida albicans* efficiently [11].

Another studies found airborne microbes collected at indoor air with filters installed in two shopping centers in Singapore. The most common microorganism appears to be several species of *Brevundimonas* (50%) [12] other study has identified *Brevundimonas diminuta*as producer of a nematicidal metabolite known as (R)-(-)-2-ethykhexan-1-ol which have a strong activity against *C. elegans* and *B. xylophilus* [13].

6.2. Drug discovery from soil microorganisms

Soil microorganisms (Figure 3), such as bacteria and fungi, play central roles in soil fertility and promotion of plant health. It is assessed that in 1 g of soil there are 4000 different bacterial "genomic units" based on culture independent identification methods. In the other hand, an estimated 1,500,000 species of fungi, but they are more difficult to cultivated by standard methods [14].

In soil there is a constant exchange of organic substances and flow of energy. Feeding, predation, degradation of macromolecular substrates and absorption of nutrients have been important in chemical processes in soil. One of the most important microorganism in drug discovery found in natural habitat mainly in soil are the actinomycetes which are very diverse family of bacteria, they are an important source of bioactive compounds with high value in pharmaceutical industry. It's have been reported that almost 80% of the world`s antibiotics come from the genera *Micromonospora* and *Streptomyces*. Beside this, the majority of the actinomycetes in soil that are potential drug sources remain uncultivable, and therefore in cannot be screened for novel antibiotic discovery [5].

Has been reported that microorganisms found in soil are a plentiful source of chemically diverse bioactive compounds, and have been an important source for the discovery of antibacterial agents including penicillins, cephalosporins, aminoglycosides, tetracyclines, and polyketides [2].

Also, from 117 actinomycetes strains isolated from the wasteland alkaline and garden soil samples in India, were found 15 actinomycetes strain that showed antimicrobial activity against at least two pathogen bacteria between them *Staphylococcus aureus*[5].

According to reference [15], environmental factors, such as carbon and energy sources, mineral nutrients, growth factors, ionic composition, available water, temperature, pressure, air composition, electromagnetic radiation, pH, oxidation–reduction potential, surfaces, spatial relationships, genetics of the microorganisms and interaction between microorganisms, can alter the microbial diversity, activity and population dynamics of microorganisms in soil. It is important to mention that almost 80–90% of the microorganisms habiting soil are on solid surfaces [15].

http://dx.doi.org/10.5772/52659

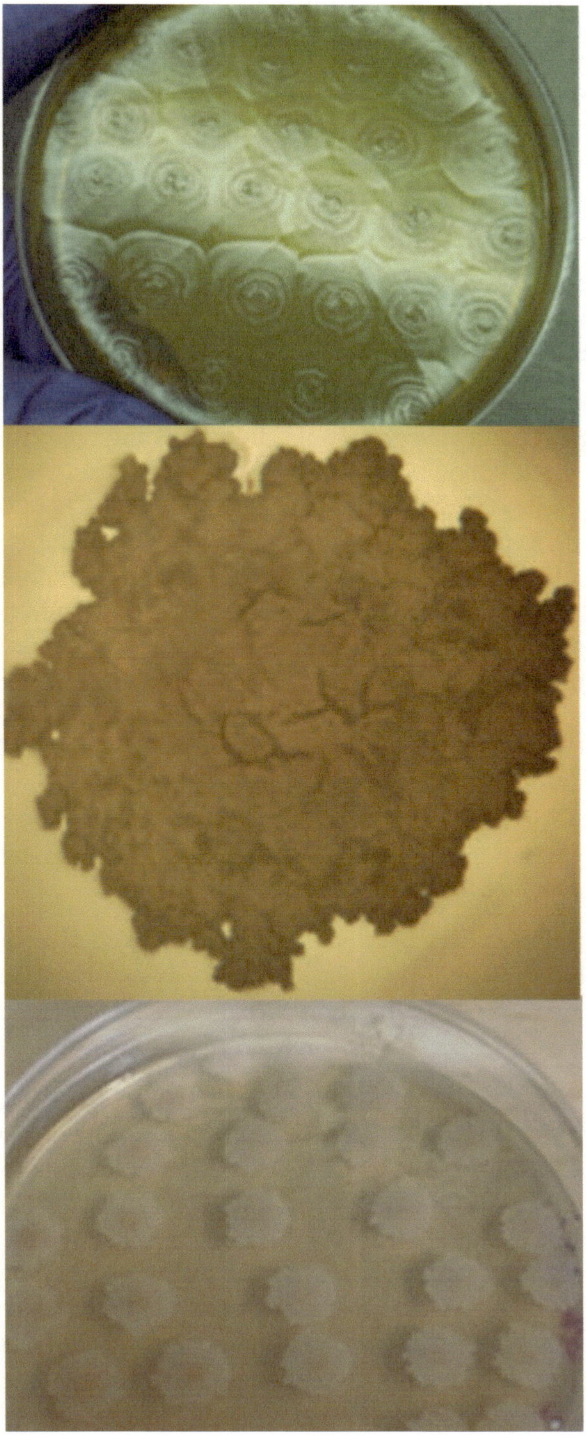

Figure 3. Bacteria strains from soil samples in Valle de las Palmas, Mexico.

6.3. Drug discovery from water microorganisms

The world's oceans comprise about 70 % of the earth's surface, where the extensive drug discovery efforts involving soil bacteria have not been extended to this ecosystem [16]. This environment have special attention since is known that typical microbial abundance of 10^6 per ml in the water column and 10^9 per ml in ocean bottom sediments. Actinobacteria is among the most dominant population and successful phyla of all environments [17]. This class takes into account 5 subclasses, 9 orders, 55 families, 240 genera and 3000 species [18].

From all actinobacteria, Marine Actinobacteria have become the most important source of secondary metabolites with medical application, such as anticancer, antibiotics, antitumor, anti-inflammatory, and antifungal compounds [16-17, 19].

Actinobacteria, called commonly actinomycetes are Gram positive bacteria having a higher guanine plus cytosine (G+C) percentage in its DNA than any other bacteria. Most of these organisms are aerobic (oxidative), some are facultative or forced anaerobes (fermentation) [20]. These microorganisms grow as networks called mycelium. They structures are filamentous. Sometimes are on the surface, for that is called aerial mycelium, or substrate mycelium if it attaches to the substrate surface [21]. The individual filaments of the mycelium or hyphae are divided into units as a result of growth of the cell wall into the hyphae at regular intervals along this structure. This process is called septation and each of the resulting septa contains one DNA molecule. The mycelium bacterium is analogous to the mycelium forming filamentous fungi [22]. Actinobacteria produce spores in specialized hyphae many of which are developed on the aerial filament, sometimes these spores are flagellated. The Actinobacteria inhabit the soil where play an important role in soil chemistry, the characteristic odor of soil is due to special metabolites that are known as Geominas [23]. Actinobacteria also inhabit aquatic environments including those marine. Actinomycetes are the most economically and biotechnologically valuable prokaryotes [24].

Almost 60 years in actinomycetes researches, more than 15000 bioactive compounds have been discovery for academic and pharmaceutical researchers many of which are used as drugs today. Fact more than half of the antibiotics discovered to date are obtained from the soil-derived actinomycete bacteria *Streptomyces* and *Micromonospora* genus spores [25].

The majority of the actinomycetes isolated from marine sources was largely of terrestrial origin and had been washed to shore and existed in the ocean as metabolically inactive spores [25]. Recently, phylogenetic analyses of the 16S rRNA genes indicate that existing new taxa widely distributed in ocean sediments [26], including some that appear to be unique and obligate marine actinomycete bacteria [27]. These strains represent the most significant source of naturally occurring microbial antibiotics [17, 28- 30] and antitumor compounds [28- 30] with specific metabolic and physiological capabilities that had not been observed in terrestrial microorganisms before [31-32]. Members of this group are producers of clinically useful antitumor drugs such as anthracyclines, glycopeptides,aureolic acids, enediynes, antimetabolites, carzinophilin, mitomycins and others [19].

The studies related with new biodiversity and drugs discovery had been examined from waters all around the world such as San Diego Bay, Bahamas, Fiji and Guam Islands among others. Recently, one study in the Gulf of California [32] found Operational Taxonomic Units (OTUs) belonging *Streptomyces* and *Actinomadura* genus and a potentially represent a new genus-level taxon in the family *Streptomycetaceae*. In addition, several previously described marine species were isolated including *Micromonospora krabiensis, Saccharomonospora marina, Streptomyces fenhuangensis, Verrucosispora maris* and *Verrucosispora sediminis* suggesting that these species may have broad geographic distributions.

The genes involved in secondary metabolism are responsible for the biosynthesis of small molecules that mediate important functional traits such as allelopathy, chemical communication and iron acquisition [33]. These compounds have been used to assess biogeographical patterns among bacteria [34].

Polyketide synthase (PKSI) genes are called Type I and are responsible for the production of many important secondary metabolites including the antibiotic erythromycin [35] and the anticancer agent epothilone [35-36].

Bacteria can maintain complex assemblies of PKS genes [37], many of which are not expressed under normal laboratory conditions [38]. Recently, a study found that HGT plays an important role in the evolution of PKSI genes and that ketosynthase (KS) domains within polyketide synthase genes are phylogenetically important making predictions about production of secondary metabolites by complex biosynthetic pathways [39-40]. Other method used for providing further evidence for endemism associated with secondary metabolites [33], is the terminal restriction fragment length polymorphism (T-RFLP) used to demonstrate that subpopulations of bacteria cluster together based on collection site [41].

According to [32] targeting KS domains provides a rapid method to assess PKS diversity and novelty within individual strains. The results revealed evidence of common pathways shared with other *Salinispora* strains but also sequences that share low levels of identity with any characterized pathways and thus may be associated with the production of new secondary metabolites. It is noteworthy that the new sequence type "L" also possesses a KS sequence that has not previously been observed in "*S. pacifica*".

Secondary metabolites are linked to an organism's fitness and therefore represent an emerging marker to study population structure and function, taxonomically meaningful patterns of secondary metabolite production have been detected in bacteria [42] and fungi [43].

Progress has also been made in drug discovery from actinomycetes by using high throughput screening and fermentation, metabolic profiling technologies, genome scanning, mining genomes for cryptic pathways, and combinatorial biosynthesis to generate new secondary metabolites related to existing pharmacophores [17, 44]. Metagenomic screening of DNA from environmental samples [45-46] provides an alternative way of discovering new antibiotic biosynthetic genes.

According to [47] recently published new web tools that provide automated methods to assess the secondary metabolite gene diversity; those are the Natural Product Domain Seeker (NaPDoS) analysis based on the phylogenetic relationships of sequence tags derived from polyketide synthase and non-ribosomal peptide synthethase (NRPS) genes. These results are compared with an internal experimentally database. NaPDoS provides a rapid mechanism used to infer the generalized structures of secondary metabolites biosynthetic gene richness and diversity within a genome or environmental sample by extract and classification of ketosynthase and condensation domains from PCR products, genomes, and metagenomic datasets increasing exponentially the investigations in this field of science with benefits in the field of drug discovery.

Table 1 shows a list of microorganisms isolated from different sources which produce antioxidant, antibacterial, anticoagulant, antiviral, anti-inflammatory, immune system, antidiabetic and nematicidal activities, as well as their action mechanisms.

Microorganism	Bioactive Compounds	Bioactivity	Mechanism	Reference	Natural Source
Brevundimonas diminuta	(*R*)-(-)-2-ethylhexan-1-ol	Nematicidal	Inhibitor against *C. elegans* and *B. xylophilus*	[48]	Air
Pasteurella haemolytica	A1-Derived Leukotoxin and Endotoxin	Inmune system	Induce Intracellular Calcium Elevation in Macrophages	[49]	Air
Streptomyces strain PM0324667	NFAT-133	Antidiabetic	induced glucose uptake in L6 skeletal muscle cells	[50]	Soil
Clostridium cellulolyticum	Closthioamide	Antibiotic	*Staphylococci* Multiresistente inhibition	[51]	Soil
Gordonia sputi DSM 43896	G48 JF905613 Compound	Antimicrobial	*C. albicans, S. aureus* inhibition	[52]	Soil
Actinomycetes	3Ba3 Compound	Antibacterial	E. amylovora, P. viridiflova, A. tumefaciens, B. subtilis ATCC 663, E. coli ATCC 29998 3 inhibition	[53]	Soil
Micromonospora sp.	Diazepinomicin/ ECO-4601	Antimicrobial	Unespecific	[54]	Soil
Eurotium Herbariorum	*E. Herbariorum* NE-4	Antioxidant	Antioxidant *in vitro*	[55]	Water
Sponge	Batzelladine L y M	Antibacterial	*S. aureus* and methicillinresistant, *S. aureus* inhibition	[56]	Water
Bivalve mollucs	Anticoagulant polypeptide (TGAP)	Anticoagulant	Inhibition of factor II tolla conversion	[56]	Water
Fungus	8′-O-Demethylnigerone	Antituberculosis	M. tuberculosis inhibition	[56]	Water
Algae	Dolabelladienetriol	Antiviral	Inhibition of HIV-1 replication	[56]	Water
Soft coral	Durumolides A-C	Anti-inflammatory	Modulation of LPS-activated murine macrophage cell line	[56]	Water
Sea cucumber	Frondoside A	Immune system	Lysosomal activity, phagocytosis and ROS activation	[56]	Water

Table 1. Microorganism isolated from natural sources that produce bioactive compounds

http://dx.doi.org/10.5772/52659

7. Conclusion

Bioactive compounds isolated from aerial, terrestrial and marine organisms have extensive past and present use in the treatment of many diseases and serve as compounds of interest both in their natural form and as templates for synthetic modification. To found new compounds useful to develop new pharmaceutical drugs, a good potential source and diverse bioactive chemicals is microorganism present in natural sources as air, soil and water.

Chemical compounds from natural sources are the major protagonists in chemical diversity for pharmaceutical discovery over the past century. The interesting chemicals identified as natural products are derived from the biodiversity in which the interactions between microbial entities and their environment formulate the diverse complex chemical entities within the organisms that enhance their survival and competitiveness. Hence, it is important to study inter and intraspecific interactions between microorganism in natural environments, this will make the screening for bioactive compounds in microbes easier.

Microbial interactions can influence the secretion of bioactive compound. Has been reported, various types of contacts among bacterial species and other organism. For example, these relations can be negative (parasitism, competition and predation) or positive (metabiosis and symbiosis) for these microorganisms. Between interactions in microorganism we can emphasize competition. Some bacteria are reduced by different species when the environmental resources are limited; therefore they produce compounds that impress negatively in their competitors [4].

Finally, air, soil and water are the home of microorganism that compete all the time to survive, resist changes in temperature, pressure, nutrient, carbon and nitrogen content, microorganisms that are obligated to produce weapons against predators, change and mutate to scape of detection of other microbes. All this, are the reason why we can find an unimaginable number and variety of chemical that are effective to be part of a pharmaceutical drug formulation.

Author details

Luis Jesús Villarreal-Gómez[1*], Irma Esthela Soria-Mercado[2], Ana Leticia Iglesias[3] and Graciela Lizeth Perez-Gonzalez[3]

*Address all correspondence to: luis.villarreal@uabc.edu.mx

1 Center of Engineering and Technology, University Autonomous of Baja California, Tijuana, BC., México

2 Marine Science Faculty, University Autonomous of Baja California, Ensenada, BC., México

3 Center of Engineering and Technology, University Autonomous of Baja California, Tijuana, BC., México

References

[1] Gordaliza M. Los compuestos naturales en el descubrimiento de fármacos. Institut ode Estudios de la Ciencia y la Tecnología. Universidad de Salamanca. 2009. http:// gredos. usal. es/jspui/bitstream/10366/22600/1/DQFA_Compuestosnaturales.pdf.

[2] Chin Y-W, Balunas MJ, Chai HB, Kinghorn AD. Drug Discovery from Natural Sources. AAPS Journal. 2006; 8(2): E239-E253. DOI: 10. 1208/aapsj080228.

[3] World Health Organization. Global Health Observatory (GHO). 2008. http://www. who. int/gho/ncd/mortality_morbidity/en/index. html.

[4] Soria-Mercado IE, Villarreal-Gómez, LJ, Guerra-Rivas, G, Ayala-Sánchez, NE. Bioactive Compounds from Bacteria Associated to Marine Algae. Biotechnology. Molecular Studies and Novel Application for Improved Quality of Human Life INTECH. 2012; 3: 25-44.

[5] Kumar N, Singh RK, Mishra SK, Singh AK, Pachouri UC. Isolation and screening of soil Actinomycetes as source of antibiotics active against bacteria. International Journal of Microbiology Research. 2010; 2(2): 12-16.

[6] Tenover FC. Mechanisms of Antimicrobial Resistance in Bacteria. The American Journal of Medicine. 2006; 119(6A): 53-510.

[7] Kim YH, Cha CJ, Cerniglia CE. Purification and Characterization of an erythromycin esterase from an erythromycin-resistant Pseudomonas sp. FEMS Microbiology Letters. 2012; 210: 239-244.

[8] http://www. wcrf. org/cancer_statistics/world_cancer_statistics. php.

[9] Bowers RM, Lauber CL, Wiedinmyer C, Hamady M, Hallar AG, Fall R, Knight R, Fierer N. Characterization of Airborne Microbial Communities at a High-Elevation Siteand Their Potential To Act as Atmospheric Ice Nuclei. Applied and Environmental Microbiology. 2009; 75 (15): 5121–5130.

[10] Flores-Tena FJ, Pardave LM, Valenzuela-Cárdenas IC. Estudio Aerobiológico de la Zona Aledaña al Relleno Sanitario "San Nicolás", Municipio de Aguascalientes. Investigacióny Ciencia. 2007; 37: 13-18.

[11] Sammer UF, Völksch B, Möllmann U, Schmidtke M, Spiteller P, Spiteller M, SpitellerD. 2-Amino-3-(Oxirane-2,3-Dicarboxamido)-Propanoyl-Valine, an Effective PeptideAntibiotic from the Epiphyte Pantoea agglomerans 48b/90. 2009; Applied Enviromental Microbiology. 1-30. doi:10. 1128/AEM. 01244-09.

[12] Tringe SG, Zhang T, Liu X, Yu Y, Lee WH, Yap J, Yao F, Suan ST, Ing SK, Haynes M, Rohwer F, Lin Wei C, Tan P, Bristow J, Rubin EM, Ruan Y. The Airborne Metagenomein an Indoor Urban Environment. PLoS ONE. 2008; 3(4): e1862. doi:10. 1371/journal. pone. 0001862.

[13] Zheng L, Li G, Wang X, Pan W, Li L, Lv H, Liu F, Dang L, Mo M, Zhang K. Nematicida lendophytic bacteria obtained from plants. Annals of Microbiology. 2008; 58 (4): 569-572.

[14] Kirk JL, Beaudettea LA, Hartb M, Moutoglisc P, Klironomosb JN, Lee H, Trevors JT. Methods of studying soil microbial diversity. Journal of Microbiological Methods. 2004; 58:169– 188.

[15] Nannipieri P, Ascher J, Ceccherini MT, Landi L, Pietramellara G, Renella G. Microbial diversity and soil functions. European Journal of Soil Science. 2003; 54: 655–670. doi: 10. 1046/j. 1365-2389. 2003. 00556. x

[16] Fenical W, Jensen PR. Developing a new resource for drug discovery: marine actinomycete bacteria. Natural Chemical Biology. 2006; 2(12): 666-673.

[17] Bull AT, Stach JEM. Marine actinobacteria: new opportunities for natural product search and discovery. Trends Microbiology. 2007; 15:491–499.

[18] Goodfellow M. Selective isolation of actinobacteria. In: Manual of industrial microbiology and biotechnology, 3rd edn. Baltz RH, Davies J, Demain AL (volume eds) Section1: Isolation and screening of secondary metabolites and enzymes, Bull AT, Davies JE (section eds). ASM Press, Washington, DC, 2010. pp 13–27.

[19] Olano C, Méndez C, Salas JA. Antitumor compounds from actinomycetes from geneclusters to new derivatives by combinatorial synthesis. Natural Products Report. 2009b;. 26:628–660.

[20] Logan N. Bacterial systematic. Blackwell scientific publications, oxford. 1994; pp. 272.

[21] Torres-Beltrán M, Cardoso-Martínez F, Millán-Aguiñaga N, Becerril-Espinosa A, Soria-Mercado IE. Evaluation of the Gulf of California as a potential source of bioactive marine actinobacteria. *Ciencias Marinas* (2012), 38(4):1CM DOI:10. 7773/cm. v38i4. 2131.

[22] Nathan A, Magarvey KJM, Bernan V, Dworkin M. Isolation and characterization ofnovel marine-derived Actinomycete taxa rich in bioactive metabolites. Applied Environmental Microbiology. 2004; 70:7520–7529.

[23] Bull AT, Ward AC, Goodfellow M. Microbiology and Molecular Biology Reviews. 2000; 64:573-604.

[24] Jemimah N, Mohana-Srinivasan SV, Subathra-Devi C. Novel anticancer compounds from marine actinomycetes: A Review Journal of Pharmacy Research. 2011; 4(4): 1285-1287. ISSN: 0974-6943.

[25] Goodfellow M, Haynes JA. In Bilogical, Biochemical, and Biomedical Aspects of Actinomycetes; Ortíz-Ortíz, L., Bojalil, L. F., Yakoleff, V., Editorals. Academic Press: Orlando. 1984. Pp 453-472.

[26] Mincer TJ, Jensen PR, Kauffman CA, Fenical, W. Widespread and persistent populations of a major new marine actinomycetes taxon in ocean sediments. Applied Environmental Microbiology. 2002. 68:5,005–5, 2011.

[27] Feling RH, Buchanan GO, Mincer TJ, Kauffman CA, Jensen PR, Fenical W. SalinosporamideA: A Highly Cytotoxic proteasome inhibitor from a novel microbia lsource, a marine bacterium of the new genus Salinospora. Angewandte Chemie International Edition 2003; 42(3) 355-357.

[28] Bhatnagar I. Immense essence of excellence: Marine microbial compounds, Mar. Drugs. 2008; 8, 2673-2701.

[29] Soria-Mercado IE, Prieto-Davó, A, Jensen PR, Fenical W. Antibiotic Terpenoid-Chloro Dihydroquinones from a new Marine Actinomycete. Journal of Natural Products. 2005; 68: 904-910.

[30] Strohl WR. In Microbial Diversity and Bioprospecting. Antimicrobials. Edited by BullAT. ASM Press; 2004; 336-355.

[31] Blunt JW, Copp BR, Munro MH, Northcote PT, Prinsep MR. Marine natural products. Natural Products Reports. 2006; 23: 26-78.

[32] Magarvey NA, Keller JM, Bernan V, Dworkin M, Sherman DH. Isolation and characterization of novel marine-derived actinomycete taxa rich in bioactive metabolites. Applied Environmental Microbiology. 2004; 70:7520-7529.

[33] Becerril-Espinosa A. Actinobacterias aisladas del sedimento marino del Golfo de California y de Bahía Todos Santos: diversidad, bioactividad y dominios cetosintetasa. PhD Dissertation, Universidad Autónoma de Baja California, México. 2011. 114 pp.

[34] Wawrik B, Kutliev D, Abdivasievna UA, Kukor JJ, Zylstra GJ, Kerkhof L. Biogeography of Actinomycete Communities and Type II Polyketide Synthase Genes in Soils Collected in New Jersey and Central Asia. Applied Environmental Microbiology. 2007; 73(9):2982. DOI:10. 1128/AEM. 02611-06.

[35] Freel KC, Edlund A, Jensen PR. Microdiversity and evidence for high dispersal rates in the marine actinomycete"*Salinispora pacifica*". Enviromental Microbes. 2012; 14(2): 480-493.

[36] Cortes J, Haydock SF, Roberts GA, Bevitt DJ, Leadlay PF. An unusually large multifunctional polypeptide in the erythromycin-producing polyketide synthase of *Saccharopolyspora erythraea*. Nature. 1990; 348: 176–178.

[37] Bollag DM, McQueney PA, Zhu J, Hensens O, Koupal L, Liesch J. Epothilones, a new class of microtubule-stabilizing agents with a taxol-like mechanism of action. Cancer Research. 1995; 55: 2325-2333.

[38] Fischbach MA, Walsh CT. Assembly-line enzymology for polyketide and nonribosomal peptide antibiotics: logic, machinery, and mechanisms. Chemistry Reviews. 2006;106:3468–3496.

[39] Bentley SD, Chater KF, Cerdeno-Tarraga AM, Challis GL, Thomson NR, James KD. Complete genome sequence of the model actinomycete Streptomyces coelicolor A3(2). Nature. 2002; 417: 141–147.

[40] Ginolhac A, Jarrin C, Robe P, PerriËre G, Vogel T, Simonet P, Nalin R. Type I polyketidesynthases may have evolved through horizontal gene transfer. Journal of Molecular Evolution. 2005; 60: 716–725.

[41] Gontang EA, GaudÍncio S, Fenical W, Jensen PR. Sequence-based analysis of secondary-metabolite biosynthesis in marine actinobacteria. Applied Environmental Microbiology. 2012; 76:2487–2499.

[42] Edlund A, Loesgen S, Fenical W, Jensen PR. Geographic distribution of secondary metabolite genes in the marine actinomycete *Salinispora arenicola*. Applied Environmental Microbiology. 2011; 77:5916–5925.

[43] Jensen PR, Williams PG, Oh DC, Zeigler L, Fenical W. Species-specific secondary metabolite production in marine actinomycetes of the genus Salinispora. Applied Environmental Microbiology. 2007; 73:1146–1152.

[44] Larsen TO, Smedsgaard J, Nielson KF, Hansen ME, Frisvad JC. Phenotypic taxonomyand metabolite profiling in microbial drug discovery. Natural Products Reports. 2005; 22:672–695.

[45] Baltz RH. Renaissance in antibacterial discovery from actinomycetes. Current Opinion in Pharmacology 2008; 8:557–563.

[46] Handelsman J. Soils—the metagenomics approach. In: Bull AT (ed) Microbial diversity and bioprospecting. ASM Press, Washington, 2004; pp 109–119.

[47] Schloss PD, Handelsman J. Metagenomics for studying unculturable microorganisms: cutting the Gordian knot. Genome Biology. 2005; 6:229–232.

[48] McAlpine JB, Banskota AH, Charan RD, Schlingmann G, Zazopoulos E, Piraee M, Janso J, Bernan VS, Aouidate M, Farnet CM, Feng X, Zhao Z, Carter GT. Biosynthesis of Diazepinomicin/ECO-4601, a *Micromonospora* Secondary Metabolite with a Novel Ring System. Journal of Natural Products. 2008; 71, 1585–1590.

[49] Zheng L, Li G, Wang X, Pan W, Li L, Lv H, Liu F, Dang L, Mo M, Zhang K. Nematicidal endophytic bacteria obtained from plants. Annals of Microbiology. 2008; 58 (4) 569-572.

[50] Mayer AMS, Rodríguez AD, Berlinck RGS, Fusetani N. Marine compounds with antibacterial, anticoagulant, antifungal, anti-inflammatory, antimalarial, antiprotozoal, antituberculosis, and antiviral activities; is affecting the immune and nervous system, and other miscellaneous mechanisms of action. Comparative Biochemistry and Physiology, Part C. Marine pharmacology in 2007–8: 2011; 153 191–222.

[51] Kulkarni-Almeida AA, Brahma MK, Padmanabhan P, Mishra PD, Parab RR, Gaikwad NV. Fermentation, Isolation, Structure, and antidiabetic activity of NFAT-133 produced by Streptomyces strain PM0324667. AMB Express. 2011; 21;1(1):42.

[52] Lincke T, Behnken S, Ishida K, Roth M, Hertweck C. Closthioamide: an unprecedented polythioamide antibiotic from the strictly anaerobic bacterium *Clostridium cellulolyticum*. Angewandte Chemie International Edition. 2010; 8; 49(11):2011-3. Air, Water and Soil: Resources for Drug Discovery http://dx. doi. org/10. 5772/52659.

[53] Lee LH, Cheah YK, Sidik SM, Ab Mutalib NS, Tang YT, Lin HP, Hong K. Molecular characterization of Antarctic actinobacteria and screening for antimicrobial metabolite production. World Journal Microbiology Biotechnology. 2012; 28:2125–2137.

[54] Oskay M, Üsame Tamer A, Azeri C. Antibacterial activity of some actinomycetes isolated from farming soils of Turkey. African Journal of Biotechnology. 2004; 3 (9): 441-446.

[55] Ziemert N, Podell S, Penn K, Badger JH, Allen E, Jensen PR. The Natural Product Domain Seeker NaPDoS: A Phylogeny Based Bioinformatic Tool to Classify Secondary Metabolite Gene Diversity. Plos one/www.plosone. org: 2012; 7(3): e34064. 9 pp.

[56] Miyake Y, Ito C, Itoigawa M, Osawa T. Antioxidants produced by *Eurotium herbariorum* of filamentous fungi used for the manufacture of karebushi, dried bonito (Katsuobushi). Bioscience Biotechnology and Biochemistry. 07/2009; 73(6):1323-7.

[57] Hsuan SL, Kannan MS, Jeyaseelan S, Y. S. Prakash, G. C. Sieck, and S. K. Maheswaran. *Pasteurella haemolytica*A1-Derived Leukotoxin and Endotoxin Induce Intracellular Calcium Elevation in Bovine Alveolar Macrophages by Different Signaling Pathways. Infection and Immunity. 1998; 66(6): 2836–2844.

Chapter 12

Transition State Analogues of Enzymatic Reaction as Potential Drugs

Karolina Gluza and Pawel Kafarski

Additional information is available at the end of the chapter

http://dx.doi.org/10.5772/52504

1. Introduction

All chemical transformations pass through an unstable structure called the transition state, which is poised between the chemical structures of the substrates and products. The transition states for chemical reactions are proposed to have lifetimes near 10^{-13} sec, the time for a single bond vibration. Thus, the transition state is the critical configuration of a reaction system situated at the highest point of the most favorable reaction path on the potential-energy surface, with its characteristics governing the dynamic behavior of reacting systems decisively. It is used primarily to understand qualitatively how chemical reactions take place.

Yet transition state structure is crucial to understanding enzymatic catalysis, because enzymes function by lowering activation energy. Linus Pauling coiled an accepted view, that incredible catalytic rate enhancements caused by enzyme is governed by tight binding to the unstable transition state structure in 1948. Because reaction rate is proportional to the fraction of the reactant in the transition state complex, the enzyme was proposed to increase the concentration of these reactive species. This proposal was further formalized by Wolfenden (1972) and coworkers, who hypothesized that the rate increase imposed by enzymes is proportional to the affinity of the enzyme to the transition state structure relative to the Michaelis complex.

Transition state structures of enzymatic targets for cancer, autoimmunity, malaria and bacterial antibiotics have been explored by the systematic application of kinetic isotope effects and computational chemistry. Today the combination of experimental and computational access to transition-state information permits the design of transition-state analogs as powerful enzymatic inhibitors and exploration of protein features linked to transition-state structure.

Molecular electrostatic potential maps of transition states serve as blueprints to guide synthesis of transition state analogue inhibitors of chosen enzymes. Substances, that ideally mimic geometric and electrostatic features of a transition state (or other intermediates of high energy) are considered as excellent enzyme inhibitors (Fig.1). They bind up to 10^8 times tighter than substrate. Thus, the goal of transition-state analogs design is to create stable chemical structures with van der Waals geometry and molecular electrostatic potential surfaces as close as possible to those of the transition state.

Although some reviews on the subject have been published, this concept has not been reviewed in detail [Wolfenden, 1999; Robertson, 2005; Schramm, 2005; Schramm, 2007; Dybała-Defratyka et al. 2008; Schramm, 2011]. In this review the current trends, alongside with appropriate case studies in designing of such inhibitors will be presented.

2. Choice of the target enzyme

The sequencing of the human genome has promised a revolution in medicine. The genome encodes 20,000- 25,000 human genes, and thousands more proteins as a result of alternative gene splicing. Many of these hold the keys to treating disease, especially numerous enzymes of undefined so far physiologic functions [Gonzaga-Jagureui et al., 2012]. Out of 1200 registered drugs over 300 act as enzyme inhibitors. Most of them are simple analogs of substrates of certain enzymatic reaction. Analogy to transition state as a mean to obtain effective inhibitors emerged in 1970s [Lienhard, 1973]. Through the 1970s and 1980s, most of the known examples were natural products [Wolfenden, 1976]. The situation has changed in 1990s when synthetic inhibitors became the predominate examples of transition-state inhibitors. In 1995, there were transition-state analogues for at least 130 enzymes [Radzicka & Wolfenden, 1995].

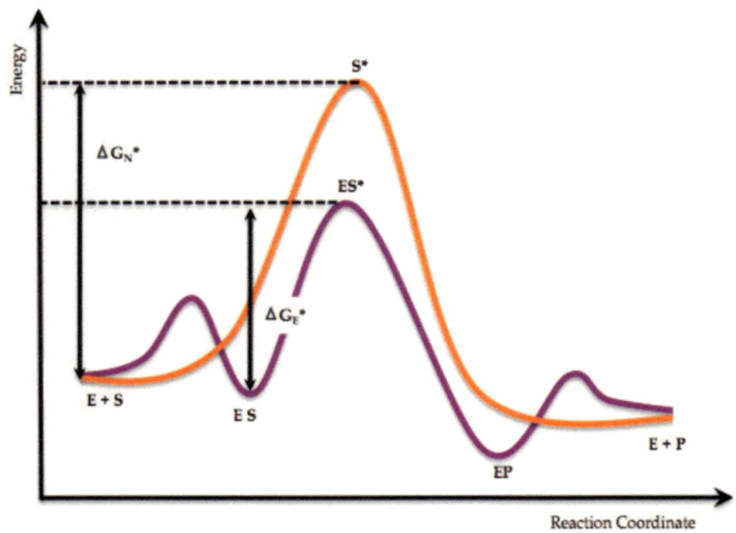

Figure 1. Progress of the enzymatic reaction versus uncatalyzed one.

The design of transition-state inhibitors is likely to become more frequent in the future, alongside with the development of theory and technology for understanding enzyme transition states. Today the sequence of information required to obtain transition state analog of enzymatic reaction considers: choice of the suitable enzyme (most likely suited to kinetic isotope effect measurement), selection of presumable mechanism(s) of catalyzed reaction, measurement of kinetic isotope effects (KIE), computer-aided calculations matching the intrinsic KIEs, construction of steric and electronic map of transition state and synthesis of stable compound(s) matching this map [Schramm, 2007]. This procedure has been developed gradually in parallel with the advances in KIE enzymology, computational chemistry, and synthetic organic chemistry.

3. Determination of transition state architecture

At present, the most reliable method to determine three-dimensional architecture of transition state is through the use of computational methods in conjunction with experimentally measured kinetic isotope effect (KIE).

Isotopic substitution is a useful technique for probing reaction mechanisms. The change of an isotope may affect the reaction rate in a number of ways, providing clues to the pathway of the reaction. The advantage of isotopic substitution is that this is the least disturbing structural change that can be effected in a molecule. Replacement of one isotope of the substrate by another at vicinity where bonds are being or re-hybridizing typically leads to a change in the rate of the reaction. Thus, kinetic isotope effects measurements compare k_{cat}/K_M values between isotope-labeled and natural abundance reactants. This provides information about which bonds are broken or formed, and identifies changes in hybridization that occur during the rate limiting step of a reaction. It is reached by conversion of atom-by-atom KIE values to a specific static model with fixed bond angles and lengths by computational matching to a quantum chemical model of the reaction of interest. Substrate, intermediate and product geometries are located as the global minima. Transition-state structures are located with a single imaginary frequency, characteristic of true potential energy saddle points.

Such an analysis was performed recently for human thymidine phosphorylase, an enzyme responsible for thymidine homeostasis, action of which promotes angiogenesis. Thus, inhibitors of this enzyme might be considered as promising anticancer agents. Its transition state was characterized using multiple kinetic isotope effect measurements applying isotopically (^{3}H, ^{14}C and ^{15}N) enriched thymidines, which were synthesized enzymatically [Schwartz et al, 2010]. A transition state constrained to match the intrinsic KIEs was found using density functional theory. In the proposed mechanism (Fig.2), departure of the thymine results in a discrete ribocation intermediate. Thymine likely leaves deprotonated at N1 and undergoes enzyme-catalyzed protonation before the next step. In the following step, the intermediate undergoes nucleophilic attack from an activated water molecule to form the products. The latter step is a reaction rate limiting step as determined by energetics of its transition state.

The transition state model predicts that deoxyribose adopts a mild 3′-*endo* conformation during nucleophilic capture (Fig. 2).

Such studies, although cumbersome and difficult, are being recently more and more popular, as demonstrated by representative studies on *Escherichia coli t*-RNA-specific adenosine deaminase [Luo & Schramm, 2008], glucoside hydrolases [Lee et al, 2004], human purine nucleoside phosphorylase [Murkin et al., 2007], *Trypasnosoma cruzi trans*-sialidase [Pierdominici-Sottile et al., 2011], *L*-dopa decarboxylase [Lin & Gao, 2011] or *cis*-prenyltransferase [Hu et al., 2010].

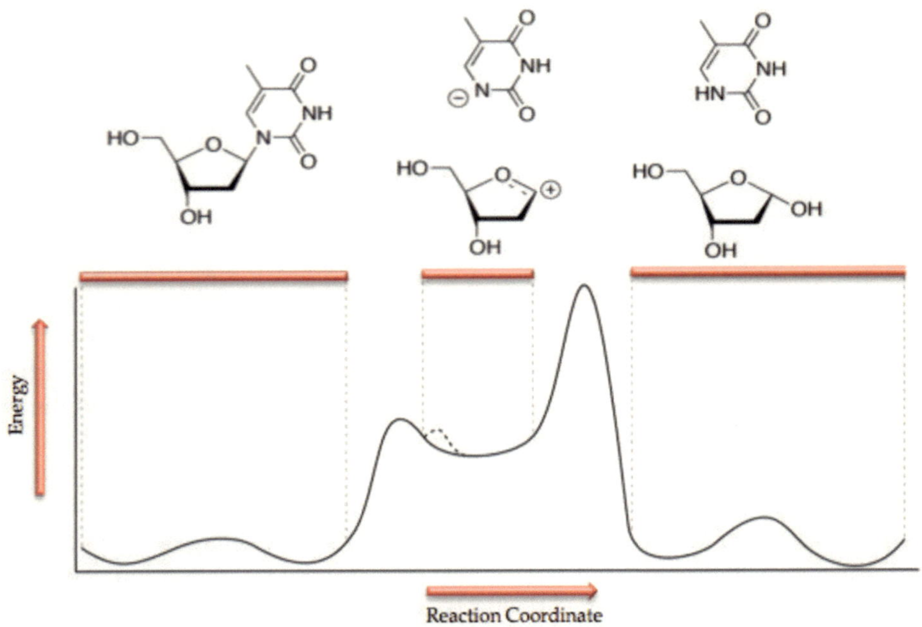

Figure 2. Mechanism of human thymidine phosphorylase catalyzed depirymidation of thymidine. The dash line represents protonation step.

Computational chemistry provides techniques for the generation and exploration of the multi-dimensional energy surfaces that govern chemical reactivity. Therefore, energy minima and saddle points can be located and characterized. The pathways that interconnect them can be determined. Thus, computational methods are increasingly at the forefront of elucidating mechanisms of enzyme-catalyzed reactions, and shedding light on the determinants of specificity and efficiency of catalysis [Kollman et al., 2002; Parks et al., 2010; Williams, 2010; Lonsdake et al., 2012].

At the beginning of a molecular modeling study choice upon the specific catalytic process to model has to be undertaken. This decision may sound simple, but it includes the nontrivial task of exhaustively searching the literature to determine what is already known about the selected enzymatic system, either from experiments or from previous computational studies. Reaction mechanisms may have already been proposed in the literature, and thus provide a logical starting point for modeling studies. The three-dimensional structure of the enzyme, preferably with a bound substrate analog, reaction product or inhibitor, is among the most critical sources of information. In practice, this usually means that a high-resolution X-ray crystal structure of a reacting enzyme complex is required.

Molecular mechanics methods are important in simulations of enzymes, even though these methods cannot model chemical reactions. For that molecular dynamics simulations, or combination of molecular mechanics with quantum mechanical methods are commonly used [Senn & Thiel, 2007; Hou & Cui, 2011; Kosugi & Hayashi, 2012; Londsdale et al., 2012]. Enzymes are large molecules consisting of thousands of atoms whereas the active site may comprise only around 100 atoms. Since quantum chemical calculations are nowadays affordable only for up to a few hundred atoms (depending on the level of accuracy) the system is split into two regions: a small region encapsulating the reaction at the active site is modeled with a quantum mechanical methods, while the rest of the enzyme alongside with surrounding water is modeled using molecular mechanics (Fig. 3.)

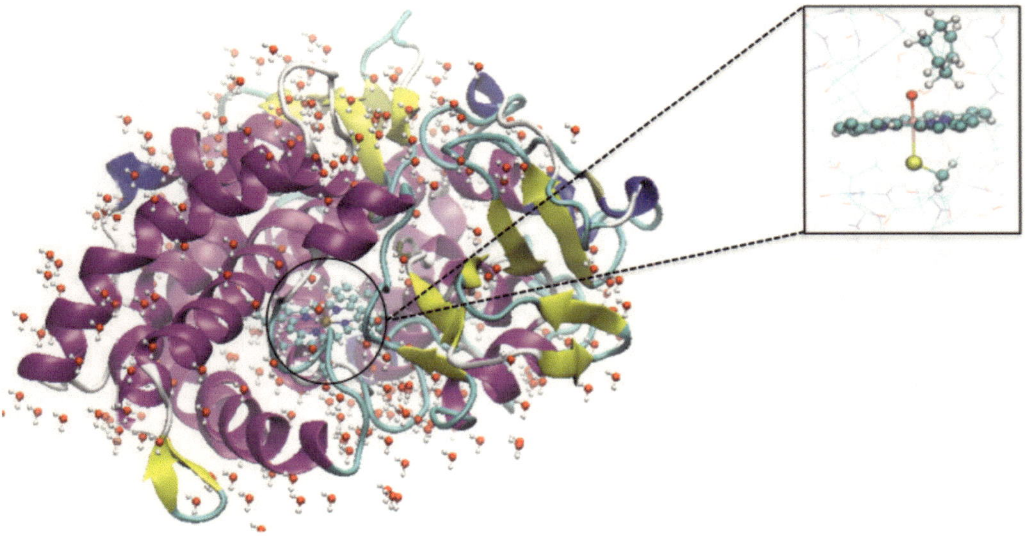

Figure 3. Quantum mechanics/molecular mechanics calculation of an enzymatic reaction illustrated by cytochrome P450 with bound cyclohexene [Lonsdake et al., 2010].

These calculations do not take in the consideration such an important factor as protein dynamic. There is an agreement that fast (at nano- or picosecond scale) protein motions couple directly to transition state formation in enzymatically catalyzed reactions and are an integral part of the reaction coordinate. Slower protein dynamic motions also influence the heights of barriers in enzymatic reactions, however detailed description of these effects require elaboration of new computational methods [Saen-oon et al., 2008].

4. Inhibitors of proteinases

First inhibitors being transition state analogs were designed for proteolytic enzymes. The design was based on the resemblance of transition state of phosphonamidates and phosphonic, phosphinic (Fig. 4) acids to the sp^3 intermediate of the hydrolysis of peptide bond. Because the lengths of oxygen-to-phosphorus and carbon-to-phosphorus bonds are significantly longer than the corresponding carbon-to-carbon and carbon-to-oxygen bonds, organophosphorus fragment of the molecule might be considered as "swollen" tetrahedral intermediate and thus can be treated similar to the transition state of this reaction.

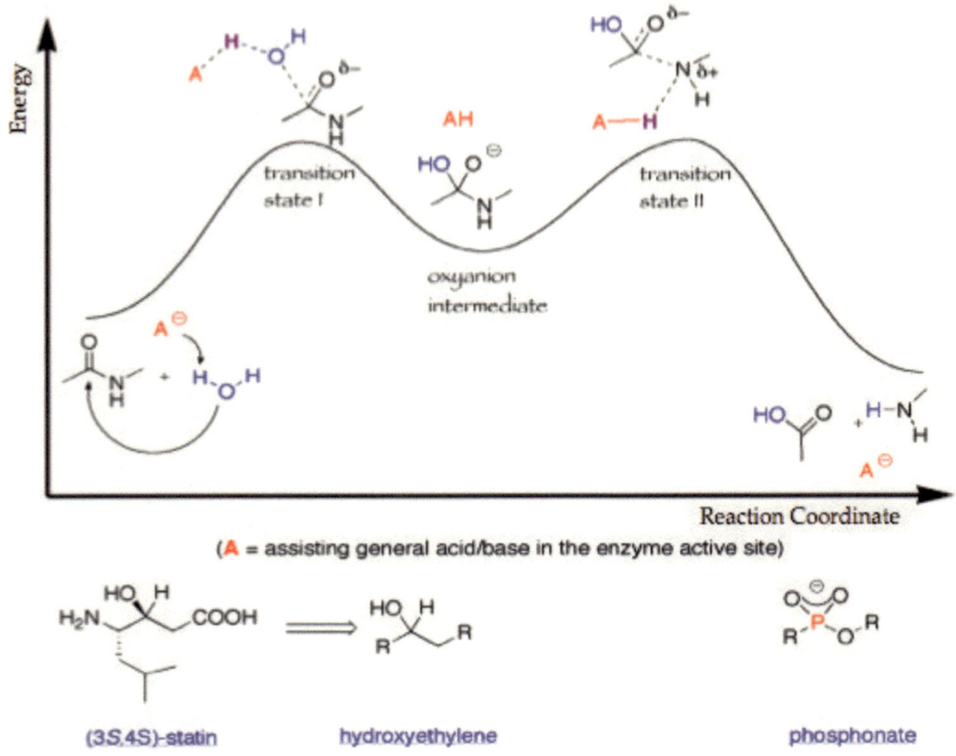

Figure 4. Organophosphoprus compounds as transition state analog inhibitors of hydrolysis of peptide bonds.

Crystallography of enzyme-inhibitor complexes and molecular modeling studies had shown that their potent inhibitory activities result from both: resemblance to the transition state and strong electrostatic interactions between positively charged active-site metal ions (predominantly zinc ions) and negatively charged phosphonic acid (or related) group [Mucha et al., 2010; Mucha et al., 2011]. Although the phosphonate/phosphinate group is a rather weak zinc complexing moiety, it offers other advantageous structural and electronic features [Collinsova & Jiráček, 2000].

http://dx.doi.org/10.5772/52504

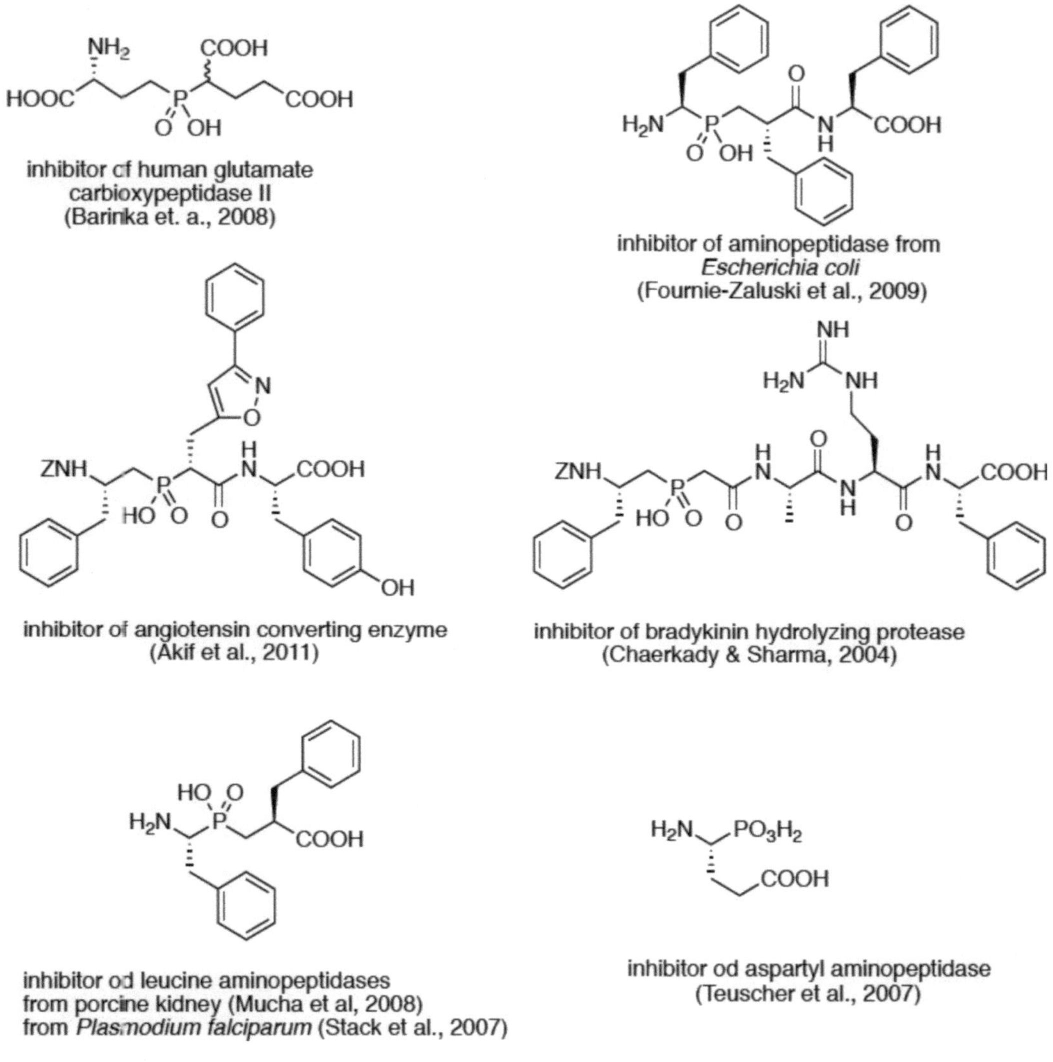

Figure 5. Representative organophosphorus inhibitors of metalloproteinases.

Simple phosphonic acid analogs of amino acids and pseudopeptides, containing phosphinate moiety replacing scissile peptide bond, are acting via this mechanism and rank amongst most potent inhibitors of metalloproteinases (Fig. 5). Inhibitors of neutral alanyl (M1) and leucine (M17) aminopeptidases are among the most recognized and most intensively studied representatives of metal-containing exopeptidases of biomedical significance [Lowther & Matthews, 2002; Grembecka et al., 2003; Vassiliou et. al. 2007]. Functions related to tumorigenesis and invasion makes these enzymes molecular targets for the development of potential anticancer drugs [Grembecka & Kafarski, 2001; Zhang & Xu, 2008; Fournié-Zaluski et al., 2009; Grzywa et al., 2010]. The recognized role of neutral aminopeptidase in the pathogenesis of hypertension provides also an opportunity for regulating arterial blood pressure by their inhibitors [Banegas et al., 2006; Bodineau et al., 2008]. Additionally, two of these pseudodipeptides appear to be excellent inhibitors when applied to *Plasmodium falciparum* M1 and M17 aminopeptidases (Fig. 5), the protozoan counterparts of neutral and leucine aminopeptidases [Stack et al., 2007; Cunningham et al, 2008; McGowan et al., 2009; McGowan et al., 2010]. They efficiently controlled the growth of *P. falciparium* in cultures, including those of malaria cells lines resistant to chloroquine, and significantly reduced malaria infections in murine model (*Plasmodium chabaudi*) [Skinner-Adams et al., 2007]. These findings positively validated *P. falciparum* M1 and M17 aminopeptidases as promising targets for a novel treatment of malaria and identify new leads with anti-parasite potential [Skinner-Adams et al., 2010; Thivierge et al., 2012].

The design and development of pseudopeptidic inhibitors of aminopeptidases are greatly facilitated by two factors. First, the results of extensive structure-activity relationship studies, available for a wide collection of fluorogenic substrates, have defined the requirements of the S1 binding pockets of these enzymes [Drag & Salvesen, 2009; Drag et al., 2010; Gajda et al., 2012; Poręba et al., 2011; Poręba 2012]. Second, computer-aided analysis of numerous crystal structures available for leucine aminopeptidase has pointed to this enzyme as a primary molecular target for extending and optimizing interactions within the S1′ pocket [Grembecka et al., 2001; Jørgensen et al., 2002; Evdokimov et al., 2007; Khandelwal et al., 2005; Khaliullin et al. 2010; Li et al., 2010].

Phosphinic pseudopeptides have also clearly revealed their potential for the regulation of matrix metalloproteinases (MMPs, matrixins), zinc-dependent endopeptidases implicated in the breakdown of the extracellular matrix [Yiotakis at al., 2004; Fisher & Mobashery, 2006]. Cleavage of the matrix component (collagen, lamanin, elastin, gelatin, etc.) is physiologically essential for tissue remodeling processes such as morphogenesis, embryogenesis and reproduction [Overall & Kleifield, 2006; Sang et. al., 2006]. Overexpression or inadequate level of matrix metalloproteinases leads to pathological states such as osteoarthritis, rheumatoid arthritis and inflammation, but it is most associated with tumor growth, invasion, and metastasis. Angiogenetic process favored by these enzymes is essential for vascoularization and growth of tumors. Thus, they were the first proteinase targets seriously considered for combating cancer. Despite that preliminary clinical/preclinical studies on MMP inhibition in tumor models brought positive results the outcome in the drug market has been so far unsatisfactory. The spectacular failure of the last-step clinical trials is mainly due to a lack of selectivity and serious side effects [Fisher & Mobashery, 2006]. The field is now resurging with careful reinvestigation of the precise roles of each particular MMP member and a focus on the development of selective inhibitors that fully discriminate between different members of the MMP family [Reiter et al., 2003; Matziari et al., 2007; Zucker & Cao, 2009; Devel et al., 2010; Johnson et al., 2011]. Such selectivity had been reached by variation of peptide scaffold by means of combinatorial pseudopeptide synthesis [Buchardt et al, 2000; Dive et al., 2004] or by application of molecular modeling based on crystallographic studies of these enzymes [Rao, 2005; Pirard, 2007; Verma & Hansch, 2007; Anzellotti & Farrell, 2008; Kalva et al., 2012]. Representative selective inhibitors of this class are shown in Figure 6.

http://dx.doi.org/10.5772/52504

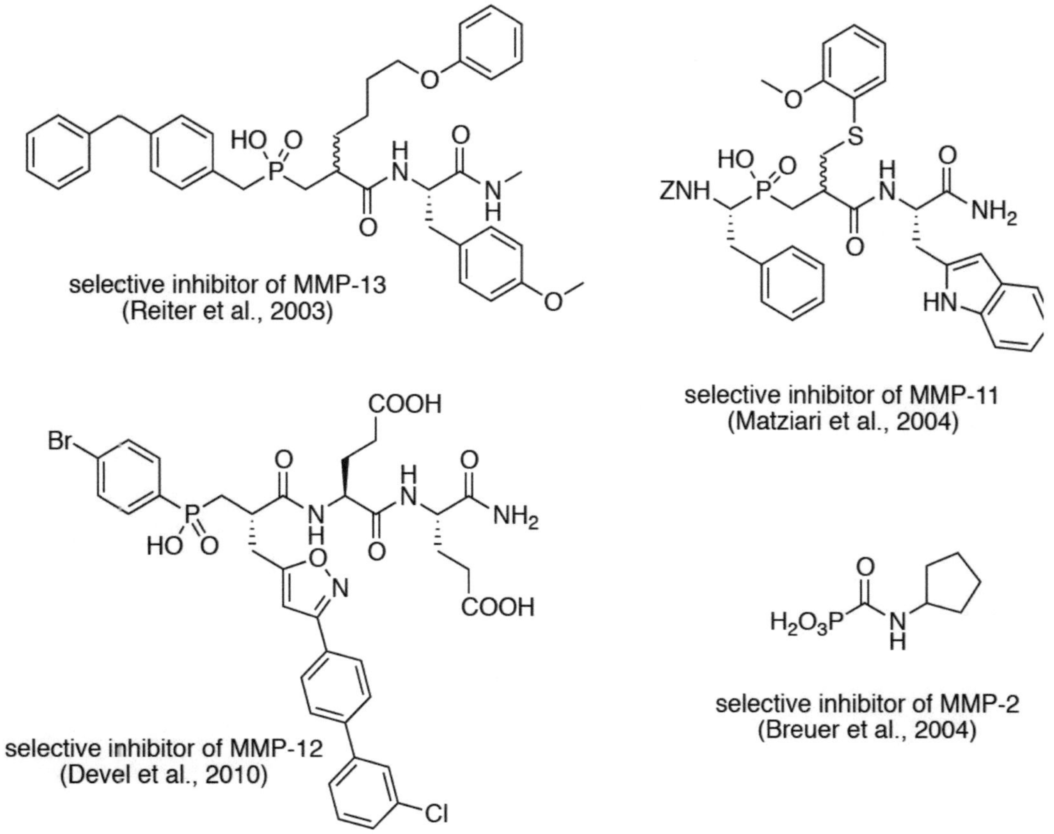

Figure 6. Representative inhibitors selective against chosen matrix metalloproteinases.

Quite interesting approach is preparation of hybrid systems as this composed of a phosphinate transition state analogue that has been incorporated within a triple-helical peptide template. The template sequence was based on the $\alpha1(V)436$-450 collagen region, which is hydrolyzed at the Gly_{439}-Val_{440} bond selectively by MMP-2 and MMP-9. In that manner highly selective inhibitor towards these two gelatinases was found [Lauer-Fields et al., 2007; Lauer-Fields et al., 2008].

Phosphinic transition state analog approach has been also recently applied for the design and synthesis of novel potent inhibitors of other proteinases of medicinal importance. Thus, inhibitors of angiotensin converting enzyme [Mores et al., 2008; Julien et al. 2010; Akif et al., 2011] are potential drugs against hypertension, aspartyl aminopeptidase as antimalarial agent [Teuscher et al., 2007], inhibitors of cathepsin C and renal dipeptidase may be considered as potential anticancer agents [Gurulingappa et al., 2003: Mucha et al., 2004], inhibitors of sortase, which is bacterial virulence protein [Kruger et al., 2004], whereas inhibition of pyroglutamyl peptidase II enhances the analeptic effect of thyrotropin [Matziari et al., 2008; Lazcano et al. 2012].

It is worth mentioning that *Monopril®*, the sodium salt of fosinopril [Fig. 7], the ester prodrug of an angiotensin-converting enzyme (ACE) inhibitor fosinoprilat, is perhaps one of the most effective implementation of transition state analogy in medicine [Powell et al., 1984].

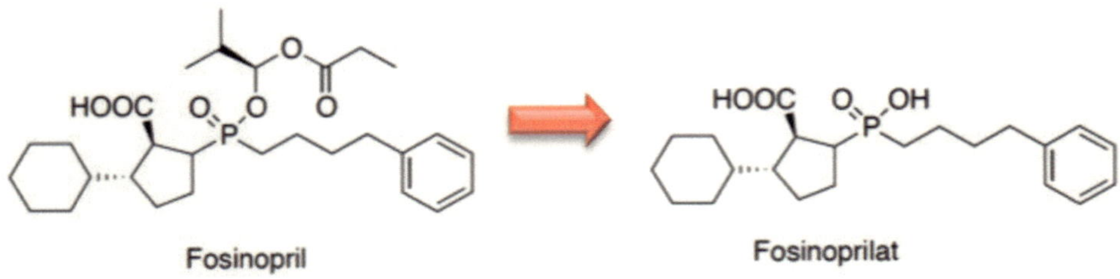

Figure 7. Fosinopril and fosinoprilat.

Sulfonamides also mimic both shape and electronic environment of the transition state of peptide bond hydrolysis. This approach was used for introduction of transition state inhibitors of HIV-protease, thermolysin and thrombine as well as haptens for generation of catalytic antibodies (Fig. 8) [Moree, et al., 1993; Moree, et al., 1995; Löwik et al., 2000; Liskamp & Kruijzer, 2004; Turcotte et al., 2012]. Unfortunately most of them appeared to be ineffective. This might be explained by non-typical bonding of potent inhibitor of this class with HIV protease (Fig. 9). It appeared that sulfonamide moiety displaces water molecule from active site and forms hydrogen bonds with two isoleucines, not as expected with catalytic aspartic acids [Meanwell, 2011]. Thus, sulfonamide group does not act as transition state analogue.

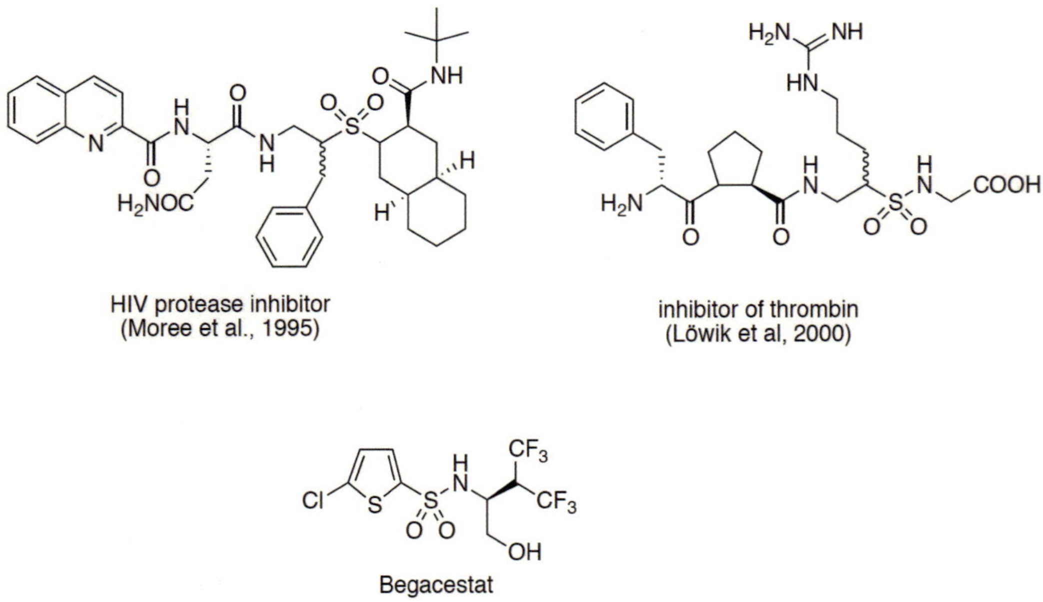

Figure 8. Sufonamides as inhibitors of proteases.

http://dx.doi.org/10.5772/52504

Begacestat (Fig. 8), an effective and potent inhibitor of γ-secretase is an exception here [Mayer et al., 2008; Martone et al., 2009]. γ-Secretase catalyzes the final step in the generation of amyloid β peptides from amyloid precursor protein. Amyloid β-peptides aggregate to form neurotoxic oligomers, senile plaques, and congophilic angiopathy, some of the cardinal pathologies associated with Alzheimer's disease. Begacestat appeared to be well tolerated in mouse and dog toxicity studies and has been advanced to human clinical trials for the treatment of this neurological disease.

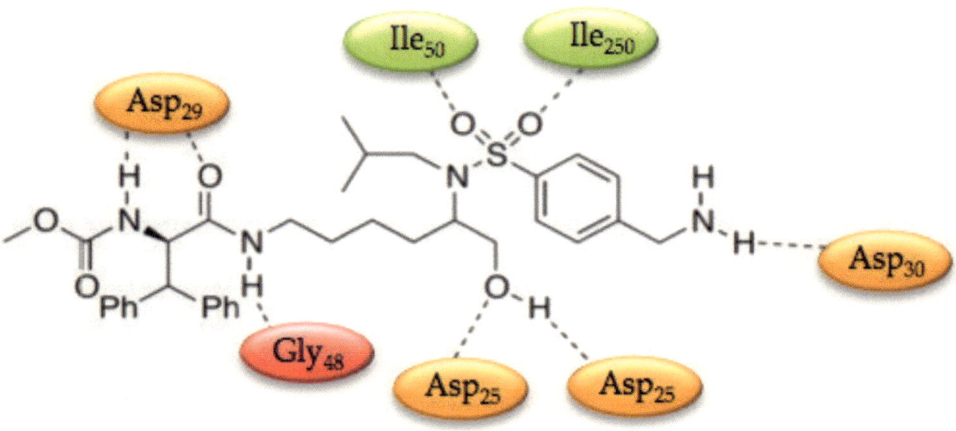

Figure 9. Mode of binding of sulfonamide HIV protease inhibitor.

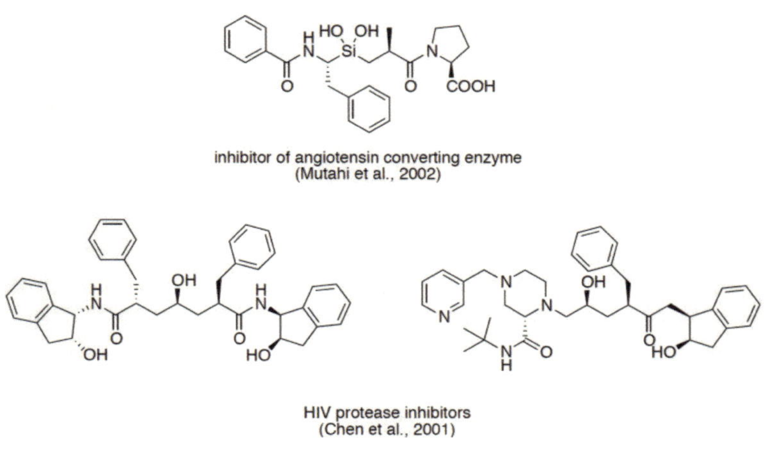

Figure 10. Si enediols as proteinase inhibitors.

Dialkylsilanediols are tetrahedral functional groups that can mimic hydrated carbonyls and thus might be also considered as „swollen" intermediates of peptide bond hydrolysis. When silanediols are embedded in a peptide-like structure, they are recognized by proteinases and act as hydrolytically stable entities. Thus, dialkylsilanol is an effective functional group for the design of active site-directed protease inhibitors. This concept has been successfully tested by replacing the presumed tetrahedral carbon of thermolysin, HIV-protease and angiotensin converting enzyme substrates with silanediol groups (Fig. 10), which resulted in potent inhibitors of these enzymes [Juers et al., 2005; Sieburth & Chen, 2006; Bo et al., 2011; Meanwell, 2011].

5. Hydroxyethylene intermediate analogs as inhibitors of proteases

Aspartic proteases generally bind 6-10 amino acid regions of their polypeptide substrates, which are typically processed with the aid of two catalytic aspartic acid residues in the active site. Thus, there is usually considerable scope for building inhibitor specificity for a particular aspartic protease by taking advantage of the collective interactions between a putative inhibitor on both sides of its scissile amide bond, and a substantial portion of the substrate-binding groove of the enzyme [Eder et al., 2007]. A very effective group of their inhibitors are simple hydroxyethylene analogs of tetrahedral oxyanion intermediates of the hydrolysis of peptide bonds. This approach is based on the structure of bestatin, a general inhibitor of aminopeptidases and aspartyl proteinases isolated in 1976 from *Streptomyces olivoreticuli* [Umezawa et al., 1976].

Today, HIV protease inhibitors constitute around 40% of available drugs against HIV. Nearly all of them contain hydroxyethylene unit as transition state analog mimic, to mention only Darunavir, Atazanavir, Fosamprenavir, Lopinavir (or Ritonavir) or the oldest one Saquinavir (Fig. 11) [Brik & Wong, 2003; Pokorna et. al, 2009].

Availability of anti-HIV drugs enabled to introduce highly active antiretroviral therapy (HAART), which resulted in dramatic decrease of the mortality and morbidity for a wide variety of opportunistic viral, bacterial, fungal and parasitic infections among HIV-infected individuals in economically developed countries [Andreoni & Perno, 2012]. Thus, the design, development and clinical success of HIV protease inhibitors represent one of the most remarkable achievements of molecular medicine. However, both the academias, as well as, the industry need to continue in their effort to develop novel, more potent compounds. This is mainly connected with HIV drug resistance, which in turn results from the high mutation rate, caused by the lack of proofreading activity of the viral reverse transcriptase. The pattern of mutations associated with the viral resistance is extremely complex as shown in Figure 12 [Pokorna et al., 2009]. Taken together, in spite of the indisputable success of the HAART and benefit to patients, new approaches to the antiviral treatment are highly desirable [Clarke, 2007; Adachi et al., 2009; Pokorna et al., 2009; Alfonso & Mozote, 2011].

Quite interestingly, small modifications of core structure of the inhibitor results in minute changes in inhibitor affinity to HIV protease as demonstrated in Figure 13 [Wu et al., 2008; Mahalingham et al., 2010].

Studies conducted in order to evaluate the influence of these antiviral drugs on the development of parasites, which are known to co-infect HIV-positive individuals, surprisingly

http://dx.doi.org/10.5772/52504

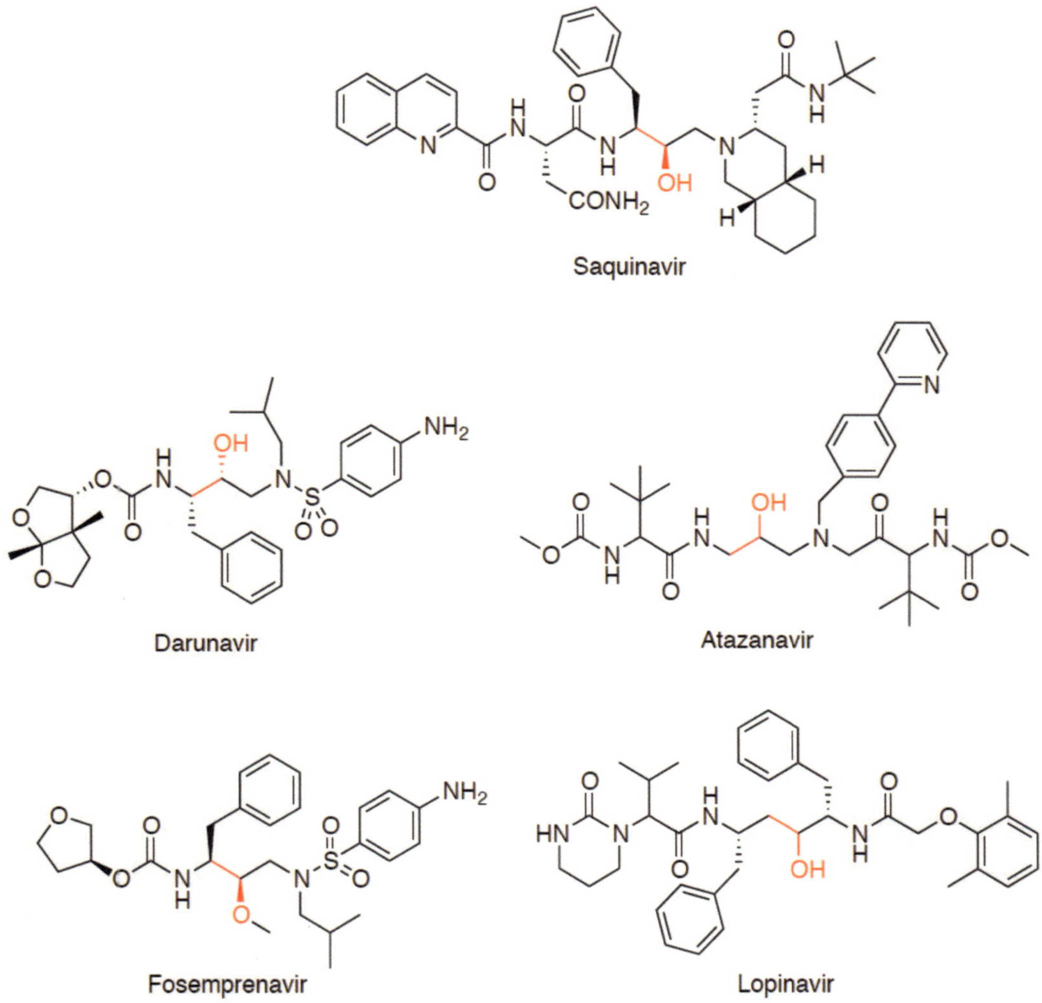

Figure 11. Representative examples of clinical HIV protease drugs.

shown, that these drugs exhibit marked antiprotozoal activity. For example Saquinavir, Lopinavir, Indinavir directly inhibited the grown of *Plasmodium falciparum* in vitro at clinically relevant concentrations. This findings suggest that some inhibitors of HIV protease are active against the most virulent human malaria parasite *P. falciparum* that is known to express number of aspartic proteases (plasmepsins) [Skinner-Adams, et al., 2004; Alfonso & Mozote, 2011].

More than 25 million people are suffering from dementia, and the annual socioeconomic worldwide costs have been estimated to exceed U.S. $200 billion. γ-Secretase, along with β - secretase produces the amyloid β-protein of Alzheimer's disease. Because of its key role in the pathogenesis γ-secretase has been a prime target for drug discovery, and many inhibitors of this protease have been developed. These enzymes are also effectively inhibited by

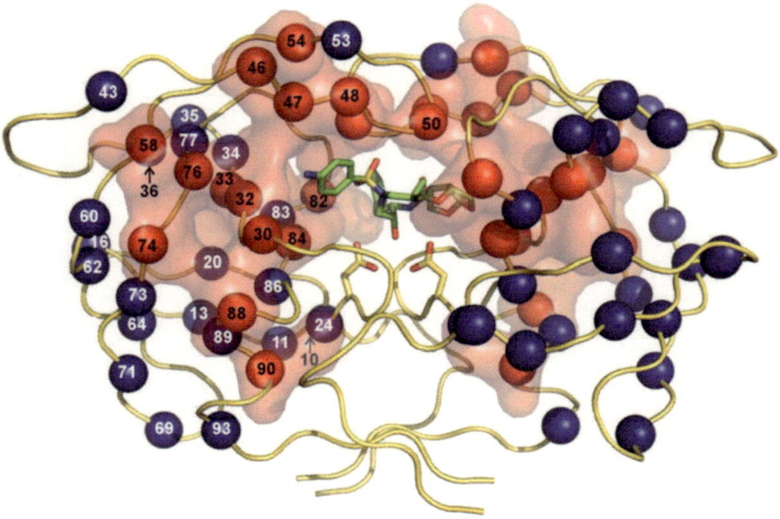

Figure 12. Three-dimensional structure of HIV protease complexed with Darunavir. Mutations associated with resistance to clinically used inhibitors are depicted as balls.

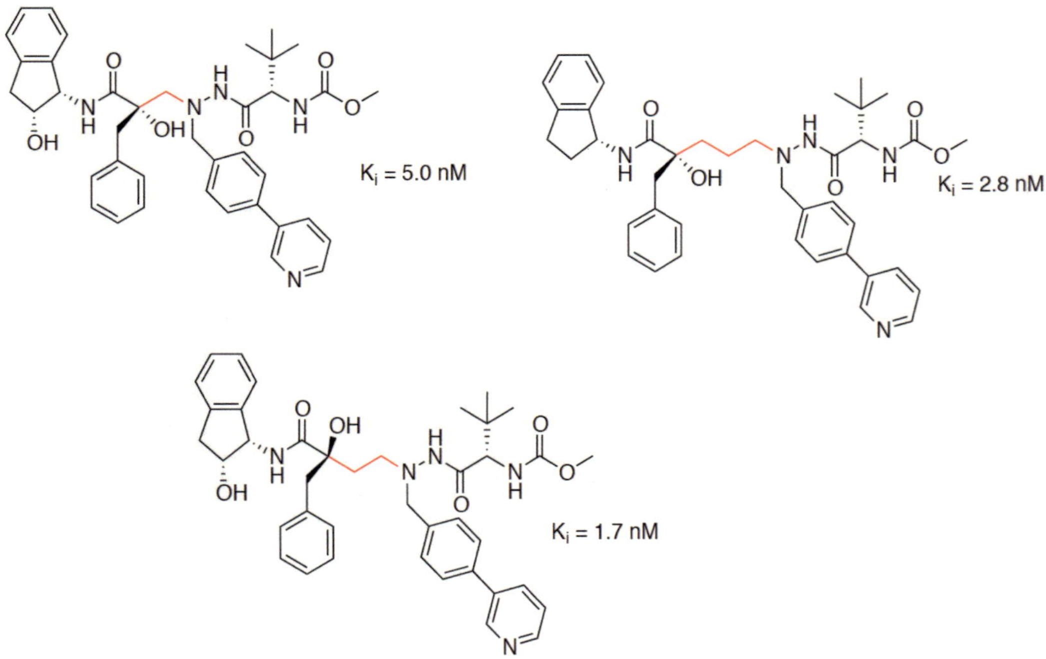

Figure 13. Influence of linker length on activity of HIV protease inhibitors.

http://dx.doi.org/10.5772/52504

peptidomimetics containing hydroxyethylene fragment replacing hydrolyzed peptide bond. Only one drug (Semagacestat, Fig. 14) reached phase III clinical studies so far, however, uncovered evidence of cognitive worsening in treated patients compared with placebo led to suspension of the trials in 2010. Anyway, design, synthesis and evaluation of new low-molecular, nanomolar inhibitors of secretases, structure of which significantly drifted away from peptidic transition state analogs (Fig. 14), is still challenging and brought new promising results [Osterman et al., 2006; Wolfe, 2012]. Due to rapid technological progress in chemistry, bioinformatics, structural biology and computer technology, computer-aided drug design plays more and more important role in this respect [Avram et al., 2006; Fujimoto et al., 2008; Xu et al., 2009; Al-Tel et al. 2011; Hamada et al., 2012].

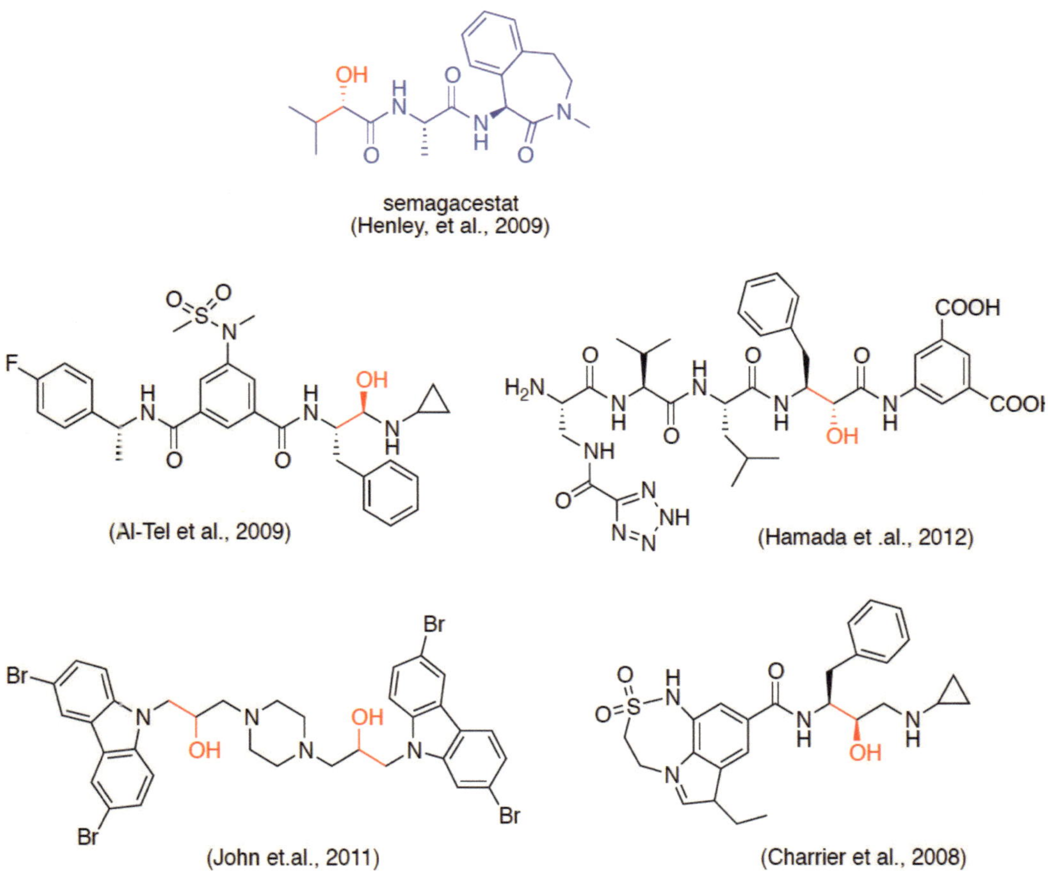

Figure 14. Inhibitors of secretases.

Hypertension is a major risk factor for cardiovascular diseases such as stroke, myocardial infarction, and heart failure, the leading causes of death in the Western world. Inhibitors of the renin–angiotensin system have proven to be successful treatments for hypertension. As renin specifically catalyses the rate limiting step of this system, it represents the optimal target for antihypertensive drugs. Aliskiren (Fig. 15), a promising drug lowering blood pressure in sodium-depleted marmosets and hypertensive human patients, was developed using a combination of crystal structure analysis of renin–inhibitor complexes and computational methods [Wood et al., 2003]. The therapy was introduced under the names Takturna and Rasilez.

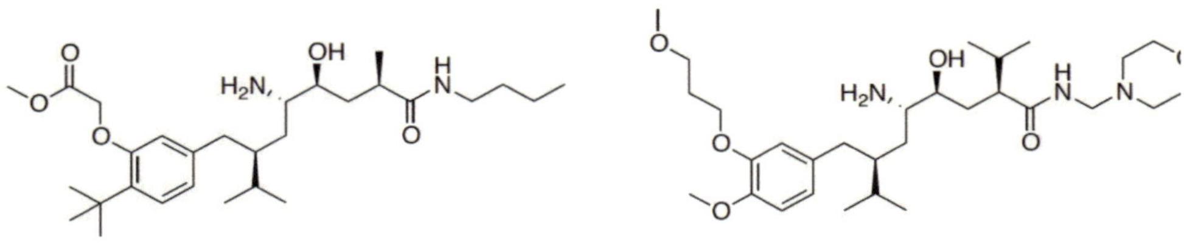

Figure 15. Aliskiren (left hand side) and its more potent analog.

Another possibility arose from use of fluoroketone derivatives. α-monofluoroketones are approximately 50% hydrated, whereas the α,α-difluoroketones are 100% hydrated in aqueous solutions (Fig. 16). The latter ones are obviously of choice because of their striking similarity to phosphinic inhibitors (two hydroxyls placed at terahedral atom). This approach is applied very rarely but gave good inhibitors of fungal endothiapepsin [Tuan et al., 2007] and matrix metalloprotease [Reiter et al., 2000] (Fig. 16).

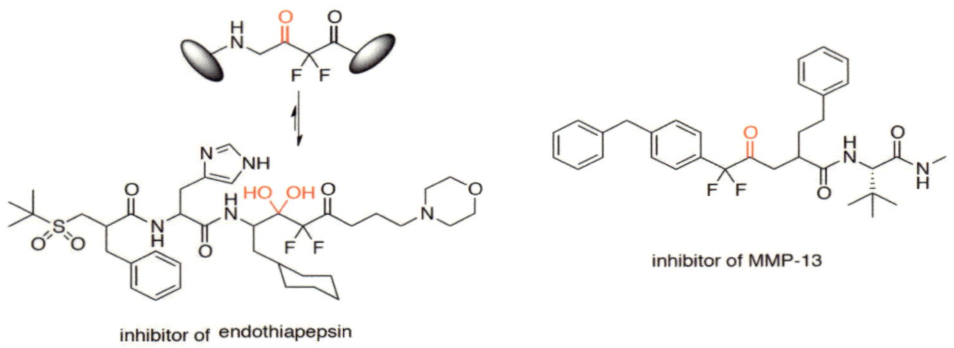

Figure 16. Difluoroketones as transition state inhibitor.

6. Suicide substrates yielding transition state analogues

Peptide aldehydes and boronic acids are inhibitors of serine and threonine enzymes forming both, hydrogen and covalent bonds in the enzyme active site. Tetrahedral adduct generated from these compounds upon their action on enzymes bear a closer relationship to the structure of the true intermediate and they may be considered as suicidal substrates. There is,

http://dx.doi.org/10.5772/52504

however, an important difference between these two types of inhibitors. The boronic acid derivative possesses a negative charge, whereas the hemiacetal adduct is neutral (Fig 17).

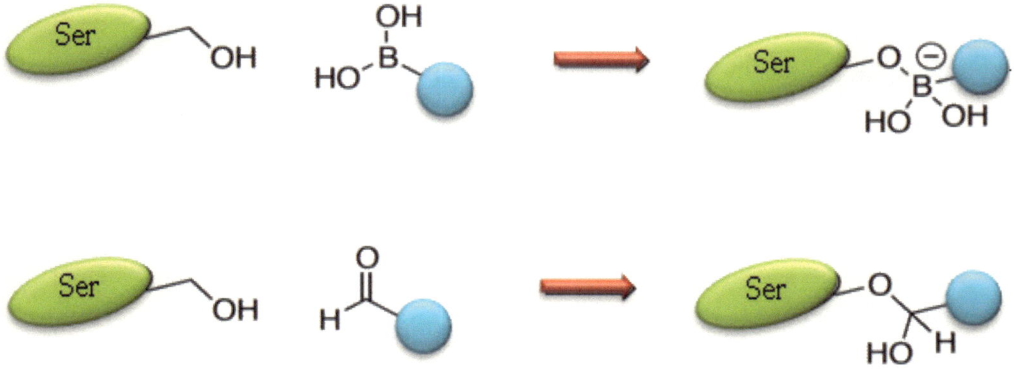

Figure 17. Suicidal substrates yielding transition state analogs

Hence, the peptidyl boronic acid adduct is a better transition state analog than the hemiacetal formed from peptidic aldehyde [Polgár, 2005]. Aldehydes typically have a low prevalence in drugs and drug candidates because of their potential chemical reactivity and susceptibility to be engaged in a reduction/oxidation pathways in vivo. Therefore peptidyl boronic acids are considered as far better drug candidates. Additionally slight changes in pH can result in release of the inhibitor from the active site, which is profitous.

In 2003, bortezomib (Fig. 18), a first-in-class therapeutic, gained approval from the US Federal Drug Administration for the treatment of relapsed multiple myeloma and mantle cell lymphoma. Approval in the UK, for multiple myeloma, followed in 2006. It possesses a unique mode of action. Bortezomib acts as inhibitor of the 26S proteasome, the key regulator of intracellular protein degradation, found in the nucleus and cytosol of all eukaryotic cells, and forming part of the critical ubiquitin-proteasome system. This inhibition results in disruption of homeostatic mechanisms within the cell that can lead to cell death.

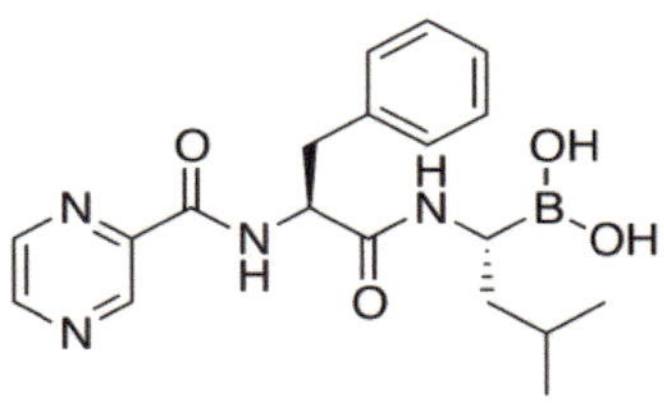

Figure 18. Structure of bortezomib.

This finding initiated intensive researches on boronic inhibitors of serine and threonine proteases [Trippier & McGuigan, 2010]. For, example recently inhibitors of Lon proteases (bacterial ATP-dependent protease conferring bacterial virulence) afforded interesting antibacterial agents [Frase and Lee, 2007], inhibitors of prostate-specific antigen for prostate cancer imaging and therapy [LeBeau et al., 2008], antifungal inhibitors of kexin (regulatory proteins from *Candida*) [Holyoak et al., 2004; Wheatley & Holyoak, 2007], inhibitor of HCV NS3 protease as potential drug against hepatitis [Zhang et al., 2003; Venkatraman et al., 2009], and anticancer and antibacterial inhibitors of proteasome [Hu et al., 2006]. Representative examples of these inhibitors are shown in Figure 19.

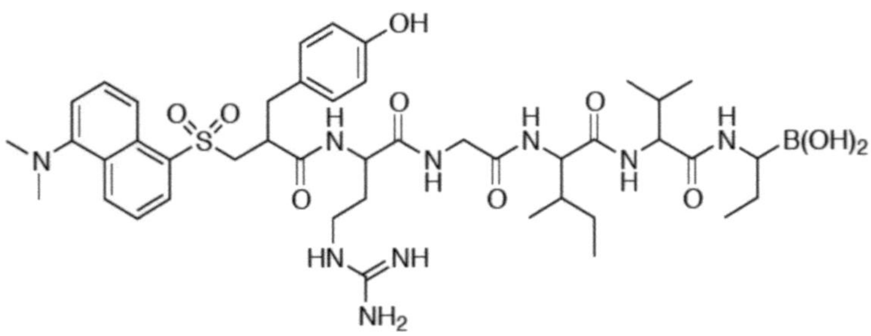

Lon protease inhibitor

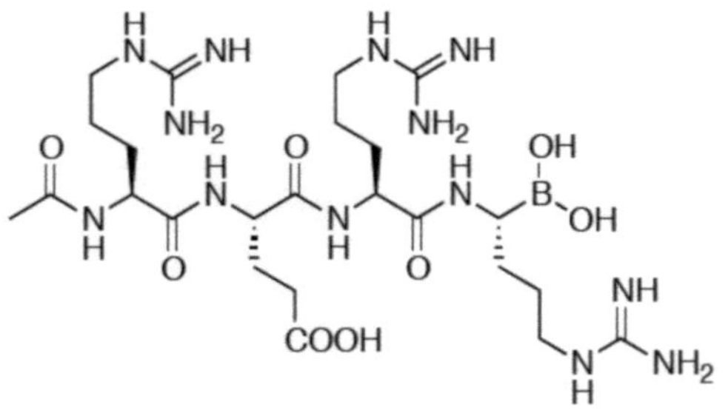

inhibitor of kexin

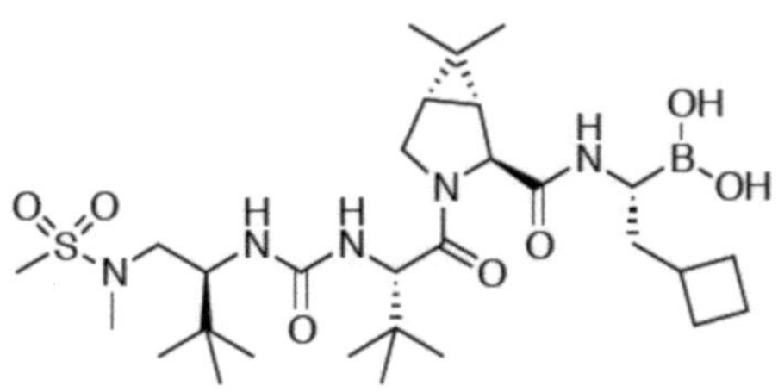

inhibitor ofHCV-NS3 protease

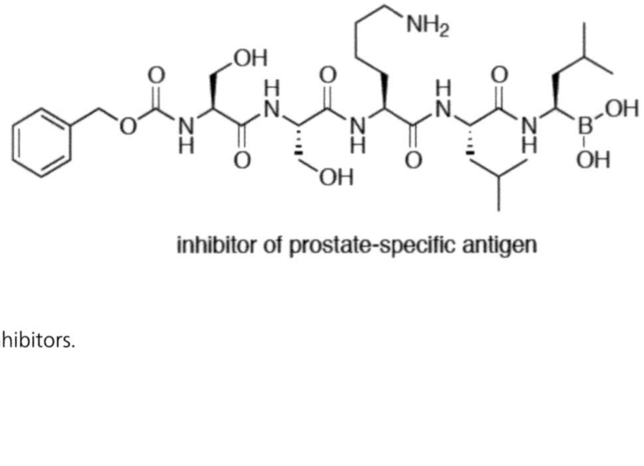

inhibitor of prostate-specific antigen

Figure 19. Boronic acid based inhibitors.

7. Other hydrolases

The data considering transition state analogue inhibitors of other hydrolases are practically limited to inhibitors of β–lactamases, arginase and urease.

Antibiotic resistance, especially to widely prescribed β-lactam antibiotics, is a serious threat to public health and is responsible for the increase in morbidity, mortality, and health care costs related to the treatment of bacterial infections. In most cases emergence of antibiotic-resistant bacteria is primarily driven by overuse of β-lactam antibiotics in food and agricultural products. The most prominent resistance mechanism is related to the expression of β-lactamases, which hydrolyze β–lactam fragment of the drug molecule. In nature, four classes of these enzymes exist. Three of them are serine-based, whereas fourth is zinc-dependent-hydrolase. To counteract β-lactamases, mechanism-based inhibitors were developed to be administered in concert with β-lactam antibiotics. Presently, there are three commercially available β-lactamase inhibitors (clavulanate, sulbactam, and tazobactam). The new approach to obtain such inhibitors is combination of structure of potent β-lactam antibiotics with a boronic [Thomson, et al., 2007; Eidam et al., 2010: Ke, et al., 2011; Chan, et al., 2012] or phosphonic [Nukaga, et al., 2004] acid moieties with the goal of mimicking the transition state and creating a high-affinity, reversible inhibitor that cannot be inactivated by β-lactamases since they do not bear hydrolyzable β-lactam ring.

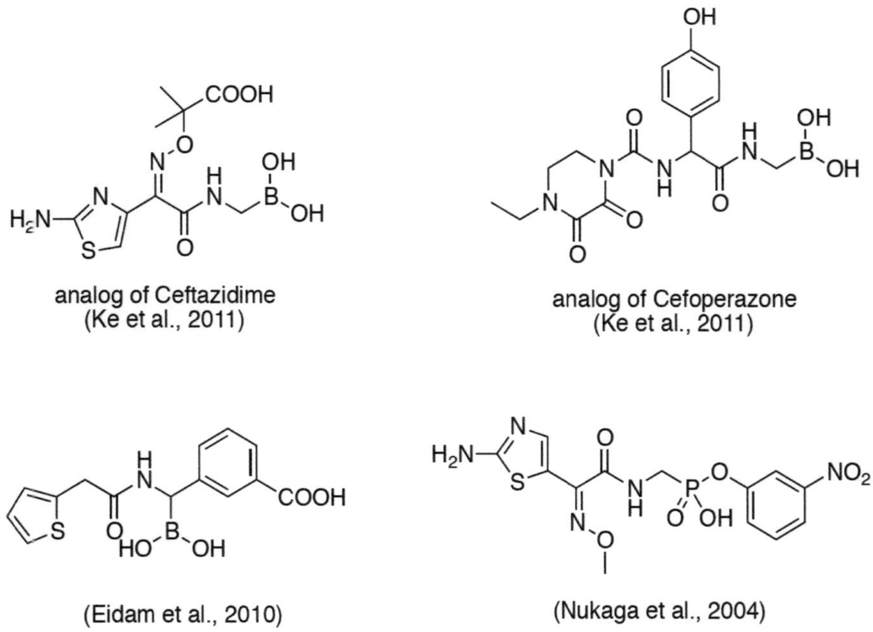

Figure 20. Transition state inhibitors of lactamases.

Arginase is a binuclear manganese metalloenzyme that serves as a therapeutic target for the treatment of asthma, erectile dysfunction, and atherosclerosis. The hydrolysis of *L*-arginine to *L*-ornithine and urea (Fig. 21) is also the final cytosolic step of the urea cycle in mammalian liver. *S*-(2-Boronoethyl)-*L*-cysteine is one of the most effective inhibitor of the enzyme (Fig 21). The specificity determinants of amino acid recognition by arginase were identified by X-Ray structure of human arginase I enzyme complexed with this inhibitor. These studies undoubtedly shown that boronate adopts tetrahedral configuration [Cama et al., 2003 & 2003a; Shishova, et al., 2009]. Also aldehydes and sulfonamides similar to boronic acids appeared to be promising inhibitors of arginases [Shin et al., 2004].

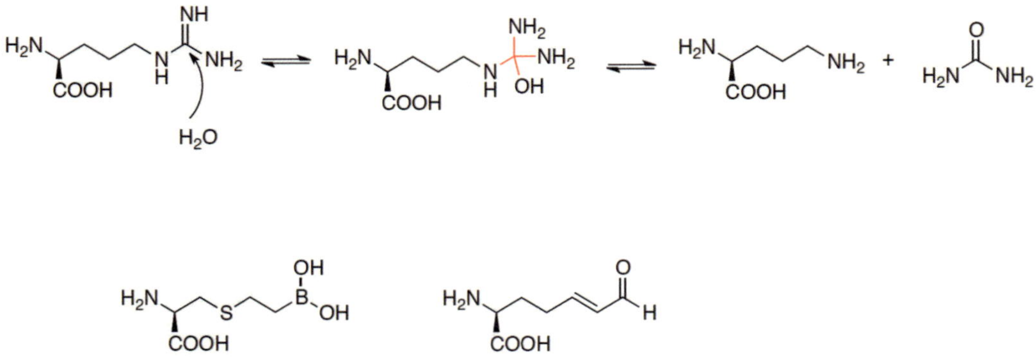

(Shishova et al., 200(9)   (Shin et al., 2004)

Figure 21. Arginase catalyzed reaction and representative inhibitors of the enzyme.

Urease catalyzes hydrolysis of urea in the last step of organic nitrogen mineralization to give ammonia and carbamate, which decomposes to give a second molecule of ammonia and bicarbonate (Fig. 22). The hydrolysis of the reaction products induces an overall pH increase that has negative implications both in human and animal health as well as in the ecosphere. Urease is a virulence factor in infections of urinary (*Proteus mirabilis, Ureaplasma urealyticum*) and gastrointestinal tracts (*Helicobacter pylori*), causing severe diseases such as peptic ulcers, stomach cancer, and formation of urinary stones. The efficiency of soil nitrogen fertilization with urea (the most used fertilizer worldwide) decreases due to ammonia volatilization and root damage caused by soil pH increase. Thus, control of the activity of urease through the use of inhibitors could counteract these negative effects [Kosikowska & Berlicki, 2011; Zambelli et al., 2011]. Di- and triamides of phosphoric acid represent a group of urease inhibitors with the highest activity. It is the direct consequence of their similarity to the tetrahedral transition state of the enzymatic reaction of urea hydrolysis. Takeda Chemicals have patented a large group of N-acyltriamido phosphates and found over 90 examples with nanomolar activity against *H. pylori* urease, with flurofamide being the most effective (Fig. 22) [Kosikowska & Berlicki, 2011].

Recently design, synthesis, and evaluation of novel ogranophosphonate inhibitors of bacterial urease have been described as an attractive alternative to known phosphoramidates. On the basis of the crystal structure of *Bacillus pasteurii* urease, several phosphinic acids and their short peptides have been designed by using the computer-aided techniques. The stepwise scheme of inhibitor design, shown in Figure 21, led to the synthesis of compounds with low structural complexity, high hydrolytic stability and satisfactory biological activity against various ureases, including cytoplasmic urease from pathogenic *Proteus* species [Vassiliou et al., 2008; Berlicki et al., 2012; Vassiliou et al., 2012].

8. Peptide bond formation by ribosome

Ribosomes are molecular machines that synthesize proteins in the cell. Recent biochemical analyses and high-resolution crystal structures of the bacterial ribosome have shown that the active site for the formation of peptide bonds – the peptidyl-transferase center – is composed solely of rRNA. Thus, the ribosome is the largest known RNA catalyst and the only natural ribozyme that has a synthetic activity. Peptide bond formation during ribosomal protein synthesis involves an aminolysis reaction between the aminoacyl α-amino group and the carbonyl ester of the growing peptide via a transition state with a developing negative charge - the oxyanion. Therefore the observed intermediates and transition states are similar to those observed in proteinases (Fig. 23). Structural and molecular dynamic studies have suggested that the ribosome may stabilize the oxyanion in the transition state of peptide bond formation via a highly ordered water molecule [Rodnina et al., 2006; Carrasco et al., 2011].

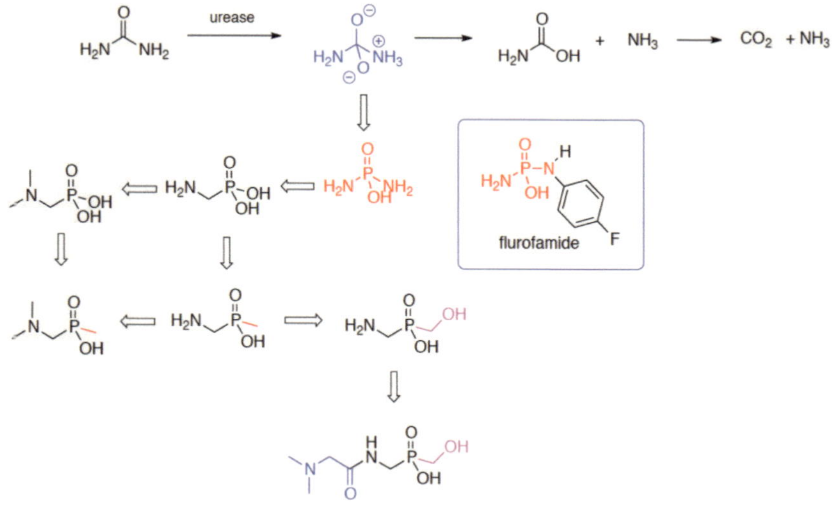

Figure 22. Urease hydrolysed reaction and evolution of the structure of its inhibitors.

To biochemically elucidate how the ribosome stabilizes the developing negative charge in the transition state of peptide bond formation, a series of tetrahedral transition state mimics were synthesized. Their relative binding affinities for the ribosomes also were measured (Fig. 23). The obtained results confirmed high affinity of predicted mechanism of ribosome action [Green & Lorsch, 2002; Weinger et al., 2004; Carrasco, et al., 2011].

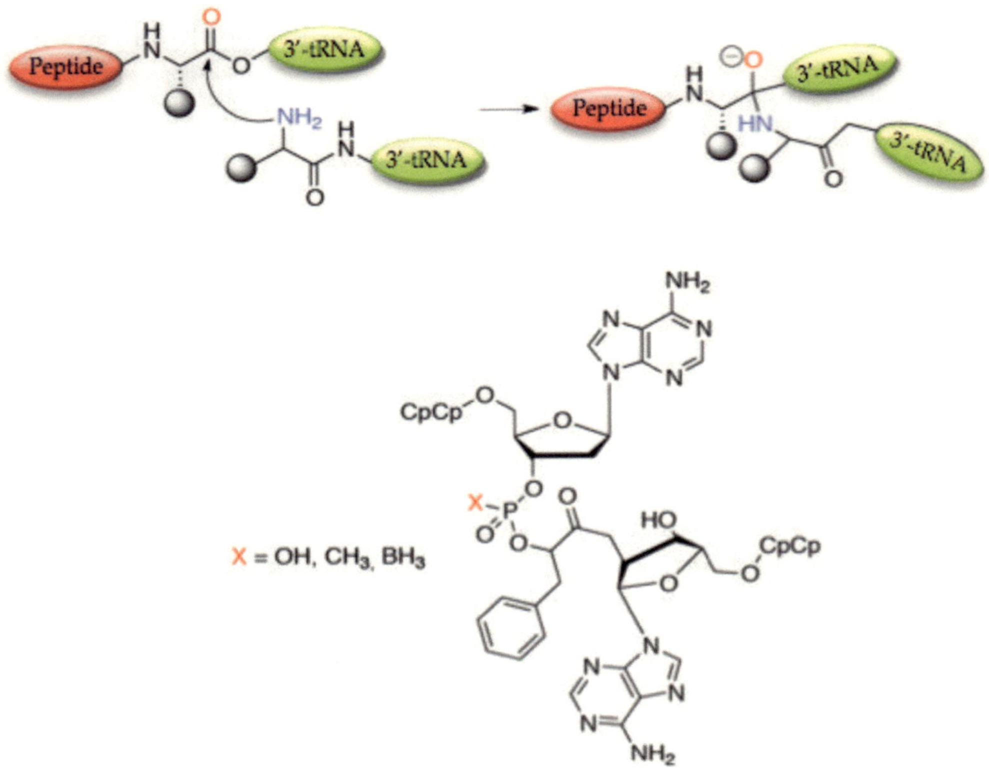

Figure 23. Transition state analog inhibitor of peptidyl transferase.

9. Enzymes forming amide and ester bonds via carboxylic-phosphate anhydride

Activation of carboxylic group of amino acid by ATP-phosphorylation yielding mixed carboxylic-phosphate anhydride is quite popular mechanism of synthesis of amide and ester bonds.

D-Alanyl-*D*-alanine ligase is one of the key enzymes in peptidoglycan biosynthesis and is an important target for antibacterial drugs. The enzyme catalyzes the condensation of two alanine molecules using ATP to produce *D*-Ala-*D*-Ala (Fig. 24), which is the terminal peptide of a peptidoglycan monomer. Analogs of *D*-Ala-*D*-Ala, in which phosphonate or phosphinate moiety replaces peptide bond appear to be potent inhibitors. As determined by kinetic [Ellsworth et al., 1996], X-Ray [Wu et al., 2008], and molecular modeling studies the inhibitor behaves as substrate and reacts with ATP to produce ADP and a tight-binding phosphorylated transition state analogue, which exerts inhibitory action against the enzyme (Fig. 24). Thus, these compounds might be rather considered as suicide substrates.

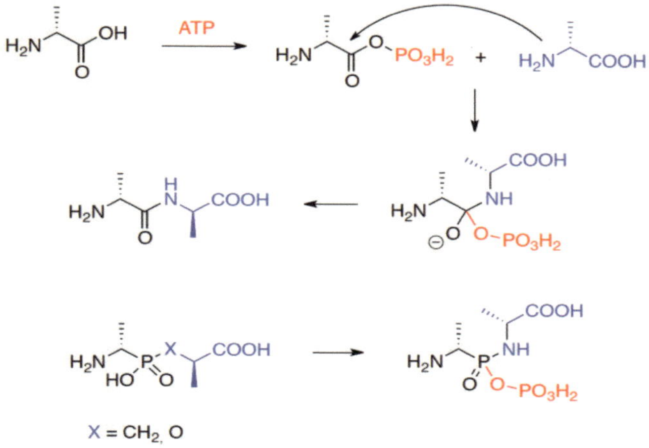

Figure 24. Mechanism of condensation of two molecules of D-Ala catalyzed by *D*-alanine-*D*-alanine ligase.

Similarly acting inhibitors have been found for glutamine synthetase (phosphinothricin and methionine sulfoximine and their analogs) [Berlicki et al., 2005; Berlicki & Kafarski 2006; Berlicki, 2008], γ-glutamylcysteine synthetase [Hibi et al., 2004], or penicillin binding proteins [Dzekieva et al., 2010; Dzekieva et al., 2012] (Fig. 25).

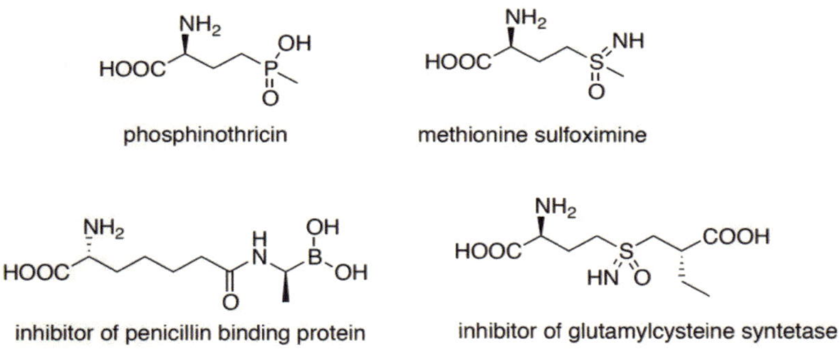

Figure 25. Inhibitors activated by ATP.

10. Nucleotide deaminases

Enzymes of the deaminase superfamily catalyze deamination of bases in nucleotides and nucleic acids across in diverse biological contexts. Representatives that act on free nucleotides or bases are primarily involved in the salvage of pyrimidines and purines, or in their catabolism in bacteria, eukaryotes and phages. Other members of the deaminase superfamily catalyze the *in situ* deamination of bases in both RNA and DNA. Such modifications play a central role in RNA editing, which is critical for generating the appropriate anti-codon sequences for decoding the genetic code, modification of the sequences of microRNA and other transcripts and alteration of the reading frames in mRNAs, defense against viruses via hypermutation-based inactivation, and somatic hypermutation or class switching of antigen receptor genes in vertebrates [Iyer et al., 2011].

Adenosine deaminase (ADA) is an enzyme present in all organisms and catalyzes the irreversible deamination of adenosine and deoxyadenosine to inosine and deoxyinosine (Fig. 26). Both adenosine and deoxyadenosine are biologically active purines that can have a deep impact on cellular physiology. For example it plays a vital role in regulating T-cell coactivation. Deficiency of this enzyme in humans causes severe combined immunodeficiency. Increased serum activity of this enzyme have been found in many infectious diseases caused by microorganisms infecting the macrophages, in leprosy, brucellosis, HIV infections, viral hepatitis, infectious mononucleosis, liver cirrhosis and tuberculosis. Its extended transition state inhibitor – conformycin was isolated from *Nocardia interforma* and *Streptomyces kaniharaensis*. Analogs of conformycin (Fig. 26) are proposed as an antineoplastic synergists and immunosuppressants [Wolfenden, 2003].

The wide potential of these inhibitors may be illustrated by the fact that deaminoformycin was recently applied to evaluate mechanisms responsible for lethality caused by genetic and herbicide-based activity of adenosine deaminase [Sabina et al., 2007], as well as identification of highly selective inhibitor of purine salvage pathway in malaria parasites [Tyler et al., 2007]. This is because of a unique feature of *Plasmodium falciparum* enzyme that catalyzes the deamination of both adenosine and 5'-methylthioadenosine.

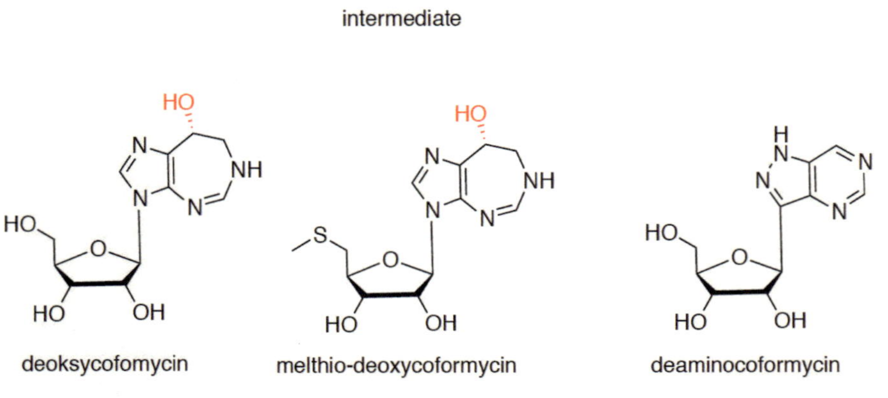

Figure 26. Inhibitors of adenosine deaminase.

Guanine deaminase is an enzyme that hydrolyzes guanine to form xanthine that is unsuitable for DNA/RNA buildup. This enzyme has been found in normal or transformed human organs and sera. One of the approaches for antiviral/anticancer therapy is to design structural mimics of natural guanine as nucleic acid building blocks, with an anticipation that such analogs would be incorporated into DNA/RNA of virus for cancer cells, interrupting their normal replicative processes. Unfortunately these potent anticancer mimics are believed to be substrates for the enzyme guanine deaminase, which converts them into their respective inactive forms. A potent inhibitor would restore the original potency of these anticancer compounds. Such an activity was determined for azepinomycin [Isshiki et al., 1987] and its analog designed as transition state of this reaction (Fig. 27) [Chakraborty et al., 2011].

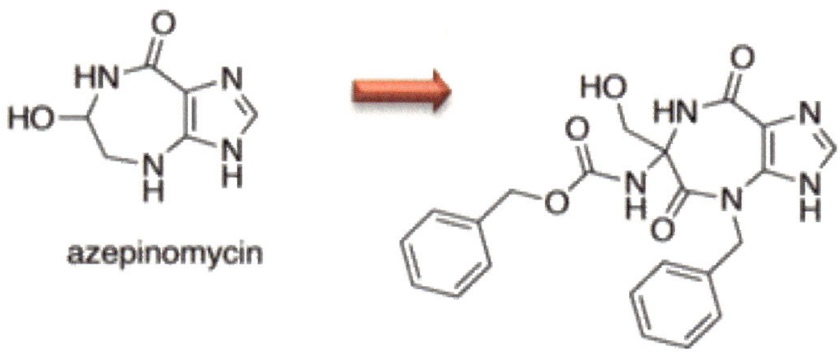

Figure 27. Apizenomycin as a template for guanine deaminase inhibitor.

11. Glycosidases and related enzymes

Glycoside hydrolases, the enzymes catalyzing hydrolysis of the glycosidic bond in di-, oligo- and polysaccharides, and glycoconjugates, are ubiquitous in Nature and fundamental to existence. The extreme stability of the glycosidic bond caused that they have evolved into highly proficient catalysts, with an estimated 10^{17} fold rate enhancement over the uncatalysed reaction. Such rate enhancements mean that enzymes bind the substrate at the transition state with extraordinary affinity [Gloster & Davies, 2010].

In the most cases of glycoside hydrolysis, the short-lived transition state possesses substantial oxocarbenium character (Fig. 27) resembling classical S_N1 reaction intermediate. Under these conditions the anomeric carbon possesses trigonal character, which causes sp^2 hybridisation predominantly along the bond between the anomeric carbon and endocyclic oxygen and significant relative positive charge accumulation on the pyranose ring [Lee et al., 2004; Biarnés et al., 2011; Davies at al., 2012].

The quest for potent and selective inhibitors of glycosidases is extremely active at present. This results from the involvement of glycosidases in lysosomal storage disorders, cancer, viral infections, diabetes and many others. Consequently a plethora of glycosidase inhibitors have been already synthesized and evaluated. The number of them is continually growing. It is outside the scope of this chapter to mention all of them in detail. One of the most appealing ways to design a transition state analog would be to incorporate both the features of geometry and charge present at the transition state. Distortion of the ring to generate compounds which may resemble the geometry of the transition state can be done by introducing a double bond in the pseudo-glycoside ring itself, whereas introduction of the charge might be done by application of sulfonium or ammonium ions [Rempel & Withers, 2008; Gloster & Davies, 2010; Sumida et al., 2012].

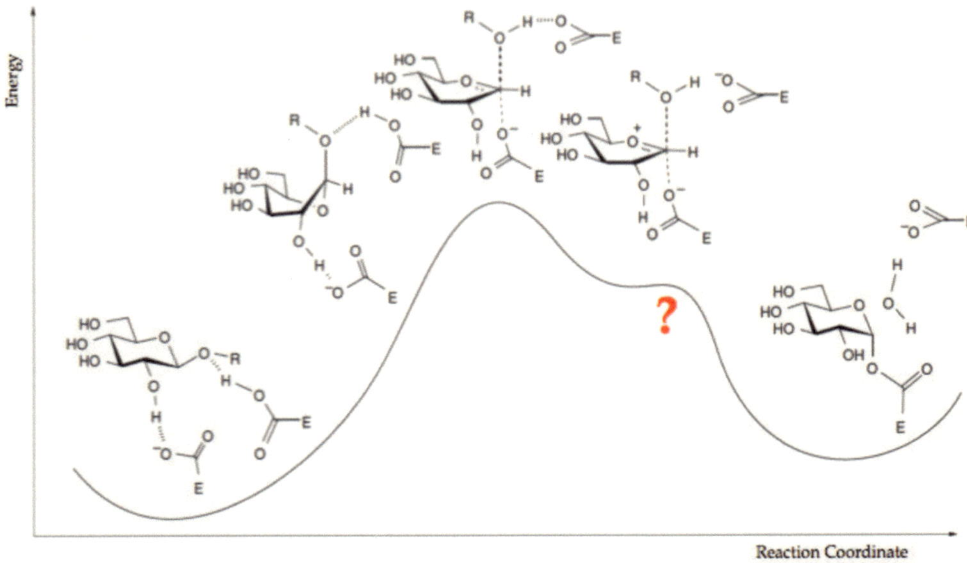

Figure 28. Mechanism of β-glucosidase action [after Vasella et al., 2002].

Some representatives, which fulfills these requirements are: salicinol, one of the active principles in the aqueous extracts of *Salacia reticulata* that is traditionally used in Sri Lanka and India for the treatment of diabetes [Ghavami et al., 2001] and its structurally variable analogues [Liu et al., 2006; Bhat et al., 2007; Mohan & Pinto, 2008].

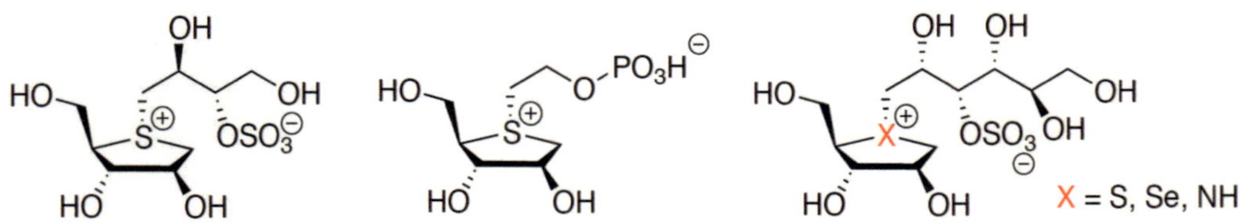

Figure 29. Salicinol and its analogs.

Sialic acids play an important role in a variety of biological processes. They are usually attached to the terminal positions of glycoproteins, glycolipids and oligosaccharides. From more than 100 different sialic acids, *N*-acetylneuraminic acid (NeuAc) is the most abundant one. Sialidases or neuraminidases are a family of exo-glycoside hydrolases that catalyze the

http://dx.doi.org/10.5772/52504

cleavage of terminal sialic acid residues from sialylated oligosaccharides, glycoproteins, and glycolipids. Aberrant expression of different human sialidases was found to associate with various pathological conditions, including lysosomal storage diseases such as sialidosis and galactosialidosis. Non-specific transition-state analog of sialidase, 2-deoxy-2,3-dehydro-*N* -acetylneuraminic acid (DANA, Fig. 30) is a good starting point for the synthesis of specific inhibitors of human enzymes [Streicher & Busse, 2006; Li et al., 2011].

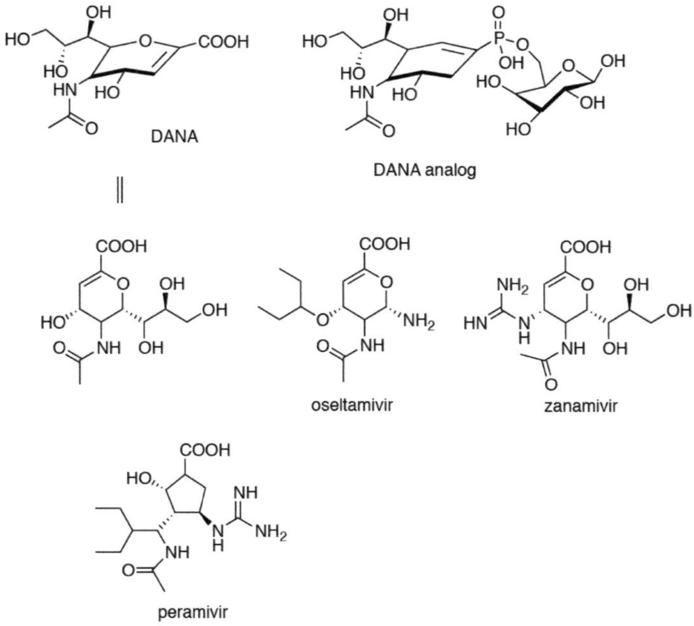

Figure 30. Chemical structures of neuraminidaze inhibitors.

Influenza viruses, in particular those of type A that can infect animals and humans, continue to represent a major threat to public health and animal health worldwide. The social and economic burden associated with a pandemic is substantial. Two viral surface glycoproteins, the sialoside-hydrolysing neuraminidase and the sialic acid-binding hemagglutinin, have become important targets for such approach. Most likely, the function of flu virus neuraminidase is to remove sialic acid receptors for the virus from the host cells, and also, perhaps more importantly, from the newly formed virus particles themselves [Nelson & Holmes, 2007; Medina & Garcia-Sastre, 2011]. Three inhibitors of neuraminidase have been successfully introduced as anti-influenza drugs, all of them being transition state analog inhibitors. They were designed by systematic reduction of DANA structure using crystallographic data and computer-aided methods [Wei, et al., 2006]. Relenza (zanamivir) was the first inhibitor to be synthesized which specifically inhibited neuraminidases of both Type A and Type B influenza viruses and is effective in controlling influenza infections. In people is given as a powder by oral inhalation [Palese et al., 1974]. Interestingly, it is weaker inhibitor of neuramidase than DANA, however, DANA inhibited influenza virus replication in tissue culture but failed to prevent disease in flu-infected animals. In order to produce a neuraminidase inhibitor, which was orally bioavailable and which was taken orally in capsules or as a suspension, Tamiflu (oseltavimir) was developed in 1997 [Kim et al.]. Third drug, which has been authorized for the emergency use of treatment of certain hospitalized patients with known or suspected 2009 H1N1 influenza, is permavir [Chand, et al., 2005]. Structures of these drugs are presented in Figure 30.

All three drugs soon became lead structures for the design and preparation of new, presumably more effective ones. Syntheses and eveluation of phosphinic analogs and significantly simplified analogs of permavir (Fig. 31) have been recently described [Kati et al., 2001; Bianco et al., 2005; Shie et al., 2007; Udommaneethanakit et al., 2009].

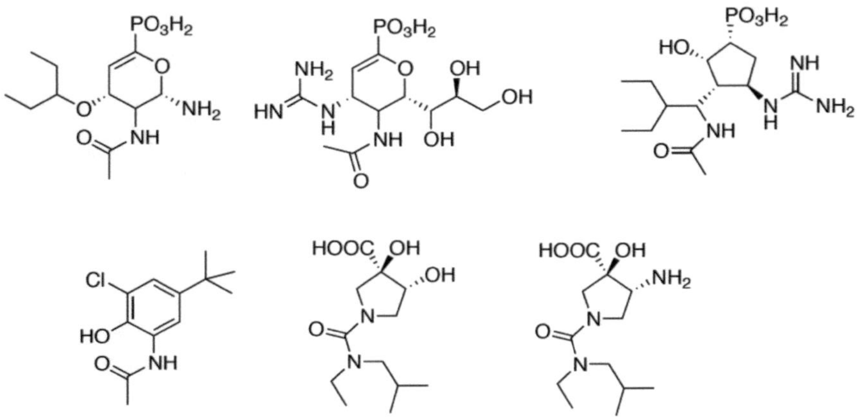

Figure 31. Second generation of influenza neuraminidase inhibitors.

Modified phosphonic analogs of oseltamivir were used to functionalize gold nanoparticles and were found to bind strongly and selectively to all seasonal and pandemic influenza virus strains, and thus could serve as prototypes for novel virus sensors. This may be helpul in fast influenza diagnosis [Stanley et al., 2012].

12. Transition state analogues of nucleic acids metabolism

N-Ribosyltransferases are a general class of enzymes that catalyze nucleophilic displacement reactions by migration of the cationic ribooxacarbenium carbon from the fixed purine to phosphate and water nucleophiles, respectively. Two major classes of these enzymes are hydrolases and phosphorylases. Hydrolases, which release the heterocycle to generate a free sugar ribosyl unit, include enzymes for DNA repair, RNA depurinations by plant toxins, and purine and pyrimidine nucleoside and nucleotide metabolism. Phosphorylases, which transfer ribosyl groups to phosphate, are also involved in the pathway for nucleoside salvage. Genetic defects in this pathway prevent normal purine catabolism in humans.

The focus on transition states for a family of *N*-ribosyltransferases roots from physiologic importance of these enzymes. Similarly as in the case of glycosidases, most sugar transferases form transition states with cationic charge at the anomeric carbon. The geometry is altered at this center from sp^3 (tetrahedral geometry) in the reactant sugar to sp^2 (trigonal planargeometry) at the transition state (Fig. 32) [Schramm, 2002; Murkin et al., 2007; Silva et al., 2011].

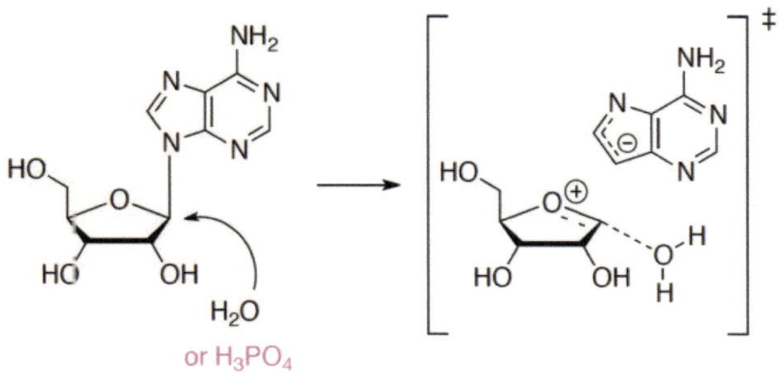

Figure 32. Course of reaction catalyzed by *N*-ribosyltransferases.

Newborns with a genetic deficiency of purine nucleoside phosphorylase are normal, but exhibit a specific T-cell immunodeficiency during the first years of development. All other cell and organ systems remain functional. Human purine nucleoside phosphorylase degrades deoxyguanosine, and apoptosis of T-cells occurs as a consequence of the accumulation of deoxyguanosine in the circulation. Thus, control of T-cell proliferation is desirable in T-cell cancers, autoimmune diseases, and tissue transplant rejection. The search for powerful inhibitors of these enzymes as anti-T-cell agents has culminated in the discovery of immucillins. The atomic replacements between inosine and immunocilin H make an insignificant change in atomic size, but a dramatic change in the molecular electrostatic potential surface (Fig. 33). Thus, analysis of the molecular electrostatic potential surface similarity between transition state and immucilin confirmed utility of this simple approach in helping to design effective inhibitor [Schramm, 2002; Schramm, 2007].

Evolution of immucilin structure, performed using standard structural analogy techniques, enabled to obtain new inhibitors of purine nucleotide phosphorylase of nano- to picomolar affinities to the enzyme (Fig. 34) [Evans et al., 2008; Edwards et al., 2009; Ho et al. 2010; Rejman et al., 2012].

Plasmodium parasites (causative agents of malaria) are purine auxotrophs and require preformed purine bases for synthesis of nucleotides, cofactors, and nucleic acids. The purine phosphoribosyltransferases catalyze transfer the 5-phosphoribosyl group from 5-phospho-α-*D*-ribofuranosyl-1-pyrophosphate to salvage hypoxanthine, guanine, or xanthine to form intracellular nucleosides. Purine salvage in *Plasmodium falciparum* uses hypoxanthine formed in erythrocytes or in parasites by the sequential actions of adenosine deaminase and purine nucleoside phosphorylase

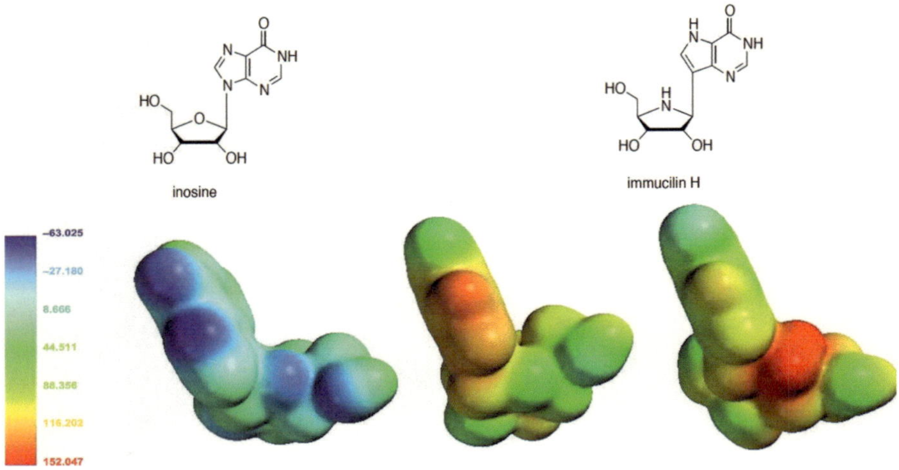

Figure 33. Molecular electrostatic potential surfaces for inosine, the transition state of purine nucleoside phosphorylase and immucilin H.

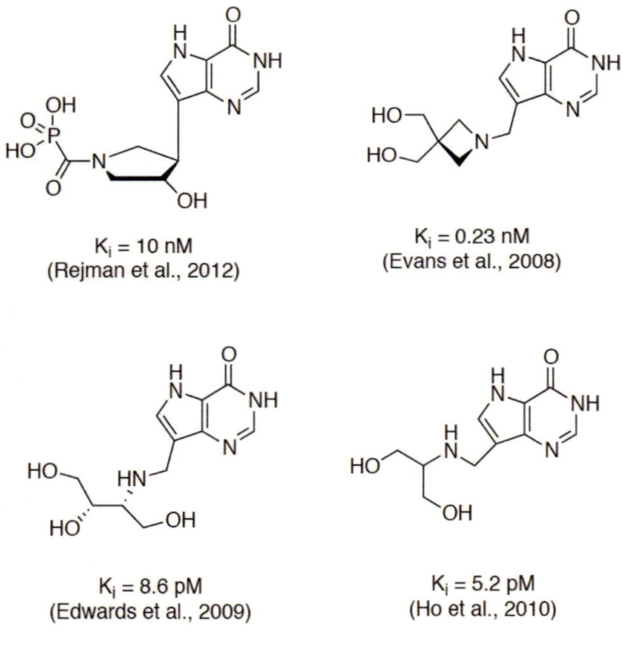

Figure 34. Effective inhibitors of purine nucleotide phosphorylase.

Therefore, effective inhibitors of both enzymes influence the life cycle of P. falciparum and these pathways have been targets for antimalarials since the discovery that *Plasmodium* parasites are purine auxotrophs.

Immunocillins HP and GP [Shi et al., 1999] and BCX4945 [Cassera et al., 2011] (Fig. 35) appear to be effective inhibitors of phosphoribosyltransferases and are also able to influence purine nucleoside phosphorylase, being dual inhibitor of the process. Especially the efficacy, oral availability, chemical stability, unique mechanism of action and low toxicity of BCX4945 demonstrate potential for combination therapies with this novel antimalarial agent. Similar studies have been also carried out for acyclic nucleoside phosphonates [Keough et al., 2009].

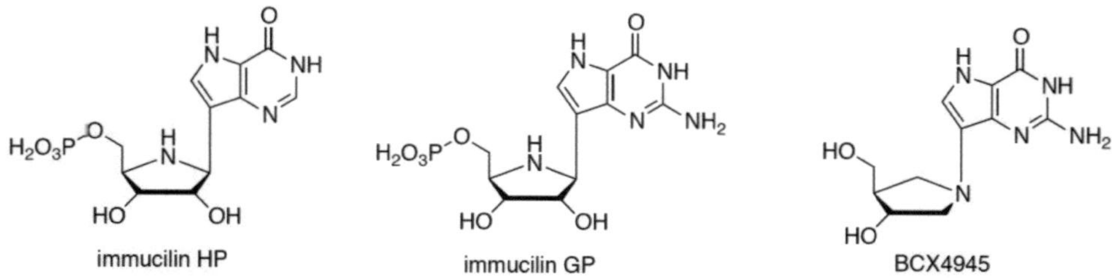

Figure 35. Antimalarial agents of dual inhibitory action.

Acknowledgements

This work is dedicated to Professor Henri-Jean Cristau from Ecole Nationale Superieure de Chimie in Mointpellier on the occasion of his 70th birthday.

Authors thank Polish Ministry of Science and Higher Education for financial support.

Author details

Karolina Gluza and Pawel Kafarski

Department of Bioorganic Chemistry, Faculty of Chemistry, Wroclaw University of Technology, Wybrzeze Wyspianskiego, Wroclaw, Poland

References

[1] Abbenante, G.; Fairlie, D. P. (2005) Protease Inhibitors in the Clinic. Medicinal Chemistry Vol. 1 (No. 1): 71-104

[2] Adachi, M.; Ohhara, T.; Kurihara, K.; Tamada, T.; Honjo, E.; Okazaki, N.; Arai, S.; Shoyama, Y.; Kimura, K.; Matsumura, H.; Sugiyama, S.; Adachi, H.; Takano, K.; Mori, Y.; Hidaka, K.; Kimura, T.; Hayashi, Y.; Kiso, Y. & Kuroki, R. (2009) Structure of HIV-1 Protease in Complex with Potent Inhibitor KNI-272 Determined by High-Resolution X-ray and Neutron Crystallography. *Proc. Natl. Acad. Sci. U.S.A.* Vol. 106 (No. 12): 4641-4646

[3] Akif, M.; Schwarger, S. L.; Anthony, C. S., Czrny, B.; Beau, F.; Dive, V.; Sturrock, E. D. & Acharya, D. L. (2011) Novel Mechanism of Inhibition of Human Angiotensin-I-Converting Enzyme (ACE) by a Highly Specific Phosphinic Tripeptide. *Biochem. J.* Vol. 436 (No. 1): 53-59

[4] Alfonso, Y. & Monzotte, L. (2011) HIV Protease Inhibitors: Effect on the Opportunistic Protozoan Parasites. *Open Med. Chem. J.* Vol. 5 (March 2011): 40-50

[5] Al-Tel, T. H.; Al-Qawasmeh, R. A.; Schmidt, M. F.; Al-Aboudi, A.; Rao, S. N.; Sabri, S. S. & Voelter, W. (2009) Rational Design and Synthesis of Potent Dibenzazepine Motifs as -Secretase Inhibitors. *J. Med. Chem.* Vol. 52 (No. 20): 6484-6488

[6] Al-Tel, T. H.; Samreen, M. H.; Al-Quawasmeh, R. A.; Schmidt, M. F.; El-Awadi, R.; Ardah, M.; Zaarour, R.; Rao, S. N. & El-Agnaf, O. (2011) Design, Synthesis, and Qualitative Structure-Activity Evaluations of Novel -Secretase Inhibitors as Potential Alzheimer's Drug Leads. *J. Med. Chem.* Vol. 54 (No. 24): 8373-8385

[7] Andreoni, M. & Perno, C. F. (2012) Positioning of HIV-Protease Inhibitors in Clinical Practice. *Eur. Rev. Med. Pharmacol. Sci.* Vol. 16 (No. 1): 10-18

[8] Anzellotti, A. I., & Farrell, N. P. (2008) Zinc Metalloproteins as Medicinal Targets. *Chem. Soc. Rev.* Vol. 37 (No. 8): 1629-1651

[9] Avram, S.; Milac, A. L.; Mihailescu, D. L.; Dabu, A. & Flonta M. L. (2006) Computer-Aided Drug Design Applied to Beta and Gamma Secretase Inhibitors-Perspectives for New Alzheimer Disease Therapy. *Curr. Enzyme Inhib.* Vol. 2 (No. 4): 311-328

[10] Banegas, I.; Prieto, I; Vives, F.; Alba, F.; deGAsparo, M.; Segarra, A. B.; Hermoso, F.; Durán, R. & Ramirez, M. (2006) Brain Aminopeptidases and Hypertension. *J. Renin Angiotensin Aldosterone Syst.* Vol. 7 (No.3): 129-134

[11] Barinka, C.; Hlouchova, K.; Rovenska, M.; Majer, P.; Dauter, M.; Hin, N.; Ko, Y.-S.; Tsukamoto, T.; Slusher, B. S.; Konvalinka, J. & Lubkowski, J. (2008) Structural Basis of Interactions between Human Glutamate Carboxypeptidase II and Its Substrate Analogs. *J. Mol. Biol.* Vol. 376 (No. 5): 1438-1350

[12] Berlicki, L.; Obojska, A.; Forlani, G. & Kafarski, P. (2005) Design, Synthesis, and Activity of Analogues of Phosphinothricin as Inhibitors of Glutamine Synthetase. *J. Med. Chem.* Vol. 48 (No. 20): 6340-6349

[13] Berlicki, L. & Kafarski P. (2006) Computer-aided Analysis of the Interactions of Glutamine Synthetase with its Inhibitors. *Bioorg. Med. Chem.* Vol. 14 (No. 13): 4578 - 4585

[14] Berlicki, L. (2008) Inhibitors of Glutamine Synthetase and Their Potential Application in Medicine. *Mini-reviews Med. Chem.*Vol. 8 (No. 9): 869 - 878

[15] Berlicki, L.; Bochno, M.; Grabowiecka, A.; Białas, A.; Kosikowska, P. & Kafarski P. (2012) N-Substituted Aminomethanephosphonic and Aminomethane-P-methylphosphinic Acids as Inhibitors of Ureases. *Amino Acids* Vol. 42 (No. 5): 1937-1942

[16] Bhat, R. G.; Kumar, N. G. & Pinto, B. M. (2007) Synthesis of Phosphate Derivatives Related to the Glycosidase Inhibitor Salacinol. *Glycomimetics* Vol. 342 (No. 12-13): 1934-1942

[17] Bianco, A.; Brufani, M.; Dri, D. A.; Melchioni, C. & Filocamo, L. (2005) Design and Synthesis of a New Furanosic Sialylmimetic as a Potential Influenza Neuraminidase Viral Inhibitor. *Lett. Org. Chem.* Vol. 2 (No. 1): 83-89

[18] Biarnés, X.; Ardèvol. A.; Iglesias-Fernández, J.; Planas, A. & Rovira, C. (2011) Catalytic Itinerary in 1,3-1,4--Glucanase Unraveled by QM/MM Metadynamics. Charge Is Not Yet Fully Developed at the Oxocarbenium Ion-like Transition State. *J. Am.Chem. Soc.* Vol. 133 (No. 50): 20301-20309

[19] Bo, Y.; Singh, S.; Duong, H. Q.; Cao, C. & Sieburtf, S. McN. (2011) Efficient, Enantioselective Assembly of Silanediol Protease Inhibitors. *Org. Lett.* Vol. 13 (No.7): 1387-1389

[20] Bodineau, L.; Fugière, A.; Marc, Y.; Inguimbert, N.; Fassot, C.; Balavoine, F.; Roques, B. & Llorens-Cortes, C. (2008) Orally Active Aminopeptidase A Inhibitors Reduce Blood Pressure A New Strategy for Treating Hypertension. *Hypertension* Vol. 51 (No. 5): 1318-1325

[21] Breuer, E.; Salomon, C. J.; Katz, Y.; Chen, W.; Lu, S.; Röschenthaler, G.-V.; Hander, R. & Reich, R. (2004) Carbamoylphosphonates, a New Class of *In vivo* Active Matrix Metalloproteinase Inhibitors. 1. Alkyl- and Cycloalkylcarbamoylphosphonic Acids. *J. Med. Chem.* Vol. 47 (No. 11): 2826-2832

[22] Brik, A. & Wong, C.-H. (2003) HIV-1 Protease: Mechanism and Drug Discovery. *Org. Biomol. Chem.* Vol. 1 (No.)1: 5-14

[23] Buchardt, J; Bruun Schiødt, K.; Krsog-Jensen, K.; Dellaise, J.-M.; Tækker Foged, N. & Meldal, M. (2000) Solid Phase Combinatorial Library of Phosphinic Peptides for Discovery of Matrix Metalloproteinase Inhibitors. *J. Comb. Chem.* Vol. 2 (No. 6): 624-6238

[24] Cama, E.; Colleluori, D. M.; Emig, F. A.; Shin, H.; Kim, S. W.; Kim, N. N.; Traish, A. M.; Ash, D. E. & Christianson, D. W. (2003) Human Arginase II: Crystal Structure and Physiological Role in Male and Female Sexual Arousal. *Biochemistry* Vol. 43 (No. 28): 8445-8451

[25] Cama, E.; Shin, H. & Christianson, D. W. (2003a) Design of Amino Acid Sulfonamides as Transition-State Analogue Inhibitors of Arginase. *J. Am. Chem. Soc.* Vol. 125 (No. 43): 13052-13057

[26] Carrasco, N.; Hiller, D. A. & Strobel S. A. (2011) Minimal Transition State Charge Stabilization of the Oxyanion During Peptide Bond Formation by the Ribosome. *Biochemistry* Vol. 50 (No. 48): 10491-10498

[27] Cassera, M. B.; Hazleton, K. Z.; Merino, E. F.; Obladia III, N.; Ho, M.-C.; Murkin, A. S.; DePinto, R.; Gutierrez, J. A.; Almo, S. C.; Evans, G. B.; Babu, Y. S. & Schramm, V.

L. (2011) Plasmodium falciparum Parasites Are Killed by a Transition State Analogue of Purine Nucleoside Phosphorylase in a Primate Animal Model, *PloS ONE* Vol. 6 (No. 11): e26916

[28] Chaerkady, R. & Sharma, K. K. (2004) Characterization of a Bradykinin-Hydrolyzing Protease from the Bovine Lens. *Invest. Ophthalmol. Vis. Sci.* Vol. 45 (No. 4): 1214-1223

[29] Chakraborty, S.; Shah, N. K.; Fishbein, J. C. & Hoschamne R. S. (2011) A Novel Transition State Analog Inhibitor of Guanase Based on Azepinomycin Ring Structure: Synthesis and Biochemical Assessment of Enzyme Inhibition. *Bioorg. Med. Chem. Lett.* Vol. 21 (No. 2): 756-759

[30] Chan, F. Y.; Neves, M. A. C.; Sun, N.; Tsang, M. W.; Leung, Y. C.; Chan. T.-H.; Abagyan, R. & Wong, K. Y. (2012) Validation of the AmpC -Lactamase Binding Site and Identificationof Inhibitors with Novel Scaffolds. *J. Chem. Inf. Model.* Vol. 52 (No. 5): 1367-1375

[31] Chand, P.; Bantia, S.; Kotian, P.; El-Kattan, Y.; Lin, T. & Babu, Y. S. (2005) Comparison of the Anti-influenza Virus Activity of Cyclopentanederivatives with Oseltamivir and Zanamivir In Vivo. *Bioorg. Med. Chem.* Vol. 13 (No. 12): 4071–4077.

[32] Charrier, N.; Clarke, B.; Cutler, L.; Demont, E.; Dingwall, C.; Dunsdon, R.; East, P.; Hawkins, J,.; Howes, C.; Hussain, I.; Jeffrey, P.; Maile, G.; Matico, R.; Mosley, J.; Naylor, A.; O'Brien, A.; Redsahw, S.; Rowland, P.; Soleil, V.; Smith, K.; Sweitzer, S.; Theobald, P,; Vesey, D.; Walter, D. S. & Wayne, G. (2008) Second Generation of Hydroxyethylamine BACE-1 Inhibitors: Optimizing Potency and Oral Bioavailability. *J. Med. Chem.* Vol 51 (no.11): 3313-3317

[33] Chen, S. A.; Sieburth S. McN.; Glekas, A.; Hewitt, G. W.; Trainor, G. L.; Erickson-Viitanen, S.; Garbor, S. S.; Cordova, B.; Jeffrey, S. & Klabe, R. M. (2001) Drug Design with a New Transition State Analog of the Hydrated Carbonyl: Silicon-based Inhibitors of the HIV Protease. *Chem. Biol.* Vol. 8 (No.12): 1161-1166

[34] Clarke, S. G. (2007) HIV Protease Inhibitors and Nuclear Lamin Processing: Getting the Right Bells and Whistles. *Proc. Natl. Acad. Sci. U.S.A.* Vol. 104 (No. 35): 13857-13858

[35] Collinsova, M. & Jiráček, J. (2000) Phosphinic Acid Compounds in Biochemistry, Biology and Medicine. *Curr. Med. Chem.* Vol. 7 (No. 6): 629-647

[36] Cunningham, E.; Drąg, M.; Kafarski, P. & Bell, A. (2008) Chemical Target Validation Studies of Aminopeptidase in Malaria Parasites Using alpha-Aminoalkylphosphonate and Phosphonopeptide Inhibitors. *Antimirob. Agnets Chemother.* Vol. 52 (No. 9): 3221 – 3228

[37] Davies, G. J.; Planas, A. P. & Rovira C. (2012) Conformational Analyses of the Reaction Coordinate of Glycosidases. *Acc. Chem. Res.* Vol. 45 (No.2): 308-316

[38] Devel, L.; Garcia, S.; Czarny B.; Beau, F.; Lajeunesse, E.; Vera, L.; Georgiadis, D.; Sture , E. & Dive, V. (2010) Insights from Selective Non-phosphinic Inhibitors of

http://dx.doi.org/10.5772/52504

MMP-12 Tailored to Fit with an S_1' Loop Canonical Conformation. *J. Biol. Chem.* Vol. 285 (No. 46): 35900-35909

[39] Dive, V.; Georgiadis, D.; Matziari, M.; Beau, F.; Cuniasse, P. & Yiotakis, A. (2004) Phosphinic Peptides as Zinc Metalloproteinase Inhibitors. *Cell. Mol. Life Sci.* Vol. 61 (No. 16): 2010-2019

[40] Drag, M. & Salvesen, G. S. (2010) Emerging Principles in Protease-based Drug Discovery. *Nature Rev. Drug. Discov.* Vol. 9 (September 2010): 690-701

[41] Drag, M.; Bogya, M.; Ellman, J. A. & Salvesen, G. S. (2010) Aminopeptidase Fingerprints, an Integrated Approach for Identification of Good Substrates and Optimal Inhibitors. *J. Biol. Chem.* Vol. 285 (No. 5): 3310-3318

[42] Dybala-Defratyka, A.; Rostkowski, M. & Paneth, P. (2008) Enzyme Mechanisms from Molecular Modeling and Isotope Effects. *Archiv. Biochem. Biophys.* Vol. 474 (No. 2): 274-282

[43] Dzhekieva, L.; Rocaboy, M.; Kerff, F.; Charlier, P.; Sauvage, E. & Pratt, R. F (2010) Crystal Structure of a Complex between the *Actinomadura* R39 DD-Peptidase and a Peptidoglycan-mimetic Boronate Inhibitor: Interpretation of a Transition State Analogue in Terms of Catalytic Mechanism. *Biochemistry* Vol. 49 (No. 30): 6411-6419

[44] Dzhekieva, L.; Kumar, I. & Pratt, R. F. (2012) Inhibition of Bacterial DD-Peptidases (Penicillin-Binding Proteins) in Membranes and in Vivo by Peptidoglycan-Mimetic Boronic Acid, *Biochemistry* Vol. 58 (No. 13): 2804-2811

[45] Eder, J.; Hommel, U.; Cumin, F.; Martoglio, B. & Gerthartz, B. (2007) Aspartic Proteases in Drug Discovery. *Curr. Pharm. Des.* Vol. 13 (No. 3): 271-285

[46] Edwards, A. A.; Mason, J. M.; Clinch, K.; Tyler, P. C.; Evans, G. B. & Schramm V. L. (2009) Altered Enthalpy-Entropy Compensation in Picomolar Transition State Analogues of Human Purine Nucleoside Phosphorylase. *Biochemistry* Vol. 48 (No. 23): 5226-5238

[47] Eidam, Oliv.; Romagnoli, C.; Caselli, E.; Babaoglu, K.; Teotico Pohlhaus, D.; Karpiak, J.; Bonnet, R.; Stoichet, B. K. & Prati, F. (2010) Design, Synthesis, Crystal Structures, and Antimicrobial Activity of Sulfonamide Boronic Acids as -Lactamase Inhibitors. *J. Med. Chem.* Vol. 53 (No.21): 7852-7863

[48] Ellsworth, B. A.; Tom, N. J. & Bartlett, P. A. (1996) Synthesis and Evaluation of Inhibitors of Bacterial D-Alanine:D-Alanine Ligases. *Chem.Biol.* Vol. 3, (No. 1): 37–44

[49] Evans, G. B.; Furneaux, R. H.; Greatrex, B.; Murkin, A. S.; Schramm, V. L. & Tyler, P. C. (2008) Azetidine Based Transition State Analogue Inhibitors of N-Ribosyl Hydrolases and Phosphorylases. *J. Med.Chem.* Vol. 51 (No. 4): 948-956

[50] Evdokimov, A. G.; Pokross, M.; Walter, R. M.; Mekel, M.; Barnett, B. L.; Amburger, J.; Seibel, W. L.; Soper, S.J.; Djung, J, F.; Fairweather, N.; Diven, C.; Rastogi, V.; Grinius, L.; Klanke, C.; Siehner, R.; Twinem, T. & Andrews, R. (2007) Serendipitous Discovery

of Novel Bacterial Methionine Aminopeptidase Inhibitors. *Proteins* Vol. 66 (No. 3): 538-546

[51] Fisher, J. F. & Mobashery S. (2006) Recent Advances in Recent MMP Inhibitor Design. *Cancer Matastasis Rev.* Vol. 25 (No. 1): 115-136

[52] Fournié-Zaluski, M-.C.; Poras, H.; Roques, B.P.; Nakajima, Y.; Ito, K. & Yoshimoto, T. (2009) Structure of Aminopeptidase N from *Escherichia coli* Complexed with the Transition-state Analogue Aminophosphinic Inhibitor PL250. *Acta Crystallogr. D* Vol. 65 (No. 8): 814-822

[53] Frase, H. F. & Lee, I. (2007) Peptidyl Boronates Inhibit *Salmonella enterica* Serovar Typhimurium Lon Protease by a Competitive ATP-Dependent Mechanism, *Biochemistry* Vol. 46 (No.22): 6647-6657

[54] Fujimoto, T.; Matsushita, Y.; Gouda, H.; Yamaotsu, N. & Hirono, S. (2008) In Silico Multi-filter Screening Approaches for Developing Novel -Secretase Inhibitors. *Bioorg. Med. Chem. Lett.* Vol. 18 (No. 9): 2771-2775

[55] Gajda, A.; Pawelczak, M. & Drag, M. (2012) Substrate Specificity Screening of Oat (*Avena sativa*) Seeds Aminopeptidase Demonstrate Unusually Broad Tolerance in S1 Pocket. *Plant Physiol. Biochem.* Vol. 54 (May 2012): 6-9

[56] Ghavami, A.; Johnston, B. D. & Pinto, B. M. (2001) A New Class of Glycosidase Inhibitor: Synthesis of Salacinol and Its Stereoisomers. *J. Org. Chem.*, Vol. 66 (No .7): 2312-2317

[57] Gloster, T. M. & Davies, G. J. (2010) Glycosidase Inhibition: Assessing Mimicry of the Transition State. *Org. Biomol. Chem.* Vol. 8 (No.): 305-320

[58] Gonzaga-Jagureui, C.; Lupski, J. R. & Gibbs, R. A. (2012) Human Genome Sequencing in Health and Disease. *Annu. Rev. Med.* Vol. 63: 35-61

[59] Green, R. & Lorsch, J. R. (2002) The Path to Perdition Is Paved with Protons. *Cell* Vol. 110 (No. 6): 665-668

[60] Grembecka, J. & Kafarski, P. (2001) Leucine Aminopeptidase as a Target for Inhibitor Design. *Mini Rev. Med. Chem.* Vol. 1 (No. 2): 133 - 144.

[61] Grembecka, J.; Mucha, A.; Cierpicki, T. & Kafarski, P. (2003) The Most Potent Organophosphorus Inhibitors of Leucine Aminopeptidase. Structure-based Design, Chemistry, and Activity. *J. Med. Chem.* Vol. 46 (No. 13): 2641 – 2655

[62] Grzywa, R.; Oleksyszyn, J.; Salvesen, G. S. & Drag, M. (2010) Identification of Very Potent Inhibitor of Human Aminopeptidase N (CD13). *Bioorg. Med. Chem. Lett.* Vol. 20 (No.8): 2497-2499

[63] Gurulingappa, H.; Buckhaults, P.; Kumar, S. K.; Kinzler K. W.; Vogelstein, B. & Khazn, S. R. (2003) Design, Synthesis and Evaluation of New RDP Inhibitors. *Tetrahedron Lett.* Vol. 44 (No. 9): 1871-1873

[64] Hamada, Y.; Tagad, H. D.; Nishimura, Y.; Ishiura, S. & Kiso, Y. (2012) Tripeptidic BACE1 Inhibitors Devised by *In-silico* Conformational Structure-based Design. *Bioorg. Med. Chem.* Vol. 22 (No. 2): 1130-1135

[65] Henley, D. B.; May, P. C.; Dean, R.A. & Siemers, R. E. (2009) Development of Semagacestat (LY450139), a Functional Gamma-secretase Inhibitor, for the Treatment of Alzheimer's Disease. *Expert Opinion Pharmacoother.* Vol. 10 (No. 10): 1657-1654

[66] Hibi, T.; Nii, H.; Nakatsu, T.; Kimura, A.; Kato, H.; Hiratake, J. & Oda, J. (2004) Crystal Structure of γ -Glutamylcysteine Synthetase: Insights Into the Mechanism of Catalysis by a Key Enzyme for Glutathione Homeostasis. *Proc. Natl. Acad. Sci. U.S.A.* Vol. 101 (No. 42): 15052-15057

[67] Holyoak, T.; Kettner, C. A.; Petsko, G. A; Fuller, R. S. & Ringe, D. (2004) Structural Basis for Differences in Substrate Selectivity in Kex2 and Furin Protein Convertases. *Biochemistry* Vol. 43 (No. 9): 2412-2421

[68] Hou, G. & Cui, Q. (2011) QM/MM Analysis Suggests that Alkaline Phosphatase (AP) and Nucleotide Pyrophosphatase/Phosphodiesterase Slightly Tighten the Transition State for Phosphate Diester Hydrolysis Relative to Solution: Implication for Catalytic Promiscuity in the AP Superfamily. *J. Am. Chem. Soc.* Vol. 134 (No. 1): 229-246

[69] Hu, G.; Lin, G.; Wang, M.; Dick, L.; Xu, R. M.; Nathan, C. & Li, H. (2006) Structure of the Mycobacterium tuberculosis Proteasome and Mechanism of Inhibition by a Peptidyl Boronate. *Mol. Microbiol.* Vol. 59 (No. 5): 1417-1428

[70] Hu, Y. P; Liu, H. G.; Teng, K. H. & Liang, P. H. (2010) Mechanism of cis-Prenyltransferase Reaction Probed by Substrate Analogues. *Biochem. Biophys. Res. Commun.* Vol. 400 (No. 4): 758-762

[71] Iyer, L. M.; Zhang, D. P. ; Rogozhin, I. B. & Aravind, L. (2011) Evolution of the Deaminase Fold and Multiple Origins of Eukaryotic Editing and Mutagenic Nucleic Acid Deaminases from Bacterial Toxin Systems. *Nucl. Acid. Res.* Vol. 39 (No. 22): 9473-9497

[72] Jeurs, D. H.; Kim, J.; Matthews, B. W. & Sieburth, S. McN. (2005) Structural Analysis of Silanediols as Transition-State-Analogue Inhibitors of the Benchmark Metalloprotease Thermolysin. *Biochemistry* Vol. 44 (No. 50): 16524-16528

[73] John, S.; Thangapandian, S.; Sakkiah, S. & Lee, K. W. (2011) Potent Bace-1 Inhibitor Design Using Pharmacophore Modeling, In Silico Screening and Molecular Docking Studies. *BMC Bioinformatics* Vol. 12 (Suppl. 1): S28

[74] Johnson, J. L.; Devel, L.; Czarny, B.; George, S. J.; Jackson, C. L.; Rogakos, V.; Beau, F.; Yiokatis, A.; Newby, A. C. & Dive, V. (2011) A Selective Matrix Metalloproteinase-12 Inhibitor Retards Atherosclerotic Plaque Development in Apolipoprotein E-knockout Mice. *Arterioscl. Tromb. Vasc. Biol.* Vol. 31 (No. 3): 528-535

[75] Jørgensen, A. T.; Norrby, P. O. & Liljefors, T. (2002) Investigation of the Metal Binding Site in Methionine Aminopeptidase by Density Functional Theory. *J. Comput. Aided Mol. Des.* Vol. 16 (No. 3): 167-179

[76] Julien, N.; Makritis, A; Georgiadis, D.; Beau, F.; Yiotakis, A. & Dive, V. (2010) Phosphinic Tripeptides as Dual Angiotensin-Converting Enzyme C-Domain and Endothelin-Converting Enzyme-1 Inhibitors. *J. Med. Chem,.* Vol. 53 (No. 1): 208-220

[77] Kalva, S.; Vadivelan, S.; Sanam, R.; Jagarlapudi, S. A. R. P. & Saleena, L. M. (2012) Lead Identification and Optimization of Novel Collagenase Inhibitors; Pharmacophore and Structure Based Studies. *Bioinformation* Vol. 8 (No. 7): 301-308

[78] Kati, W. M.; Montgomery, D.; Maring, C.; Stoll, V. S.; Giranda, V.; Chen, X.; Laver, W. G.; Kohlbrenner, W. & Norbeck, D. W. (2001) Novel - and -Amino Acid Inhibitors of Influenza Virus Neuraminidase. *Antimicrob. Agents Chemither.* Vol. 45 (No. 9): 2563-2570

[79] Ke, W.; Sampson, J. M.; Ori, C.; Prato, F.; Drawz, S. E.; Bethel, C. R.; Bonomo, R. A.; & van den Akken, F. (2011) Novel Insights into the Mode of Inhibition of Class A SHV-1 -Lactamases Revealed by Boronic Acid Transition State Inhibitors. *Antimicrob. Agents Chemother.* Vol. 55 (No. 1): 174-183

[80] Keough, D. T.; Hoćkova, D.; Holy, A.; Naesenes, L. M. J.; Skinner-Adams, T. S.; de Jersey, J.; & Guddat, L. W. (2009) Inhibition of Hypoxanthine - Guanine Phosphoribosyltransferase by Acyclic Nucleoside Phosphonates:A New Class of Antimalarial Therapeutics. *J. Med. Chem.* Vol. 52 (No.): 4391-4399

[81] Khaliullin, I. G.; Suplatov, D. A.; Dalaeva, D. L.; Otsuka, M.; Asano, Y. & Švedas, V. K. (2010) Bioinformatic Analysis, Molecular Modeling of Role of Lys65 Residue in Catalytic Triad of D-aminopeptidase from Ochrobactrum anthropi. Acta Naturae Vol. 2 (No. 2): 66-71

[82] Khandelwal, A.; Lukacova, V.; Comez, D.; Kroll, D. M.; Raha, S. & Balaz, S. (2005) A Combination of Docking, QM/MM Methods, and MD Simulation for Binding Affinity Estimation of Metalloprotein Ligands. *J. Med. Chem.* Vol. 48 (No. 17): 5437-5447

[83] Kim, C. U.; Williams, M. A.; Lui, H.; Zhang, L.; Swaminathan, S.; Bischofberger, N.; Chen, M. S.; Mendel, D.B.; Tai, C. Y.; Laver, W. G. & Stevens, R. C. (1997). Influenza Neuraminidase Inhibitors Possessing a Novel Hydrophobic Interaction in the Enzyme Active Site: Design, Synthesis and Structural Analysis of Carbocyclic Sialic Acid Analogues with PotentAanti-influenza Activity. *J. Am. Chem. Soc.* Vol. 119 (No. 4) 681–690.

[84] Kollman, P. A.; Kuhn, B. & Peräkylä, M. (2002) Computational Studies of Enzyme-Catalyzed Reactions: Where Are We in Predicting Mechanisms and in Understanding the Nature of Enzyme Catalysis? *J. Phys. Chem. B* Vol. 106 (No. 7): 1537-1542

[85] Kosikowska, P. & Berlicki, L. (2011) Urease Inhibitors as Potential Drugs for Gastric and Urinary Tract Infections: a Patent Review. *Expert Opin. Ther. Patents* Vol. 21 (No. 6): 945-957

[86] Kotsugi, T. & Hayashi, S. (2012) Crucial Role of Protein Flexibility in Formation of a Stable Reaction Transition State in an -Amylase Catalysis. *J. Am. Chem. Soc.* Vol. 134 (No. 16): 7045-7055

[87] Kruger, R. G.; Barkallah, S.; Frankel, B. A. & Mc Cafferty, B. G. (2004) Inhibition of the *Staphylococcus aureus* Sortase Transpeptidase SrtA by Phosphinic Peptidomimetics. *Bioorg. Med. Chem.* Vol. 12 (No.13): 3723-3729

[88] Lauer-Fields, J. L.; Brew, K.; Whitehead, J. K.; Li, S.; Hammer, R. P. & Fields, G.B. (2007) Triple-Helical Transition State Analogues: A New Class of Selective Matrix Metalloproteinase Inhibitors. *J. Am. Chem. Soc.* Vol. 129 (No. 30): 10408-10417

[89] Lauer-Fields, J. L.; Whitehead, J. K.; Li, S.; Hammer, R. P. ; Brew, K. & Fields, G.B. (2008) Selective Modulation of Matrix Metalloproteinase 9 (MMP-9) Functions via Exosite Inhibition. *J. Biol. Chem.* Vol. 283 (No.29): 20087-20095

[90] Lazcano, I.; Uribe, R. M.; Martinez-Cháves, E.; Vargas, M. A.; Matziari, M.; Joseph-Bravo P. & Charli, J. M. (2012) Pyroglutamyl Peptidase II Inhibition Enhances the Analeptic Effect of Thyrotropin-Releasing Hormone in the Rat Medial Septum. *J. Pharmacol. Exp. Ther.* Vol. 342 (No. 1): 222-231

[91] Lebeau, A.; Singh, P.; Isaacs, J, & Denmeade, S. R. (2008) Potent and Selective Peptidyl Boronic Acid Inhibitors of the Serine Protease Prostate-Specific Antigen. *Chem. Biol.* Vol. 15 (No. 7): 665-674

[92] Lee, J. K.; Bain, A. D. & Berti, P. J. (2004) Probing the Transition States of Four Glucoside Hydrolyses with ^{13}C Kinetic Isotope Effects Measured at Natural Abundance by NMR Spectroscopy. *J. Am. Chem. Soc.* Vol. 126 (No. 12): 3769-3776

[93] Li, X.; Hayik, S. A. & Merz Jr, K. M. (2010) QM/MM X-Ray Refinement of Zinc Metalloenzymes. *J. Inorg. Biochem.* Vol. 104 (No. 5): 512-522

[94] Li, Y.; Cao, H.; Hai, Y.; Chen, Y.; Lau, K.; Qu, J.; Thon, V.; Sugirato, G. & Chen, X. (2011) Identifying Selective Inhibitors Against Human Cytosolic Sialidase NEU2 by Substrate Specificity Studies. *Mol. Biosyst.* Vol. 7 (No. 4): 1060-1072

[95] Lienhard, G. E. (1973) Enzymatic Catalysis and Transition-state Theory, *Science* Vol. 180 (No. 4082): 149-154

[96] Lin, Y.-L & Gao, J. (2011) Kinetic Isotope Effects of *L*-Dopa Decarboxylase, *J. Am. Chem. Soc.* Vol,. 133 (No. 12): 4398-4403

[97] Lipscamp, R. M. J. & Kruijtzer J. A. W. (2004) Peptide Transformation Leading to Peptide-peptidosulfonamide Hybrids and Oligo Peptidosulfonamides. *Mol. Divers.* Vol. 8 (No. 2): 787-97

[98] Liu, H.; Sim. L.; Rose, D. L. & Pinto, B. M. (2006) A New Class of Glucosidase Inhibitor: Analogues of the Naturally Occurring Glucosidase Inhibitor Salacinol with Different Ring Heteroatom Substituents and Acyclic Chain Extension. *J. Org. Chem.* Vol. 71 (No. 8): 3007-3013

[99] Lonsdale, R.; Harvey, J. N. & Mulholland, A. J. (2010) Compound I Reactivity Defines Alkene Oxidation Selectivity in Cytochrome P450cam. *J. Phys. Chem. B* Vol.114, (No. 2): 1156–1162

[100] Lonsdale, R.; Harvey, J. N. & Mulholland, A. J. (2012) A Practical Guide to Modelling Enzyme-Catalysed Reactions. *Chem. Soc. Rev.* Vol. 41 (No. 8): 3025–3038

[101] Löwik, D. W. P. M. and Liskamp, R. M. J. (2000) Synthesis of - and -Substituted Aminoethane Sulfonamide Arginine-Glycine Mimics. *Eur. J.Org. Chem.*, Vol. 2000 (No. 7): 1219-1228

[102] Lowther, W. T. & Matthews, B. W. (2002) Metalloaminopeptidases: Common Functional Themes in Disparate Structural Surroundings. *Chem. Rev.* Vol. 102 (No.12): 4581-4607

[103] Mahalingham, A. K.; Axelsson, L.; Ekegren, J. K.; Wanneberg, B.; Kihlström, J.; Unge, T,; Wallberg, H.; Samuelsson, B.; Larhed, M. & Hallberg, A (2010) HIV-1 Protease Inhibitors with a Transition-State Mimic Comprising a Tertiary Alcohol: Improved Antiviral Activity in Cells. *J. Med. Chem.* Vol. 53 (No. 2): 607-615

[104] Martone, R. L.; Zhou, H.; Atchison, K.; Comery, T.; Xu, J. Z.; Huang, X.; Gong, X.; Jin, M.; Kreft, A.; Harrison, B.; Mayer, S. C.; Aschmies, S.; Gonzales, C.; Zaleska, M. M.; Riddel, D. R.; Wagner, E.; Lu, P.; Sun, S.-C.; Sonnenberg-Reines, J.; Oganesian, A.; Adkins, K.; Leach, M.W.; Clarke, D. W.; Huryn, D.; Abou-Gharbia, M.; Magolda, R.; Bard, J.; Frick, G.; Raje, S.; Forlow, S. B.; Balliet, C.; Burczynski R. E.; Reinhart, P. H.; Wan, H. I.; Pangalos, M. N. & Jacobsen, J. S. (2009) Begacestat (GSI-953): A Novel, Selective Thiophene Sulfonamide Inhibitor of Amyloid Precursor Protein -Secretase for the Treatment of Alzheimer's Disease. *J. Parmacol. Exp. Ther.* Vol. 331 (No. 2): 598-608

[105] Matziari, M.; Beau, F.; Cuniasse, P.; Dive, V. & Yiotakis, A. (2004) Evaluationof P1'-Diversified Phosphinic Peptides Leads to the Development Ofhighly Selective Inhibitors of MMP-11. *J. Med. Chem.* Vol. 47 (No. 2): 325-336

[106] Matziari, M.; Dive, V. & Yiotakis, A. (2007) Matrix Metalloproteinase 11 (MMP-11; Stromelysin-3) and Synthetic Inhibitors. *Med. Res. Rev.* Vol. 27 (No. 4): 528-552

[107] Matziari, M.; Bauer, K.; Dive, V. & Yiotakis, A. (2008) Synthesis of the Phosphinic Analogue of Thyrotropin Releasing Hormone. *J. Org. Chem.* Vol. 73 (No. 21): 8591-8693

[108] Mayer, S. C.; Kreft, A. S.; Harrison, B.; Abou-Gharbia, M.; Antane, M.; Aschmies, S.; Atchison, K.; Chlenov, M.; Cole, D. C.; Comery, T.; Diamantis, G.; Ellingboe, J.; Fan, K.; Gallante, R.; Gonzales, K.; Ho, D. M.; Hoke, M. E.; Hu, Y.; Huryn, D.; Jain, U.; Jin, M.; Kremer, K.; Kubrak, D.; Lin, M.; Lu, P.; Magolda, R.; Martone, R.; Moore, W.; Oganesian, A.; Pangalos, M. N.; Porte, A.; Reinhart, P.; Resnick, L.; Riddel, D. R.; Sonnenberg-Reines, J.; Stock, J. R.; Sun, S.-C.; Wagner, E.; Wang, T.; Woller, K.; Xu, Z.; Zaleska, M. M.; Zeldis, J.; Zhang, M.; Zhou, H. & Jacobsen J. S. (2008) Discovery of Begacestat, a Notch-1-Sparing -Secretase Inhibitor for the Treatment of Alzheimer's Disease. *J. Med. Chem.* Vol. 51 (No. 23): 7348-7351

[109] McGowan, S.; Oellig, C. A.; Birru, W. A.; Caradoc-Davies, T. T.; Stack, C. M.; Lowther, J.; Skinner-Adams, T.; Mucha, A.; Kafarski, P.; Grembecka, J.; Trenholme, K. R.; Buckle, A. M.; Gardiner, D. L.; Dalton, J. P. & Whisstock, J. C. (2010) Structure of the *Plasmodium falciparum* M17 Aminopeptidase and Significance for the Design of Drugs Targeting the Neutral Exopeptidases. *Proc. Natl. Acad. Sci. U.S.A.* Vol. 107, (No. 6), 2449 – 2454

[110] McGowan, S.; Porter, C. J.; Lowther. J.; Stack, C. M.; Golding, S. J.; Skinner-Adams, T. S.; Trenholme, K. R.; Teuscher, F.; Donnelly, S. M.; Grembecka, J.; Mucha, A.; Kafarski, P.; Degori, R.; Buckle, A. M.; Gardiner, D. L.; Whisstock, J. C. & Dalton, J. P. (2009) Structural Basis for the Inhibition of the Essential Plasmodium falciparum M1 Neutral Aminopeptidase. *Proc. Natl. Acad. Sci. U.S.A.* Vol. 106 (No. 8): 2537 – 2542

[111] Medina, R. A. & Garcia-Sastre, A. (2011) Influenza A Viruses: New Research Developments. *Nat. Rev. Microbiol.* Vol. 9 (August 2011): 590-603

[112] Meanwell, N. A. (2011) Synopsis of Some Recent Tactical Application of Bioisosteres in Drug Design. *J. Med. Chem.* Vol. 54 (No. 8): 2529-2591

[113] Mohan, S. & Pinto, B. M. (2008) Zwitterionic Glycosidase Inhibitors: Salacinol and Related Analogues. *Carbohydr. Res.* Vol. 342 (No. 12-13): 1551-1580

[114] Moree, W. J.; Van Gent, L. C.; Van Der Marel, G. A. & Liskamp,R. M. J., (1993) Synthesis of Peptides Containing a Sulfinamide or a Sulfonamidetransition State Isostere. *Tetrahedron* Vol. 49 (No.5): 1133-1150

[115] Moree, W. J.; Van Der Marel, G. A. & Liskamp, R. M. J. (1995) Synthesis of Peptidosulfinamides and Peptidosulfonamides Containing the Sulfinamide or Sulfonamide Transition-state Isostere. *J. Org. Chem.*, Vol. 60 (No. 16): 5157-5169

[116] Mores, A.; Matziari, M.; Beau, F.; Cuniasse, P.; Yiotakis, A. & Dive, V,.(2008) Development of Potent and Selective Phosphinic Peptide Inhibitors of Angiotensin-Converting Enzyme 2. *J. Med. Chem.* Vol. 51 (No.7): 2216-2226

[117] Mucha, A.; Pawelczak, M.; Hurek, J. & Kafarski, P. (2004) Synthesis and Activity of Phosphinic Tripeptide Inhibitors of Cathepsin C. *Bioorg. Med. Chem. Lett.* Vol. 14 (No. 12) 3113 – 3116

[118] Mucha, A.; Lämmerhoffer, M.; Lindner, W.; Pawelczak, M. & Kafarski, P. (2008) Individual Stereoisomers of Phosphinic Dipeptide Inhibitor of Leucine Aminopeptidase. *Bioorg. Med. Chem. Lett.* Vol. 18 (No. 5): 1550-1554

[119] Mucha, A.; Drag, M.; Dalton, J. P. & Kafarski, P. (2010) Metallo-Aminopeptidase Inhibitors. *Biochimie* Vol. 92 (No. 11): 1509 - 1529.

[120] Mucha, A.; Kafarski, P. & Berlicki, L. (2011) Remarkable Potential of the -Aminophosphonate/Phosphinate Structural Motif in Medicinal Chemistry. *J. Med. Chem.* Vol. 54 (No. 17): 5955-5980

[121] Muo, L. & Schramm, V. L. (2008) Transition State Structure of E. coli tRNA-Specific Adenosine Deaminase. *J. Am. Chem. Soc.* Vol. 130 (No. 8): 2649-2655

[122] Murkin, A. S.; Birck, M. R.; Rinaldo-Matthis, A.; Shi, W.; Taylor, E. A.; Almo, S. C. & Schramm, V. L. (2007) Neighboring Group Participation in the Transition State of Human Purine Nucleoside Phosphorylase. *Biochemistry* Vol. 26 (No. 17): 5038-5049

[123] Mutahi, M.; Nittoli, T.; Guo, L.; Sieburth, S. McN. (2002) Silicon-based Metalloprotease Inhibitors: Synthesis and Evaluation of Silanol and Silanediol Peptide Analogues as Inhibitors of Angiotensin-converting Enzyme. *J. Am. Chem. Soc.* Vol. 124 (No. 25): 7363-7365

[124] Nelson, M. I. & Holmes, E. C. (2007) The Evolution of Epidemic Influenza, *Nat. Rev, Genet.* Vol. 8 (March 2007): 196-205

[125] Neuhaus, F. C. (2010) Role of Arg301 in Substrate Orientation and Catalysis in Subsite 2 of D-Alanine:D-alanine (D-Lactate) Ligase from Leuconostoc mesenteroides: A Molecular Docking Study. J. *Mol. Graphics Model.* Vol. 28 (No. 8): 728–734

[126] Nukaga, M.; Kumar, S.; Nukaga, K.; Pratt, R. F. & Knox, J. R. (2004) Hydrolysis of Third-generation Cephalosporins by Class C -Lactamases. *J. Biol. Chem.* Vol. 10 (No. 5): 9344-9352

[127] Osterman, N.; Eder, J.; Eidhoff, U.; Zink, F.; Hassiepen, U.; Worpenberg, S.; Mainbaum, J. Simic, O.; Hommel, U. & Gerhartz, B. (2006) Crystal Structure of Human BACE2 in Complex with a Hydroxyethylamine Transition-state Inhibitor. *J. Mol. Biol.* Vol. 355 (No.)2: 249-261

[128] Overall, C. M. & Kleifield O. (2006) Validating Matrix Metalloproteinases as Drug Targets and Anti-targets for Cancer Therapy *Nat. Rev. Cancer* Vol. 6 (No. 3): 227-239

[129] Palese, P.; Schulman, J. N.; Bodo, G. &Meindl, P. (1974). Inhibition of Influenza and Parainfluenza Virus Replication in Tissue culture by 2-Deoxy-2,3-dehydro-N-trifluoroacetylneuraminic Acid (FANA). *Virology* Vol. 59 (No. 2) 490–498.

[130] Parks, J. M., Imhof, P. & Smith, J. C. (2010) Understanding Enzyme Catalysis Using Computer Simulation. *Encyclopedia of Catalysis 2nd Ed.* John Wiley & Sons 2010

[131] Pauling, L. (1949) Achievement and Hope for the Future. *Am. Sci.* Vol. 36: 50-58

[132] Pierdominici-Sottile, G.; Horenstein, N. A. & Roitberg A. E. (2011) Free Energy Study of the Catalytic Mechanism of T*rypanosoma cruzi trans*-Sialidase. From the Michaelis Complex to the Covalent Intermediate. *Biochemistry* Vol. 22 (No. 46): 10150-10158

[133] Pirard, B. (2007) Insight Into the Structural Determinants for Selective Inhibition of Matrix Metalloproteinases. *Drug Discovery Today* Vol. 12 (No.15/16): 640-646

[134] Pokorná, J.; Machala, L.; Řezáčova, P. & Konvalinka, J. (2009) Current and Novel Inhibitors of HIV Protease. *Viruses* Vol. 1 (No. 3): 1209-1239

[135] Polgár, L. (2005) The catalytic triad of serine peptidases. *Cell. Mol. Life Sci.* Vol. 62 (No. 19-20): 2161-2172

[136] Poreba, M.; Gajda, A.; Picha, J.; Jiráček, J.; Marschner, A.; Klein, C. D., Salvesen, G. S. & Drag, M. (2011) S1 Pocket Fingerprints of Human and Bacterial Methionine Aminopeptidases Determined Using Fluorogenic Libraries of Substrates and Phosphorus Based Inhibitors. *Biochimie* Vol. 94 (No. 3): 704-710

[137] Poreba M.; McGowan, S.; Skinner-Adams, T. S.; Trenholme, K. S.; Gardiner, D. L.; Whisstock, J. C.; To, J.; Salvesen, G. S.; Dalton, J. P. & Drag, M. (2012) Fingerprinting the Substrate Specificity of M1 and M17 Aminopeptidases of Human Malaria, *Plasmodium falciparum. PLOS One* Vol. 7 (No. 2): e31938

[138] Powell, J. R.; DeForrest, J. M.; Cushman, D. W.; Rubin, B. & Petrillo, E. W. (1984) Antihypertensive Effects of a New ACE Inhibitor, SQ. 28555. *Fed. Proc.* Vol. 43 (No. 3): 733

[139] Radzicka, A., and Wolfenden, R. (1995) Transition State and Multisubstrate Analog Inhibitors, *Methods Enzymol.* Vol. 249: 284-312

[140] Reiter, L. A.; Martinelli, G. J.; Reeves, L. A. & Mitchell, P. G. (2000) Difluoroketones as Inhibitors of Matrix Metalloprotease-13. *Bioorg. Med. Chem. Lett.* Vol. 10 (No.14): 1581-1584

[141] Reiter, L. A.; Mitchell, P. G.; Martinelli, G. J.; Lopresti-Morrow, L. L.; Yocum, S. A. & Escra, J. D. (2003) Phosphinic Acid-Based MMP-13 Inhibitors That Spare MMP-1 and MMP-3. *Bioorg. Med. Chem. Lett.* Vol. 13 (No. 14): 2331-2336

[142] Rejman, D.; Panova, N.; Klener, P.; Maswabi, B.; Pohl, R. & Rosenberg, I. (2012) N-Phosphonocarbonylpyrrolidine Derivatives of Guanine: A NewClass of Bi-Substrate Inhibitors of Human Purine Nucleoside Phosphorylase. *J. Med. Chem.* Vol. 55 (No. 4): 1612-1621

[143] Rempel, B. R. & Withers, S. G. (2008) Covalent Inhibitors of Glycosidases and Their Applications in Biochemistry and Biology. *Glycobiology* Vol. 18 (No 8): 570-586

[144] Robertson, J. G. (2005) Mechanistic Basis of Enzyme-Targeted Drugs. *Biochemistry* Vol. 44 (No. 15): 5561-5571

[145] Rodnina, M. V.; Beringer, L. & Wintermeyer, W. (2006) How Ribosomes Make Peptide Bonds. *Trends Biochem. Sci.* Vol 31 (No.1): 20-26

[146] Sabina, R. L.; Paul, A.-L.; Ferl, R. J.; Laber, B. & Lindell, S. D. (2007) Adenine Nucleotide Pool Perturbation Is a Metabolic Trigger for AMP Deaminase Inhibitor-Based Herbicide Toxicity. *Plant Physiol.* Vol. 143 (No. 4): 1752-1760

[147] Saen-oon, S.; Quaytman-Machleder, S.; Schramm, V. L. & Schwartz, S. D. (2008) Atomic Detail of Chemical Transformation at the Transition State of an Enzymatic Reaction. *PNAS* Vol. 105 (No. 43): 16543-16545

[148] Sang, Q.-X. A.; Jin, Y.; Newcomer, R. G.; Monroe, S. C.; Fang, X.; Hurst, D. R.; Lee, S.; Cao, Q. & Schwartz, M. A. (2006) Matrix Metalloproteinase Inhibitors as Prospective Agents for the Prevention and Treatment of Cardiovascular and Neoplastic Diseases. *Curr. Top. Med. Chem.* Vol. 6 (No. 4): 289-316

[149] Schramm, V. L. (2002) Development of Transition State Analogues of Purine Nucleoside Phosphorylase as Anti-T-cell Agents. *Biochim. Biophys. Acta* Vol. 1587 (No. 2-3): 107-117

[150] Schramm, V. L. (2005) Enzymatic Transition States and Transition State Analogues. *Curr. Opin. Struct. Biol.* Vol. 15 (No. 7): 604-613

[151] Schramm, V. L. (2007) Enzymatic Transition State Theory and Transition State Analogue Design. *J. Biol. Chem.* Vol. 282 (No. 39): 28297-28300

[152] Schramm, V. L. (2011) Enzymatic Transition States, Transition-State Analogs, Dynamics, Thermodynamics, and Lifetimes. *Annu. Rev. Biochem.* Vol. 80: 703-732

[153] Schwartz, P. A.; Vetticatt, J. & Schramm V. L. (2010) Transition State Analysis of Thymidine Hydrolysis by Human Thymidine Phosphorylase. *J. Am. Chem. Soc.* Vol. 132 (No. 38): 13425-13433

[154] Senn, H. M. & Thiel, W. (2007) QM/MM Studies of Enzymes. *Curr. Opin. Chem. Biol.* Vol. 11 (No. 2): 182-187

[155] Shi, W.; Wu, C. M.; Tyler, P.C.; Furmeaux, R. H.; Cahill, S. M.; Girvin, M. E.; Grubmeyer, C.; Schramm, V. L & Almo, S.C. (1999) The 2.0 Å Structure of Malarial Purine Phosphoribosyltransferase in Complex with a Transition-State Analogue Inhibitor. *Biochemistry* Vol. 38 (No. 31): 9872-9880

[156] Shie, J. J.; Fang, J. M.; Wang, S. Y.; Tsai, K. C.; Chemg, Y.-S. E.; Yang, A. S.; Hsiao, S. C.; Su, C. Y. & Wong C. H. (2007) Synthesis of Tamiflu and its Phosphonate Congeners Possessing Potent Anti-Influenza Activity. *J. Am. Chem. Soc.* Vol. 129 (No. 39): 11892-11893

[157] Shin, H.; Cama, E. & Christianson, D. W. (2004) Design of Amino Acid Aldehydes as Transition-State Analogue Inhibitors of Arginase. *J. Am. Chem. Soc.* Vol. 126 (No. 33): 10278-10284

[158] Shishova, E. Y.; Di Costanzo, L.; Emig, S. A.; Ash, D. E. & Christianson, D. W. (2009) Probing the Specificity Determinants of Amino Acid Recognition by Arginase. *Biochemistry* Vol. 48 (No. 1): 121-131

[159] Sieburth, S. McN. & Chen, C.-A. (2006) Silanediol Protease Inhibitors: From Conception to Validation. *Eur. J. Org. Chem.* Vol. 2006 (No. 2): 311-322

[160] Skinner-Adams, T.; McCarthy, J. S.; Gardiner, D. L.; Hilton, P. M.& Andrews, K. T. (2004) Antiretrovirals as Antimalarial Agents. *J. Infect. Dis.* Vol. 190 (No. 11); 1998-2000

[161] Skinner-Adams, T. S.; Lowther, J.; Teuscher, F.; Stack, C. M.; Grembecka, J.; Mucha, A.; Kafarski, P.; Trenholme, K. R.; Dalton, J. P.; & Gardiner, D. L.(2007) Identification of Phosphinate Dipeptide Analog Inhibitors Directed Against the *Plasmodium falciparum* M17 Leucine Aminopeptidase as Lead Antimalarial Compounds. *J. Med. Chem.* Vol. 50 (No. 24): 6024 - 6031.

[162] Skinner-Adams, T. S.; Stack, C. M.; Trenholme, K. R.; Brown, C. L.; Grembecka, J.; Lowther, J.; Mucha, A.; Drag, M.; Kafarski, P.; McGowan, S.; Whisstock, J. C.; Gardiner, D. L. & Dalton, J. P. (2010) *Plasmodium falciparum* Neutral Aminopeptidases: New Targets for Anti-malarials. *Trends Biochem. Sci.* Vol. 35 (No. 1): 53 – 61

[163] Silva, R. G.; Hirschi, J. S.; Ghanem, M.; Murkin, A. S.; & Schramm, V. L. (2011) Arsenate and Phosphate as Nucleophiles at the Transition States of Human Purine Nucleoside Phosphorylase. Biochemistry, Vol. 50 (No.): 2701-2709

[164] Stack, C. M.; Lowther, J.; Cunningham, E.; Donnelly, S.; Gardiner, D. L.; Trenholme, K. R.; Skinner-Adams, T. S.; Teuscher, F.; Grembecka, J.; Mucha, A.; Kafarski, P.; Lua, L.; Bell, A. & Dalton, J. P. (2007) Characterization of the *Plasmodium falciparum* M17 Leucyl Aminopeptidase. A Protease Involved in Amino Acid Regulation with Potential for Antimalarial Drug Development. *J. Biol. Chem.* Vol. 282 (No. 3): 2069 – 2080

[165] Stanley, M.; Cattle, N.; McCauley, J.; Martin, S. R.; Rashid, A.; Field, R. A.; Carbain, B. & Streicher, H. (2012) 'TamiGold': Phospha-oseltamivir-Stabilised Gold Nanoparticles as the Basis for Influenza Therapeutics and Diagnostics Targeting the Neuraminidase (Instead of the Hemagglutinin). *MedChemComm* doi: 10.1039/c2md20034a

[166] Streicher, H. & Busse, H. (2006) Building a Successful Structural Motif into Sialylmimetics - Cyclohexenephosphonate Monoesters as Pseudo-sialosides with Promising Inhibitory properties. *Bioorg. Med. Chem.* Vol. 14 (No. 4): 1047-1057

[167] Sumida, T.; Stubbs, K. A.; Ito, M. & Yokohama, S. (2012) Gaining Insight into the Inhibition of Glycoside Hydrolase Family 20 exo--N-Acetylhexosaminidases Using a Structural Approach. *Org. Biomol. Chem.*Vol. 10 (No. 13): 2607-2612

[168] Teuscher, F.; Lowther, J.; Skinner-Adams, T.S.; Spielmann, T.; Dixon, M.W.A.; Stack, C.M.; Donnelly, S.; Mucha, A.; Kafarski, P.; Vassiliou, S.; Gardiner, D.L.; Dalton, J.P.; Trenholme, K. (2007) The M18 Aspartyl Aminopeptidase of the Human Malaria Parasite *Plasmodium falciparum*. *J. Biol. Chem.* Vol. 282 (No. 42): 30817 – 30826

[169] Thivierge, K.; Mathew, R. T.; Nsangou, D. N. N.; Da Silva, F.; Cotton, S. Skinner-Adams, T. S.; Trenholme, K. R.; Brown, C. L.; Stack, C. M.; Gardiner D. M. & Dalton, J. P. (2012) Anti-malaria Drug Development Targeting the M1 Alanyl and M17 Leucyl Aminopeptidases. ARKIVOC 2012 (No. 4): 330-346

[170] Thomson, J. M.; Prati, F.; Bethel, C. R. & Bonomo, R. A. (2007) Use of Novel Boronic Acid Transition State Inhibitors To Probe SubstrateAffinity in SHV-Type Extended-Spectrum -Lactamase. *Antimicrob. Agents Chemother.* Vol. 51 (No. 4): 1577-1579

[171] Trippier P. C. & McGuigan, C. (2010) Boronic Acids in Medicinal Chemistry: Anticancer, Antibacterial and Antiviral Applications. *Med. Chem. Commun.* Vol. 1 (No. 3): 183-198

[172] Tuan, H. F.; Erskin, P.; Langan, P. Cooper, J. & Coates, L. (2007) Preliminary neutron and ultrahigh-resolution X-ray diffraction studies of the aspartic proteinase endothiapepsin cocrystallized with a gem-diol inhibitor. *Acta Crystallogr.* Vol. 63 (No. 12): 1080-1083

[173] Turcotte, S.; Bouayad-Gervais, H. & Lubell, W. (2012) N-Aminosulfamide PeptideMimic Synthesis by Alkylation of Aza-sulfurylglycinyl Peptides. *Org. Lett.* Vol. 14 (No. 5): 1318-1321

[174] Tyler, P. C.; Taylor, E. A.; Fröhlich, F. R. G. & Schramm, V. L. (2007) Synthesis of 5'-Methylthio Coformycins: Specific Inhibitors for Malarial Adenosine Deaminase. *J. Am. Chem. Soc.* Vol. 129 (No. 21): 6872-6879

[175] Udommaneethanakit, T. Rungrotmongkol, T.; Bren, U.; Frecer, V. & Miertus, S. (2009) Dynamic Behavior of Avian Influenza A Virus Neuraminidase Subtype H5N1 in Complex with Oseltamivir, Zanamivir, Peramivir, and Their Phosphonate Analogues. *J. Chem. Inf.Model.* Vol. 49 (No.10): 2323-2332

[176] Umezawa, H.; Aoyagi, T.; Suda, H.; Hamada, M. & Takeuchi, T. (1976) Bestatin, an Inhibitor of Aminopeptidase B, Produced by Actinomycetes. Journal of Antibiotics (Tokyo) Vol. 29 (No. 1): 97-99

[177] Vasella, A.; Davies, G. J. & Böhm, M (2002) Glycosidase Mechanisms. *Curr. Opin. Chem. Biol.* Vol. 5 (No. 6): 619-629

[178] Vassiliou, S.; Xeilari, M.; Yiotakis, A.; Grembecka, J.; Pawelczak, M.; Kafarski, P. & Mucha, A. (2007) A Synthetic Method for Diversification of the P1' Substituent in Phosphinic Dipeptides as a Tool for Exploration of the Specificity of the S1' Binding Pockets of Leucine Aminopeptidases. *Bioorg. Med. Chem.* Vol. 15 (No. 9): 3187 – 3200

[179] Vassiliou, S.; Grabowiecka, A.; Kosikowska, P.; Yiotakis, A.; Kafarski, P. & Belicki, Ł. (2008) Design, Synthesis, and Evaluation of Novel Organophosphorus Inhibitors of Bacterial Ureases. *J. Med. Chem.* Vol. 51 (No. 18): 5736-5744

[180] Vassiliou, S.; Grabowiecka, A.; Kosikowska, P. & Berlicki, L. (2012) Three Component Kabachnik-Fields Condensation Leading to Substituted Aminomethane-P-hydroxymethylphosphonic Acids as a Tool for Screening of Bacterial Urease Inhibitors. *ARKIVOC* Vol. 2012 (No. 4): 33-43

[181] Weinger, J. S.; Kitchen, D.; Scaringe, S. A.; Strobel, S. A. & Muth, G. W. (2004) Solid Phase Synthesis and Binding Affnity of Peptidyl Transferase Transition State Mimics Containing 2'-OH at P-site Position A76. *Nucl. Acids Res.* Vol. 32 (No. 4):1502-1511

[182] Venkatraman, S.; Wu, W.; Prongay, A.; Girijavallabhan, V. & Njoroge, F. G. (2009) Potent Inhibitors of HCV-NS3 Protease Derived from Boronic Acids. *Bioorg. Med. Chem. Lett.* Vol. 19 (No. 1): 180-183

[183] Verma, R. P. & Hansch, C. (2007) Matrix Metalloproteinases (MMPs): Chemical–Biological Functions and (Q)SARs. *Bioorg. Med. Chem.* Vol. 15 (No. 6): 2223-2268

[184] Wei, D.-Q.; Du, Q.-S.; Sun, H. & Chou, K. H. (2006) Insights from Modeling the 3D Structure of H5N1 Influenza Virus Neuraminidase and its Binding Interactions with Ligands. *Biochem. Biophys. Res. Commun.* Vol. 344 (No. 3): 1048-1055

[185] Wheatley, J. L. & Holyoak, T. (2007) Differential P1 Arginine and Lysine Recognition in the Prototypical Proprotein Convertase Kex2. *Proc. Natl. Acad. Sci. U.S.A.* Vol. 104 (No. 16): 6626-6631

[186] Williams, I. H. (2010) Catalysis: Transition-state Molecular Recognition? *Beilstein J. Org. Chem.* Vol. 6: 1026-1034

[187] Wolfe, M. S. (2012) -Secretase Inhibitors and Modulators for Alzheimer's Disease. *J. Neurochem.* Vol. 120 (Suppl. 1): 89-98

[188] Wolfenden, R. (1972) Analogue Approaches to the Structure of the Transition State in Enzyme Reactions. *Acc. Chem. Res.* Vol. 5: 10-18

[189] Wolfenden, R. (1976) Transition State Analog Inhibitors and Enzyme Catalysis, *Annu. Rev. Biophys. Bioeng.* Vol. 5: 271-306

[190] Wolfenden, R. (1999) Conformational Aspects of Inhibitor Design: Enzyme-Substrate Interactions in the Transition State. *Bioorg. Med. Chem. Lett.* Vol. 7 (No. 5): 647-652

[191] Wolfenden, R. (2003) Thermodynamic and Extrathermodynamic Requirements of Enzyme Catalysis. *Biophys. Chem.* Vol. 105 (No. 2-3): 559-572

[192] Wood, J. M.; Maibaum, J.; Rahuel, J.; Grütter, M. G.; Cohen, N. C.; Rasetti, V.; Rüger, H.; Göschke, R.; Stutz, S.; Fuhrer, W.; Schilling, W.; Rigollier, P.; Yamaguchi, Y.; Cumin, F.; Baum, H.-P.; Schnell, C. R.; Herold, P.; Mah, R.; Jensen, C.; O'Brien, E.; Stanton, A. & Bedigian, M. P. (2003) Structure-based Design of Aliskiren, a Novel Orally Effective Renin Inhibitor. *Biochem. Biophys. Res. Commun.* Vol. 308 (No.4): 698-705

[193] Wu., X.; Öhrngren, P.; Ekegren, J. K.; Unge, J.; Unge, T.; Wallberg, H.; Samuelssom, B.; Hallberg, A. & Larhed, M. (2008) Two-Carbon-Elongated HIV-1 Protease Inhibitors with a Tertiary-Alcohol-Containing Transition-State Mimic. *J. Med. Chem.* Vol. 51 (No.): 1053-1057

[194] Wu, D.; Zhang, L.; Kong, Y.; Du, J.; Chen, S.; Chen, J.; Ding, J.; Jiang, H. & Shen, X. (2008a) Enzymatic Characterization and Crystal Structure Analysis of the D-Alanine-D-alanine Ligase from Helicobacter pylori. *Proteins* Vol. 72, (No. 4): 1148–1160

[195] Xu, W.; Cheng, G.; Liew, O. W.; Zuo, Z.; Jiang, H. & Zhu, W. (2009) Novel Non-peptide -Secretase Inhibitors Derived from Structure-based Virtual Screening and Bioassay. *Bioorg. Med. Chem. Lett.* Vol. 19 (No. 12): 3188-3192

[196] Yiotakis, A.; Georgiadis, D.; Matziari, M. & Dive, V. (2004) Phosphinic Peptides: Synthetic Approaches and Biochemical Evaluation as Zn-Metalloprotease Inhibitors. *Curr. Org. Chem.* Vol. 8 (No. 12): 1135-1158

[197] Zambelli, B.; Musialini, F., Benini, S. & Ciurli, S. (2011) Chemistry of Ni^{2+} in Urease: Sensing, Trafficking, and Catalysis. *Acc. Chem. Res.*Vol. 44 (No. 7): 520-530

[198] Zhang, X.; Schmitt, A. C.; Jiang, W.; Wasserman, Z. & Decicco, C. P. (2003) Design and Synthesis of Potent, Non-peptide Inhibitors of HCV NS3 Protease. *Bioorg. Med. Chem. Lett.* Vol. 13 (No.6): 1157-1160

[199] Zhang, X. & Xu, W. (2008) Aminopeptidase N (APN/CD13) as a Target for Anti-cancer Agent Design. *Curr. Med. Chem.* Vol. 15 (No.27): 2850-2865

[200] Zucker, S. & Cao, J. (2009) Selective Matrix Metalloproteinase (MMP) Inhibitors in Cancer Therapy. *Cancer Bio. Ther.* Vol. 8 (No. 24): 2371-2323

Chapter 13

Suppression of Pro-Inflammatory Cytokines via Targeting of STAT-Responsive Genes

Charles J. Malemud

Additional information is available at the end of the chapter

http://dx.doi.org/10.5772/52506

1. Introduction

The Janus Kinase/Signal Transducers and Activators of Transcription (JAK/STAT) signaling pathway play a fundamental role in regulating chronic systemic inflammatory responses in rheumatoid arthritis (RA) [1-5], based on compelling evidence that JAK/STAT is activated by many of the pro-inflammatory cytokines such as interleukin-1β (IL-1β), IL-2, IL-3, IL-6, IL-12, IL-17, IL-18, IL-19/IL-20, interferon-α/γ (IFN-α/γ) and oncostatin M (OSM) which are well-known to regulate, in part, immune-mediated inflammation in several autoimmune diseases, including RA [6-10]. However, complicating matters is the fact that some of the anti-inflammatory cytokines, which are known to dampen inflammatory responses induced by pro-inflammatory cytokines, including, IL-4, IL-10 and IL-13 also activate JAK/STAT [11-14]. In this regard, Müller-Ladner *et al.* [15] showed that synovial tissue obtained from RA patients contained significant amounts of constitutively activated IL-4/STAT. Therefore it will be necessary to understand more precisely the extent to which pro- and/or anti-inflammatory cytokine gene expression is deregulated in RA and which of the STAT-responsive genes known to alter immune-mediated inflammation in response to these cytokines may be amenable to therapeutic intervention.

2. JAKs

JAKs are non-receptor tyrosine kinases that are pre-associated with the membrane-proximal site of cytokine receptors [16]. Four mammalian JAK isoforms, JAK1, JAK2 and JAK3 and TYK2 have been described to date mainly from the results of gene structural analysis [17]. All of the JAK isoforms share a common structure known as the JAK homology (JH) domain. Leonard and O'Shea [18] identified a proline-rich conserved region in the cytokine receptors, called Box1, that associated with JH7 whereas the catalytic phosphotyrosine kinase site, called YY was determined to correspond to the other JH domains (Figure 1).

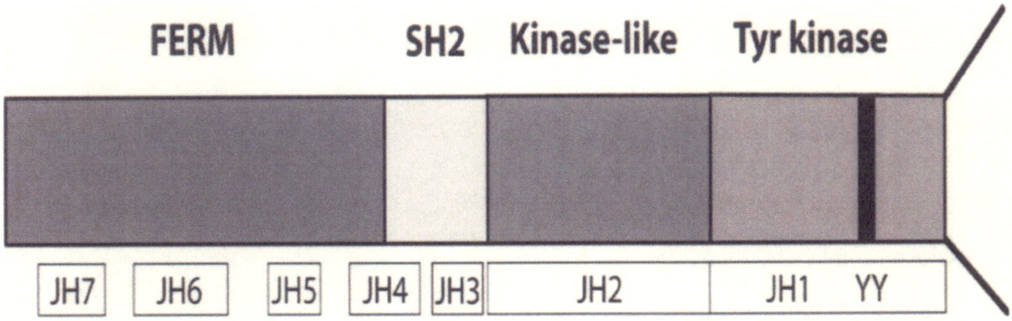

Figure 1. JH domains and phosphorylation sites of JAK3: Structural analysis combined with functional studies of JAK3 showed that the JH4-JH7 region contained band 4.1 also known as the Four-point-one, Ezrin, Radixin, Moesin (FERM) domain. Reprinted by permission from [16].

Additional structural analysis predicted that the JH2 domain was more than likely to be a pseudosubstrate domain [19]. In view of this latter finding the structural requirements for JAK activation was further clarified. Thus, the JH3-JH4 domain which shows a Src-homology-2-like structure had a shared homology with JH2. This finding indicated that the JH4-JH7 domains were, indeed, the critical regions required for regulating the interactions between the various JAK isoforms and other protein kinases. JH4-JH7 were also found to be essential for receptor binding, catalytic function, JAK autophosphorylation and even in some cases, inhibition of JAK activity.

3. Stat proteins

Gene analysis has revealed the existence of at least 6 STAT protein isoforms, namely, JAK1, JAK2, JAK3, JAK5A, JAK5B and JAK6 [20]. In normal homeostasis, phosphorylation of these STAT proteins is achieved via phosphorylation (i.e. activation) of specific JAK isoforms following the interaction of various cytokines and growth factors with their specific receptors [16, 21]. In this manner, cytokine receptor-mediated JAK activation results in the conversion of latent cytoplasmic un-phosphorylated STAT (U-STAT) proteins into phosphorylated STAT (p-STAT) proteins which can form homo- or heterodimers and are then translocated to the nucleus where these activated STAT protein dimers act as potent transcription factors [17-20]. Although phosphorylation of specific STAT-tyrosine residues remains the primary requisite mechanism for p-STAT protein dimer formation, a second phosphorylation site was also recognized at a serine in the C-termini domain of the STAT protein [20, 22].

An amplification loop with potential major clinical significance in RA involves the transcriptional activity of p-STAT proteins which further regulate the expression of pro-inflammatory and anti-inflammatory cytokine genes as well as other genes of significance in cancer and autoimmune diseases [23-28]. In addition, p-STAT proteins can regulate other signaling pathways necessary for lymphocyte development, as well as the aberrant survival of activated dendritic cells, monocytes, lymphocytes and synoviocytes in disorders of the immune system [29-33].

It is noteworthy that during normal homeostasis, activation of STAT proteins induced the expression of Suppressor of Cytokine Signaling (SOCS) and Cytokine-Inducible SH-2 (CIS) proteins and it has been concluded that this is the negative feedback loop that underlies one of the mechanisms responsible for inhibiting JAK-mediated signaling by cytokines [34-38]. Thus, results of recently published experiments with human endothelial cells are germane to this point since the data in this paper provided a direct connection between the silencing of STAT3 with STAT3-specific silencing RNA and the suppression of SOCS3 [39].

The extent to which negative regulation of JAK-mediated signaling by SOCS/CIS may be inactivated in autoimmune diseases is a focus of current studies. In that regard, recent advances in unraveling the details of mechanism(s) governing negative regulation of cytokine signaling by SOCS/CIS proteins have shed additional light on the extent to which SOCS/CIS-mediated down-regulation of pro- and/or anti-inflammatory cytokine JAK/STAT signaling may be compromised in inflammatory arthritis [40]. However, the results of some recent studies with osteoarthritic human cartilage have not clarified this issue. For example, one study showed that the level of SOCS2 and CIS-1, but not SOCS1 and SOCS3, were reduced in femoral head cartilages from subjects with osteoarthritis [41], whilst the results of another study [42] indicated that SOCS3, but not SOCS1 expression, was elevated in chondrocytes obtained from osteoarthritic cartilage compared to chondrocytes from cartilage obtained from patients who had femoral neck fracture.

The status of the activity of certain other negative regulators such as protein tyrosine phosphatases, including SHP-1,-2 [43] and CD45 [44] and the 'Protein Inhibitor of Activated STAT' (PIAS) proteins [16, 45, 46] are also not precisely known in autoimmune diseases. These proteins could very likely suppress the activity of phosphorylated JAKs and p-STAT proteins by dephosphorylation or by interacting with p-STAT proteins in normal cells. However, these pathways may be compromised or markedly suppressed in arthritis.

It is also critical for gaining a further understanding of what alterations may occur in cytokine signaling in RA to recognize the fact that activation of JAK/STAT by any of the relevant cytokines can also activate other intracellular signaling pathways via the "cross-talk" mechanism. Thus, "cross-talk" between JAK/STAT and other signaling pathways [16] can cause activation of the Stress-Activated Protein Kinase/Mitogen-Activated Protein Kinase (SAPK/MAPK) pathway, the Phosphatidylinositol-3-Kinase/Akt/mammalian Target of Rapamycin (PI3K/Akt/mTOR) pathway [47], activation of signaling via Toll-like receptors [47, 48] and immunoreceptor tyrosine-based activation motifs (ITAMs) [49] as well as the NF-κB pathway [50]. These alternative signaling pathways which are all connected to inflammation have also been shown to significantly modulate many of the survival and/or apoptosis-signals required to perpetuate abnormal proliferation and/or to cause the death of activated dendritic cells, lymphocytes, macrophages, synoviocytes and chondrocytes.

Evidence from a genome-wide analysis study (GWAS) of STAT-target genes showed that many of these genes regulated cellular proliferation, angiogenesis and metastasis in cancer cells [51]. These results when coupled with the data from another recent study [52] which highlighted the nature of the several forms of STAT-interacting proteins that bind to DNA suggested that GWAS could be employed to identify pro-inflammatory and/or anti-inflammatory cytokine STAT-target gene structures and potentially additional STAT-interacting proteins present in RA joint tissues. Thus GWAS may be considered the next step in the development of future therapies for RA based on targeting STAT-responsive genes. This could be especially useful depending on the status of the activity of the SOCS/CIS protein family acting on cytokine-receptor-mediated signaling. For example, if SOCS/CIS activity is dampened or deregulated in RA then it would be unlikely that this negative regulator pathway for controlling cytokine signaling would be able to inhibit the amplification of pro-inflammatory cytokine-induced JAK/STAT signaling. To illustrate this point, Isomäki et al. [40] showed that although SOCS-1 and SOCS-2 were up-regulated in T-cells recovered from peripheral blood, that SOCS-3 was found in peripheral blood monocytes and a significant number of synovial tissue macrophages expressed SOCS-1 and SOCS-3 proteins, the majority of T-cells in RA synovium were 'SOCS negative.'

For further discussion, this chapter will focus on the recent progress that has been made in furthering our understanding of how cytokine gene expression is regulated by both U-STAT and p-STAT proteins. The long-term prospect arising from the results of these studies would be to exploit this new knowledge to reduce the level of pro-inflammatory cytokines or to raise the level of anti-inflammatory cytokines in RA. By doing so this could potentially restore the balance between these cytokine families and retard ongoing synovial joint damage whilst also ameliorating RA clinical signs and symptoms.

4. Stat-DNA promoter-binding motifs

Defining transcription factor binding sites was critical for revealing the structure of cis-regulatory motifs that regulated transcriptional activity [53]. However, microarray analysis using different cell types determined that although several hundred genes were potential STAT3-target gene sites, only a small fraction of those STAT3-target gene sites turned out to be true direct STAT3-target genes [54].

As previously indicated, p-STAT proteins do not act independently of one another and U- and p-STAT-protein interactions take various forms which enable them to bind efficiently to DNA [55]. These activated STAT-protein interaction types include, 1) the direct binding of activated STAT homodimers to DNA; 2) the interaction of activated STATs with non-STAT proteins to form activated STAT/non-STAT protein complexes which bind to DNA; and 3) activated STAT proteins interacting with other non-STAT transcription factors or co-activator proteins which bind to DNA [16, 53]. In addition, several novel mechanisms were described for the binding of U-STAT3 and U-STAT1 to DNA [54, 55]. In that regard, Cheon et al. [56] showed that U-STAT3 can drive expression of proteins not induced by p-STAT3, whereas U-STAT1 was shown to extend and up-regulate the expression of a subset of genes initially responsive to p-STAT1 (e.g., interferon, IL-6), that result in more prolonged antiviral and/or immune responses. Thus, the results of these studies provided novel information regarding the functional significance for U-STAT1 and U-STAT3 acting as transcriptional activators and organizers of chromatin. These events have been shown to be important cellular mechanisms for regulating gene transcription in the nuclei of cells of the immune system and cancer cells.

The results of DNA sequencing studies originally demonstrated specific DNA-binding sites for STAT1 and STAT3 [57]. Boucheron et al. [58] then demonstrated that specific DNA binding sites existed for STAT5A and STAT5B homodimers despite the fact that STAT5A and STAT5B are evolutionarily conserved and encoded by 2 genes with a 91% homology in amino acid structure [59]. Moreover, targeted gene deletion of STAT5A and STAT5B in mice resulted in distinctive phenotypes [60]. This finding suggested a structural dissimilarity in the DNA-binding motifs for these two STAT proteins. The results of studies reported in [60] were later confirmed using the IL-3-dependent early pre-B cell line, Ba/F3 [61]. Here it was shown that both STAT isoforms bound to all of the promoters tested, but STAT5A and STAT5B bound with differing kinetics [62]. This result suggested that DNA binding activity was likely at the root of any differences in the biological activity of these two STAT protein isoforms.

Ehret et al. [63] compared the specificity of STAT-DNA binding sites in specific STAT gene knockout mice showing distinct phenotypes with the STAT-DNA binding sites in a variety of cultured cells. From the *in vitro* analysis, Ehret et al. [63] also demonstrated that DNA binding site motifs for STAT1, STAT5A, STAT5B and STAT6 were essentially the same with only minor differences in DNA binding site specificity. However, STAT5A DNA-binding specificity was much more similar to STAT6 than was the preferential DNA-binding site for STAT1. Thus, the preferential DNA binding site for STAT6 contained a 4 base pair spacer (i.e. TTCNNNNGAA) (N_4) which was defined as the weak DNA binding site. However, additional analyses showed that STAT6 bound to TTCNNNG-AA (N_3) sites (i.e. the strong binding site) as well [63]. The binding of STAT1 and STAT5 to the N_3 site was distinct from STAT5A which preferred N_4. Of note, most of the STAT6 binding sites were found in IL-4 responsive promoters in the N_4 sites [64-67]. These results reported by Ehret et al. [63] were extended by the findings of Moucadel and Constantinescu [64] who showed that STAT5B bound to chromatin at both the N_3 and the N_4 site.

5. Stat-responsive cytokines genes

This overview covering the specificity of STAT-DNA binding becomes especially important for improving our understanding of which cytokine gene expressional events are altered by p-STAT and U-STAT proteins. This section analyzes our current interpretation of several cytokines relevant to RA and other autoimmune diseases, namely, IL-2, IL-3, IL-4, IL-6, IL-15, IL-17, IL-19 and INF-γ, all of which have been shown to activate the JAK/STAT pathway [16]. Moreover, activation of JAK/STAT signaling by these cytokines was shown to result in altered patterns of transcriptional activity which lead to changes in the expression of the following cytokine or cytokine-related genes, IL-2R, IL-3, IL-4, IL-6, IL-6ST (gp130), IL-10, IL-18R1, INF-γ, oncostatin M (OSM) and TNF-α (Table 1).

STAT Responsive Cytokine/Protein	STAT Activator[1]	Activated STAT(s)[2]	Major Function(s) of STAT-Responsive Genes[3]	Involvement of STAT activator in RA	Representative Reference
IL-2Rα	IL-4	STAT6	Complexes with IL-2Rβ/IL-2Rγ→high affinity IL-2R	Anti-inflammatory Cytokine	[81]
					[73]
IL-10	IL-2, IL-3	STAT5, STAT5A, STAT5B	Activator of JAK3, I-SRE-4/IL-10 gene	↑ T-Cell Growth	[207] [127]
IL-18R1	IL-4	STAT6	↑ T_{reg} Cell Development IL18/IL-18R1	↑ T-Cell Development Inducer of TNF-α, GM-CSF, IFN-γ	
IL-6	IL-6/IL-17	STAT3/STAT1	Activator of JAK3	Promotes T_h17 Cell Production;	[9]
	IL-3	STAT5			[174]
	IL-12	STAT4			[140]
	IL-19	STAT3			
	IL-10/IL-13	STAT4		↑MMP Synthesis	[207]
				↑MMP Synthesis	[140]
IL-6ST(gp130)[4]	IL-6/IL-17/OSM	STAT3/STAT4/STAT5A	Heterodimer between gp130/LIFR[5] forms the OSMR[6]	Promotes T_h17 Cell Production	[100]
IL-4	IL-2	STAT3/STAT4/STAT5A	↑T_h2 Differentiation		[118]
INF-γ	IFN-γ	STAT1/STAT4/STAT5/STAT6	Activator of multiple protein kinases	Inhibitor of Anti-Inflammatory Cytokine IL-4 and IL-10 Production	[86]
	IL-3				[207]
	IL-2	STAT5			[207]
	IL-12	STAT5 STAT4			[113]
OSM	IL-2/IL-3	STAT5	Activator of JAK2	↑ Monocyte Trafficking	[122]
		STAT3		↑ MMP-2 ↑ VEGF	[125]
TNF-α	IL-3	STAT5	Activator of JAK3;	Activator of NF-κB	[200]
	IL-6/IL-19	STAT3/STAT5			[86]
	IL-15 IL-22	STAT1/STAT3/STAT5	Activator of p38[7], JNK[8]		[186]

[1]Cytokines that activate this STAT protein

[2]Activated STAT that becomes a transcription factor for the STAT-responsive cytokine/protein

[3]Function(s) of STAT-responsive cytokine/protein

[4]IL-6 Signal Transducer

[5]Leukemia Inhibitory Factor Receptor

[6]Oncostatin M Receptor

[7]p38 kinase

[8]C-Jun-N-terminal kinase

Table 1. STAT-Responsive Pro-Inflammatory Cytokine Gene Expression

http://dx.doi.org/10.5772/52506

6. T_h1/T_h2 Cells, T_{reg} Cells, IL-2R, and IL-15

Up-regulation of the T_h1 and T_h17 T-cell subsets and reduced levels of human T-regulatory (T_{reg}) cells are known to occur in autoimmune diseases [16, 68]. In addition, T_{reg} cells are a critical contributor to T-cell development in the thymus as well as being the T-cell subset that regulates the genesis and maintenance of immune tolerance [16].

The IL-2Rα/IL-2Rβ subunits in complex with the common IL-2γ subunit make up the high-affinity IL-2 receptor, whereas homodimeric IL-2Rα results in a low-affinity receptor [69]. The functional significance of blocking the high-affinity IL-2R with the small molecule inhibitor (SMI), SP4206 (K_d ~70nM) in response to IL-2 (K_d~10nM) was that JAK/STAT activation was inhibited [70]. This result could provide the impetus for development of the next generation SMI designed to efficiently inhibit the IL-2/IL-2R pathway and this task should be facilitated by employing recently developed technologies based on the principles of protein-protein interactions [71].

As indicated previously, the interaction of IL-2 with the high-affinity IL-2R causes activation of JAK/STAT with STAT5A and STAT5B, the principally activated STAT proteins. However, the eventual change in STAT5-gene responsiveness following IL-2 activation of STAT5 was shown to be dependent on the complexity of the promoter regions of those STAT5-target genes [72]. Interestingly, Tsuji-Takayama et al. [73] showed that IL-2-mediated JAK/STAT activation up-regulated the production of IL-10 by T_{reg} cells. The production of IL-10 arose from the interaction of STAT5 with a STAT5-responsive element within intron 4, designated I-SRE-4 of the IL-10 locus which was considered to be an interspecies conserved enhancer sequence (Table 1). Of note, the clustered CpG regions around I-SRE-4 were under-methylated in IL-10-producing T_{reg} cells, but not in other T-cell subsets. This result confirmed previous results which showed that expression of Foxp3, a member of the forkhead/winged-helix family of transcription factors and a biomarker for the development and function of T_{reg} cells [47, 74] was also IL-2/STAT5-dependent [75]. Thus, development of T_{reg} cells was regulated by the methylation status of CpG residues because methylation of CpG residues suppressed Foxp3 expression [76].

Chen et al. [77] identified a novel set of IL-4/STAT6-target genes in mice that regulated the proliferation of activated T-cells. In addition, these genes were shown to regulate the production of the T_h2 lineage as evinced by the finding that the cells isolated from wild-type mice produced T_h2 whereas cells from STAT6$^{-/-}$ mice did not. Later, Lund et al. [78] showed that the IL-4/STAT6 pathway was also critical for the commitment of naïve T-cells to become either the T_h1 or T_h2 subset. In that regard, the ratio of T_h1 to T_h2 produced from naïve T-cells was found to be dependent on a set of STAT6-responsive genes which included the transcription factors STATB1, Bcl-6, and TCF7 [78, 79]. Moreover, the IL-4/STAT6-mediated pathway was also shown to be a strong modulator of human T_{reg} cell production from either T_h1 or T_h17 cells [80].

Wurster et al. [81] were among the first to demonstrate that IL-4-mediated activation of STAT6 could also up-regulate IL-2Rα gene expression (Table 1). Because IL-2 is the major growth-promoting cytokine for T-cells [81], elevated production of IL-2Rα in response to activated STAT6 is considered instrumental in facilitating the proliferation of activated T-cells in cancer as well as in several types of autoimmune diseases. In that regard, the high level of expression of IL-2Rα in tumors correlated with a poor prognosis in cancer patients [82]. Thus, it will be interesting to determine if the same relationship holds true for RA patients as well, including what role IL-2Rα polymorphisms [83, 84] might play in determining the level of the expression of IL-2Rα. For example, IL-15, a pro-inflammatory cytokine which interacts with two receptor subunits similar to IL-2Rα/β drives the production of the memory CD8$^+$ T-cell phenotype [85]. Experimental therapies focusing on inhibiting the binding of IL-15 to the IL-2Rα/β receptor complex were a decade ago considered to be a potential target for autoimmune diseases [85]. However, since then considerable evidence has accumulated showing a robust relationship between IL-15/IL-2Rα/β-mediated signaling, osteoclastogenesis and boney erosions in RA joints [3]. In addition, González-Alvaro et al. [86] showed that IL-15 stimulated production of TNF-α by monocytes derived from RA patients including, the induction of the CD69 monocyte biomarker, and synthesis of IFN-γ protein by natural killer (NK) cells. Of note, the results of a clinical study showed that IL-15 expression in RA synovial tissue persisted even after TNF-α blockade, the latter treatment resulting in a positive clinical response and reduced disease activity [87]. However, treating mononuclear cells *in vitro* with HuMax-IL-15 f $(ab')_2$ neutralized the effect of IL-15 on these cells. Furthermore, treatment with HuMax-IL-15 $f(ab')_2$ caused a significant improvement in RA disease activity as measured by the American College of Rheumatology (ACR) clinical response criteria [88]. This finding may be particularly important for future drug development because the results of a recently completed clinical trial showed that high levels of serum IL-15 in patients with early arthritis predicted a more progressive and severe clinical course which may call for early and aggressive drug therapy [89].

6.1. IL-6/gp130/IL-17

The IL-6/IL-6R/gp130 pathway is one of the strongest inducers of STAT3 activation [9] (Table 1) so much so that many studies have been devoted to the activation of the JAK/STAT pathway by IL-6 because IL-6 is critical to the progression of joint damage in RA [16]. In fact, the development of the anti-IL-6R monoclonal antibody, tocilizumab, appears to have been predicated on this emerging evidence such that this drug is now considered useful in the armamentarium of drug therapies for RA [90, 91]. Most compelling was recent evidence that tocilizumab in conjunction with methotrexate retarded the progression of joint damage in RA patients [92], an effect of this drug regimen that was apparently independent of the capacity of tocilizumab to modify several clinical biomarkers of inflammation and concomitant RA disease activity.

Recent results have also emerged which have focused attention on the extent to which other pro-inflammatory cytokines, such as IL-17, activate JAK/STAT and the mechanism by which IL-17 modifies the production of IL-6 and other pro-inflammatory cytokines [9]. In that regard, the results of a study by Jovanovic et al. [93] was extremely informative because it provided evidence that IL-17 was capable of activating additional signaling pathways other than JAK/STAT which resulted in elevated production of IL-1β and TNF-α. Therefore, it has become obvious that suppressing the activity of IL-17 could bring about a reduction of these pro-inflammatory cytokines as well, although this point must be rigorously reexamined in view of the results from Dragon et al. [94] who showed that IL-17A significantly decreased GM-CSF-induced neutrophil/granulocyte apoptosis by suppressing activation of p38 kinase, extracellular-regulated kinase 1/2 and STAT5B.

Inhibiting aberrant T-cell survival in RA may ultimately hinge on the development of a therapeutic strategy directed specifically at STAT3 since STAT3 was shown to inhibit T-cell proliferation by up-regulating the Class O Forkhead transcriptions factors (Fox) via the binding of STAT3 to FoxO1and FoxO3a promoters [95]. Potentially, STAT3 may also protect T-cells from apoptosis [30, 96] in RA by suppressing IL-2 activity, although the results [95] indicated that STAT3 increased T-cell proliferation and their survival through the up-regulation of OX-40 (CD134), a member of the TNFR-superfamily of receptors and bcl-2 and by suppressing FasL and Bad expression.

Perhaps the most intriguing aspect of the clinical studies with tocilizumab performed in RA patients is the extent to which neutralization of the IL-6/IL-6R/gp130 pathway using this drug together with the putative suppression of IL-6 and gp130 gene expression in response to inhibition of the STAT3 activation rebalances the skewed ratio of T_h17/T_{reg} in favor of T_{reg} [97, 98], the elevated serum levels of T_h17-associated cytokines, IL-17, IL-23, IL-6 and TNF-α, and the depressed level of T_{reg} cells with its associated growth factor, transforming growth factor-β (TGF-β) [99]. What is pertinent to these events are the results of a recent study which showed that treatment of RA patients with tocilizumab in combination with methotrexate resulted in a significant decrease in the percentage of T_h17 cells (from 0.9% at baseline to 0.45%) and a significant increase in T_{reg} cells (from 3.05% to 3.94%) whilst maintaining their functional activity [98].

The extent to which gp130 gene expression is altered in response to inhibition of the JAK/STAT pathway activation is also an area of immense importance because deregulated over-expression of gp130 in RA patients should not be neutralized by anti-IL-6R therapy. Importantly, O'Brien and Manolagas [100] showed that IL-6 or oncostatin M (OSM), a member of the IL-6 protein superfamily, stimulated the activity of the gp130 (Table 1) promoter in which the cytokine response element contained a cis-acting motif for activated STAT complexes, including activated STAT1 and STAT3 homo- and heterodimers. Furthermore, it can be conjectured that other pro-inflammatory cytokine members of the IL-6 protein superfamily, such as ciliary neutrotrophic factor (CNTF), leukemia inhibitory factor (LIF) and cardiotropin-1 which use gp130 as their primary signal transducer protein [9, 101] may provide an alternate mechanism resulting in constitutive JAK/STAT activation. Under those conditions STAT protein activation may not be inhibited any of the anti-IL-6R agents which retain up-regulated gp130 gene expression. Of note, constitutive activation of STAT proteins is one of the signature events in the development and progression of various cancers [102, 103] with a similar phenomenon having been described in RA synovial tissue [15]. Constitutively activated STAT proteins could also be predictive of a more aggressive form of RA [96].

6.2. INF-α/IFN-γ

The interferon protein family in conjunction with the interferon-regulated gene (IRG) pathway plays an important role in RA, SLE and other autoimmune diseases because the IRG pathway is a critical mediator of autoimmune-dependent inflammation [104-106]. INF-γ is known to be one of the strongest activators of JAK/STAT and Tyk2 resulting in IRG-mediated responses [16, 107, 108]. INF-γ has also been shown to play a role in the epigenetic regulation of specific gene activation as evinced by the finding of an association of pJAK2 and IFN-γ receptor in the nucleus with histone H3 in IFN-γ-treated human amnionic (WISH; American Tissue Culture Collection; CCL 25) cells *in vitro* [109]. AG-490 a JAK2 inhibitor, also down-regulated STAT1 gene expression and AG-490 inhibited prolactin-induced IFN-γ, TNF-α, IL-1β and IL-12p40 synthesis in mouse peritoneal macrophages *in vitro* [110]. Of note, inhibition of JNK activity with the SMI, SP600125, also resulted in down-regulating IFN-γ and TNF-α indicating that both the JAK/STAT and MAPK pathways contributed to alterations in the expression of these cytokines. Although the importance of these results in providing a rationale for manipulating signal transduction pathways in human RA remains to be fully elucidated, the fact that the expression of several pro-inflammatory cytokines relevant to RA pathology are potentially controlled by cross-talk between JAK/STAT and MAPK appears to be significant [47, 111, 112].

Three DNA-binding sites related to STAT protein-DNA binding have been recognized within the IFN-γ promoter. These DNA binding sites include an IL-12-mediated STAT4/DNA binding site, an IL-2-induced STAT5/DNA binding site and a CD2-mediated STAT/IFN-γ binding site [113]. Thus, CD2-mediated activation of human peripheral blood mononuclear cells was shown to result in STAT/DNA binding to a 3.6kb DNA motif within the IFN-γ promoter which occurred principally via STAT5A binding and less so by STAT5B, with both being independent of IL-2.

Induction of some of the IFN-regulatory factors (Irfs), including those gene responses brought about by activation of irf9 via IFN-α were found to be STAT protein-independent [114]. In addition, results from other studies showed that Akt activity was also involved in key IFN-α, -γ gene responses [115]. Moreover, regulation of IFN-α, -γ-mediated responses required the direct control of mTOR [116] beginning with the initiation of protein translation [117].

In RA, the depressed level of IL-4 and IL-10 in mononuclear phagocytes is, in part, responsible for the imbalance in T_h1/T_h2 cytokines [3, 16]. The primary model employed to describe the relationship between IFN-γ and IL-4/IL-10 is dependent on several factors. This view was originally proposed by Hamilton et al. [118] as follows; IL-4 was shown to markedly suppress the transcriptional activity of IFN-γ because the promoter sequence between IL-4 and IFN-γ were essentially identical. Proof of this came from the results of experiments that showed that IFN-γ/STAT1 and IL-4/STAT6 both formed complexes at the same regulatory sequence, but whereas activated STAT1 promoted IFN-γ transcription, activated STAT6 did not. However, activated STAT6 was required to suppress the transcriptional up-regulation of IL-4. Thus, in the model, IL-4 appeared to be necessary to reduce IFN-γ gene expression (Table 1) and was related to a competition between activated STAT1 and activated STAT6 for binding to the IFN-γ promoter. In keeping with this model, the expression of IL-10 is also known to be suppressed by INF-γ

[119]. Thus, it was shown that when transfected RPMI 8226.1 B-cells were incubated with IFN-γ followed by lipopolysaccharide (LPS), IFN-γ reduced LPS-induced IL-10 promoter activity which was independent of the irf, but dependent on an activated STAT-motif. Further analyses indicated that IFN-γ down-regulated IL-10 gene expression via displacement of the trans-activated STAT3 by STAT1 induced by IFN-γ.

Experimental strategies could be designed to increase the mononuclear cell expression of IL-4/IL-10 by manipulating the ultra-sensitive INF-γ promoter region with various activated STAT protein types. Another strategy for potentially improving the level of IL-10 in RA would involve manipulating natural T_{reg} cells in a cell-based therapy mode because T_{reg} cells are a rich source of IL-10 [120, 121]. However, as pointed out by Nandakumar et al. [121] one must be mindful that the antigen specificity of natural T_{reg} cells must be carefully regulated to protect against the development of self-reactive effector T-cells or for that matter, T_{reg} cells with inappropriate antigen specificity.

6.3. OSM

Recent advances have assigned OSM, a member of the IL-6 protein superfamily an important role in the pathogenesis and progression of RA and OA [101]. In that regard, one of the more important experimental results involving OSM were reported by Hams et al. [122] who compared the inflammatory responses in wild-type mice to IL-6-deficient and mice deficient in the OSM receptor β (OSMRβ). They showed that the OSMRβ knockout mice showed enhanced trafficking of monocytes to sites of inflammation when these mice were compared to the wild-type or IL-6-knockout mice. However, the OSMRβ knockout mice did not demonstrate any differences in neutrophil or lymphocyte migration to inflamed tissue when compared to their wild-type or IL-6-deficient counterparts. These results suggested that the OSM/OSMRβ-pathway probably regulated chemokine production and chemokine function. Indeed this proved to be the case when the up-regulated chemokine in response to the activation of the OSMRβ-pathway was eventually identified as CCL5. CCL5 has been shown to be a critical chemokine for regulating the recruitment and retention of monocytes in inflamed RA synovial joints [3]. Although the evidence was indirect, these results suggested that a drug with the capacity to neutralize the interaction between IL-6 and IL6R in arthritic joints would not alter OSM/OSMRβ-mediated STAT activation [9]. This view was supported by the results from several previous studies which showed that 1) although the OSMR consisted of a heterodimer of the LIF receptor and gp130, the alternative form of OSMR, namely, OSMRβ, was activated only by OSM and not by LIF [123]; 2) OSM, but neither IL-6 nor LIF induced tyrosine phosphorylation in the Shc adaptor protein p52 and p66 isoforms which in association with growth factor receptor-bound protein 2 (Grb2) were both recruited to OSMR, but not to gp130 [124]; and 3) at least in human or canine osteosarcoma cell lines, treatment with OSM phosphorylated JAK2/STAT3 and Src, each of which was shown to be involved in an OSM dose-dependent-mediated increase in expression of the MMP-2 gene (i.e. 72kDa gelatinase) and vascular endothelial growth factor (VEGF) gene [125]. Of note, the STAT3 SMI, LLL3, inhibited MMP-2 and VEGF gene expression indicating that MMP-2 and VEGF were genes targeted by activated STAT3. Importantly, Clarkson et al. [126] showed that another one of the activated STAT-responsive genes in mammary epithelial cells was OSMR. This finding was critical for completing the circle which showed that activation of OSMRβ was central to the upstream activation of the OSM-mediated pathway as well as to the downstream increase in the expression of the OSMRβ gene, both events involving STAT proteins.

7. Other cytokines/cytokine receptors

The role played by activated STAT proteins in various aspects of autoimmune diseases and in oncogenesis is best exemplified by the many genes and transcription factors that have been shown to be STAT protein-responsive [51, 127]. Many of these STAT-regulated genes include additional pro-inflammatory cytokine and cytokine receptor genes besides those previously discussed. In this section we will analyze the contributions of these cytokine and cytokine receptor genes to the pathology of RA.

7.1. IL-18

IL-18 is structurally similar to IL-1 and the IL-18 receptor is a member of the IL-1R/TLR protein superfamily [128]. However, the function of IL-18 differs considerably from that of IL-1 and, in fact unlike IL-1, IL-18 is produced by a variety of immune as well as non-immune cells. Although IL-18 in its role as a stimulator of T_h1 responses is well known by its activity as an immune defense cytokine against microbial infection, the over-production of IL-18 can result in autoimmune disease via its capacity to modify and accentuate adaptive immunological responses such as those seen in RA [129-132]. However, paradoxically IL-18 can also stimulate T_h2-related cytokine responses as well [128]. Thus, its putative role in altering the T_h1/T_h2 cytokine repertoire cannot be dismissed.

Particularly important with regard to the role played by IL-18 in RA were results of a study by Gracie et al. [133] who first identified abundant IL-18 in RA synovial tissue. These findings are relevant when coupled with those from other studies by Tanaka et al. [134] who also found elevated IL-18 and the IL-18 receptor α/β in RA synovial tissue. They also demonstrated that IL-18 was a co-factor and regulatory cytokine in stimulating the synthesis of IFN-γ by T-cells in RA synovial tissue, the latter also requiring IL-12, thus implicating the up-regulation of IL-18 gene expression as an important component of RA disease progression.

Activated STAT3 was identified as the JAK/STAT-related transcription factor responsible for the increased synthesis of IL-18 [127]. In that regard, TNF-α was shown to increase IL-18 gene expression in RA synoviocyte cultures suggesting the possibility that TNF-α, a known activator of p38 kinase and JNK may also activate STAT3 in synoviocyte and chondrocyte cultures. Indeed, recent results from our laboratory showed that recombinant human TNF-α activated STAT3 in normal human chondrocyte cultures and TNF-α activated STAT3, p38 kinase and JNK in cultured chondrocytes derived from human osteoarthritic knee cartilage [Malemud et al. submitted]. Thus, it was instructive to learn that treating RA patients with the combination therapy of infliximab and methotrexate reduced the level of IL-18 in serum whilst the level of the chemokine, CXCL12 was unaltered [135]. Moreover, synovial fluid from these RA patients had higher levels of IL-18 (as well as TNF-α and IL-15) prior to beginning combination therapy with infliximab and methotrexate compared to the level of these cytokines in a patient's sera. In addition, the level of IL-18/TNF-α in synovial fluid was strongly correlated with a patient's high Disease Activity Score-28 [136]. Thus, it may be informative going forward to assess the level of activated STAT3 and IL-18 in the synovial fluid and sera of RA patients before and after treatment with TNF antagonists or other biological drugs that neutralize the activation of JAK/STAT and MAPK pathways to determine the extent to which the level of activated STAT3, p38 kinase or JNK is correlated with IL-18 gene expression by synovium and cartilage *ex vivo*.

7.2. IL-12

IL-12 is made up of 2 disulfide-linked protein subunits, termed IL-12p35 and IL-12p40 linked in a heterodimer configuration [137, 138]. Whilst the IL-12p40 subunit has structural similarities with cytokine receptors, the IL-12p35 component is structurally similar to IL-6 and granulocyte-colony stimulating factor (G-CSF) [139]. Of note, if IL-12p35 and IL-12p40 are produced by the same cell, the bioactive heterodimer is termed, IL-12p70 [140].

IL-12 is synthesized by many cell types of the innate and adaptive immune systems, including, monocytes, macrophages, dendritic cells and neutrophils. IL-12 is a minor product of B-cells [140]. Although IL-12p35 is constitutively expressed at low levels by many of these cells, the expression of IL-12p40 is limited to those phagocytic cells that synthesize IL-12p70.

The connection between IL-12 and activation of the JAK/STAT pathway stems from the finding that IL-12 production was positively regulated by IFN-γ, the latter cytokine which is also induced by IL-12. Thus, IFN-γ regulates IL-12 gene expression and vice versa. By contrast, two of the anti-inflammatory cytokines, namely, IL-10 and IL-13 which also activate JAK/STAT, suppressed IL-12 production [140] (Table 1). In addition, the type I interferon proteins, exemplified by IFN-β, which activates STAT1 [141] was shown to inhibit IL-12 gene expression in mice [142].

The main immune functions of IL-12 involve the regulation of T_h1 differentiation via the activation of STAT4 which induces the synthesis of the T-bet transcription factor [143]. T-bet was shown to regulate IFN-γ expression and $CD8^+$ suppressor T-cell development which had been characterized as principally IFN-γ/STAT1-dependent, and IL-12/STAT4 independent. In fact, expression of T-bet was shown to require activated STAT4 to achieve total IL-12-dependent T_h1 cell-fate determination [143]. However, Yang et al. [144] showed that the effect of IL-12/STAT4 was more complex. Thus, IL-12 -induced activated STAT4 bound to a distant but highly conserved STAT-responsive T-bet enhancer region where it induced IFN-γ-activated STAT1 independent T-bet gene expression in $CD8^+$ cells. Importantly, IL-4-induced STAT6 activation regulates the development and effector functions, not of T_h1 cells, but rather of T_h2 cells in peripheral tissues such as skin, lung and gut [145]. However, T_h2 cell produced in lymph nodes did not require IL-4-mediated activation of STAT6 [145].

In summary, cell-fate determination induced by the IL-12-mediated activation of STAT4, IL-4-mediated activation of STAT6, transforming growth factor-β (TGF-β), IL-6 plus TGF-β and IL-27 activation of STAT3 profoundly influence the balance of T_h1 and T_h2 cells, T_h17 cells and T_{reg} cell production, respectively [80, 146-149]. This conclusion must, however, be tempered by results of recent studies which also showed that formal interplays occurred between IL-4-induced STAT6 phosphorylation, the GATA-binding protein-3 ($GATA_3$) zinc-finger transcription factor [150] and the T_{reg} cell transcription factor, FoxP3 as well. Importantly, $GATA_3$ was revealed as the key transcription factor in this complex interplay because $GATA_3$ could 1) directly inhibit T_h1 differentiation through its capacity to block upregulation of the IL-12β2 receptor; 2) inhibit the activity of STAT4; and 3) neutralize the activity of runt-related transcription factor 3 (runx3), via its capacity to induce protein-protein interactions [150]. Thus, by modulating the activities of IL-4/STAT6, $GATA_3$/STAT4 and runx3 one could potentially alter the activity of pro-inflammatory and anti-inflammatory cytokines as well as overcome immune tolerance.

7.3. IL-21

IL-21 is a member of the Type I cytokine superfamily of cytokine receptors. In this group, the common γ cytokine receptor complex is the functional component for receptor-mediated signal transduction of IL-2, IL-4, IL-7, IL-9 and IL-15 [151-153]. Although IL-21 has strong structural homology to IL-15, IL-21 interacts with a unique receptor, termed, IL-21Rα, which pairs with the γ-common cytokine receptor chain (i.e. CD132) to form the active IL-21 receptor complex [154].

IL-21-mediated events affect the functions of NK cells, T-cells and B-cells. Although development of T_{reg} cells from the T_h17 lineage is generally considered to require IL-6 because IL-6 reciprocally controls T_h17 and T_{reg} cell development through its ability to inhibit TGF-β-induced FoxP3 and by inducing RORγ, in fact, IL-21 can also induce RORγ and T_h17 development in the absence of IL-6. However, evidence also showed that the number of T_h17 cells, the recruitment of T_h17 cells to inflamed tissues and the development of autoimmune encephalitis and myocarditis did not differ between IL-21R and IL-21 deficient mice compared to their wild-type counterparts [155, 156]. More importantly, IL-6 was the more potent inducer of T_h17 differentiation compared to IL-21 thus calling into question, whether IL-21 was even required for T_h17 development.

Despite the emerging controversies regarding how important IL-21 is in T-cell development and immune responses, a therapeutic intervention designed to limit the responses of immune cells to IL-21 has long been considered for treating cancer and autoimmune diseases [157]. In addition, because the binding of IL-21R induces activation of several of the JAK isoforms [153], it became apparent that it would be necessary to elucidate which cellular events were controlled by STAT proteins activated by phosphorylated JAKs in response to IL-21/IL-21R. Attempting to address this point, Habib et al. [151] found that IL-21 induced proliferation of pro-B-lymphoid cells *in vitro* which was dependent on both γc and the γc-associated JAK3 complex. However, a monoclonal antibody reactive only with γc was effective in limiting the proliferation of BaF3/IL21R α cells [151] indicating that neutralization of γc alone could cause inhibition of JAK activation by IL-21/IL-21R.

http://dx.doi.org/10.5772/52506

Implying a role for IL-21 in the development and progression of RA would also depend on finding an elevated level of IL-21 in human RA tissues and by demonstrating an involvement of IL-21 in the pathogenesis of CIA or inflammatory arthritis in other animal models. Thus the results of a study by Young et al. [158] were noteworthy in this regard for several reasons. First and foremost, treating DBA mice with CIA with an antibody to IL-21R (i.e. IL-21R.Fc) reduced the severity of arthritis. The reduction in hind paw swelling was accompanied by lower levels of IL-6 in the hind paw but also in the sera of mice treated with IL-21R.Fc suggesting that one of the downstream events regulated by IL-21 was IL-6 gene expression. Of note, the level of INF-γ was increased in the hind paws of mice with CIA. Furthermore, the cultured cells from the lymph nodes of mice with CIA treated with IL-21R.Fc showed an increased level of IFN-γ *ex vivo*. These findings (i.e. reduced IFN-γ; increased IL-6) were mirrored *ex vivo* using Type II collagen-specific spleen cells from CIA mice treated with IL-21R.Fc. Most importantly from the perspective of potentially using an anti-IL-21R antibody as a therapeutic agent for RA was the finding that treating Lewis rats with adjuvant –induced arthritis therapeutically with IL-21R.Fc "reversed" the swelling in inflamed joints and tissues from these joints whilst the tissues showed improvement using a well-validated histological scoring system. More recently, Yuan et al. [159] showed that IL-21R mRNA was found in human RA synovial tissue samples. In addition, this group also confirmed the results of the Young et al. study [158] since they showed that an anti-IL-21R antibody ameliorated the severity of arthritis in CIA which was accompanied by reduced cytokine levels in cells derived from the anti-IL-21R antibody-treated mice. Interestingly, IL-21R-deficient K/BxN mice [160] failed to develop arthritis; a result which suggested that IL-21R played a critical role in the pathogenesis of K/BxN serum-induced arthritis.

There now are several lines of evidence that showed that the IL-21/IL-21R pathway plays a functional role in regulating inflammatory responses in autoimmune arthritis. In that regard, anti-IL-21 blockade should also be considered for future drug development for RA. However, what would also be crucial to improving our understanding of the role of IL-21 in RA would be to discover which pro-inflammatory cytokine levels are altered in response to the JAK/STAT activation by IL-21/IL21R. This could provide a novel paradigm for reducing pro-inflammatory cytokine levels in RA.

8. The extended IL-10 cytokine superfamily

IL-19, IL-20, IL-22, IL-24 (melanoma differentiation-associated gene 7; mda-7), and IL-26 (AK155) are all structurally similar to IL-10 and these interleukins constitute members of the extended IL-10 cytokine superfamily [161-163]. Three additional members of the IL-10 cytokine superfamily have recently been added to this list, namely, IL-28A, IL-28B and IL-29 which now comprise the IFN-λ cytokine subfamily [164-166].

IL-19 and IL-20 are α-helical proteins. They have similar cysteine sites; their amino acid sequences are approximately 30% identical. In the human genome, the genes encoding these IL-10 superfamily members are located in two clusters; one cluster comprises the genes for

IL-10, IL-19, IL-20, and IL-24/mda-7 which are located on chromosome 1q31-32 [167]. IL-19 and IL-20 were predominately expressed in monocytes, as well as non-immune cells under inflammatory conditions [168], whereas IL-22 and IL-26 was only produced by T-cells, especially T_h1 cells and NK cells, whilst IL-24 synthesis was restricted to monocytes and T-cells [169].

Both IL-20 and IL-24 bind to the IL-20R complex which is made up of the cytokine receptor family 2-8/IL-20Rα (IL-20R1) [170], although it was previously shown that IL-19/IL-19 receptor binding was similar to IL-20/IL-24 receptor binding [170]. IL-19 was also shown to interact with a DIRS1-like element which is composed of tyrosine recombinase-encoding transposons/IL-20Rβ (IL-20R2) [170-172].

In all cases, the binding of IL-19, IL-20 or IL-24 to these receptors caused activation of STAT3 and activation of a minimal promoter region containing those sequences identified as STAT-binding sites. Importantly, absent either of the R1 proteins in the two types of receptor complexes, IL-20R1/IL-20R2 and IL-22R1/IL-22R2 reduced the affinity of IL-19 or IL-24 for these receptors. Furthermore, IL-20R2, and not IL-20R1, was identified as the high affinity receptor chain for these cytokines [173].

The functional significance of the IL-10-related cytokines, IL-19, IL-20, IL-21, IL-22 and IL-24 in terms of the pathophysiology of RA and other autoimmune diseases is systematically being elucidated. In most cases, the role played by these cytokines has been inferred from measurements in sera of RA patients before and/or after medical therapy.

8.1. IL-19

Sakurai et al. [174] showed that IL-19 was produced by cells of human RA synovial tissue. The majority of IL-19 positive cells were vimentin- and CD68-positive, indicating that fibroblasts and macrophages were the main sources of IL-19 in RA synovium. From a functional perspective, synovial tissue lining and sublining layers were both identified with anti-IL-20R1 and anti-IL-20R2 antibodies.

IL-19 activated synoviocyte STAT3 and, downstream, STAT3 activation caused up-regulation of IL-6 and IL-19 gene expression whilst decreasing synoviocyte apoptosis induced by serum-starvation [174], a change which may predict the role of IL-19 in the development of synovial hyperplasia [30, 96]. However, the role of IL-19 in RA relative to its activation of signal transduction was further complicated by the findings of Alanärä et al. [175] who showed that IL-1β, an activator of the MAPK pathway [176], also increased the level of IL-19 in peripheral blood mononuclear cells *in vitro*. Combined with other data this result showed that in RA joints IL-19 expression was the highest of all of the IL-10 family cytokines. Furthermore, these results suggested that IL-19 played a significant role in synovial tissue inflammation, with the caveat that further consideration of IL-19 as a target for intervention in in RA must focus on the relative level of JAK/STAT activation of JAK/STAT versus activation of the other signaling pathways.

IL-19 was highly expressed in synovial tissue and, in particular, expressed in fibroblasts isolated from rats with collagen-induced arthritis (CIA) [177]. Of note, treating these rats with a anti-IL-19 antibody, 1BB1, reduced arthritis severity which was accompanied by the lower level of boney erosions and an improvement in the quality of subchondral bone. Moreover, treatment of rats with CIA with 1BB1 reduced the expression of TNF-α, IL-1β, IL-6 and Receptor Activator of Nuclear Factor Kappa-B Ligand (RANKL) genes in synovial tissue and also lowered IL-6 levels in serum. Synovial fibroblasts isolated from rats with CIA responded to treatment with IL-19 in a similar fashion seen with synovial tissue *in situ* where increased synthesis of TNF-α, IL-1β, IL-6 and RANKL was detected.

There is now compelling evidence that IL-19-mediated activation of STAT3 was associated with the development and progression of inflammatory arthritis which was characterized by the elevated expression of many of the pro-inflammatory cytokines pertinent to human RA joint destruction. These data also showed that the rat CIA model could be further exploited to determine the extent to which specific dampening or up-regulation of STAT-responsive cytokine genes would ameliorate inflammatory responses associated with CIA.

8.2. IL-20

IL-20 interacts with IL-20R1/IL-20R2 to activate the JAK/STAT pathway [166] and IL-20 has been implicated in the pathogenesis of autoimmune diseases [178]. However, IL-20R2 signaling was shown to blunt mouse CD4 and CD8 T-cell responses to antigen *in vitro* and *in vivo* [179]. Thus, it remains to be determined the extent to which IL-20 promotes or suppresses immune-mediated inflammation.

In the CIA model in the rat, treatment with an anti-IL-20 antibody 7E, either alone, or in combination with the TNF blocker, etanercept was compared to etanercept alone for their capacity to 1) ameliorate cartilage damage; 2) stabilize bone mineral density; and 3) alter cytokine production [180]. In addition, the effect of antibody 7E on expression of various genes implicated in the progression of CIA was evaluated on rat synovial fibroblasts *in vitro*. Treatment with 7E or etanercept or the combination of 7E and etanercept significantly reduced the severity of arthritis as measured by rat hind paw thickness and swelling. These treatments also prevented cartilage degradation and bone loss whilst reducing the level of synovial tissue IL-20, IL-1β, IL-6, RANKL and MMPs. Of note, IL-20 induced the expression of TNF-α in synovial fibroblasts isolated from rats with CIA. Moreover, IL-20 induced RANKL production in synovial fibroblasts, osteoblasts and T_h17 cells. In another study, antibody 7E was shown to inhibit mouse osteoclast differentiation induced by macrophage-CSF and RANKL [181]. These results [181] coupled with results from the CIA model [180] indicated that IL-20 was likely to have promoted the increased bone loss in CIA by promoting osteoclast differentiation and the activity of osteoclast-mediated bone resorption.

Correlative human studies of IL-20-mediated responses in RA are just emerging. However, the results have differed somewhat from those seen in the CIA model. Thus, Kragstrup et al. [182] showed that plasma IL-20 levels were increased in RA compared to OA patients with the elevated level of IL-20 primarily localized to mononuclear cells and neutrophils. Stimulating mononuclear cells isolated from RA synovium with recombinant IL-20 resulted in the increased secretion of the chemoattractant CCL2/MCP-1. However, at variance with findings in the CIA model, recombinant IL-20 did not alter the expression of TNF-α or IL-6 by mononuclear cells *in vitro*.

8.3. IL-22

IL-22 binds to the class II cytokine receptor family, IL-22R and IL-10Rβ [183]. IL-22 was shown to activate STAT-1, -3 and -5 in H4IIE rat hepatoma cells by inducing the phosphorylation of JAK1 and Tyk2, but not JAK1 [184]. However, H4IIE failed to respond to IL-10 via activation of JAK1 and Tyk2 indicating a distinct signaling pathway for IL-22 versus IL-10. IL-22 also failed to inhibit pro-inflammatory cytokine gene expression by monocytes in response to LPS although IL-22 did blunt the inhibitory effects of IL-4 produced from T_h2 cells, a finding distinct from the activity of IL-10.

A role for IL-22 in inflammation was inferred from its involvement as an inducer of pancreatitis-associated protein by pancreatic acinar cells [185] and by the elevated serum levels of IL-22 in patients with active Crohn's disease [186]. With regard to activating various signaling mechanisms, Lejeune et al. [187] showed that IL-22 activated JAK/STAT. However, IL-22 also activated ERK, JNK and p38 kinase indicating that IL-22 could activate all of the 3 major MAPK pathways. Brand et al. [186] then showed that treating intestinal epithelial cells with TNF-α, IL-1β or LPS significantly increased IL-22R1 gene expression without altering IL-10R2 mRNA. IL-22 also activated STAT1/STAT3, Akt, ERK 1/2 and JNK and, most importantly IL-22 increased the expression of SOCS3, TNF-α, IL-8 and human-defensin-2 mRNAs. Because IL-22 was shown to activate several disparate signaling pathways it is conjecture that up-regulation of pro-inflammatory gene mRNAs by IL-22 involves 'cross-talk' between all three pathways. Thus, experiments employing specific SMIs added either individually or together to cells in culture will have to be performed to determine the extent to which any or all of these signaling pathways are involved in regulating TNF-α, IL-8 or IL-1β gene expression in response to IL-22.

IL-22 is elevated in RA synovial tissue with the lining and sublining layers of RA synovium expressing the highest levels of IL-22R1 [188]. Recently, Leipe et al. [189] showed that about 50% of the RA patients studied had elevated serum IL-22 compared to a group of healthy subjects. The level of serum IL-22 closely correlated with the extent of bone erosions as determined from radiographic analysis. However serum IL-22 did not correlate with the presence or absence of either rheumatoid factor (RF) or anti-cyclic citrullinated peptide antibodies nor was IL-22 associated with disease activity. CD4 T-cells were identified as the main source of IL-22 in these RA patients. However, in another study, de Rocha Jr et al. [190] showed that elevated serum IL-22 did correlate with the Disease Activity Score-28 (DAS-28) and the Clinical Disease Activity Index, a positive titer for RF and the extent to which bone was eroded. The findings from this study [190] agreed with the results from another recently published study [191] the latter showing that plasma IL-22 was increased in 30 patients with established RA (i.e. mean disease duration of 10.7 years), even in those patients receiving immunomodulatory therapy. Thus, any discrepancies between the results of these various clinical studies relative to establishing a relationship between IL-22, RA disease activity and RF levels may involve differences in terms of the types and duration of the immunotherapies employed or in the proportion of RA patients who were in the early or late stage of disease. The relationship between IL-22 and the presence of RF could also correlate with the immunological status of B-cells since, unlike IL-10, IL-22 does apparently not regulate the induction of Ig by activated B-cells [192].

8.4. IL-24/mda-7

The apoptosis-inducing activity of IL-24/mda-7 has made this unique member of the extended IL-10 cytokine family a target for cancer therapeutics [193-195] in view of the finding that IL-24/mda-7 could kill cancer cells specifically without affecting the vitality off normal cells or tissues [196]. Receptor binding of IL24/mda-7 to IL-20R activates STAT1 and STAT3 although additional signaling pathways have been shown to be modulated by cells over-expressing IL-24/mda-7 which did not involve JAK/STAT activation [193]. Besides the interest in IL-24/mda-7 as a tumor suppressor cytokine, mda-7/IL-24 has also been implicated in regulating some of components of RA and psoriasis immunopathology [197]. However, some of the details of the mechanism(s) by which IL-24/mda-7 could alter pro-inflammatory cytokine gene expression in RA via JAK/STAT have not been fully elucidated, although epigenetic and other transcriptional factor activity beyond activated STAT proteins have been postulated to play critical roles. Thus, it is of interest that Sahoo et al. [198] recently showed that STAT6 and c-Jun binding to the IL-24 promoter locus in T_h2 cells caused trans-activation of the IL-24 gene. Finding a relationship between the activators of STAT6 and c-Jun that are relevant to RA which leads to IL-24 gene transcription may hold the key to increasing local IL-24/mda-7 levels by T_h2 cells. This, in turn, could help overcome the 'apoptosis-resistance' of RA synovium [96].

8.5. IL-3

IL-3 is one of several major cytokines that drive the differentiation of cells of the hematopoietic lineage. The interaction between IL-3 and its cognate receptor activates several signaling pathways, including, JAK/STAT, PI3K/Akt/mTOR and the Ras/Raf/MAPK pathways [199]. Downstream events that are regulated by IL-3 which are germane to RA and autoimmunity, in general, include the findings that depending on the conditions in the microenvironment, IL-3 can alter cell proliferation, survival or induce cell death by apoptosis [30].

IL-3 was identified as an activator of JAK2 and STAT5 [200] and the expression of the pro-apoptotic protein, c-myc. This finding provided the initial evidence that cell proliferation and apoptosis was regulated, in part, by activated STAT5. However, a subsequent study by Chaturvedi et al. [201] provided evidence to the contrary in that the interaction of IL-3 with its receptor activated STAT3 via the phosphorylation of tyr^{701}. Moreover, the results of this study [201] also showed that myeloid cell proliferation was regulated by IL-3-activated Src kinase and not by IL-3-actiivated JAK3. This conclusion was based on the following results. Inhibition of c-Src kinase activation using a dominant-negative (dn) Src mutant also blocked STAT3 activation and, this in turn, inhibited proliferation of the 32Dcl3 myeloid cell line in response to IL-3. Moreover, expression of a dn-JAK2 mutation increased apoptosis in 32Dcl3 cells in the absence of IL-3 which also involved the concomitant down-regulation of ERK-2. Taken together these results indicated that Src kinase activation of STAT proteins regulated myeloid cell proliferation whereas JAKs controlled the activation of ERK-2 and associated anti-apoptotic signals [202].

The results of another study [203] showed that IL-3 played an important role in regulating SOCS3 and PIAS proteins [16, 20, 21] both of which are important in regulating cytokine signaling as well as the fine-tuning of the survival and/or cell death pathways for immune and non-immune cells in general. IL-3 plays a particularly critical role in regulating these events in mast cells [203], plasmacytoid dendritic cells [204], osteoclast-like cells, [205] and osteoclasts [206, in particular. All of these cell types are involved in some aspect of RA pathology.

To further illustrate this point, Gupta et al. [206] showed that osteoclasts treated with IL-3 were diverted to the dendritic cell lineage which may also be related to the finding that that IL-3 dampened human osteoclast-mediated bone resorption. Most recently, Srivastava et al. [207] showed that IL-3 increased the number of functionally active T_{reg} cells by stimulating the production of IL-2 by non-T_{reg} cells the latter being dependent on the dose of IL-3. Of note, treating mice with CIA with IL-3 significantly reduced the severity of arthritis and also increased the frequency of T_{reg} cells found in the thymus, lymph nodes and spleen. Although this study [207] did not directly measure the status of activated STAT proteins in the CIA mice treated with IL-3, these additional results showed that treatment of CIA with IL-3 decreased production of IL-6, IL-17A, TNF-α and IL-1 whilst increasing IFN-γ and IL-10 (Table 1).

8.6. IL-7

IL-7 was shown to be a fundamental contributor to thymocyte development as well as a regulator of T-cell homeostasis in peripheral blood. IL-7 activates both the PI3K/Akt/mTOR and JAK/STAT pathways suggesting that IL-7 regulates the survival and/or death of T-cells [208].

The IL-7 receptor provides an indicator of the biological activity of IL-7. IL-7R is composed of a γC and Rα polypeptide. JAK3 associates with γC. The binding of JAK3 to γC allows IL-7 dimer formation to occur between γC and Rα so that JAK3 can phosphorylate Rα and/or JAK1 [209]. In most cases, activation of JAK3 causes STAT5 to be phosphorylated.

With respect to relationship between IL-7 and RA, Kim et al. [210] showed that the levels of IL-1β and TNF-α found in the synovial fluid of RA patients could typically increase IL-7 production by stromal cells in culture. In addition, IL-7 was also a strong inducer of RANKL production by T-cells, independent of TNF-α [210]. Interestingly, van Roon et al. [211] showed that TNF-α blockade in RA patients reduced IL-7 production. However, high levels of IL-7 persisted in RA patients who failed to respond to antagonists of TNF-α.

Hartgring et al. [212] found significantly higher amounts of IL-7Rα in the synovial fluid of RA patients as well as in synovial fluid from patients with undifferentiated arthritis. IL-7 level strongly correlated with the number of activated $CD3^+$ T-cells. IL-7Rα was also identified on B-cells and macrophages from RA patients, but importantly IL-7Rα-expressing T-cells did not co-express, FoxP3. *Ex vivo* studies performed on monocytes collected from RA patients revealed that recombinant human IL-7Rα inhibited IL-7 induced T-cell proliferation and IFN-γ production suggesting that blockade of IL-7Rα in RA patients reduced the expression of the STAT-responsive gene, IFN-γ.

With respect to the putative role of IL-7 in regulating certain aspects of cartilage responses in arthritis, Yammani et al. [213] reported that IL-7, IL-6 or IL-8 stimulated the production of the Ca^{2+}-binding protein, S100A4, by cultured human articular chondrocytes. Importantly, IL-7 increased the synthesis of S100A4 to a greater extent than either IL-6 or IL-8 with IL-7-stimulated S100A4 resulting from JAK3/STAT3 activation. In that regard, pre-treating chondrocytes with the experimental JAK3, inhibitor, WHI-P154, or with cyclohexamide blocked S100A4 synthesis which also inhibited the production of MMP-13. Because S100A4 has been implicated as significantly contributing to pannus-mediated destruction of cartilage in RA inflammation [214], blockade of IL-7R may be useful for down-regulating the expression of S100A4 and MMP-13 with associated blunting of pannus invasion into cartilage.

The interaction between S100A4 and the tumor suppressor p53 protein was purported to be related to the role of S100A4 as a promoter of cancer metastasis [215]. IL-7 via S100A4 was also shown to induce the expression of MMP-13 as well as MMP-1, MMP-9 and S100A4 was also shown to be involved in the neoangiogenesis and aberrant cell proliferation of rheumatoid synovium [216]. Importantly a selective inhibitor of MMP-13 reduced the level of cartilage destruction in 2 of 3 animal models of RA, including the SCID-mouse co-implantation model and CIA, but not adjuvant arthritis. [217]. Thus, evidence has gradually accumulated to show that up-regulation of S100A4 via activation of STAT3 significantly alters the progression of inflammatory arthritis.

9. Experimental therapies that inhibit activated stat proteins: Is cytokine gene expression altered?

The results of a Phase 2B RA clinical trial have recently been published which showed that the JAK3-specific SMI, tofacitinib (CP690, 550) had clinical efficacy as measured by the ACR response criteria [218]. However, there has been less progress on developing novel strategies to directly inhibit activated STAT proteins or dampen STAT gene responses. Noteworthy have been proof-of-principle studies that activated STAT proteins can be experimentally 'deactivated' which result in the inhibition of STAT/DNA binding. Thus, JNK-mediated phosphorylation of the STAT6 ser^{707} decreased the DNA binding capacity of IL-4-stimulated STAT6 resulting in the inhibition of STAT6-responsive genes [219]. Using immunosuppressive STAT oligodeoxynucleotides (ODN) to inhibit activated STAT proteins have also been relatively successful. These ODN have been shown to interfere with the phosphorylation of STAT1 and STAT4 [220] and STAT1 and STAT3 [221]. Lastly, administration of a single dose of a STAT1 decoy ODN suppressed joint swelling and the histological appearance of acute and chronic adjuvant-induced experimental arthritis in the mouse [222]. Electrophoretic mobility shift analysis of the nuclear extracts from synoviocytes from the STAT1 decoy ODN-treated animals incubated with the STAT-1 decoy ODN inhibited STAT-1 binding to DNA. Of note, STAT-1 decoy ODN also inhibited the expression of macrophage CD40 suggesting that interference with CD40-mediated signaling by macrophages may be the mechanism responsible for the attenuation of arthritis by the STAT-1 decoy ODN.

10. Conclusion

The medical therapy of RA was revolutionized with the introduction of biological drugs, including TNF antagonists, the IL-6R antagonist, tocilizumab, the T-cell co-stimulatory factor inhibitor, abatacept, the B-cell inhibitor, rituximab and the IL-1 receptor antagonist, anakinra as well as the use of first-line therapy with disease-modifying anti-rheumatic drugs (DMARDs) such as methotrexate and anti-malarial drugs [223]. Nevertheless, the long-term and chronic use of these drugs for treating RA patients is not without potential deleterious consequences for those RA patients who use them. Thus, RA patients prescribed DMARDs and/or biological drugs need to be continuously monitored for changes in liver enzyme levels, ocular and/or kidney toxicities, infections and to a lesser extent malignancies such as lymphoma [224]. Just as important is the fact that some RA patients fail to respond to one or several of these biological drugs or become refractory to their action [225].

Development of JAK-specific SMIs was originally predicated on their use as a treatment for suppressing organ transplant rejection. However, JAK-SMIs were also considered as a potential adjunctive therapy for overcoming issues of long-term use of biological drugs for the therapy of RA [7, 11, 16, 17]. Now only time will tell whether or not the JAK-specific SMI, tofacitinib [218, 225], will be aggressively employed in the treatment of RA, or whether tofacitinib will be used in RA patients who only have exhibited a moderate or inadequate response to biological drugs or DMARDs.

Presently, there has been little attention paid, comparatively speaking, on acquiring data from RA patients in the general population who have been treated over several years with biological drugs to determine the extent to which the pro-inflammatory and/or anti-inflammatory cytokine repertoires have been altered from baseline. In addition, there are hardly any systematic studies, with the exception of some analyses conducted (often as a minor component of an RA clinical trial) with respect to which of several biological drugs restore the imbalance between T_h1 and T_h2 cytokines, suppress the activity of T_h17-producing cytokines, or improve the biological activity of dysfunctional T_{reg} cells [225]. Truly, the possibility exists that treating RA patients with biological drugs only partially inhibit over-expression of the pro-inflammatory cytokines that have been shown to mainly contribute to the progression of RA, namely, IL-6, IFN-γ and TNF-α (Table 1). This 'take-home' point appears to adequately justify a continual search for alternative cellular mechanisms that are active in determining whether clinical remission in RA patients is sustained or not. In conclusion, determining how STAT-responsive cytokine genes are regulated at the molecular and cellular level offers the potential going forward for developing yet another treatment modality designed to suppress the clinical activity and progression of RA pathology.

http://dx.doi.org/10.5772/52506

Acknowledgments

The Arthritis Research Laboratory at Case Western Reserve University School of Medicine was supported by an investigator-initiated project grant from Takeda Pharmaceuticals of North America (Deerfield, IL) and is presently supported by an investigator-initiated project grant from Genentech/Roche Group, (South San Francisco, CA).

Author details

Charles J. Malemud*

Address all correspondence to: cjm4@cwru.edu

Arthritis Research Laboratory, Division of Rheumatic Diseases, Case Western Reserve University School of Medicine, Cleveland, Ohio, USA

The author declares no conflict of interest.

References

[1] Ivashkiv LB, Hu X. Signaling by STATs. Arthritis Research & Therapy 2004; 6(4) 159-168.

[2] Walker JG, Ahern MJ, Coleman M et al. Expression of Jak3, STAT1, STAT4 and STAT6 in inflammatory arthritis: unique Jak3 and STAT4 expression in dendritic cells in seropositive rheumatoid arthritis. Annals of the Rheumatic Diseases 2006; 65(2) 149-156.

[3] Malemud CJ, Reddy SK. Targeting cytokines, chemokines and adhesion molecules in rheumatoid arthritis. Current Rheumatology Reviews 2008; 4(4) 219-234.

[4] Imboden JB. The immunopathogenesis of rheumatoid arthritis. Annual Review of Pathology 2009; 4 417-434.

[5] Stritesky GL, Kaplan MH. Changing the STATus quo in T helper cells. Transcription 2011; 2(4) 179-182.

[6] Hanada T, Yoshimura A. Regulation of cytokine signaling and inflammation. Cytokine & Growth Factor Reviews 2002; 13(4-5) 413-421.

[7] Hebenstreit D, Horejs-Hoeck J, Duschl A. JAK/STAT-dependent gene regulation by cytokines. Drug News Perspective 2005; 18(4) 243-249.

[8] Schindler C, Plumlee C. Interferons pen the JAK-STAT pathway. Seminars in Cell and Developmental Biology 2008; 19(4) 311-318.

[9] Malemud CJ. Recent advances in neutralizing the IL-6 pathway in arthritis. Open Access Rheumatology Research & Reviews 2009; 1: 133-150.

[10] Goenka S, Kaplan MH. Transcriptional regulation by STAT6. Immunologic Research 2011; 50(1) 87-96.

[11] Heim MH. The Jak-STAT pathway: cytokine signalling from the receptor to the nucleus. Journal of Receptor Signal Transduction Research 1999; 19(1-4) 75-120.

[12] Jiang H, Harris MB, Rothman P. IL-4/IL-13 signaling beyond JAK/STAT. Journal of Allergy & Clinical Immunology 2000; 105(6 Pt 1) 1063-1070.

[13] Hebenstreit D, Wirnsberger G, Horejs-Hoeck J, Duschl A. Signaling mechanisms, interaction partners, and target genes of STAT6. Cytokine & Growth Factor Reviews 2006; 17(3) 173-188.

[14] Tuomela S, Rautajoki KJ, Moulder R, Nyman TA, Lahesmaa R. Identification of novel Stat6 regulated proteins in IL-4-treated mouse lymphocytes. Proteomics 2009; 9(4): 1087-1098.

[15] Müller-Ladner U, Judex M, Ballhorn W et al. Activation of the IL-4 STAT pathway in rheumatoid synovium. Journal of Immunology 2000; 164(7) 3894-3901.

[16] Malemud CJ, Pearlman E. Targeting JAK/STAT signaling pathway in inflammatory diseases. Current Signal Transduction Research 2009; 4 201-221.

[17] Darnell JE Jr. STATS and gene regulation. Science 1997; 277(5332) 1630-1635.

[18] Leonard WJ, O'Shea JJ. Jaks and STATs: biological implications. Annual Review of Immunology 1998; 16 293-322.

[19] Giordanetto P, Kroemer RT. Prediction of the structure of human Janus kinase2 (JAK2) comprising JAK homology domains 1 through 7. Protein Engineering 2002; 15(9) 727-737.

[20] Decker T, Korvarik P. Serine phosphorylation of STATs. Oncogene 2000; 19(21) 2628-2637.

[21] Malemud CJ. Differential activation of JAK enzymes in rheumatoid arthritis and autoimmune disorders by pro-inflammatory cytokines: potential drug targets. International Journal of Interferon, Cytokine & Mediator Research 2010; 2(1) 97-111.

[22] Zhu J, Cote-Sierra J, Guo L, Paul WE. Stat5 activation plays a critical role in Th2 differentiation. Immunity 2003; 19(5) 739-748.

[23] Hennighausen L, Robinson GW. Interpretation of cytokine signaling through the transcription factors STAT5A and STAT5B. Genes & Development 2008; 22(6) 711-721.

[24] Radtke S, Wüller S, Xang XP et al. Cross-regulation of cytokine signalling: pro-inflammatory cytokines restrict IL-6 signalling through receptor internalisation and degradation. Journal of Cell Science 2010; 123 (Pt 6) 947-959.

[25] Santos CI, Costa-Pereira AP. Signal transducers and activators of transcription-from cytokine signaling to cancer biology. Biochimica et Biophysica Acta 2011; 1816(1) 38-49.

[26] Stark GR, Darnell JE Jr. The JAK-STAT pathway at twenty. Immunity 2012; 36(4) 503-514.

[27] Wang X, Liu Q, Ihsan A et al. JAK/STAT pathway plays a critical role in the proinflammatory gene expression and apoptosis of RAW264.7 cells induced by trichothecenes as DON and T-2 toxin. Toxicological Sciences 2012; 127(2) 412-424.

[28] Buitenhuis M, Coffer PJ, Koenderman L. Signal transducer and activator of transcription 5 (STAT5). International Journal of Biochemistry & Cell Biology 2004; 36(11) 2120-2124.

[29] Kasperkovitz PV, Verbeet NL, Smeets TJ et al. Activation of the STAT1 pathway in rheumatoid arthritis. Annals of the Rheumatic Diseases 2004; 63(3) 233-239.

[30] Malemud CJ, Gillespie HJ. The role of apoptosis in arthritis. Current Rheumatology Reviews 2005; 1(1) 131-142.

[31] Walker JG, Ahern MG, Coleman M et al. Changes in synovial tissue Jak-STAT expression in rheumatoid arthritis in response to successful DMARD treatment. Annals of the Rheumatic Diseases 2006; 65(12) 1558-1564.

[32] Walker JG, Ahern MG, Coleman M et al. Characterisation of a dendritic cell subset in synovial tissue which strongly expresses Jak/STAT transcription factors from patients with rheumatoid arthritis. Annals of the Rheumatic Diseases. 2007; 66 (8) 992-999.

[33] Stritesky GL, Muthukrishnan R, Sehra S et al. The transcription factor STAT3 is required for T helper 2 cell development. Immunity 2011; 34(1) 39-49.

[34] Krebs DL, Hilton DJ. SOCS proteins: negative regulators of cytokine signaling. Stem Cells 2001; 19(5) 378-387.

[35] Giordanetto F, Kroemer RT. A three-dimensional model of Suppressor of Cytokine Signaling 1 (SOCS-1). Protein Engineering 2003; 16(2) 115-124.

[36] Yoshimura A, Naka T, Kubo M. SOCS proteins, cytokine signalling and immune regulation. Nature Reviews Immunology 2007; 7(6) 454-465.

[37] van de Geijn GJ, Gits J, Touw IP. Distinct activities of suppressor of cytokine signaling (SOCS) proteins and involvement of the SOCS box in controlling G-CSF signaling. Journal of Leukocyte Biology 2004; 76(1) 237-244.

[38] Bruun C, Heding PE, Rønn SG et al. Suppressor of cytokine signalling-3 inhibits tumor necrosis factor-alpha induced apoptosis and signalling in beta cells. Molecular & Cellular Endocrinology 2009; 311(1-2) 32-38.

[39] Pirvulescu M, Manduteanu I, Gan AM et al. A novel pro-inflammatory mechanism of action of resistin in human endothelial cells: upregulation of SOCS3 expression

through STAT3 activation. Biochemical & Biophysical Research Communications 2012; 422(2) 321-326.

[40] Isomäki P, Alanärä T, Isohanni P et al. The expression of SOCS is altered in rheumatoid arthritis. Rheumatology (Oxford) 2007; 46(10) 1538-1546.

[41] de Andrés MC, Imagawa K, Hashimoto K et al. Suppressors of cytokine signaling (SOCS) are reduced in osteoarthritis. Biochemical & Biophysical Research Communications 2011; 407(1) 54-59.

[42] van de Loo FA, Veenbergen S, van den Brand B et al. Enhanced suppressor of cytokine signaling-3 in arthritic cartilage dysregulates human chondrocyte function. Arthritis & Rheumatism 2012; 64(10) 3313-3323.

[43] Zhang J, Somani AK, Siminovitch KA. Roles of SHP-1 tyrosine phosphatases in the negative regulation of cell signaling. Seminars in Immunology 2000; 12 (4) 361-378.

[44] Alexander DR. The CD45 tyrosine phosphatase: a positive and negative regulator of immune cell function. Seminars in Immunology 2000; 12(4) 349-359.

[45] Shuai K. Regulation of cytokine signaling pathways by PIAS proteins. Cell Research 2006; 16(2) 196-202.

[46] Tahk S, Liu B, Chernishof V, Wong KA, Wu H, Shuai K. Control of specificity and magnitude of NF-κB and STAT1-mediated gene activation through PIASy and PIAS1 cooperation. Proceedings of the National Academy of Sciences United States of America 2007; 104(28) 11643-11648.

[47] Malemud CJ. Dsyfunctional immune-mediated inflammation in rheumatoid arthritis dictates that development of anti-rheumatic drugs target multiple intracellular signaling pathways. Anti-Inflammatory & Anti-Allergy Agents in Medicinal Chemistry 2011; 10(1) 78-84.

[48] Hu X, Chen J, Wang L, Ivashkiv LB. Crosstalk among JAK-STAT, Toll-like receptor, and ITAM-dependent pathways in macrophage activation. Journal of Leukocyte Biology 2007; 82(2) 237-243.

[49] Ivashkiv LB. Cross-regulation of signaling by ITAM-associated receptors. Nature Immunology 2009; 10(4) 340-347.

[50] Lawrence T. The nuclear factor NF-κB pathway in inflammation. Cold Spring Harbor Perspectives in Biology 2009; 1(6) e001651.

[51] Alvarez JV, Frank DA. Genome-wide analysis of STAT target genes. Elucidating the mechanism of STAT-mediated oncogenesis. Cancer Biology & Therapy 2004; 3(11) 1045-1050.

[52] Oh YM, Kim JK, Choi S, Yoo JY. Identification of co-occurring transcription factor binding sites from DNA sequence using clustered position weight matrices. Nucleic Acids Research 2012; 40(5) e38.

[53] Snyder M, Huang XY, Zhang JJ. Identification of novel direct Stat3 target genes for control of growth and differentiation. Journal of Biological Chemistry 2008; 283(7) 3791-3798.

[54] Shuai K. Modulation of STAT signaling by STAT-interacting proteins. Oncogene 2000; 19(21) 2638-2644.

[55] Timofeeva OA, Chasovskikh S, Lonskaya I et al. Mechanisms of unphosphorylated STAT3 transcription factor binding to DNA. Journal of Biological Chemistry 2012; 287(17) 14192-14200.

[56] Cheon H, Yang J, Stark GR. The functions of signal transducers and activators of transcriptions 1 and 3 as cytokine-inducible proteins. Journal of Interferon & Cytokine Research 2011; 31(1) 33-40.

[57] Horvath CM, Wen Z, Darnell JE Jr. A STAT protein domain that determines DNA sequence recognition suggests a novel DNA-binding domain. Genes & Development 1995; 9(8) 984-994.

[58] Boucheron C, Dumon S, Santos SC et al. A single amino acid in the DNA binding regions of STAT5A and STAT5B confers distinct DNA binding specificities. Journal of Biological Chemistry 1998; 273(51) 33936-33941.

[59] Basham B, Sathe M, Grein J et al. In vivo identification of novel STAT5 target genes. Nucleic Acids Research 2008; 36(11) 3802-3818.

[60] Grimley PM, Dong F, Rui H. Stat5a and Stat5b: fraternal twins of signal transduction and transcription activation. Cytokine & Growth Factor Reviews 1999; 10(2) 131-157.

[61] Chang Y, Spicer DB, Sonenshein GE. Effects of IL-3 on promoter usage, attenuation and antisense transcription of the c-myc oncogene in the IL-3-dependent Ba/F3 early pre-B cell line. Oncogene 1991; 6(11) 1979-1982.

[62] Nelson EA, Walker SR, Alvarez JV, Frank DA. Isolation of unique STAT5 targets by chromatin immunoprecipitation-based gene identification. Journal of Biological Chemistry 2004; 279(52) 54724-54730.

[63] Ehret GB, Reichenbach P, Schindler U et al. DNA binding specificity of different STAT proteins. Comparison of *in vitro* specificity with natural target sites. Journal of Biological Chemistry 2001; 276(9) 6675-6688.

[64] Moucadel V, Constantinescu SN. Differential STAT5 signaling by ligand-dependent and constitutively active cytokine receptors. Journal of Biological Chemistry 2005; 280(14) 13364-13373.

[65] Rickert M, Wang X, Boulanger MJ, Goriatcheva N, Garcia KC. The structure of interleukin-2 complexed with its alpha receptor. Science 2005; 308(5727) 1477-1480.

[66] Kanai A, Suzuki K, Tanimoto K, Mizushima-Sugano J, Suzuki Y, Sugano S. Characterization of STAT6 target genes in human B cells and lung epithelial cells. DNA Research 2011; 18(5) 379-392.

[67] Thanos CD, DeLano WL, Wells JA. Hot-spot mimicry of a cytokine receptor by a small molecule. Proceedings of the National Academy of Sciences of the United States of America. 2006; 103(42) 15422-15427.

[68] Quaglino P, Bergallo M, Ponti R et al. Th1, Th2, Th17 and regulatory T cell patterns in psoriatic patients: modulation of cytokines and gene targets induced by etanercept treatment and correlation with clinical responses. Dermatology 2011; 223(1) 57-67.

[69] Delphin S, Stavnezer J. Characterization of an interleukin 4 (IL-4) responsive region in the immunoglobulin heavy chain germline epsilon promoter: regulation by NF-IL-4, a C/EBP family member and NF-kappa B/p50. Journal of Experimental Medicine 1995; 181(1) 181-192.

[70] Kotanides H, Reich NC. Interleukin-4-induced STAT6 recognizes and activates a target site in the promoter of the interleukin-4 receptor gene. Journal of Biological Chemistry 1996; 271(41) 25555-25561.

[71] Morelli X, Bourgeas R, Roche P. Chemical and structural lessons from recent successes in protein-protein interaction inhibition (2P2I). Current Opinion in Chemical Biology 2011; 15(4) 475-481.

[72] Lin JX, Leonard WJ. The role of Stat5a and Stat5b in signaling by IL-2 family cytokines. Oncogene 2000; 19(21) 2566-2576.

[73] Tsuji-Takayama K, Suzuki M, Yamamoto M et al. The production of IL-10 by human regulatory T cells is enhanced by IL-2 through a STAT5-responsive intronic enhancer in the IL-10 locus. Journal of Immunology 2008; 181(6) 3897-3905.

[74] Ochs HD, Gambineri E, Torgerson TR. IPEX, FOXP3 and regulatory T-cells: a model for autoimmunity. Immunologic Research 2007; 38(1-3) 112-121.

[75] Murawski MR, Litherland SA, Clare-Salzler MJ, Davoodi-Semiromi A. Upregulation of Foxp3 expression in mouse and human Treg is IL-2/STAT dependent: implications for the NOD STAT5B mutation in diabetes pathogenesis. Annals of the New York Academy of Sciences 2006; 1079 198-204.

[76] Lai G, Bromberg JS. Epigenetic mechanisms of regulation of Foxp3 expression. Blood 2009; 114(18) 3727-3735.

[77] Chen Z, Lund R, Aittokallio T, Kosonen M, Nevalainen O, Lahesmaa R. Identification of novel IL-4/STAT6-regulated gene in T lymphocytes. Journal of Immunology 2003; 171(7) 3627-3635.

[78] Lund R, Ahlfors H, Kainonen E, Lahesmaa AM, Dixon C, Lahesmaa R. Identification of genes involved in the initiation of human Th1 or Th2 cell commitment. European Journal of Immunology 2005; 35(11) 3307-3319.

[79] Maier E, Hebenstreit D, Posselt G, Hammerl P, Duschl A, Horejs-Hoeck J. Inhibition of suppressive T cell factor (TCF-1) isoforms in naïve CD_4^+ T cells is mediated by IL-$_4$/STAT6 signaling. Journal of Biological Chemistry 2011; 286(2) 919-928.

http://dx.doi.org/10.5772/52506

[80] Chapoval S, Dasgupta P, Dorsey NJ, Keegan AD. Regulation of the T helper cell type 2 (Th2/T regulatory cell (Treg) balance by IL-4 and STAT6. Journal of Leukocyte Biology 2010; 87(6) 1011-1018.

[81] Wurster AL, Tanaka T, Grusby MJ. The biology of Stat4 and Stat6. Oncogene 2000; 19(21) 2577-2584.

[82] Kuhn DJ, Dou QP. The role of interleukin-2 receptor alpha in cancer. Frontiers in Bioscience 2005; 10 1462-1474.

[83] Kurreeman FA, Daha NA, Chang M et al. Association of IL2RA and IL2RB with rheumatoid arthritis: a replication study in a Dutch population. Annals of the Rheumatic Diseases 2009; 68(11) 1789-1790.

[84] Raychaudhuri S. Recent advances in the genetics of rheumatoid arthritis. Current Opinion in Rheumatology 2010; 22(2) 109-118.

[85] Waldmann TA. The IL-2/IL-15 receptor systems: targets for immunotherapy. Journal of Clinical Immunology 2002; 22(2) 51-56.

[86] González-Álvaro I, Domínguez-Jiménez C, Ortiz AM et al. Interleukin-15 and interferon-γ participate in the cross-talk between natural killer and monocytic cells required for tumor necrosis factor production. Arthritis Research & Therapy 2006; 8(4) R88.

[87] Ernestam S, af Klint E, Catrina AI et al. Synovial expression of IL-15 in rheumatoid arthritis is not influenced by blockade of tumor necrosis factor. Arthritis Research & Therapy 2006; 8(1) R18.

[88] Baslund B, Tvede N, Danneskiold-Samsoe B et al. Targeting interleukin-15 in patients with rheumatoid arthritis: a proof-of-concept study. Arthritis & Rheumatism 2005; 52(9) 2686-2692.

[89] González-Álvaro I, Ortiz AM, Álvaro-Gracia JM et al. Interleukin-15 levels in serum may predict a severe disease course in patients with early arthritis. Public Library of Science One 2011; 6(12) e29492.

[90] Navarro-Millán I, Singh JA, Curtis JR. Systematic review of tocilizumab for rheumatoid arthritis: a new biologic agent targeting the interleukin-6 receptor. Clinical Therapy 2012; 34(4) 788-802.e3.

[91] Ogata A, Hirano T, Hishitani Y, Tanaka T. Safety and efficacy of tocilizumab for the treatment of rheumatoid arthritis. Clinical Medicine Insights in Arthritis & Musculoskeletal Disorders 2012; 5 27-42.

[92] Smolen JS, Avila JC, Aletaha D. Tocilizumab inhibits the progression of joint damage in rheumatoid arthritis irrespective of its anti-inflammatory effects: dissociation of the link between inflammation and destruction. Annals of the Rheumatic Diseases 2012; 71(5) 687-693.

[93] Jovanovic DV, Di Battista JA, Martel-Pelletier J et al. IL-17 stimulates the production and expression of proinflammatory cytokines, IL-1β and TNF-α, by human macrophages. Journal of Immunology 1998; 160(7) 3513-3521.

[94] Dragon S, Saffar AS, Shan L, Gounni AS. IL-17 attenuates the anti-apoptotic effects of GM-CSF in human neutrophils. Molecular Immunology 2008; 45(1) 160-168.

[95] Oh HM, Yu CR, Golestaneh N et al. STAT3 protein promotes T-cell survival and inhibits interleukin-2 production through up-regulation of Class O Forkhead transcription factors. Journal of Biological Chemistry 2011; 286(35) 30888-30897.

[96] Malemud CJ. Apoptosis-resistance in rheumatoid arthritis synovial tissue. Journal of Clinical & Cellular Immunology 2012; S3-006; doi: 10.4172/21559899.

[97] Kimura A, Kishimoto T. IL-6: regulator of Treg/Th17 balance. European Journal of Immunology 2010; 40(7) 1830-1835.

[98] Samson M, Audia S, Janikashvili N et al. Inhibition of IL-6 function corrects Th17/Treg imbalance in patients with rheumatoid arthritis. Arthritis & Rheumatism 2012; 64(8) 2499-2503

[99] Niu Q, Cai B, Huang ZC, Shi YY, Wang LL. Disturbed Th17/Treg balance in patients with rheumatoid arthritis. Rheumatology International 2012; 32(9) 2731-2736.

[100] O'Brien CA, Manolagas SC. Isolation and characterization of the human gp130 promoter. Regulation by STATs. Journal of Biological Chemistry 1997; 272(23) 15003-15010.

[101] Malemud CJ. Anticytokine therapy for osteoarthritis. Evidence to date. Drugs & Aging 2010; 27(2) 95-115.

[102] Wang T, Niu G, Kortylewski M et al. Regulation of the innate and adaptive immune responses by Stat-$_3$ signaling in tumor cells. Nature Medicine 2004; 10(1) 48-54.

[103] Costa-Pereira AP, Bonito NA, Secki MJ. Dysregulation of janus kinases and signal transducers and activators of transcription in cancer. American Journal of Cancer Research 2011; 1(6) 806-816.

[104] Sozzani D, Bosisio D, Scarsi M, Tincani A. Type I interferons in systemic autoimmunity. Autoimmunity 2010; 43(3) 196-203.

[105] Biswas PS, Bhagat G, Pernis AB. IRF4 and its regulators: insights into the pathogenesis of inflammatory arthritis? Immunologic Reviews 2010; 233(1) 79-96.

[106] Pramanik R, Jørgensen TN, Xin H, Kotzin BL, Choubey D. Interleukin-6 induces expression of lfi202, an interferon-inducible candidate gene for lupus susceptibility. Journal of Biological Chemistry 2004; 279(16) 16121-16127.

[107] Christova R, Jones T, Wu PJ et al. P-STAT1 mediates higher-order chromatin remodeling of the human MHC response to IFNγ. Journal of Cell Science 2007; 120(Pt 18) 3262-3270.

[108] Vogl C, Flatt T, Fuhrmann B et al. Transcriptosome analysis reveals a major impact of JAK protein tyrosine kinase (Tyk2) on the expression of interferon-responsive and metabolic genes. Biomedical Central Genomics 2010; 11 199.

[109] Noon-Song EN, Ahmed CM, Dabelic R, Canton J, Johnson HM. Controlling nuclear JAKs and STATs for specific gene activation by IFNγ. Biochemical & Biophysical Research Communications 2011; 410(3) 648-653.

[110] Tripathi A, Sodhi A. Prolactin-induced production of cytokines in macrophages in vitro involves JAK/STAT and JNK MAPK pathways. International Immunology 2008; 20(3) 327-336.

[111] David M, Petricoin E III, Benjamin C, Pine R, Weber MJ, Larner AC. Requirement of MAP kinase (ERK2) activity in interferon α and interferon β-stimulated gene expression through STAT proteins. Science 1995; 269(5231) 1721-1723.

[112] Aznar S, Valéron PF, del Rincon SV, Peréz LF, Perona R, Lacal JC. Simultaneous tyrosine and serine phosphorylation of STAT3 transcription factor is involved in Rho A GTPase oncogenic transformation. Molecular & Cellular Biology 2001; 12(10) 3282-3294.

[113] Gonsky R, Deem RL, Bream J, Young HA, Targan SR. Enhancer role of STAT5 in CD2 activation of IFN-γ gene expression. Journal of Immunology 2004; 173(10) 6241-6247.

[114] Tsuno T, Mejido J, Zhao T, Schmeisser H, Morrow A, Zoon KC. IRF9 is a key factor for eliciting the antiproliferative activity of IFN-α. Journal of Immunotherapy 2009; 32(8) 803-816.

[115] Kaur S, Uddin S, Platanias LC. The PI3′ kinase pathway in interferon signaling. Journal of Interferon & Cytokine Research 2005; 25(12) 780-787.

[116] Kaur S, Sassano A, Dolniak B et al. Role of the Akt pathway in mRNA translation of interferon-stimulated genes. Proceedings of the National Academy of Sciences of the United States of America 2008; 105(12) 4808-4813.

[117] Kaur S, Katsoulidis E, Platanias LC. Akt and mRNA translation by interferons. Cell Cycle 2008; 7(14) 2112-2116.

[118] Hamilton TA, Ohmori Y, Tebo JM, Kishore R. Regulation of macrophage gene expression by pro- and anti-inflammatory cytokines. Pathobiology 1991; 67(5-6) 241-244.

[119] Schaefer A, Unterberger C, Frankenberger M et al. Mechanism of interferon-gamma mediated down-regulation of interleukin-10 gene expression. Molecular Immunology 2009; 46(7) 1351-1359.

[120] Torgerson GR. Regulatory T cells in human autoimmune diseases. Springer Seminars in Immunopathology 2006; 28(1) 63-76.

[121] Nandakumar S, Miller CW, Kumaraguru U. T regulatory cells: an overview and intervention techniques to modulate allergy outcome. Clinical & Molecular Allergy 2009; 12(7) 5.

[122] Hams E, Colmont CS, Dioszeghy V et al. Oncostatin M receptor-β signaling limits monocyte cell recruitment in acute inflammation. Journal of Immunology 2008; 181(3) 2174-2180.

[123] Mosley B, De Imus C, Friend D et al. Dual oncostatin M (OSM) receptors. Cloning and characterization of an alternative signaling subunit conferring OSM-specific receptor activation. Journal of Biological Chemistry 1996; 271(51) 32635-32643.

[124] Hermanns HM, Radkte S, Schaper F, Heinrich PC, Behrmann I. Non-redundant signal transduction of interleukin-6-type cytokines. The adaptor protein Shc is specifically recruited to the oncostatin M receptor. Journal of Biological Chemistry 2000; 275(52) 40742-40748.

[125] Fossey SL, Bear MD, Kisseberth WC, Pennell M, London CA. Oncostatin M promotes STAT3 activation, VEGF production and invasion of osteosarcoma cell lines. Biomedical Central Cancer 2011; 11 125.

[126] Clarkson RWE, Boland MP, Kritikou EA et al. The genes induced by signal transducers and activators of transcription (STAT)3 and STAT5 in mammary epithelial cells define the roles of these STATs in mammary development. Molecular Endocrinology 2006; 20(3) 675-685.

[127] STAT Gene Regulatory Network. rulai/cshl.edu/TRED/GRN/STAT.htm

[128] Nakanishi K, Yoshimoto T, Tsutsui H, Okamura H. Interleukin-18 regulates both Th1 and Th2 responses. Annual Review of Immunology 2001; 19 423-474.

[129] Liew FY, McInnes IB. Role of interleukin 15 and interleukin 18 in inflammatory response. Annals of the Rheumatic Diseases 2002; 61(Suppl 2) ii100-ii102.

[130] McInnes IB, Liew FY, Gracie JA. Interleukin-18: a therapeutic target in rheumatoid arthritis? Arthritis Research & Therapy 2005; 7(1) 38-41.

[131] Matsui K, Tsutsui H, Nakanishi K. Pathophysiological roles for IL-18 in inflammatory arthritis. Expert Opinion on Therapeutic Targets 2003; 7(6) 701-724.

[132] Lotito AP, Silva CA, Mello SB. Interleukin-18 in chronic joint diseases. Autoimmunity Reviews 2007; 6(4) 253-256.

[133] Gracie JA, Forsey RJ, Chan WL et al. A proinflammatory role for IL-18 in rheumatoid arthritis. Journal of Clinical Investigation 1999; 104(10) 1393-1401.

[134] Tanaka M, Harigai M, Kawaguchi Y et al. Mature form of interleukin-18 is expressed in rheumatoid arthritis synovial tissue and contributes to interferon-gamma production by synovial T-cells. Journal of Rheumatology 2001; 28(8) 1779-1787.

[135] Van Oosterhout M, Levarht EWN, Sont JK, Huizinga TWJ, Toes REM, van Laar JM. Clinical efficacy of infliximab plus methotrexate in DMARD naïve and DMARD re-

fractory rheumatoid arthritis is associated with decreased synovial expression of TNFα and IL-18 but not CXCL12. Annals of the Rheumatic Diseases 2005; 64(4) 537-543.

[136] Petrovic-Rackov I, Pejnovic N. Clinical significance of IL-18, IL-15, IL-12 and TNF-α measurement in rheumatoid arthritis. Clinical Rheumatology 2006; 25(4) 448-452.

[137] Trinchieri G, Scott P. Interleukin-12: a proinflammatory cytokine with immunoregulatory functions. Research in Immunology 1995; 146(7–8) 423–431.

[138] Trinchieri G, Scott P. Interleukin-12: basic principles and clinical applications. Current Topics in Microbiology & Immunology 1999; 238 57–78.

[139] Merberg DM, Wolf SF, Clark SC. Sequence similarity between NKSF and the IL-6/G-CSF family. Immunology Today 1992; 13(2) 77–78.

[140] Watford WT, Moriguchi M, Morinobu A, O'Shea JJ. Mini review. The biology of IL-12: coordinating innate and adaptive immune responses. Cytokine & Growth Factor Reviews 2003; 14 361–368.

[141] Yen JH, Kong W, Ganea D. IFN-β inhibits dendritic cell migration through STAT-1-mediated transcriptional suppression of CCR7 and matrix metalloproteinase 9. Journal of Immunology 2010; 187(7) 3478-3486.

[142] Tuohy VK, Yu M, Yin L, Mathisen PM, Johnson JM, Kawczak JA. Modulation of the IL-10/IL-12 cytokine circuit by interferon-β inhibits the development of epitope spreading and disease progression in murine autoimmune encephalomyelitis. Journal of Neuroimmunology 2000; 111(1-2) 55-63.

[143] Thieu VT, Yu Q, Chang HC et al. Signal transducer and activator of transcription 4 is required for the transcription factor T-bet to promote T helper 1 cell-fate determination. Immunity 2008; 29(5) 679-690.

[144] Yang Y, Ochando JC, Bromberg JS, Ding Y. Identification of a distant T-bet enhancer responsive to IL-12/Stat4 and IFNγ/Stat1 signals. Blood 2007; 110(7) 2494-2500.

[145] Forbes E, van Panhuys N, Min B, Le Gros G. Differential requirements for IL-4/STAT6 signalling in CD4 T-cell fate determination and the Th2-immune effector responses. Immunology and Cell Biology 2010; 88(3) 240-243.

[146] Huber M, Steinwald V, Guralnik A et al. IL-27 inhibits the development of regulatory T cells via STAT3. International Immunology 2008; 20(2) 223-234.

[147] Afzali B, Lombardi G, Lechler RI, Lord GM. The role of T helper 17 (Th17) and regulatory T cells (Treg) in human organ transplantation and autoimmune disease. Clinical & Experimental Immunology 2007; 148(1) 32-46.

[148] Peck A, Mellins ED. Plasticity of the T-cell phenotype and function: the T helper type 17 example. Immunology 2010; 129(2) 147-153.

[149] Chen Z, O'Shea JJ. Th17 cells: a new fate for differentiating helper T cells. Immunologic Research 2008; 41(2) 87-102.

[150] Yagi R, Zhu J, Paul WE. An updated view on transcription factor $GATA_3$-mediated regulation of T_h1 and T_h2 cell differentiation. International Immunology 2011; 23(7) 415-420.

[151] Habib T, Senadheera S, Weinberg K, Kaushansky K. The common γ chain (γc) is a required signaling component of the IL-21 receptor and supports IL-21-induced cell proliferation via JAK3. Biochemistry 2002; 41(27) 8725-8731.

[152] Mehta DS, Wurster AL, Grusby MJ. Biology of IL-21 and the IL-21 receptor. Immunologic Reviews 2004; 202 84-95.

[153] Ma J, Ma D, Ji C. The role of IL-21 in hematological malignancies. Cytokine 2011; 56(2) 133-139.

[154] Collins M, Whitters MJ, Young DA. IL-21 and IL-21 receptor: a new cytokine pathway modulates innate and adaptive immunity. Immunologic Reviews 2003; 28(2) 131-140.

[155] Sonderegger I, Kisielow J, Meier R, King C, Kopf M. IL-21 and IL-21R are not required for development of Th17 cells and autoimmunity in vivo. European Journal of Immunology 2008; 3897 1833-1838.

[156] Coquet JM, Chakravarti S, Smyth MJ, Godfrey DI. Cutting edge: IL-21 is not essential for Th17 differentiation or experimental autoimmune encephalomyelitis. Journal of Immunology 2008; 180(11) 7097-7101.

[157] Davis ID, Skak K, Smyth MJ, Kristjansen PE, Miller DM, Sivakumar PV. Interleukin-21 signaling: functions in cancer and autoimmunity. Clinical Cancer Research 2007; 13(23) 6926-6932.

[158] Young DA, Hegen M, Ma HL et al. Blockade of the interleukin-21/interleukin-21 receptor pathway ameliorates disease in animal models of rheumatoid arthritis. Arthritis & Rheumatism 2007; 56(4) 1152-1163.

[159] Yuan FL, Hu W, Lu WG et al. Targeting interleukin-21 in rheumatoid arthritis. Molecular Biology Reports 2011; 38(3) 1717-1721.

[160] Wooley PA. What animal models are best to test novel rheumatoid arthritis therapies? Current Rheumatology Reviews 2008; 4(4) 277-287.

[161] Dumoutier L, Louahed J, and Renauld JC. Cloning and characterization of IL-10-related T cell-derived inducible factor (IL-TIF), a novel cytokine structurally related to IL-10 and inducible by IL-9. Journal of Immunology 2000; 164(4) 1814-1819.

[162] Blumberg H, Conklin D, Xu WF et al. Interleukin 20: discovery, receptor identification and role in epidermal function. Cell 2001; 104(1) 9-19.

[163] Zenewicz LA, Flavell RA. Recent advances in IL-22 biology. International Immunology 2011 23(3) 159-163.

[164] Donnelly RP, Sheikh F, Kotenko SV, Dickensheets H. The expanded family of class II cytokines that share the IL-10 receptor-2 (IL-10R2) chain. Journal of Leukocyte Biology 2004; 76(2) 314-321.

[165] Commins S, Steinke JW, Borish L. The extended IL-10 superfamily: IL-10, IL-19, IL-20, IL-22, IL-24, IL-26, IL-28 and IL-29. Journal of Allergy & Clinical immunology 2008; 121(5) 1108-1111.

[166] Trivella DB, Ferreira-Júnior JR, Dumoutier L, Renauld JC, Polikarpov I. Structure and function of interleukin-22 and other members of the interleukin-10 family. Cellular & Molecular Life Sciences 2010; 67(17) 2909-2935.

[167] Asadullah K, Sterry W, Volk HD. Interleukin-10 therapy – review of a new approach. Pharmacological Reviews 2003; 55(2) 241-269.

[168] Sabat R, Wallace E, Endesfelder S, Wolk K. IL-19 and IL-20: two novel cytokines with importance in inflammatory diseases. Expert Opinion on Therapeutic Targets 2007; 11(5) 601-612.

[169] Wolk K, Kunz S, Asadullah K, Sabat R. Cutting edge: Immune cells as sources and targets of the IL-10 family members. Journal of Immunology 2002; 168(11) 5397-5402.

[170] Parrish-Novak J, Xu W, Brender T et al. Interleukins 19, 20, and 24 signal through two distinct receptor complexes. Differences in receptor-ligand interactions mediate unique biological functions. Journal of Biological Chemistry 2002; 277(49) 47517-47523.

[171] Dumoutier L, Leemans C, Lejeune D, Kotenko SV, Renauld JC. Cutting edge: STAT activation by IL-19, IL-20 and mda-7 through IL-20 receptor complexes of two types. Journal of Immunology 2001; 167(7) 3545-3549.

[172] Kunz S, Wolk K, Witte E et al. Interleukin (IL)-19, IL-20 and IL-24 are produced and act on keratinocytes and are distinct from classical ILs. Experimental Dermatology 2006; 15(12) 991-1004.

[173] Zdanov A. Structural features of the interleukin-10 family of cytokines. Current Pharmaceutical Design 2004; 10(31) 3873-3884.

[174] Sakurai N, Kuroiwa T, Ikeuchi H et al. Expression of IL-19 and its receptors in RA: potential role for synovial hyperplasia formation. Rheumatology (Oxford) 2008; 47(6) 815-820.

[175] Alanärä T, Karstila A, Moilanen T, Silvennoinen O, Isomäki P. Expression of IL-10 family cytokines in rheumatoid arthritis: elevated levels of IL-19 in joints. Scandinavian Journal of Rheumatology 2010; 39(2) 118-126.

[176] Malemud CJ. MAP kinases. In: OA, Inflammation and Degradation: A Continuum: Biomedical and Health Research - Vol 70. Buckwalter J, Lotz M, Stoltz J-F. (eds). Amsterdam: IOS Press; 2007. p 99-117.

[177] Hsu YH, Hsieh PP, Chang MS. Interleukin-19 blockade attenuates collagen-induced arthritis in rats. Rheumatology (Oxford) 2012; 51(3) 434-442.

[178] Leng RX, Pan HF, Tao JH, Ye DQ. IL-19, IL-20 and IL-24: potential therapeutic targets for autoimmune diseases. Expert Opinion on Therapeutic Targets 2011; 15(2) 119-126.

[179] Wahl C, Müller W, Leithäuser F et al. IL-20 receptor signaling down-regulates antigen-specific T cell responses. Journal of Immunology 2009; 182(2) 802-810.

[180] Hsu YH, Chang MS. Interleukin-20 antibody is a potential therapeutic agent for experimental arthritis. Arthritis & Rheumatism 2010; 62(11) 3311-3321.

[181] Hsu YH, Chen WY, Chan CH, Wu CH, Sun ZJ, Chang MS. Anti-IL-20 monoclonal antibody inhibits the differentiation of osteoclasts and protects against osteoporotic bone loss. Journal of Experimental Medicine 2011; 208(9) 1849-1861.

[182] Kragstrup TW, Otkjaer K, Holm C et al. The expression of IL-20 and IL-24 and their shared receptors are increased in rheumatoid arthritis and spondyloarthropathy. Cytokine 2008; 41(1) 16-23.

[183] Kotenko SV, Izotova LS, Mirochnitchenko OV et al. Identification of the functional Interleukin-22 (IL-22) receptor complex. The IL-10R2 chain (IL-10Rβ) is a common chain of both the IL-10 and IL-22 (IL-10-related T cell-derived inducible factor, IL-TIF) receptor complexes. Journal of Biological Chemistry 2001; 276(4) 2725-2732.

[184] Xie MH, Aggarwal S, Ho WH et al. Interleukin (IL)-22, a novel human cytokine that signals through the interferon receptor-related proteins CRF2-4 and IL-22R. Journal of Biological Chemistry 2000; 275(40) 31335-31339.

[185] Aggarwal S, Xie MH, Maruoka M, Foster J, Gurney AL. Acinar cells of the pancreas are a target of interleukin-22. Journal of Interferon & Cytokine Research 2001; 21(12) 1047-1053.

[186] Brand S, Beigel F, Olszak T et al. IL-22 is increased in active Crohn's disease and promotes proinflammatory gene expression and intestinal cell migration. American Journal of Physiology-Gastrointestinal and Liver Physiology 2006; 290(4) G827-G-838.

[187] Lejeune D, Dumoutier L, Constantinescu S, Kruijer W, Schuringa JJ, Renauld J-C. Interleukin-22 (IL-22) activates the JAK/STAT, ERK, JNK, and p38 MAP kinase pathways in a rat hepatoma cell line. Pathways that shared with and distinct from IL-10. Journal of Biological Chemistry 2002; 277(37) 33676-33682.

[188] Ikeuchi H, Kuroiwa T, Hiramatsu N et al. Expression of interleukin-22 in rheumatoid arthritis. Potential role as a proinflammatory cytokine. Arthritis & Rheumatism 2005; 52(4) 1037-1046.

[189] Leipe J, Schramm MA, Grunke M et al. Interleukin 22 serum levels are associated with radiographic progression in rheumatoid arthritis. Annals of the Rheumatic Diseases 2011; 70(8) 1453-1457.

[190] da Rocha LF Jr, Duarte AL, Dantas AT et al. Increased serum interleukin-22 in patients with rheumatoid arthritis and correlation with disease activity. Journal of Rheumatology 2012; 39(7) 1320-1325.

[191] Zhang L, Li JM, Liu XG et al. Elevated Th22 cells correlated with Th17 cells in patients with rheumatoid arthritis. Journal of Clinical Immunology 2011; 31(4) 606-614.

[192] Lécart S, Morel F, Noraz N et al. IL-22, in contrast to IL-10, does not induce Ig production, due to absence of a functional IL-22 receptor on activated human B cells. International Immunology 2002; 14(11) 1351-1356.

[193] Gopalkrishnan RV, Sauane M, Fisher PB. Cytokine and tumor cell apoptosis inducing activity of mda-7/IL-24. International Immunopharmacology 2004; 4(5) 635-647.

[194] Dent P, Yacoub A, Hamed HA et al. The development of MDA-7/IL-24 as a cancer therapeutic. Pharmacology & Therapeutics 2010; 128(2) 375-384.

[195] Dent P, Yacoub A, Hamed A et al. MDA-7/IL-24 as a cancer therapeutic: from bench to bedside. Anticancer Drugs 2010; 21(8) 725-731.

[196] Dash R, Bhutia SK, Azab B et al. mda-7/IL-24: a unique member of the IL-10 gene family promoting cancer-targeted toxicity. Cytokine & Growth Factor Reviews 2010; 21(5) 381-391.

[197] Sahoo A, Sim SH. Molecular mechanism governing IL-24 gene expression. Immune Network 2012; 12(1) 1-7.

[198] Sahoo A, Lee CG, Jash A et al. Stat6 and c-Jun mediate Th2 cell-specific IL-24 gene expression. Journal of Immunology 2011; 186(7) 4098-4109.

[199] Yen JJ, Yang-Yen HF. Transcription factors mediating interleukin-3 survival signals. Vitamins & Hormones 2006; 74 147-163.

[200] Mui AL, Wakao H, Kinoshita T, Kitamura T, Miyajima A. Suppression of interleukin-3-induced gene expression by a c-terminal Stat5. European Molecular Biology Organization Journal 1996; 15(10) 2425-2433.

[201] Chaturvedi P, Reddy MV, Reddy EP. Src kinases and not JAKs activates STATs during IL-3-induced myeloid cell proliferation. Oncogene 1998; 16(13) 1749-1758.

[202] Reddy EP, Korapati A, Chaturvedi P, Rane S. IL-3 signaling and the role of Src kinases, JAKs and STATs: a covert liaison unveiled. Oncogene 2000; 19(21) 2532-2547.

[203] Morales JK, Falanga YT, Depcrynski A, Fernando J, Ryan JJ. Mast cell homeostasis and the JAK-STAT pathway. Genes & Immunity 2010; 11(8) 599-608.

[204] Cavanagh LL, Boyce A, Smith L et al. Rheumatoid arthritis synovium contains plasmacytoid dendritic cells. Arthritis Research & Therapy 2005; 7(2) R230-R240.

[205] Barton BE, Mayer R. IL-3 induces differentiation of bone marrow precursor cells to osteoclast-like cells. Journal of Immunology 1989; 143(10) 3211-3216.

[206] Gupta N, Barhanpurkar AP, Tomar GB et al. IL-3 inhibits human osteoclastogenesis and bone resorption through downregulation of c-Fms and diverts the cells to dendritic cell lineage. Journal of Immunology 2010; 185(4) 2261-2272.

[207] Srivastava RK, Tomar GB, Barhanpurkar AP et al. IL-3 attenuates collagen-induced arthritis by modulating the development of $Foxp3^{+}$ regulatory T cells. Journal of Immunology 2011; 186(4) 2262-2267.

[208] Khaled AR, Durum SK. Death and Baxes: mechanism of lymphotropic cytokines. Immunologic Review 2003; 193 48-57.

[209] Malemud CJ. The discovery of novel experimental therapies for inflammatory arthritis. Mediators of Inflammation doi: 10.1155/2009/698769.

[210] Kim HR, Hwang KA, Park SH, Kang I. IL-7 and IL-15: Biology and roles in T-cell immunity in health and disease. Critical Reviews in Immunology 2008; 28(4) 325-339.

[211] van Roon JA, Hartgring SA, Wenting van Wijk M. Persistence of interleukin-7 activity and levels on tumour necrosis factor α blockade in patients with rheumatoid arthritis. Annals of the Rheumatic Diseases 2007; 66(5) 664-669.

[212] Hartgring SA, van Roon JA, Wenting van Wijk M. Elevated expression of interleukin-7 receptor in inflamed joints mediates interleukin-7-induced immune activation in rheumatoid arthritis. Arthritis & Rheumatism 2009; 60(9) 2595-2605.

[213] Yammani RR, Long D, Loeser RF. Interleukin-7 stimulates secretion of S100A4 by activating the JAK/STAT signaling pathway in human articular chondrocytes. Arthritis & Rheumatism 2009; 60(3) 792-800.

[214] Senolt L, Grigorian M, Lukanidin E et al. S100A4 is expressed at site of invasion in rheumatoid arthritis synovium and modulates production of matrix metalloproteinases. Annals of the Rheumatic Diseases 2006; 65(12) 1645-1648.

[215] Grigorian M, Andresen S, Tulchinsky E et al. Tumor suppressor p53 protein is a new target for the metastasis-associated Mts1/S100A4 protein. Functional consequences of their interaction. Journal of Biological Chemistry 2001; 276(25) 22699-22708.

[216] Senolt L, Grigorian M, Lukanidin E et al. S100A4 (Mts1): Is there any relation to the pathogenesis of rheumatoid arthritis? Autoimmune Reviews 2006; 5(2) 129-131.

[217] Jüngel A, Ospelt C, Lesch M et al. Effect of oral application of a highly selective MMP-13 inhibitor in three different animal models of rheumatoid arthritis. Annals of the Rheumatic Diseases 2010; 69(5) 898-902.

[218] Fleischmann R, Cutolo M, Genovese MC et al. Phase IIB dose-ranging study of the oral JAK inhibitor tofacitinib (CP650,550) or adalimumab monotherapy versus placebo in patients with active rheumatoid arthritis with an inadequate response to DMARDs. Arthritis & Rheumatism 2012; 64(3) 617-629.

[219] Shirakawa T, Kawazoe Y, Tsujikawa T, Jung D, Sato S, Uesugi M. Deactivation of STAT6 through serine 707 phosphorylation by JNK. Journal of Biological Chemistry 2011; 286(5) 4003-4010.

[220] Klinman DM, Tross D, Klaschik S, Shirota H, Sato T. Therapeutic applications and mechanisms underlying the activity of immunosuppressive oligonucleotides. Annals of the New York Academy of Sciences 2009; 1175 80-88.

[221] Lührmann A, Tschernig T, von der Leyen H, Hecker M, Pabst R, Wagner AH. Decoy oligodeoxynucleotides against STAT transcription factors decrease allergic inflammation in a rat asthma model. Experimental Lung Research 2010; 36(2) 85-93.

[222] Hückel M, Schurigt U, Wagner AH et al. Attenuation of murine antigen-induced arthritis by treatment with a decoy oligodeoxynucleotide inhibiting signal transducer and activator of transcription-1 (STAT-1). Arthritis Research & Therapy 2006; 8(1) R17.

[223] Feely MG, Erickson A, O'Dell JR. Therapeutic options for rheumatoid arthritis. Expert Opinion on Pharmacotherapy 2009; 10(13) 2095-2106.

[224] Malemud CJ. Inhibitors of JAK for the treatment of rheumatoid arthritis: rationale and clinical data. Clinical Investigation 2012; 2(1) 39-47.

[225] Malemud CJ. Molecular mechanisms in rheumatic diseases: rationale for novel drug development – Introduction. Anti-Inflammatory & Anti-Allergy Agents in Medicinal Chemistry 2011; 10 73-77.

Chapter 14

Coupled Enzyme Activity and Thermal Shift Screening of the Maybridge Rule of 3 Fragment Library Against *Trypanosoma brucei* Choline Kinase; A Genetically Validated Drug Target

Louise L. Major, Helen Denton and Terry K. Smith

Additional information is available at the end of the chapter

http://dx.doi.org/10.5772/52668

1. Introduction

Infectious diseases caused by parasitic protozoa affect approximately 15% of the global population, and more than 65% of the population in the Third and developing world, yet current drug therapies for protozoal infections are woefully inadequate. As protozoal infections take their toll predominantly in the developing world, market forces are insufficient to promote the development of novel anti-protozoal drugs. In 2000, only ca. 0.1% of global investment in health research was spent on drug discovery for tropical diseases [1].

One such neglected parasitic disease is Human African Trypanosomiasis (HAT) or African sleeping sickness, which is caused by the protozoan parasite *Trypanosoma brucei* and is transmitted by the bite of the Tsetse fly. The WHO estimates that HAT constitutes a serious health risk to 60 million people in sub-Saharan Africa, 300,000-500,000 of whom become infected each year, with an estimated 10,000 fatalities. The related disease in cattle, Cattle Trypanosomiasis or Nagana, also represents a major health concern due to its devastating economic, social and nutritional impact on African families, estimated by the WHO as an annual economic loss of ~US$ 4 billion. As such, the total burden of Trypanosomiasis translates into 1,598,000 Disability-Adjusted Life Years, this is on a par with big killers such as *Mycobacterium tuberculosis* and Malaria [2, 3].

Treatment of HAT is dependent upon four drugs: suramin, melarsoprol, pentamidine and eflornithine.These therapies are often toxic, difficult to administer and increasingly have an acquired drug resistance [4, 5].Developed before the 1950s suramin and melarsoprol are used for chemotherapy of early stages of the disease, as is pentamidine. The arsenical melarsoprol is extremely toxic, with death for ~1 in 20 of cases and treatment failures as high as 30% in certain areas [4, 6]. Treatment of the second stage of the disease, where the parasites cross the blood-brain barrier and invade the central nervous system, is limited to melarsoprol and eflornithine [7].The WHO as a desperate measure recently introduced nifurtimox-eflornithine combination therapy for the treatment of HAT. This is despite nifurtimox, a drug often used to treat Chagas' disease (caused by the related protozoan the South American *Trypanosoma cruzi*), having low efficacy against HAT [8].

Hence there is an urgent need for new, more effective, less toxic, cheap and easy to administer therapeutic agents to treat African sleeping sickness and other closely related parasitic diseases, e.g. Chagas' disease and Leishmaniasis, whose current treatments suffer from similar limitations.

T. brucei is able to survive and multiply in the harsh environment of a mammalian hosts' bloodstream. This is due to the parasite's dense cell-surface coat of the glycosylphosphatidylinositol anchored variant surface glycoprotein (5 X 10^6 dimers/cell) [9-11], which protects the parasite in two ways. Firstly by acting as a diffusion barrier, such that complement is unable to reach and attack the plasma membrane of *T. brucei.* Secondly *T. brucei* is able to undergo antigenic variation, where by it is able to express a new variant surface glycoprotein from a repertoire of more than 1000 different genes, before the hosts' innate immune system is able to catch up [12, 13]. This antigenic variation is why a vaccine against this parasite is not a viable option as a therapy.

Phospholipids account for ~80% of total lipids in *T. brucei* with a significant proportion of these containing a choline-phosphate headgroup; phosphatidylcholine (PC) (~48%) and sphingomyelin (~15%) [14,15]. Sphingomyelin is made from PC via the sphingomyelin synthases transferring the choline-phosphate headgroup from PC to a ceramide lipid moiety [16]. These lipids contribute to the structural integrity of the membrane and in addition determine membrane fluidity and cell surface charge. Unsurprisingly, the biosynthesis and utilisation of these choline-containing molecules are implicated in a variety of cellular processes, including signaling, intracellular cellular protein sorting and transport [reviewed in 16]. Phosphocholine has been reported to be a required mitogen for DNA synthesis induced by growth factors [17]. Recently we have shown that the essential *T. brucei* neutral sphingomyelinase is actively involved in post Golgi sorting of the glycosylphosphatidylinositol anchored variant surface glycoprotein mentioned earlier [18].

Most eukaryotes have three alternative pathways by which PC can be synthesised [19 and reviewed in 20]. The first two pathways both involve three consecutive methylations of PE by S-adenosyl-L-methionemethyltransferases [20]. The PE can be derived from two alternative pathways, either from the concerted actions of the CDP-DAG dependantphosphatidylserine synthase and phosphatidylserine decarboxylase, or via the CDP-ethanolamine branch of the Kennedy pathway. This involves phosphorylation of ethanolamine by an ethanolamine kinase, its activation to CDP-ethanolamine by an ethanolamine-phosphate cytidyltransferase and its transfer to diacylglycerol by an ethanolamine phosphotransferase. The presence of this branch of the Kennedy pathway was demonstrated in *T. brucei* [22], however only recently have the constituent enzymes been characterized [23].

The trypanosomal genomes have revealed that *T. brucei* does not contain homologues for any methyltransferase(s) required to convert PE to PC [24] (neither does *T. cruzi*, but *Leishmania* do). *Plasmodium falciparum* have an alternative single plant-like S-adenosyl-L-methionemethyltransferase [25-27], responsible for phosphoethanolamine conversion to phosphocholine, however there are no trypanosomatid homologues. This rather surprising absence of PE to PC methylation has been confirmed by *in vivo* labellings by ourselves and others [15, 22, 28].

The third alternative pathway for *de novo* synthesis of PC, and the only pathway by which *T. brucei* can *de novo* synthesise PC, utilises the CDP-choline branch of the Kennedy pathway [19, 29-33]. This involves the phosphorylation of choline by a choline kinase, its activation to CDP-choline by a choline-phosphate cytidyltransferase and its transfer to diacylglycerol by a choline phosphotransferase. Biochemical characterisation of the two choline/ethanolamine kinases involved in the initial steps of the Kennedy pathway show that unusually amongst eukaryotes only one of the kinases is able to phosphorylate choline [23].

Collectively this evidence of an absence of redundancy of *de novo* PC synthesis in *T. brucei*, compared with other organisms (including humans), suggests *T. brucei* has a vulnerability to inhibition of their only way to synthesise PC, i.e. the Kennedy pathway. Recently we have exploited this fact by genetically validating the only *T. brucei* choline kinase (*Tb*CK) as a drug target both in culture and in an animal model [34]. Chemical intervention of the *Tb*CK enzyme activity is likely to interfere with the parasite's biology in multiple ways and *Tb*CK is therefore of interest as a target for novel chemotherapeutics.

In this study we interrogate ~630 compounds of the Maybridge Rule of 3 Fragment Library for compounds that interact with, and inhibit *Tb*CK.The Maybridge Rule of 3 Fragment Library is a small collection of quantifiable diverse [35, 36], pharmacophoric rich, chemical entities that comply with the following criteria; MW ≤ 300, cLogP ≤ 3, H-Bond Acceptors ≤ 3, H-Bond Donors ≤ 3, Rotatable bonds (Flexibility Index) ≤ 3, Polar Surface Area ≤ 60 Å^2 and aqueous solubility ≥ 1 mM using LogS and high purity (≥ 95%). Comparisons between two different screening methods, a coupled enzyme activity assay and differential scanning fluorimetry,has allowed identification of compounds that interact and inhibit the *T. brucei* choline kinase, several of which possess selective trypanocidal activity.

2. Experimental

2.1. Materials

All materials unless stated were purchased either from Sigma/Aldrich or Invitrogen. An in house Maybridge Rule of 3 Fragment Library kept in master plates at 200 mM in DMSO (100%), was transferred into working plates with compounds occupying the central 80 wells of a 96-well plate, at 10 mM in 5% DMSO, allowing the two outside columns for positive and negative controls.

2.2. Recombinant expression and purification of *Tb*CK

Large-scale recombinant expression and purification of *Tb*CK was conducted using the construct pET-15bTEV-*Tb*CK in BL21 Rosetta (DE3) cells as described previously [23], except the cells were grown in tryptone phosphate broth [37], harvested by centrifugation at 3500 g for 20 min at 4°C and affinity purified with either a HisTrap™ FF crude column (enzyme activity assay) or a HisTALON Cartridge (thermal shift analysis).

Briefly, pelleted cells were suspended in buffer A (50 mMTris/HCl, pH 8.0, 300 mMNaCl and 10 mM imidazole) and lysed in the presence of DNase I by sonication. The lysate was cleared by centrifugation at 35000 g for 30 min at 4°C and applied to a 1 ml HisTrap™ FF crude column column (GE Healthcare) pre-loaded with Ni^{2+}. Unbound proteins were removed by washing the column with 15 column volumes of buffer A containing 32.5 mM imidazole and *Tb*CK was eluted with 250 mM imidazole in the same buffer. Using a PD10 column, *Tb*CK was buffer exchanged into 50 mMTris/HCl, pH 8.0, 300 mMNaCl, glycerol (15% w/v) and stored at -80°C.

Alternatively, pelleted cells were suspended in 50 mMTris/HCl, pH 8.0, 300 mMNaCl and 5 mM imidazole and lysed by sonication. The lysate was cleared by centrifugation at 35000 g for 30 min at 4°C and applied to a 1 ml HisTALON Cartridge (Clontech).Unbound proteins were removed by washing the column with 10 column volumes of loading buffer, *Tb*CK was eluted with 15 mM imidazole and a final clearing wash of 250 mM imidazole in the same buffer. Using a PD10 column, *Tb*CK was buffer exchanged into 50 mM HEPES pH 8.0, 300 mMNaCl and 15% glycerol prior to storage at -80°C.

Typical yields were > 10 mg per litre of bacterial culture,*Tb*CK was stable and freeze thawing did not lead to any significant loss of activity.

2.3. *T. brucei* choline kinase activity assay

High throughput screening of the Maybridge Rule of 3 Fragment Library was carried out at a final test concentration of 0.5 mM in 96-well plates (final assay volume 200 µl) using a spectrophotometric assay that has been described previously [23]. The screened library working plates consisted of compounds arrayed in 96 well plates at 10 mM in 5% DMSO; columns 1 and 12 contained 5% DMSO only. For high throughput screening, 10 µl from each well of the working plates was added to 110 µl of buffer containing 50 mM MOPS (pH 7.8), 150 mMKCl and 6 mM $MgCl_2$. 3 µg of purified *Tb*CK was added to each well in 30 µl of the same buffer and the plates were mixed and incubated for 5 min at room temperature. A further 30 µl of buffer containing PEP (1 mM final), ATP (0.5 mM final), NADH (0.5 mM final) and pyruvate kinase and lactate dehydrogenase(PK/LDH) (5 units/ml final) was added, and the reaction was started by addition of 30 µl choline (0.5 mM final) to rows 1-11, 30 µl buffer alone was added to row 12 (negative control) and this was used as an intra-plate control (background rate) in conjunction with row 1 (maximal rate). Following mixing the change in absorbance at 341 nm was monitored for 10 min at room temperature. For testing inhibition of the coupling enzymes (PK/LDH), standard buffer conditions were used but the assay contained 1 mM PEP, 0.1 mM ADP and 0.5 mM NADH. The PK/LDH was titrated to give a change in absorbance of approximately 0.05 absorbance units/min in the absence of inhibitor.

2.4. Differential scanning fluorimetry with *Tb*CK

Differential scanning fluorimetry was set up in 96 well PCR plates using a reaction volume of 100 μL. Samples contained 2.1 μM *Tb*CK, 6 mM $MgCl_2$, 50 mM HEPES pH 8.0, 80 mMNaCl, 5.25% glycerol (v/v) and 1.4 x Sypro Orange (Invitrogen), Maybridge Ro3 compounds were screened at 1 mM concentration with a final DMSO concentration of 0.5% (v/v).Two controls with eight repetitions per plate were used for the thermal shift experiments: 0.5% DMSO; 0.5 mM ATP, 0.5% DMSO.

Differential fluorimetric scans were performed in a realtime PCR machine (Stratagene Mx3005P with software MxPro v 4.01) using a temperature scan from 25°C to 95°C at 0.5°C min^{-1}.Data were then exported to Excel for analysis using "DSF analysis" modified from the template provided by Niesen et al. [38].T_m values were calculated by non-linear regression, fitting the Boltzmann equation to the denaturation curves using GraFit. *Tb*CK T_m, in the presence of 6 mM $MgCl_2$ and 0.5% DMSO, 41.21 ± 0.03°C (n > 60), T_m for *Tb*CK and 0.5 mM ATP = 44.46 ± 0.05°C (n > 60).

3. Results and discussion

Screening for inhibitors of the genetically validated drug target *Tb*CK is problematic due to the difficulty in following the reaction either continuously or directly. A direct choline kinase activity assay assessing the production of phosphocholine, utilising a modified method of Kim *et. al.* [39], using *Tb*CK and radiolabelled choline has been performed previously [23]. However this is not suitable for screening purposes, so choline kinase activity was measured by a spectrophotometric coupled assay (Figure 1). This coupled enzyme assay utilises regeneration of ATP from the ADP by-product of the choline kinase by pyruvate kinase, and subsequent oxidation of NADH as the resulting pyruvate is converted to lactate, by lactate dehydrogenase. This assay using coupled enzymes is also problematic, as a compound could potentially inhibit the coupled enzymes giving rise to a false positive.

An alternative approach for screening is differential scanning fluorimetry (Figure 2), allowing identification of compounds that interact with the *Tb*CK protein, either to stabilise or destabilise it, therefore influencing the protein's T_m (melting point) [38-40].

Initially *Tb*CK was subjected to differential scanning fluorimetry to ascertain if this approach was possible. Known components required for enzyme activity were tested to see if thermal shifts were observed.In the presence of 6 mM $MgCl_2$, a T_m of 41.2°C was obtained (Figure 1C, solid dark line). The addition of 0.5 mM ATP resulted in a > 3°C T_m shift for *Tb*CK(Figure 1C, dashed-line). These encouraging results showed *Tb*CK was amenable to differential scanning fluorimetry and allowed validation of this screening method.It is worth noting the surprising low T_m of *Tb*CK, considering that these parasites live within the bloodstream of a mammalian host, i.e. 37°C, or higher with a fever. However, the presence of physiological

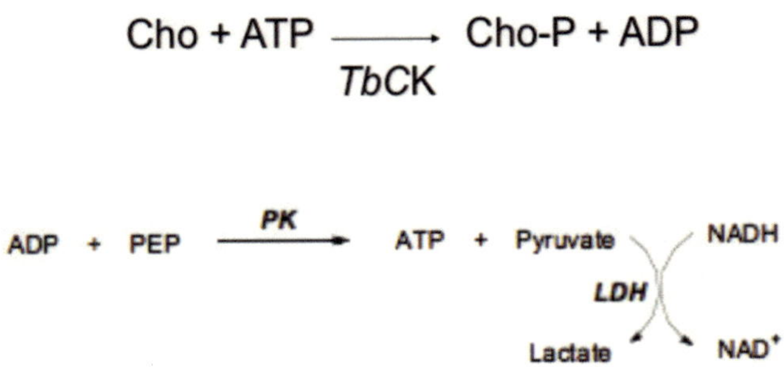

Figure 1. Schematic of the *Tb*CK reaction and coupled assay.

T. brucei choline kinase (*Tb*CK) catalyses the ATP dependent phosphorylation of choline, the ADP is converted back to ATP by pyruvate kinase (PK), which converts phosphoenolpyruvate (PEP) to pyruvate in the process. The resulting pyruvate is reduced to lactate by the NADH dependent lactate dehydrogenase (LDH). The resulting conversion of NADH to NAD^+ is monitored, by measuring the reduction in absorbance at 341 nM.

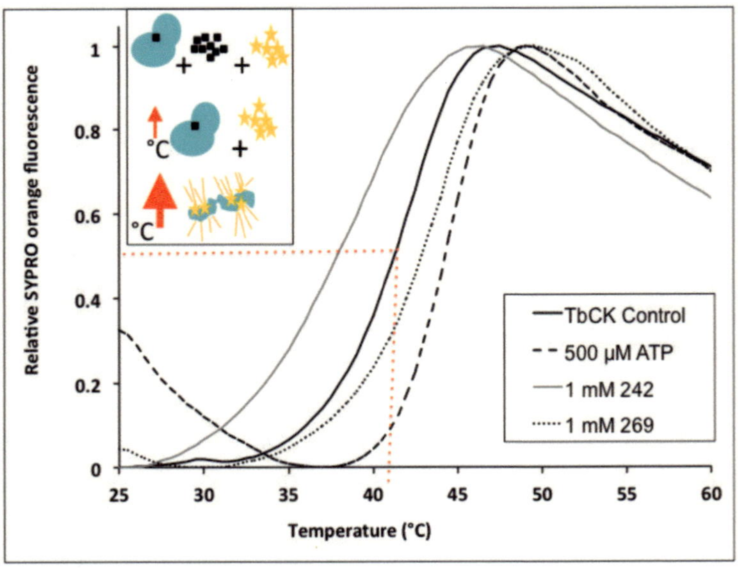

Figure 2. Thermal shift assay; typical differential fluorimetry scans of TbCK.

Differential fluorimetric scans were performed and analysed as described in Experimental. *Tb*CK + DMSO (control) solid dark line, *Tb*CK + 0.5 μM ATP (positive control) dashed line, *Tb*CK + 1 mM compound 242, solid light line, *Tb*CK + 1 mM compound 269, dotted line.T_m of *Tb*CK in the presence of 0.5%DMSO is 41.21 ± 0.03°C (control); T_m of *Tb*CK and 0.5 mM ATP is 44.46 ± 0.05°C (positive control). Insert: schematic representation of the thermal shift assay.A protein will unfold exposing hydrophobic domains as it is denatured due to the increasing temperature. Dyes such as sypro orange (star) are able to bind to these exposed hydrophobic areas giving rise to fluorescence. A plot of this increased fluorescence versus temperature allows determination of T_m (melting point) of the protein. If a compound (squares) is able to interact with the protein it may alter the protein's T_m and thus a library of compounds can be screened to see if they stabilise (increase in T_m) or destabilise (decrease in T_m) the target protein.

An alternative approach for screening is differential scanning fluorimetry (Figure 2), allowing identification of compounds that interact with the *Tb*CK protein, either to stabilise or destabilise it, therefore influencing the protein's T_m (melting point) [38-40].

Initially *Tb*CK was subjected to differential scanning fluorimetry to ascertain if this approach was possible. Known components required for enzyme activity were tested to see if thermal shifts were observed. In the presence of 6 mM $MgCl_2$, a T_m of 41.2°C was obtained (Figure 1C, solid dark line). The addition of 0.5 mM ATP resulted in a > 3°C T_m shift for *Tb*CK(Figure 1C, dashed-line). These encouraging results showed *Tb*CK was amenable to differential scanning fluorimetry and allowed validation of this screening method.It is worth noting the surprising low T_m of *Tb*CK, considering that these parasites live within the bloodstream of a mammalian host, i.e. 37°C, or higher with a fever. However, the presence of physiological relevant levels of ATP does stabilize *Tb*CK by > 3 °C, which may prolong the half-life of the protein in the parasite.

The respective controls in both assay types allowed Z-factors to be determined for all of the plates screened (Figure 3). Both the coupled enzyme activity assay and the thermal shift analysis showed Z-factors to be above 0.5 for all plates, except for plate 5 for the thermal shift assay (but still above 0.45), this is indicative of good reliable assays, with meaningful results [41].

The MayBridge Rule of 3 Fragment Library was distributed over 9 plates (80 compounds per plate) providing space for adequate positive and negative controls, allowing Z-factors to be determined. This was done for each plate for both the choline kinase assay (+) and thermal shift analysis (x). A Z-factor above 0.4 is acceptable and validates the data on that plate as being reliable.

The ~630 compounds from the MayBridge Rule of 3 Fragment Library were assessed for their ability to inhibit the *Tb*CK coupled enzyme activity assay at a single concentration of 0.5 mM (Figure 4A). At this relative high concentration only 9 of the compounds (1.4%) showed > 70% inhibition. These primary hits were retested in triplicate at 0.5 mM (Table 1), 2 of the 9 (compounds 320 and 635) were confirmed as being false positives, while the remaining 7 were confirmed to show good inhibition (80-100%) against the *Tb*CK coupled enzyme activity assay. These 7 compounds were then tested against just the coupled enzymes, some inhibition was observed for some of the compounds, but this was insufficient to account for the strong inhibition against the *Tb*CK, thus these 7 compounds were believed to show true *Tb*CK inhibition.

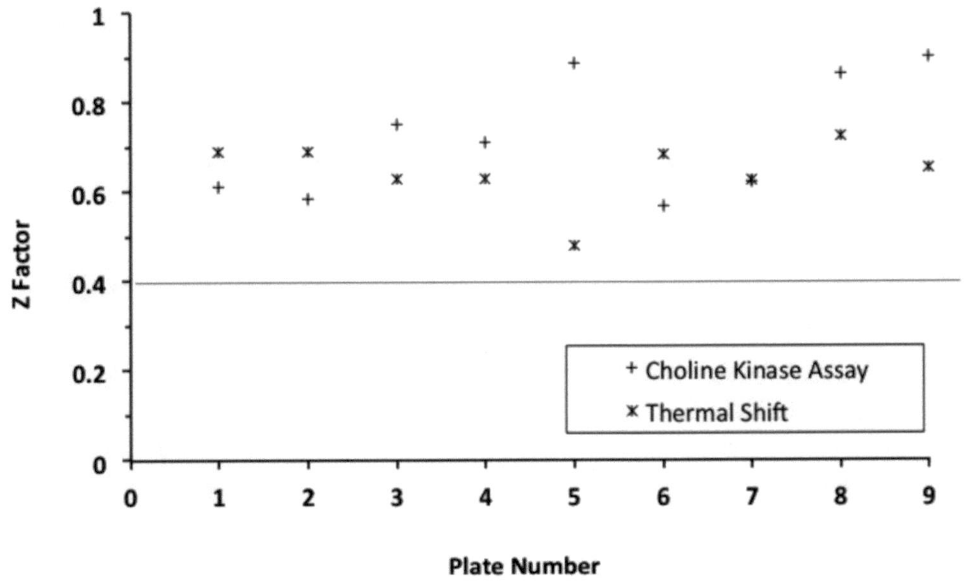

Figure 3. Quality control (Z factors) for the *Tb*CK thermal shift analysis and coupled enzyme activity assay.

It is worth noting the lack of false positives arising from significant inhibition of either of the coupling enzymes, pyruvate kinase and lactate dehydrogenase this is encouraging when screening other ATP utilizing enzymes.

Thermal shift analysis of *Tb*CK with the ~630 compounds from the MayBridge Rule of 3 Fragment Library showed that the vast majority of compounds had little or no affect on the T_m of *Tb*CK (Figure 4B). Relatively few compounds showed an increase in T_m (stabilisation), and only a handful of these showing an increase in T_m> 1°C, i.e. compound 269 (Figure 2, dotted line), this was rather surprising given that ATP stabilises *Tb*CK by > 3°C. Significantly more compounds showed a destabilisation affect, with 3 compounds having > 10°C decrease in the Tm, i.e. compound 242 (Figure 2, solid light line). Most of the compounds observed in this screen that show significant destabilisation of *Tb*CK, do not cause similar destabilisation affects with other enzymes that we have screened in a similar manner, the only exceptions are compounds 68 (2-aminothiophene-3-carbonitrile) and 565 (4-(2-amino-1,3-thiazol-4-yl)phenol) (Table 1).

Several drug discovery style studies have shown that an increase in the thermal stability of a protein is proportional to the concentration and affinity of the ligand to the protein in keeping with the equilibrium associated with ligand-protein binding [38, 41-44]. On those occasions where this interaction destabilizes a protein, i.e. lowering T_m, a thermodynamic model has been proposed which explains the how the same ligand can stabilise and destabilise different proteins [42]. While the same protein may be stabilized and destabilized by very similar ligands, this was exquisitely demonstrated by the changes in thermal stability of Acyl-CoA thioesterase, upon incubation with either CoA (destabilise) or Acyl-CoA (stabilise) [45].

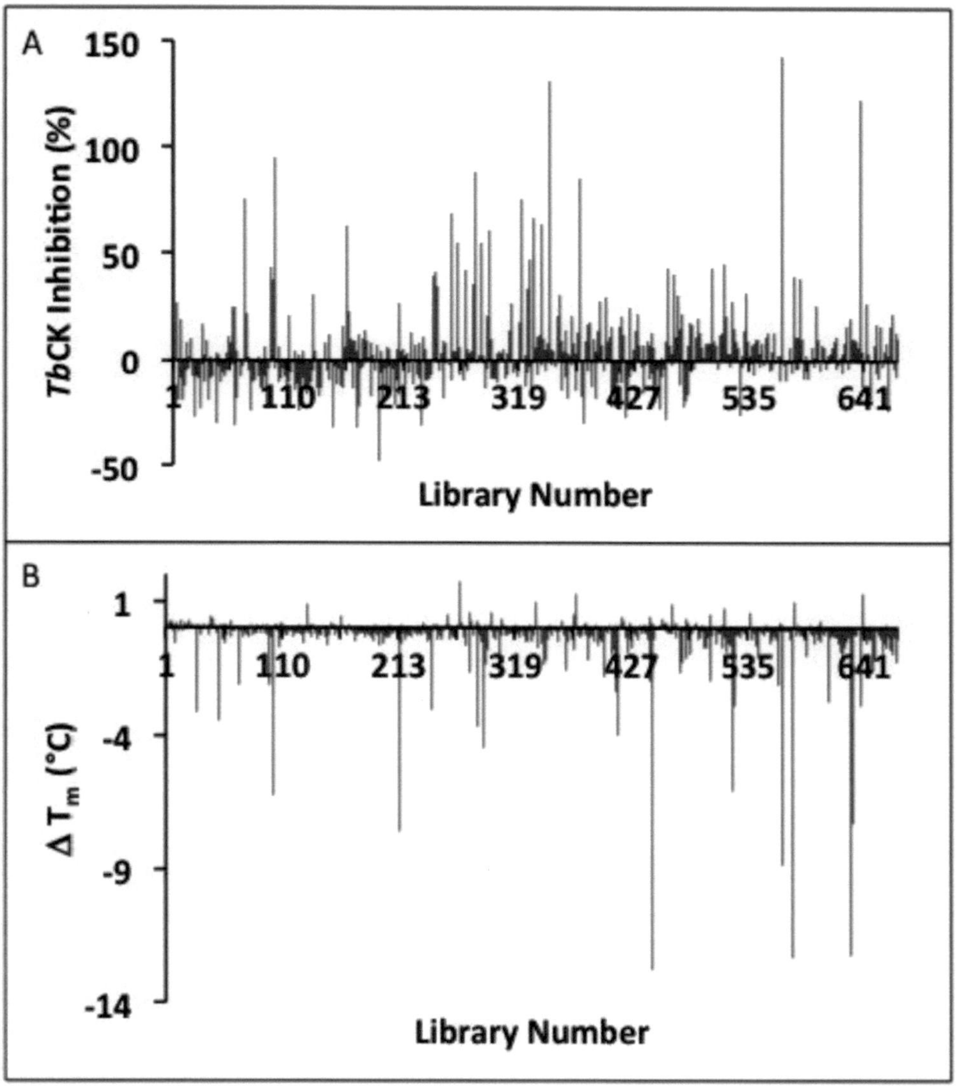

Figure 4. A) Percentage inhibition of *Tb*CK enzyme activity assay for each of the compounds tested. B) Observed thermal shifts of *Tb*CK for each of the compounds tested

Library number[a]	CAS number[b]	Molecular Structure	Compound Name	*Tb*CK activity % inhibition at 500µM Mean ± SD (*n*=3)	*TbCK IC50 (υM)*	PK/LDH % inhibition at 500 υM mean (n=2)	*TbCK* T_m*Shift*[c]	*T. brucei % survival*[d]
68	4651-82-5	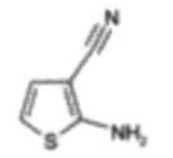	2-aminothiophene-3-carbonitrile	101 ± 3	~758	40	-2.15 ± 0.08	10.3 ± 11
95	933-67-5	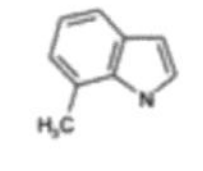	7-methyl-1H-indole	84 ± 4	~380	49	-2.16 ± 0.14	4.1 ± 5.2
257	59147-02-3	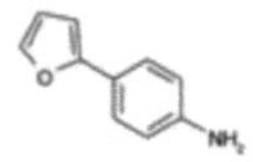	4-(2-furyl)aniline	80 ± 3	~234	63	0.46 ± 0.08	9.3 ± 8.5
278	199590-00-6	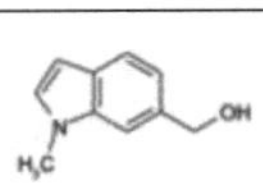	(1-methyl-1H-indol-6-yl)methanol	101 ± 2	25.45 ±1.16	28	0.26 ± 0.09	8.8 ± 10.8
320	39270-39-8	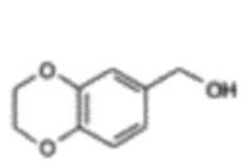	2,3-dihydro-1,4-benzodioxin-6-ylmethanol	6 ± 4	ND	ND	-0.17 ± 0.07	63.1 ±9.5
346	57976-57-5	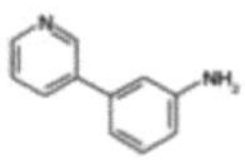	3-pyridin-3-ylaniline	100 ± 0	12.35 ± 0.64	68	-1.18 ± 0.06	15.6 ±9.3
372	143426-51-1	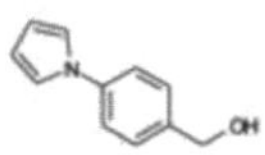	[4-(1H-pyrrol-1-yl) phenyl] methanol	80 ± 1	109.7 ± 10.6	26	1.24 ± 0.04	27 ± 14
565	57634-55-6	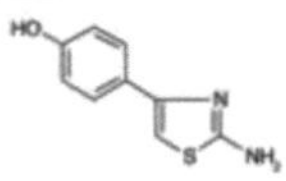	4-(2-amino-1,3-thiazol-4-yl)phenol	100 ± 0	~120	85	-8.91 ± 0.49	28.7±19.3
635	64354-50-3	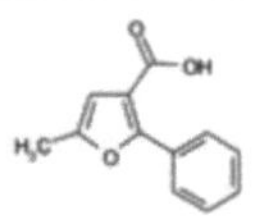	5-methyl-2-phenyl-3-furoic acid	23 ± 4	ND	ND	-2.94 ± 0.16	20.5 ± 7.4

[a] Arbitrary library number

[b] CAS numbers are unique identifiers assigned by the "Chemical Abstracts Service" to describe every chemical described in open access scientific literature.

[c] Tm shift in °C, observed for TbCK in the presence of compound (1mM), value is mean ± SD from the Boltzman curve fitting, see Experimental for details.

[d] Cytotoxicity studies, see Major and Smith 2011 for details, values are percentage of controls in the absence of compound, either mean ± SD (n=3) or mean ± SE (n=2), the latter being in bold.

Table 1. The compounds from the Maybridge Rule of 3 library that show >70% inhibition of TbCK.

All of the compounds in the two data sets (the coupled enzyme activity assay and the thermal shift analysis), were compared to assess any correlation between the two very different methods. In other words looking for compounds that showed a significant change in T_m and a significant inhibition in *Tb*CK enzyme activity (Figure 5A). The vast majority of compounds showed little or no inhibition and little or no shift in T_m. Compounds showing < 40% inhibition of the enzyme activity were removed for clarification (Figure 5B), this highlighted that the majority of compounds that show *Tb*CK enzyme inhibition do not significantly alter the T_m of *Tb*CK. The exceptions are compound 565 with a decrease in T_m~9°C, and compound 68 and 95 with a decrease in T_m~2°C respectively, all show complete inhibition at 0.5 mM (Table 1). Twenty-one compounds showed > 40% enzyme inhibition, 9 of these (43%) displayed > 1°C change in *Tb*CK T_m. This is a substantial enrichment compared to the 7% of compounds with T_m shifts > 1°C observed for the entire library.

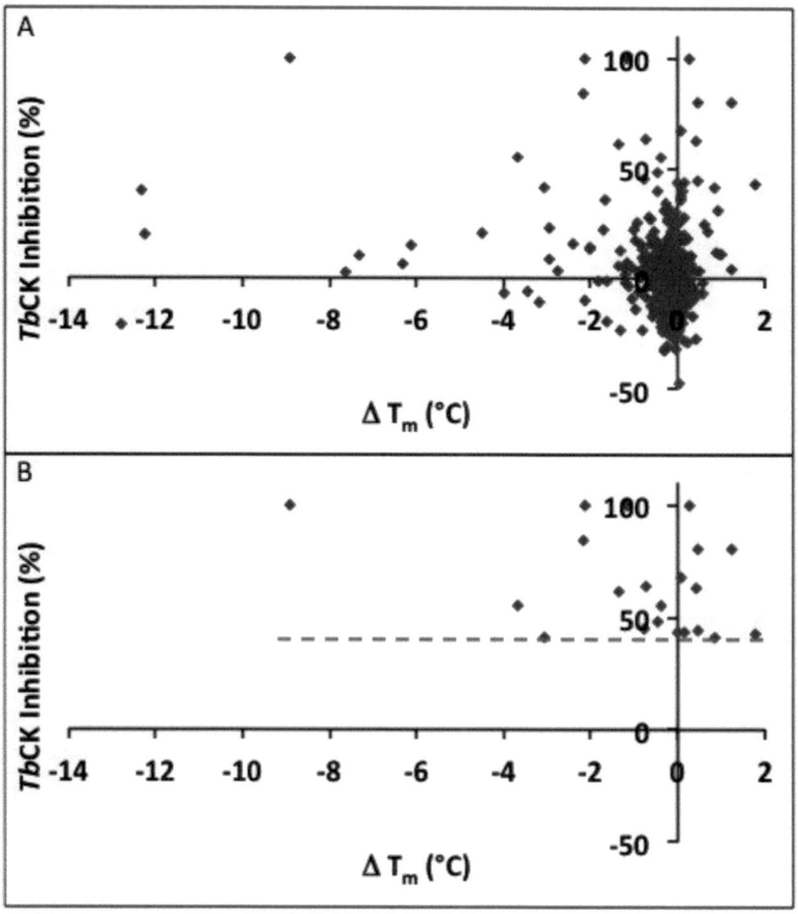

Figure 5. Scatter graph representation showing the correlation between the observed thermal shifts and percentage inhibition of *Tb*CK enzyme activity. A) All of the compounds from the MayBridge Rule of 3 Fragment Library tested. B) For those compounds with > 40% (dotted line) inhibition of *Tb*CK enzyme activity.

Of the compounds identified that alter the T_m of *Tb*CK by > 1°C, ~20% of them inhibit *Tb*CK enzyme activity by > 40%. This suggests that for *Tb*CK thermal shift analysis has allowed significant enrichment, but not total capture of the potential inhibitors of *Tb*CK. However, if a direct assay for a potential drug target was very problematic, prior thermal shift analysis could significantly streamline the number of compounds to be screened, thereby increasing the potential to identify lead compounds. Thermal shift analysis has the disadvantage that good inhibitors could be missed if they do not significantly alter the T_m of the protein.

This raises an interesting question, is it a viable option to target compounds that specifically destabilise an enzyme, causing a decrease in enzyme activity? One could argue this is exactly what pharmaceutical companies are focusing their research efforts upon, but with a slightly different approach. Some of their therapeutic targets rely on finding compounds that disrupt various interactions; hetero- or homo-oligomeric protein-protein, DNA-binding protein and RNA polymerases, many of these are associated with signaling events. Success stories include the identification of HDM2 antagonists associated with P53 activation [46], the identification of anti-cancer agent for the BCL-X_L protein-protein complex and several others, reviewed by Wells and McClendon [47] and more recently by Coyne and colleagues [48].

The techniques utilized to study the formation / disruption of protein-protein complexes are driven by high throughput drug discovery, including fragment based approaches, these include X-ray crystallography, NMR, dynamic light scattering, differential static light scattering, differential scanning fluorimetry [42-50].

In summary, destabilisation by a ligand could affect the oligomeric state of a protein, or in the case of a monomer disrupt intra-molecular interactions, i.e. between stacking α-helixes or β-sheets, causing partial unfolding and thus destabilisation.In the case of *Tb*CK, which we know exists as a dimer, one of several potential mechanisms of destabilisation could be disruption of the dimer interface, whereby a ligand is able to bind to freshly exposed hydrophobic surfaces on the protein, and this interaction allows further destabilisation of the monomer structure.

As it was clear that compounds that inhibit *Tb*CK enzyme activity do not necessarily show a significant increase or decrease in T_m, it was decided to compare inhibition of *Tb*CK enzyme activity with previously determined trypanocidal activities for the compounds [51]. From this comparison (Figure 6) a group of compounds above a threshold of > 70% inhibition of *Tb*CK showed significant trypanocidal activity (circled), suggesting a direct correlation.

Compounds from the May Bridge Rule of 3 Fragment Library with greater than 70% inhibition (dotted line) of the TbCK enzyme activity are circled and numbered. Numbers correspond to arbitrary compound library numbers; see Table 1 for chemical structures and extra data. *T. brucei* survival data was previously determined [51].

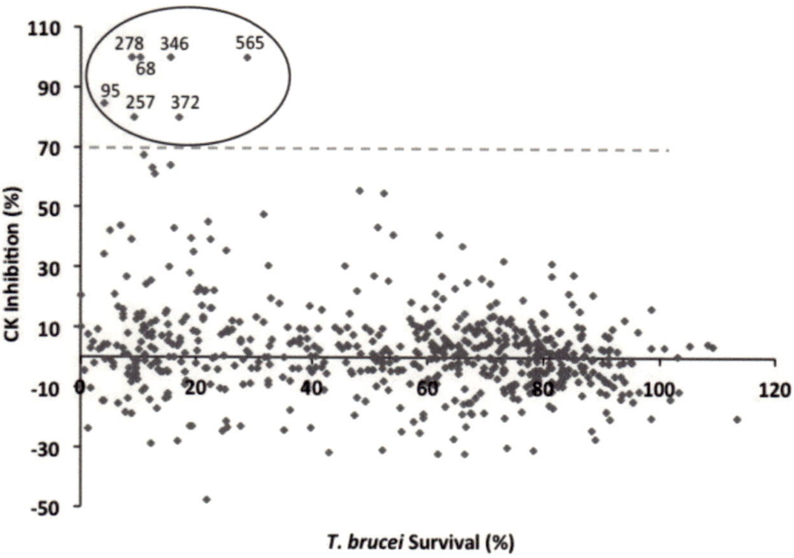

Figure 6. Correlation of the percentage inhibition of *Tb*CK enzyme activity assay and *T. brucei* survival.

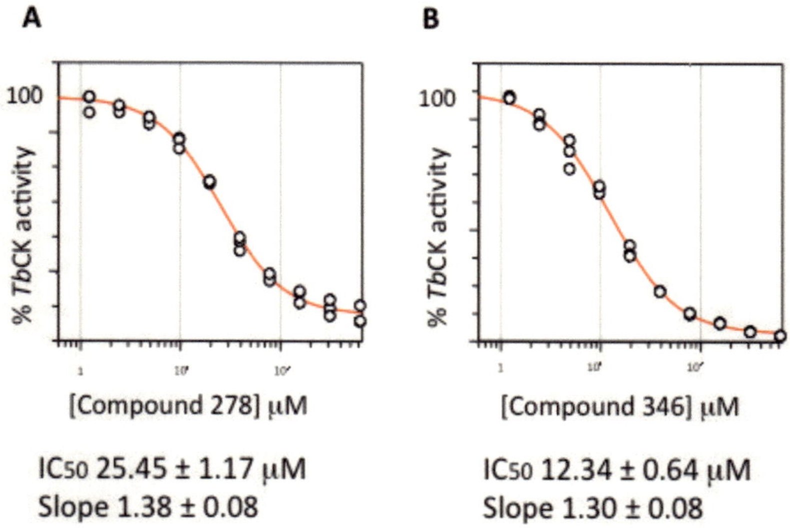

Figure 7. IC50 curves of the promising compounds (278 and 346) that show significant TbCK inhibition.

IC50 values were determined for these compounds (Table 1, Figure 7) ranging from 100s of μM to low μM. For example, compound 278 (1-methyl-(1H-indol-6-yl)methanol) has an IC50 value of 25.45 ± 1.16 μM however the selectivity index is not very good, while compound 346 (3-pyridin-3-ylaniline) has an IC50 value of 12.35 ± 0.64 μM with a high selectivity index.

One of the strengths of the Maybridge Rule of 3 Fragment Library is the chemical diversity, additionally a range of analogous structures can normally be found within it allowing initial structure activity relationships to be formulated. There are several close analogues of compound 278 (1-methyl-(1H-indol-6-yl)methanol), which highlight that the N-methyl indole moiety seems necessary to have any *Tb*CK inhibition and the methanol portion of the molecule can not be replaced by a carboxylic acid. Investigation of the CHEMBL database for similar compounds identified 1-Methyl-1H-pyrrolo[2,3-c]pyridine (CHEMBL594467) which was screened as one of a library of tricyclic and bicyclic analogues of indoloquinoline alkaloids against a variety of protozoan parasites. The analogue mentioned here showed weak trypanocidal activity (624 μM) against *Trypanosoma brucei rhodesiense*, but significantly better (37 μM) against *Plasmodium falciparum* [52].

Another analogue, 1-Methyl-1H-indole (CHEMBL19912) has been shown to interact with human intracellular adhesion molecules and highlights the importance of selectivity [53]. 1H-indol-5-yl-methanol (CHEMBL1650258) has previously been screened against *Leishmania* as a potential PTR1 inhibitor but was shown to be inactive at 500 μM [54]

For the relatively simple compound 346 (3-pyridin-3-ylaniline), there are several analogous structures in the library, including compound 262 (2-(1H-imidazo-1-yl)aniline) which shows ~55% *Tb*CK enzyme inhibition and is trypanocidal. Compound 347 (4-pyridin-3-ylaniline) is a structural isomer of 346 but shows no *Tb*CK enzyme inhibition and is not trypanocidal. The only related structure in the CHEMBL database was 3-(pyridin-3-yl)benzenaminium (CHEMBL1778131) which was shown to be a weakinhibitor of metallo-β–lactamase IMP-1 [55].

4. Conclusions

In this study, screening of a comparatively small fragment library by two different screening methods has allowed identification of several compounds that interact with and inhibit *Tb*CK, a genetically validated drug target against African sleeping sickness. Some of the inhibitory fragments were also selectively trypanocidal, considering these are relatively simple molecules with no optimization, finding low μM inhibitors is very encouraging. Moreover some of the morphological phenotypes of these trypanocidal compounds include cell-cycle arrests similar to those observed for the *Tb*CK conditional knockout grown under permissive conditions.

This study highlights that if faced with a drug target that is problematic to screen, prior thermal shift analysis could significantly triage the number of compounds to be screened, thereby significantly increasing the potential to identify lead compounds. This approach obviously has the limitation that potential inhibitors could be missed if they do not significantly alter the T_m of the protein.

Future follow up work with *Tb*CK will include expanding the structure activity relationship of our most promising hits identified by this study. Their trypanocidal mode of action will be investigated by undertaking various *in vivo* biochemical phenotyping experiments to ascertain if they are inhibiting *Tb*CK, thus causing a lack of *de novo* PC synthesis, known to be essential for the parasite.

The ultimate goal is to identify new easy to make, affordable, easy to administer, drugs in the fight against African sleeping sickness and other closely related protozoan transmitted Third World diseases.

Acknowledgements

This work was supported in part by a Wellcome Trust Senior Research Fellowship (067441) and Wellcome Trust project grants 086658 and 093228. We thank the late and sorely missed Dr Rupert Russell (St Andrews), supported by SUSLA, for access to the May Bridge Rule of 3 Fragment Library.

Author details

Louise L. Major, Helen Denton and Terry K. Smith

Biomedical Sciences Research Centre, The North Haugh, The University, St. Andrews, Fife, Scotland, U.K.

References

[1] WHO web site: http://www.who.int/topics/trypanosomiasis_african/en/

[2] Steverding, D. Parasites & vectors 2010, 3, 15.

[3] Priotto, G.; Kasparian, S.; Mutombo, W.; Ngouama, D.; Ghorashian, S.; Arnold, U.; Ghabri, S.; Baudin, E.; Buard, V.; Kazadi-Kyanza, S.; Ilunga, M.; Mutangala, W.; Pohlig, G.; Schmid, C.; Karunakara, U.; Torreele, E.; Kande, V. Lancet 2009, 374, 56.

[4] Delespaux, V.; de Koning, H. P. Drug resistance updates : reviews and commentaries in antimicrobial and anticancer chemotherapy 2007, 10, 30.

[5] Baker, N.; Alsford, S.; Horn, D. MolBiochemParasit 2011, 176, 55.

[6] Bouteille, B., O. Oukem, S. Bisser, and M. Dumas. 2003. Treatment perspectives for human African trypanosomiasis. Fundam. Clin. Pharmacol. 17:171

[7] Priotto, G., C. Fogg, M. Balasegaram, O. Erphas, A. Louga, F. Checchi, S. Ghabri, and P. Piola. 2006. Three drug combinations for late-stage *Trypanosoma brucei gambiense* sleeping sickness: a randomized clinical trial in Uganda. PLoSClin. Trials 1:e39

[8] Priotto, G., S. Kasparian, W. Mutombo, D. Ngouama, S. Ghorashian, U. Arnold, S. Ghabri, E. Baudin, V. Buard, S. Kazadi-Kyanza, M. Ilunga, W. Mutangala, G. Pohlig, C. Schmid, U. Karunakara, E. Torreele, and V. Kande. 2009. Nifurtimox-eflornithine combination therapy for second-stage African *Trypanosoma brucei gambiense* trypanosomiasis: a multicentre, randomised, phase III, non-inferiority trial. Lancet 374:56-64

[9] M. A. Ferguson; G. A. Cross Myristylation of the membrane form of a *Trypanosoma brucei* variant surface glycoprotein. J. Biol. Chem. 1984, 259, 3011-3015.

[10] M. A. Ferguson; M. G. Low; G.A. Cross Glycosyl-sn-1,2-dimyristylphosphatidylinositol is covalently linked to *Trypanosoma brucei* variant surface glycoprotein. J. Biol. Chem. 1985, 260, 14547-14555.

[11] Ferguson, M.A.J., Brimacombe, J.S., Brown, J.R., Crossman, A., Dix, A., Field, R.A., Guther, M.L.S., Milne, K.G., Sharma, D.K. and Smith, T.K., (1999). The GPI biosynthetic pathway as a therapeutic target for African sleeping sickness. Biochim. Biophys. Acta 1455, 327-340.

[12] G. A. M. Cross Antigenic variation in trypanosomes: Secrets surface slowly. BioEssays 1996, 18, 283-287.

[13] N. Aitcheson; S. Talbot; J. Shapiro; K. Hughes; C. Adkin; T. Butt; K. Sheader; G. Rudenko VSG switching in *Trypanosoma brucei*: antigenic variation analysed using RNAi in the absence of immune selection. MolMicrobiol. 2005, 57, 1608-1622.

[14] Smith, T.K, &Bütikofer, P. (2010) Phospholipid biosynthesis in Trypansomabrucei. Mol Bio Para 172:66-79.

[15] Richmond, G.S,Gibellini, F., Young, S.A., Major, L., Denton, H. Lilley, A. and Smith T.K (2010) Lipidomic Analysis of bloodstream and procyclic form *Trypanosoma brucei* Parasitology 137 (9) l: 1357-1392.

[16] Young SA, Mina JG, Denny PW, Smith TK.(2012) Sphingolipid and ceramide homeostasis, potential therapeutic targets Biochem Res Int. 2012;2012:248135.

[17] Li, Z. and Vance, D.E. (2008) Phosphatidylcholine and choline homeostatis J Lipid Res. 49: 1187-1194.

[18] Young, S.A & Smith, T.K, (2010) The essential neutral sphingomyelinase is involved in the trafficking of the variant surface glycoprotein in the bloodstream form of *Trypanosoma brucei*. Molecular Microbiology 76(6): 1461-1482.

[19] Kennedy E.P., and Weiss, S.B. (1956) The function of cytidine coenzymes in the biosynthesis of phospholipids. J. Biol. Chem. 222:193-214

[20] Gibellini, F & Smith T.K (2010) Critical Review on the Kennedy Pathway for IUBMB Life 62: 414-428.

[21] Kanipes, M.I. and S.A. Henry, 1997 The phospholipid methyltransferases in yeast. BiochimBiophysActa. 1348(1-2): p. 134-41.

[22] Rifkin, M.R., C.A. Strobos, and A.H. Fairlamb, 1995 Specificity of ethanolamine transport and its further metabolism in *Trypanosoma brucei*. J Biol Chem. 270(27): p. 16160-6.

[23] Gibellini. F., Hunter W. N. & Smith, T.K, (2008) Biochemical characterisation of the initial steps of the Kennedy pathway in *Trypanosoma brucei*- the ethanolamine and choline kinases BJ 415 135-144.

[24] Choi, J.Y., W.E. Martin, R.C. Murphy, and D.R. Voelker, 2004 Phosphatidylcholine and N-methylated phospholipids are nonessential in Saccharomyces cerevisiae. J Biol Chem. 279(40): p. 42321-30.

[25] Pessi, G., J.Y. Choi, J.M. Reynolds, D.R. Voelker, and C.B. Mamoun, 2005 In vivo evidence for the specificity of Plasmodium falciparum phosphoethanolamine methyltransferase and its coupling to the Kennedy pathway. J Biol Chem. 280(13): p. 12461-6.

[26] Pessi, G., G. Kociubinski, and C.B. Mamoun, 2004 A pathway for phosphatidylcholine biosynthesis in Plasmodium falciparum involving phosphoethanolamine methylation. ProcNatlAcadSci U S A. 101(16): p. 6206-11.

[27] Witola, W.H., G. Pessi, K. El Bissati, J.M. Reynolds, and C.B. Mamoun, 2006 Localization of the phosphoethanolaminemethyltransferase of the human malaria parasite Plasmodium falciparum to the Golgi apparatus. J Biol Chem. 281(30): p. 21305-11.

[28] Cornell, RB and Northwood, I.C. (2000) Regulation of CTP:phosphocholinecytidyltransferase by amphitropism and relocalization. TIBS 25 441-447

[29] Jackowski, S. and P. Fagone, 2005 CTP: Phosphocholine cytidylyltransferase: paving the way from gene to membrane. J Biol Chem. 280(2): p. 853-6.

[30] Kent, C., 1997 CTP:phosphocholinecytidylyltransferase. BiochimBiophysActa. 1348(1-2): p. 79-90.

[31] Weinhold, P.A. and D.A. Feldman, 1992 Choline-phosphate cytidylyltransferase. Methods Enzymol. 209: p. 248-58.

[32] McMaster, C.R. and R.M. Bell, 1997 CDP-choline:1,2-diacylglycerol cholinephosphotransferase. BiochimBiophysActa. 1348(1-2): p. 100-10.

[33] Carman, G.M.andZeimetz, G.M (1996) Regulation of phospholipid biosynthesis in the yeast Saccharomyces cerevisiae. J. Biol. Chem. 271, 13293-13296.

[34] Simon Young, Federica Gibellini, Keith R. Mathews, William N. Hunter & Terry K. Smith (2012) In the mammalian bloodstream, *Trypanosoma brucei* is totally dependent upon its only choline kinase for survival. Pending submission.

[35] R. A. E. Carr, M. Congreve, C. W. Murray, and D. C. Rees, "Fragment-based lead discovery: leads by design," DrugDiscovery Today, vol. 10, no. 14, pp. 987–992, 2005.

[36] www.maybridge.com/images/pdfs/ro3frag.pdf

[37] J.T. Moore, A. Uppal, F. Maley, G.F. Maley (1993) Overcoming Inclusion Body Formation in a High-Level Expression System. Protein Expression and Purification, 4: 160-163

[38] Niesen, F. H., Berglund, H. and Vedadi, M. (2007) The use of differential scanning fluorimetry to detect ligand interactions that promote protein stability. Nature Protocols, 2, 2212-2221.

[39] Kim, K., Kim, K.H., Storey, M.K., Voelker, D.R. and Carman, G.M. (1999) Isolation and characterization of the *Saccharomyces cerevisiae* EKI1 gene encoding ethanolamine kinase. *JBiolChem* 274: 14857-14866

[40] M. C. Lo, A. Aulabaugh, G. Jin et al., "Evaluation of fluorescence-based thermal shift assays for hit identification in drug discovery," Analytical Biochemistry, vol. 332, no. 1, pp. 153–159, 2004.

[41] Zhang, J,H., Chang, T.D. and Oldenberg, K.R. A simple statistical parameters for use in evaluation and validation of high throughput screening assays 1999 J Biomol Screen 4: 67-73.

[42] Kopen, J. And Schneider, G. Comparison of fluorescence and light scattering based methods to assess formation and stability of protein-protein complexes 2011 J Structural Biology 175: 211-223.

[43] Pantoliano MW, Petrella EC, Kwasnoski JD, Lobanov VS, Myslik J, Graf E, Carver T, Asel E, Springer BA, Lane P, Salemme FR. High-density miniaturized thermal shift assays as a general strategy for drug discovery. J Biomol Screen. 2001 Dec;6(6):429-40.

[44] PiotrasCimmperman, LinaBaranauskienė, SimonaJachimovičiūtė, JelenaJachno, JolantaTorresan, VilmaMichailovienė, JurgitaMatulienė, JolantaSereikaitė, VladasBumelis, DaumantasMatulis

A Quantitative Model of Thermal Stabilization and Destabilization of Proteins by Ligands Biophysical Journal 2008 (Vol. 95, Issue 7, pp. 3222-3231)

[45] Marfori M, Kobe B, Forwood JK. Ligand-induced conformational changes within a hexameric Acyl-CoA thioesterase. J Biol Chem. 2011 Oct 14 ;286(41):35643-9

[46] Grasberger BL, Lu T, Schubert C, Parks DJ, Carver TE, Koblish HK, Cummings MD, LaFrance LV, Milkiewicz KL, Calvo RR, Maguire D, Lattanze J, Franks CF, Zhao S, Ramachandren K, Bylebyl GR, Zhang M, Manthey CL, Petrella EC, Pantoliano MW, Deckman IC, Spurlino JC, Maroney AC, Tomczuk BE, Molloy CJ, Bone RF Discovery and cocrystal structure of benzodiazepinedione HDM2 antagonists that activate p53 in cells.J Med Chem. 2005;48(4):909-12.

[47] Wells, J.A. and McClendon, C.L. Reaching for high-hanging fruit in drug discovery at protein-protein interfaces 2007 450: pp1001-1009

[48] Coyne A.G, Scott, D.E and Abell, C. Drugging challenging targets using fragment-based approaches 2010 Current opinions in Chemical Biology 14:299-307.

[49] Murray C.W. and Rees D.C. The rise of fragment-based drug discovery Nature Chemistry 2009 1:1187-192

[50] Shuker S.B., Hajduk P.J., Meadows R.P. and Fesik, S.W. Discovering high-affinity ligands for proteins SAR by NMR 1996 Science 274: 5292, pp 1531-1534.

[51] Louise L. Major & Terry K. Smith (2011) Screening of the MayBridge Rule of 3 Fragment Library for trypanocidal compounds that interact with the myo-inositol-3-phosphate synthase from *Trypanosoma brucei* Molecular Biology International Vol 2011, Article ID 389364,doi:10.4061/2011/389364).

[52] Van Baelen G, Hostyn S, Dhooghe L, Tapolcsanyi P, Matyus P, Lemiere G, Dommisse R, Kaiser M, Brun R, Cos P, Maes L, Hajos G, Riedl Z, Nagy I, Maes BU, Pieters LStructure-activity relationship of antiparasitic and cytotoxic indoloquinoline alkaloids, and their tricyclic and bicyclic analogues.Bioorg. Med. Chem. (2009) 17:7209-7217

[53] Liu G, Huth JR, Olejniczak ET, Mendoza R, DeVries P, Leitza S, Reilly EB, Okasinski GF, Fesik SW, von Geldern TW Novel p-arylthiocinnamides as antagonists of leukocyte function-associated antigen-1/intracellular adhesion molecule-1 interaction. 2. Mechanism of inhibition and structure-based improvement of pharmaceutical properties.J. Med. Chem. (2001) 44:1202-1210

[54] Stefania Ferrari, Federica Morandi, DomantasMotiejunas, Erika Nerini, Stefan Henrich, Rosaria Luciani, Alberto Venturelli, Sandra Lazzari, SamueleCalò, Shreedhara Gupta, Veronique Hannaert, Paul A. M. Michels, Rebecca C. Wade, and M. Paola Costi Journal of Medicinal Chemistry 201154 (1), 211-221

[55] Vella P, Hussein WM, Leung EW, Clayton D, Ollis DL, Mitic N, Schenk G, McGeary RP The identification of new metallo-BETA-lactamase inhibitor leads from fragment-based screening. Bioorg. Med. Chem. Lett. (2011) 21:3282-3285

Chapter 15

Colon Cancer: Current Treatments and Preclinical Models for the Discovery and Development of New Therapies

Samuel Constant, Song Huang,
Ludovic Wiszniewski and Christophe Mas

Additional information is available at the end of the chapter

http://dx.doi.org/10.5772/53391

1. Introduction

More than 10 years after the first sequencing of the human genome and despite major advances in scientific and technological expertise into drug research and development processes (R&D), the fact remains that we are facing a dearth of new drugs. Indeed, the number of drugs approved by the US Food and Drug Administration (FDA) has roughly fallen to 50% over the last ten years [1]. Unfortunately for pharmaceutical companies, at present this attrition in drug discovery combined with the expiration of major product patents logically lead to the development of generics. Facing both a major medical need and an obvious economical challenge, there is an urgent need to make significant improvements in the research output.

Analyses of the clinical trials landscape reveal that a large number of promising drug leads fail in late stages, mainly in phase II, with an overall failure rate of 67% (Fig. 1a). All studies agree on the reasons by pinpointing either insufficient efficacy (~55%) or safety issues (~20%) as major causes of human trials failure [2, 3]. Remarkably, the therapeutic area showing the largest number of failures is oncology, with only 29% of success rate in Phase II and 34% in Phase III (Fig.1b). Within oncology indications, the status of colorectal cancer (CRC) is the most dramatic with an overall drug approval of only 3% (Fig.1c) over the last 10 years! More surprisingly, more than half of the drugs currently approved to treat CRC work through the general inhibition of DNA synthesis and cellular division, instead of targeting molecular processes specifically involved in CRC progression (Table 1). These observations highlight the necessity to both reduce failure rates in the clinic and shorten the time required for developing innovative therapies.

From this perspective, one of the obvious strategies would be:

1. to directly target the key regulators of CRC cancers
2. to streamline the critical Phase II and Phase III to obtain faster and more reliable responses regarding the drug's efficacy.

This strategy may save years of efforts and millions of dollars, giving that the average usual time for developing a new drug is ten years and with a total cost amount to billions of dollars.

But in contrast, because a new drug has to show a benefit compared to an already approved treatment, the number of patients involved in a pivotal trials is increasing more and more in order to reach significance, and a similar trend is noted for the duration of the trial, that is directly linked to safety. Therefore, regarding the constraints imposed by regulatory authorities nowadays, it seems difficult to save on size and length of clinical trials.

In the mid-1990s, the pharmaceutical community has already attempted to increase R&D productivity by embarking in a technological shift. That was the time of the inevitable high-throughput screening, which combined with the "all-Omics" supposed to reduce costs and blew up success rates [4]. As we have seen, this approach, maybe too reductionist in the sense that it does not allow getting an idea of the full biological properties (ADME, toxicity,etc…) of a compound at an early stage, has favored the quantity instead of quality and has not kept its promises [1].

Today, efforts have to be made to clearly address the early clinical discovery steps, with the goal to better qualify "leads" to increase the signal-to-noise ratio of drugs entering into clinical trials. This point of view is supported by the important failure rate subsisting in Phases III (Fig1b), suggesting an overestimation of the efficacy of candidate molecules during preclinical tests. One of the important reasons may be the use of irrelevant models or models not predictive enough. Therefore, the development of relevant and predictive models is key to increase the quality of preclinical researches and to increase the success rate of new drugs.

Consequently, the foundations of the drug discovery process have to be reconsidered by giving definitively more emphasis to the quality of preclinical validations and by encouraging the design of new pertinent models, including human 3D (three dimensional) *in vitro* cell models and tissue explants.

This article is intended to give an overview of the current knowledge about CRC and the different models commonly used to study CRC, in order to identify the most suitable biosystems for optimal development of new CRC therapies. The first part will describe the pathology and its molecular basis, and the various drugs that are currently in clinical use or under development. Then, in the second part we will review and discuss the use of cancer cell line collections, genetically engineered mouse models (GEM), primary human tumors xenografts (PDX) and *ex vivo* organotypic cultures (EVOC) to identify and validate anticancer colon therapeutics.

http://dx.doi.org/10.5772/53391

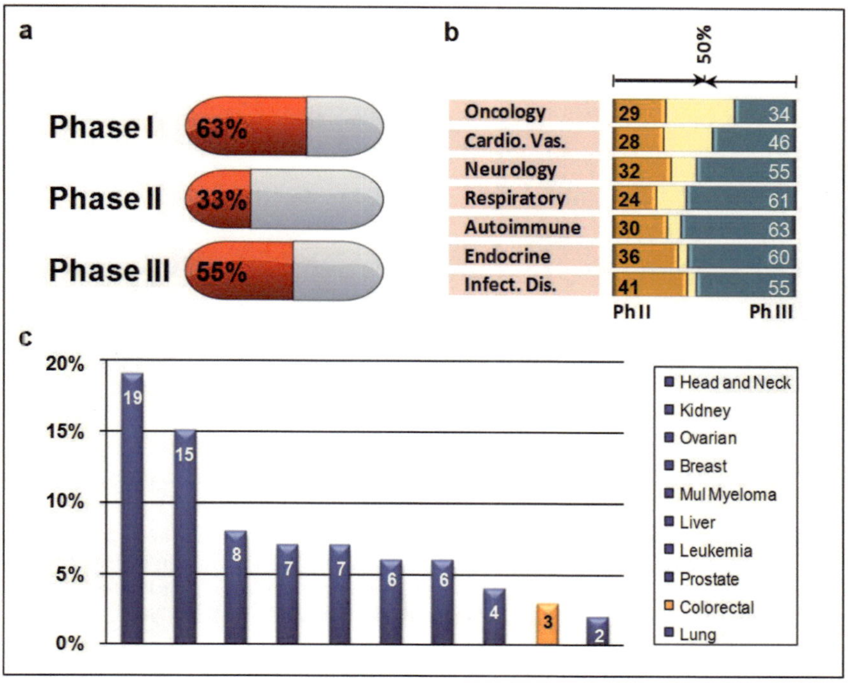

Figure 1. Success rate of drug development. Overall success rate of clinical trials for phases I-III from 2003 to 2010 corresponding to 4275 drugs and 7300 indications (a), success rate for phase II and III divided according to therapeutic areas (b) and overall success rate within specific oncologic areas (c). Source: Hay et al, 13th BIO CEO & Investor Conference, 201˙, New-York.

2. Colorectal Cancer

Colorectal cancer is one of the major health concerns in the Western world. CRC is the second most frequently diagnosed cancer in men and women, right after lung cancer. It represents the second leading cause of cancer-related deaths, both in the United States and in Europe, with a significant rate of 9% and 13% of total cancer deaths, respectively (Fig.2). The vast majority (~75%) of colon cancers are sporadic adenocarcinomas, arising from mutations in the epithelial cells lining the wall of the intestine that is in continuous renewal. CRC often begins as an adenomatous polyp, a benign growth on the interior surface of the organ. Most of polyps remain benign, but over the years some of them become progressively more dysplastic, accumulate mutations and progress to carcinoma and ultimately, to metastasis.

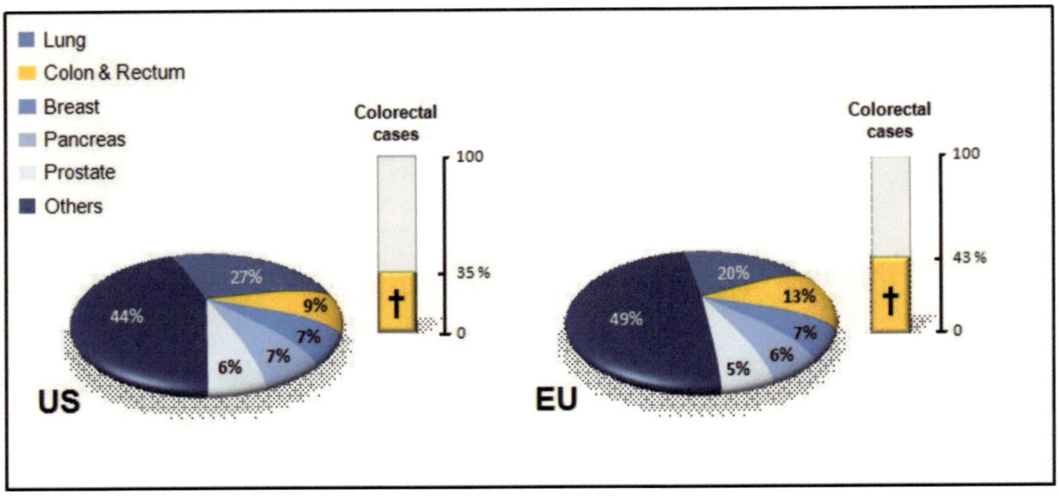

Figure 2. Cancer deaths anticipated in 2011. Estimated leading cancer sites mortality in US and in European Union (EU-27) for the year 2011 expressed as percent of total cancer deaths. Column diagrams highlight the mortality rate within the population specifically affected by colon cancer. Rates are standardized to the World Standard Population. Source: American Cancer Society and Malvezzi et al, Annals of oncology, 2011, 22(4):947-56.

2.1. Molecular mechanisms

Loss of APC function is the initial molecular event that leads to adenoma formation. Indeed, germline mutations in the gene APC have been identified as the cause of familial adenomatous polyposis (FAP), an inheritable intestinal cancer syndrome [5], and APC is mutated in more than 80% of all sporadic cancers [6]. APC belongs to the WNT signaling pathway (Figure 3) where it interacts with other proteins like AXINS and GSK3β to make a complex that down-regulates the cellular levels of β-CATENIN (see [7] for review). Activating mutations in β-CATENIN gene have also been observed in more than 10% of CRC [8]. When activated, β-CATENIN interacts in the nucleus with the transcriptional complex LEF/TCF to induce the expression of growth promoting genes, like MYC and CYCLIN D1. Additional waves of genetic and epigenetic alterations (KRAS, P53, etc…) will follow this early set of molecular changes to sustain the progression of the transformation process until carcinoma and metastasis stages.

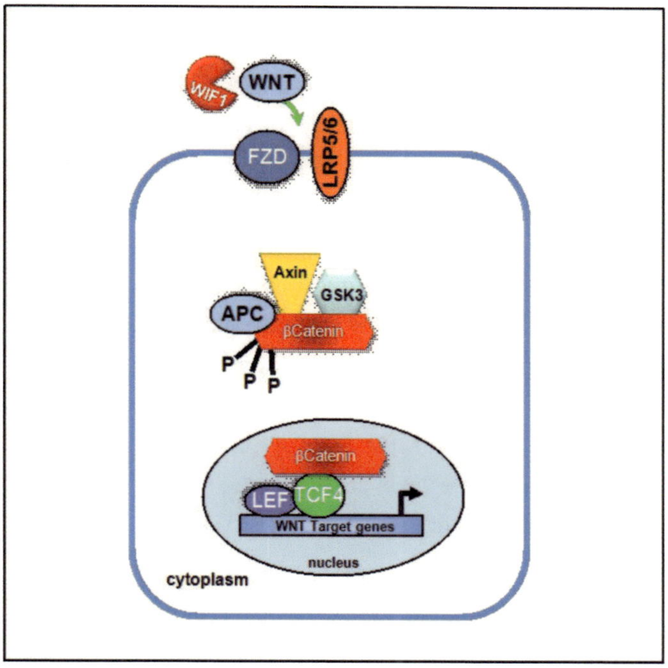

Figure 3. Shematic representation of the WNT signaling pathway. WNT proteins bind to receptors of the Frizzled and LRP families on the cell surface. Through several cytoplasmic components, the signal is transduced to β-CATENIN, which enters the nucleus and forms a complex with LEF and TCF4 to activate transcription of WNT target genes. Mutations in APC, Axin and β-CATENIN genes lead to constitutive activation of WNT signaling and ultimately to cancer development.

2.2. Clinical management

It is commonly accepted that CRC results from complex interactions between inherited and environmental factors, with a large contribution of dietary and life style factors as suggested by wide geographical risk variations. However, the primary risk factor of CRC is age, as 90% of the cases are diagnosed over the age of 50 years [9]. Surgical removal remains the most efficient treatment for early stage colorectal cancer, and may be curative for cancers that have not spread. Patients whose cancer is detected at an early, localized stage present a 5-year survival around 90% [9]. For these reasons, US and European Union have implemented preventive screening programs that have contributed to slightly reduce morbidity and mortality [10].

Unfortunately, as in many other forms of cancer, colon cancer does not display too many symptoms, develops slowly over a period of several years, and only manifests itself when the disease begins to extend. Adjuvant chemotherapy in combination with surgery or radiation is then the usual treatment. However, 5 of the 9 anti-CRC drugs approved by the FDA today are basic cytotoxic chemotherapeutics that attack cancer cells at a very fundamental level (i.e. the cell division machinery) without specific targets, resulting in poor effectiveness and strong side-effects (e.g., oxaliplatin; Table 1).

Moreover, in more advanced cases, when CRC has spread to distant organs in the form of metastasis and escape any surgical therapy, the 5-year survival dramatically drops to 12% [9]. These figures underline the urgent need to expand the standard therapy options by turning to more focused therapeutic strategies. In recent years, combination of basic chemotherapies with targeted therapies, in the form of humanized monoclonal antibodies directed against the vascular endothelial growth factor VEGF (Bevacizumab) to prevent the growth of blood vessels to the tumor, or directed against the EGF receptor (Cetuximab, Panitumumab) to block mitogenic factors that promote cancer growth, have been introduced as possible therapeutic protocol and used routinely to treat standard CRCs, as well as metastatic CRCs (Table 1). During the preparation of this manuscript (August 2012), another recombinant protein active against angiogenesis, Aflibercept, has been approved by the FDA for the treatment of metastatic CRC in second-line therapy (Table 1). This new VEGF inhibitor has demonstrated a significant advance over currently available therapy in a Phase III study (improvement in response rate and in overall survival; [11]).

Nonetheless, CRC remains a devastating disease since nearly 35-40% of all patients diagnosed will die from the disease (Fig.2). Accordingly, the expansion and the development of new path of therapy, like drugs specifically targeting the self-renewal of intestinal cancer stem cells - a tumor cell population from which CRC is supposed to relapse [12] – remains relevant.

Generic	Trade Name	Type	Class	Target
▶ Capecitabine	Xeloda	small molecule	antineoplastic prodrug (Fluorouracil)	DNA synthesis
▶ Fluorouracil	Efudex Adrucil Fluoroplex	small molecule	antineoplastic	DNA synthesis
▶ Irinotecan	Camptosar	small molecule	antineoplastic prodrug (Camptothecin)	DNA synthesis
▶ Leucovorin	Wellcovorin	small molecule	antineoplastic adjunct	DNA synthesis
▶ Oxaliplatin	Eloxatin	small molecule	antineoplastic	DNA synthesis
▶ Aflibercept	Zaltrap	Recombinant protein	antiangiogenesis	VEGF
▶ Bevacizumab	Avastin	mAb	antiangiogenesis	VEGF
▶ Cetuximab	Erbitux	mAb	antineoplastic	EGFr
▶ Panitumumab	Vectibix	mAb	antineoplastic	EGFr

Table 1. Anti-cancer colorectal drugs approved by the Food and Drug Administration. Drugs are presented sorted by type, i.e. small molecule or biologics (including recombinant protein and monoclonal antibody, noted mAb). Source: National Cancer Institute database, 2012.

http://dx.doi.org/10.5772/53391

2.3. Designing new therapies

A classical approach of drug design in oncology is to identify modulators of specific signal transduction pathways that are important for tumor growth, survival, invasion, and metastasis. Because aberrant WNT signaling has been shown to drive the earliest step of colorectal tumorigenesis (see before), the WNT/β-CATENIN pathway appears critical for CRC and therefore represents a target of choice for the development of CRC therapeutics.

2.3.1. *Oncogenic WNT/β-CATENIN pathway as a therapeutic target*

Many experiments have demonstrated that disruption of the WNT signaling pathway lead to consistent growth inhibition and apoptosis of CRC cell lines and effective inhibition of tumor growth in CRC animal models. These results can be achieved by modulating the pathway at different levels, from the membrane receptor to the final nuclear transcription factors (Figure 3). A significant number of proof of principle studies have already been published, including targeted inhibition of WNT1-2, FZD or LRP5/6 receptors by antibodies or inhibitory fusion proteins [13-15], inactivation of the pathway by re-expression of WIF1 (WNT-inhibitory factor-1) or through restoration of tumor suppressors APC and Axin expression [16], expression of a dominant-negative mutant to block the transcription factor TCF4 [17], and finally direct inhibition of β-CATENIN using RNA interfering technologies *in vitro* and *in vivo* [18, 19]. Taken together, these data provide a strong biological rationale for drugging the WNT/β-CATENIN signaling pathway.

In addition, recent evidence also points to a role for WNT/β-CATENIN signaling in the modulation of cancer stem cells. It is now well documented that a number of critical pathways regulating stem cell maintenance and normal developmental processes (e.g. HEDGEHOG-GLI, NOTCH, TGF) are also involved in the self-renewal and differentiation of cancer stem cells whose tumors are initiated [20]. Consequently, in a way similar to the HEDGEHOG-GLI pathway [21], a large number of high-throughput cell-based screening strategies, mainly designed to disrupt TCF/β-CATENIN interaction, have led to the identification of promising molecules as inhibitors of WNT/β-CATENIN pathway (reviewed by [22]).

However, currently few of these compounds have progressed beyond the preclinical stages. To date, the only compound designed to specifically disrupt β-CATENIN is developed for the treatment of Familial Adenomatous Polyposis (FAP), an inherited form of colon cancer. This new RNAi-based therapeutic known as CEQ508 consists of a modified E.coli bacterium that is able to express and deliver a shRNA to the epithelial cells of the gastrointestinal mucosa after ingestion by the patient [23]. CEQ508, which has shown efficiency in silencing β-CATENIN and preventing polyp formation in the APC^{min} FAP mouse model, is now in a Phase I clinical trial (Table 2).

Alternatively, a possible way of interfering with the WNT/β-CATENIN cascade, even if not direct, may reside in the manipulation of KLF4 levels. KLF4 (Kruppel-like factor 4) is a tumor suppressor factor which is typically deficient in a variety of cancers, including colorectal cancer. In addition to controlling the cell cycle regulator cyclin D1, KLF4 has also been shown to inhibit the expression of β-CATENIN [24]. Therefore, the modulation of KLF4 expression may represent a novel therapeutic approach for β-CATENIN-driven malignancies. LOR-253 [25], a compound that stimulates KLF4 through the inhibition of the human metal-regulatory transcription 1 (MTF1), is currently in a Phase I clinical study (Table 2).

It is noteworthy that despite the significance of this signaling axis for the treatment of sporadic colorectal cancer, none of the therapies engaged to date in CRC clinical trials are directly targeting WNT/β-CATENIN pathway members. Nonetheless, considering the huge effort done at the research level to identify potential antagonists and the few candidate already engaged into preclinical studies, no doubt that innovative therapies will emerge from this promising pathway in a near future.

2.3.2. *Acquired tumor resistance and targeted therapies*

In the recent years, a cohort of oncogenes, including BRAF, KRAS, NRAS, PI3K, PTEN and SMAD4, have been found mutated in CRC with significant frequencies ranging from 6% (NRAS) to 40% (KRAS) [26]. These observations pinpoint one of the most challenging aspects of anticancer therapy that is intrinsic or acquired drug resistance. Indeed, several studies have shown that these mutations are associated with the lack of response to Cetuximab and Panitumumab (anti-EGFR therapies) observed in a subset of chemorefractory metastatic CRCs, suggesting that the corresponding deregulated signaling pathways are responsible for the occurrence of resistance of the tumor to the clinical treatment [27-28]. As a result, downstream key components (mostly protein kinases) of these constitutively activated growth-related signaling cascades have become targets for drug development. Small molecules inhibitors of BRAF (ARQ 736), MEK (Selumetinib, PD-0325901), PI3K (PX-866, BEZ235, BKM120), and MET (Tivantinib) that were able to reverse resistance to EGFR inhibitor therapy in pre-clinical studies [29-31] are currently in CRC Phase II clinical studies (Table 2). This new class of drugs appears therefore as a promising third-line therapeutic strategy for colon cancer patients, especially after recurrence of tumor resistance. However, a recent publication reporting the apparition of resistance to PI3K and AKT inhibitors mediated by β-CATENIN overactivation, may temper this enthusiasm. Depending on the tumor status, from pro-apoptotic tumor suppressor, PI3K or AKT inhibitors could become metastatic inducers [32]. Similar side effect induction mechanisms have also been reported in CRC for the BRAF(V600E) inhibitor Vemurafenib that triggers paradoxical EGFR activation [33]. All together, the complexity of these results supports the arrival of a personalized medicine, where a careful profiling of tumors will be useful to stratify patient population in order to test drugs sensitivity and combination with the ultimate goal to make treatments safer and more effective.

2.3.3. *New anti-angiogenesis therapies*

As previously mentioned, until recently the humanized monoclonal antibody Bevacizumab against VEGF was the only anti-angiogenesis agent approved by FDA. It is now completed by Aflibercept, a recombinant protein consisting of the key domains of VEGF receptors 1 and 2. The compound captures and blocks all isoforms of VEGF-A and VEGF-B growth factors, as well as placental growth factors [34]. Due to improvement in the understanding of the critical role of angiogenesis in the maintenance of CRC tumors and the spread of their metastasis, anti-angiogenesis has become an area of active investigation [35]. However, the recent failure in Phase III first-line studies of two promising compounds (Sunitunib in 2009 and Cediranib in 2010) has cast serious doubt on that strategy. Therefore, the approval of Aflibercept provides timely support to the further development of anti-angiogenics as treatment for metastatic CRC. Today, 4 additional therapeutic agents that target VEGF, Ramucirumab [36], Icrucumab [37], Regorafenib [38] and Vatalanib [39-40] are under clinical evaluation (Table 2). This battery of anti-angiogenics is supplemented by AMG386, a recombinant peptide-antibody fusion protein (peptibody) which targets another signaling pathway involved in tumoral angiogenesis, the angiopoietin axis [41]. AMG386, which inhibits the interaction between the ligands ANGIOPOIETIN-1 and ANGIOPOIETIN-2 with their TIE2 receptor, is currently in Phase II. Finally, a phase III trial was also recently initiated (May 2012) to evaluate TAS-102, a combination agent composed of the cytotoxic pyrimidine analog TFT and a thymidine phosphorylase inhibitor (TPI) with antineoplastic activity (Table 2). TAS-102 mechanism of action is based on the inhibition of the thymidine phosphorylase (TYMP) also known as the platelet-derived endothelial cell growth factor, a potent angiogenic factor [42]. In this context, it is important to point out that differences in the efficiency to block angiogenesis and tumor progression have been observed between preclinical models and clinical trials, when comparing antibodies with small molecules [35]. These discrepancies in clinical outcome underline the necessity to validate compounds on relevant models, preferentially based on human tissues, very early during drug development process.

2.3.4. *Other cellular mechanisms under target*

Modifications in the epigenetic landscape are commonly associated with cancer, but on the contrary to genetic mutations, these changes are potentially reversible and therefore druggable. Most of the epigenetic drugs discovered to date modulate DNA methylation or histone acetylation. Four epigenetic drugs have already been approved by FDA for use in clinic against various cancers. An additional one, the histone deacetylase (HDAC) inhibitor Resminostat [43] is currently being studied in patients with CRC, in a phase I/II trial (Table 2).

Drug	Company	Type	Target	Status
▶ ARQ 736	ArQule	small molecule	BRAF	Phase I
▶ Selumetinib	Array BioPharma	"	MEK	Phase II
▶ PD-0325901	Pfizer	"	MEK	Phase I
▶ PX-866	Oncothyreon	"	PI3K	Phase II
▶ BEZ235	Novartis	"	PI3K	Phase I
▶ BKM120	Novartis	"	PI3K	Phase II
▶ Tivantinib	ArQule	"	MET	Phase II
▶ Brivanib	BMS	"	VEGFR2 PDGFRβ	Phase III
▶ Regorafenib	Bayer	"	VEGFR2-3 PDGFRβ FGFR	Phase III
▶ Vatalanib	Bayer / Novartis	"	VEGFR1-3	Phase III
▶ LOR-253	Lorus Therapeutics	"	MTF1 inhibitor	Phase I
▶ TAS-102	Taiho Pharma	"	TYMS TYMP	Phase III
▶ Resminostat	4SC	"	HDAC inhibitor	Pasel/II
▶ CEQ508	Marina Bio	biologics (shRNA)	βCATENIN	Phase I/II
▶ Icrucumab	ImClone Systems	biologics (humanized mAb)	VEGFR-1	Phase II
▶ Ramucirumab	ImClone Systems	"	VEGFR-2	Phase II
▶ AMG 386	Amgen	biologics (peptibody)	Tie-2R	Phase II
▶ GL-ONC1	Genelux	biologics (oncolytic virus)	Tumoral cells	Phase I/II
▶ ColoAd1	PsiOxus	"	"	Phase I/II
▶ NV1020	Medigene	"	"	Phase II
▶ Reolysin	Oncolytics	"	"	Phase I/II
▶ JX594	Jennerex	"	"	Phase I/II

Table 2. Anti-cancer drugs in colorectal clinical trials. This table gives an overview of the main colorectal cancer therapies being currently evaluated in clinical trials. Drugs are presented sorted by type, i.e. small molecule or biologics. For each compound, the pathway target and clinical status is provided. Source: National Cancer Institute database, 2012 and the clinical database of the *Journal of Gene Medicine* (http://www.wiley.com/legacy/wileychi/genmed/clinical).

2.3.5. Unconventional approaches

Oncolytic viral therapy represents an appealing alternative therapeutic strategy for the treatment of CRC, both as single agent or in combination with existing clinical regimens. Oncolytic viruses, like the vaccinia virus (a virus previously used for worldwide vaccination against smallpox), have the property to selectively infect and destroy tumor cells with limited or no toxicity to normal tissues. These viruses efficiently replicate in tumor tissue, cause tumor lyses and stimulate antitumor immune response. During the last decade, numerous mutants have been engineered to improve their tumor specificity and antitumor efficacy, and to allow tracking of viral delivering by non-invasive imaging [44]. No less than five oncolytic virotherapies are currently evaluated in clinical trials for metastatic CRC indication, including ColoAd1, derived from an adenovirus [45], NV1020, derived from an Herpes simplex virus [46], Reolysin, a reovirus [47], and JX-594 [48] and GL-ONC1 [49] both derived from vaccinia viruses, reflecting the many hopes carried by this emerging treatment modality. However, it is noteworthy to mention that there are still some difficulties to viral infection. Solid tumors have a complex microenvironment that includes disorganized surrounding stroma, poor vascular network as well as high interstitial fluid pressure. All these parameters will limit viral delivery since viral penetration directly depends on cellular packing density and adhesion between cancer cells [50]. Moreover, hypoxia reduces viral replication, and therefore oncolytic efficiency, without affecting tumoral cells viability [51]. These observations highlight how choosing the right experimental validation model, e.g. 3D cell cultures or spheroids *in vitro*, or patient primary-derived xenografts that retain tumoral architecture complexity *in vivo*, will be critical for future clinical success.

This inventory of new drugs for the treatment of colorectal cancer highlights the diversity of approaches being considered to combat the disease. Whether based on small molecules, humanized antibodies or modified viruses, their success in further clinical assessment is largely related to the quality of their preclinical evaluation. This is why both the choice of appropriate existing model systems and the development of more clinically relevant and predictive pre-clinical models appear critical in overcoming the high attrition rates of compounds entering clinical trials.

Current research is also focusing on the development of biomarkers that will be useful for the early detection of CRC, as well as for fine-tuning drug regimen and following efficacy during trials and treatments. To date, only a few markers have been recommended for practical use in clinic [52] but large-scale genomics technology combined with advanced statistical analyses should generate soon new biomarker panels for CRC diagnosis [53]. Then, it will be interesting to see how these biomarkers could be implemented in preclinical stages to improve drug selection.

3. Preclinical models

3.1. Colon cancer cell lines

It is worth mentioning that most of our understanding of the molecular mechanisms involved in CRC come from studies done on mouse or human cell lines that represent only a highly selected fraction of the original tumor and that may have acquired *in vitro* additional genetic abnormalities. Moreover, isolated cells grown on plastic dish flooded with growth factors appear retrospectively as a very poor model system to elucidate human CRC biology, especially with regard to the importance of growth signaling pathways (EGF/FGF) and tumor/stroma interactions in CRC progression. Clearly, the scientific community has taken into account these limitations, as shown by the growing interest for more complex models (e.g. 3D spheroids). However, although imperfect, colon cancer cell lines still represent a unique resource that can be extremely valuable in term of genetic manipulation and high-throughput screening, with cell viability, cell proliferation or promoter specific reporter activity being the usual endpoints followed. Several initiatives have been launched to maximize their utility in large scale drug discovery programs.

3.1.1. NCI-60 cancer cell lines collection

The NCI60 is a collection of 59 human cancer cell lines derived from diverse tissues, including colon (HT-29, COLO-205, HCT-15), which was established in the early 1990s by the Sanger institute (http://www.sanger.ac.uk/genetics/CGP/NCI). In an attempt to identify new active molecules, over 100,000 chemical compounds were pharmacologically tested in this cell line set. But disappointingly, most of the selected positive candidates were typical cytotoxics, affecting cancer cells via general fundamental cellular processes, like cell cycle regulation. These cell lines are under further characterization by sequencing for mutations in known human oncogenes. Interestingly, this resource can be screened on demand for any chemical or biological agent. As an example, the NCI60 has been recently used to determine the permissivity of standard cancer cell lines to VACV infection and replication, with the aim to better characterize viral oncolytic therapeutic strategies [54].

3.1.2. The Cancer Genome Project

The emergence of tumor acquired resistance to pharmacological inhibitors linked to mutations in driver oncogenes has recently revived the interest for cancer cell lines. Indeed, an extensive characterization of cell lines at the genomic and genetic levels will allow determining a genetic profile predictive of drug sensitivity. Such a signature will help to stratify patient population and identify efficient therapeutics combination, as long as cell lines reflect real tumor biology. In this perspective, the Sanger Cancer Institute has started the genetic characterization of a panel of 800 cancer cell lines (The Cancer Genome Project, http://www.sanger.ac.uk/genetics/CGP). Using current high throughput techniques this program intends to provide information on mutations, copy number variations, single nucleotide polymorphisms (SNPs) and microsatellite instability of usual cancer cell lines.

3.1.3. The Cancer Cell Line Encyclopedia

Similarly, the cancer cell line encyclopedia project is a joint initiative between The Novartis Institutes for Biomedical research and scientists from the Broad Institute (http://www.broadinstitute.org/ccle/home) to provide a detailed genetic and pharmacologic characterization of a panel of 1000 human cancer cell lines, including more than 60 CRC cell lines. Again, the ultimate purpose of this project is to establish genetic maps that would predict anticancer drug sensitivity [55].

http://dx.doi.org/10.5772/53391

3.1.4. Biomimetic cell culture models

The derivation of a cancer cell line from the primary tumor is not an obvious process, and for many cancers, few if any cell line can be obtained. A success rate of less than 10% has been reported for the establishment of human colon cancer cell lines grew immediately *in vitro* from fresh tumors [56]. Elasticity of the surrounding microenvironment has been pointed out as a critical parameter of *in vitro* cell growth. Indeed, culture plastic dishes are much more rigid than the epithelial wall of the intestine (10000 kPa vs 40 kPa). More importantly, depending on the stiffness of the substrate, cells can be differentially sensitive to drugs in term of spreading and apoptosis-induction, notably because of the expression and presentation of surface receptors [57]. Therefore, the choice of an appropriate biomimetic substrate that will preserve the *in vivo* phenotype appears decisive not only for cell survival but also for clinical relevance. Soft polymer surface, with different degrees of stiffness reproducing the original tumor environment have been engineered (ExCellness Biotech) and are now available to improve 2D or 3D cultures.

3.1.5. Colon cancer stem cell models

Cancer stem cells (CSCs) are a discrete self-renewing tumor cell subpopulation that can differentiate into multiple lineages, drive tumor growth and metastasis. Moreover, CSCs are thought to be responsible for tumor recurrence after chemotherapy and radiotherapy. One of the characteristic of the CSCs is their ability to form spherical cell colonies when they are cultured in chemically defined serum-free medium at a relative low density [58]. This model, also called colonospheres, constitutes a unique *in vitro* system to elaborate therapeutic strategies that specifically target colon CSCs, like oncolytic adenoviruses developed to target specific CSCs antigens (e.g. CD44 or LGR5). In addition, sorting of CSCs based on specific surface epitopes expression has also been used to enrich culture in tumor initiating cells in order to increase the success rate of cell line establishment and therefore improve cell line representation for CRC.

3.2. Multicellular Spheroid models

Early stage development of novel anti cancer treatment requires *in vitro* methods able to deliver fast, reliable and predictive results. To select the most active molecule lead in a library, pharmaceutical industry has turned its attention to High Throughput Screening (HTS) tests which mimic human tissues. Furthermore, 3-Dimensional (3D) test system has been widely accepted as being more informative and relevant than classical 2D cell systems. Combination of HTS and 3D models such as the multicellular tumor spheroid model has been pointed out having the potential to increase predictability of clinical efficacy from *in vitro* validation therefore contributing savings in both development cost and time [59]. Advantages of spheroids compared to classical 2D cell line culture have been reported [60]. Indeed, proteomic analysis of multicellular spheroids versus monolayers cultures identifies differential protein expression relevant to tumor cell proliferation, survival, and chemoresistance.

Consequently, spheroids strategy has been used for the screening of new anticancer agents, like compounds that modulate apoptosis pathways [61].

Standardized spherical microtissue production in a 96 or 384-well hanging-drop multiwell plate format on robotic platform has been successfully achieved by 3D Biomatrix and Insphero AG. Formation of standardized spheroids rely on the use of A431.H9, a human epithelial carcinoma cells, [62] or the colon cancer cell line HCT116 [63]. Interestingly, loss of cancer drug activity in HCT-116 cells during spheroid formation in a 3D spheroid cell culture system has been reported [64]. Spheroid cell models also enable the study of colon cancer chemoresistance and metastasis [65].

3.3. Colon cancer animal models

3.3.1. Chemically induced animal models

Colon cancer can be induced in mouse by specific carcinogens like 1,2-dimethylhydrazine (DMH) and azoxymethane (AOM). Exposure of the mouse intestine to these chemicals triggers rapid and reproducible tumor induction which recapitulates the adenoma-carcinoma sequence that occurs in human sporadic CRCs, with the notable exception however of the invasive and metastatic stage. The application of colon carcinogenesis treatment to CRC mouse model, like the $Apc^{min/+}$ animals, results in an increased tumor incidence by up to 6 fold. Interestingly, differences in genetic mutations that arise in chemically induced colon tumor models are largely carcinogen specific. K-Ras mutations are predominant in the DMH model, while AOM treated mice exhibit tumors with activating mutations in the β-catenin gene [66]. These models could therefore be useful to assess therapies targeting specific CRC signaling axis.

3.3.2. Apc $^{min/+}$ mice

The multiple intestinal neoplasia (Min) mouse was identified following random mutagenesis with ethylnitrosourea [67]. A mutation in the Apc gene was identified as the cause of the disease, like in the human Familial Adenomatous Polyposys (FAP). However, Although $Apc^{min/+}$ mice spontaneously form a large number of benign adenomas in the small intestine, colon tumors develop in fewer than half of the animals, in contrast to human FAP patients which routinely develop invasive carcinomas.

3.3.3. Genetically Engineered Mouse models (GEMs)

The main purpose for developing genetically engineered mice is to model the human disease in order to first better understand the biological processes underlying normal and malignant cell physiology, and second to establish a reliable preclinical model mimicking the true biology of human cancer and useful for drug discovery. In an attempt to accurately model the phenotype observed in FAP or sporadic CRC patients, a constellation of Apc genetically engineered mice, all based on the loss of the wild-type Apc allele, have been created (see [68] for review). To date, GEMs have been extensively used to demonstrate the function of candidate genes in CRC tumorigenesis, and the fact that tumors occur and develop naturally in the host constitutes undeniably an advantage of transgenic models compare to xenograft models.

The main disadvantage, except the time and the cost required to generate and maintain such animals, lies in the fact that none of these Apc mouse models consistently display metastasis, while treating metastasis is the current challenge.

3.4. Xenograft Models

The development of cancer xenograft models allows *in vivo* testing required for the predictive assessment of the clinical tolerability and efficacy of therapeutic agents. For decades, xenografts have been generated from human tumor cell lines that have been selected by *in vitro* culture.

3.4.1. Subcutaneous xenografts

As standard, tumor cells are implanted subcutaneous in the hindflank region of immunodeficient mice (e.g. Nude, NSG) to prevent rejection. Tumor growth during the treatment period is monitored either by measuring the tumor mass on the animals using Vernier calipers or by recording the activity of specific markers, like luminescent (Luciferase) or fluorescent (GFP) reporters, using non invasive imaging. At the end of the experiment, animals are euthanized and tumors are collected for histological or genetic analyses. Many applications are possible: complex growth competition assays can be performed inside a same tumor by injecting a mix of genetically modified tumor cell population, each expressing a specific reporter (Red/Green assay). These assays allow the identification of new oncogenic targets, revealed by growth advantage, and therefore critical for tumor development [69]. Subcutaneous xenografts are useful for the study of tumor / stroma / vascular network interactions, which is not possible in cell lines. Nonetheless, this heterotypic human/mouse model has its limitations since some murine ligands are not able to activate human receptors (e.g. HGF/MET, [70]). In addition, some CRC cell lines, even if implanted subcutaneous, can produce distant metastasis to the lung or the lymphatic nodes, allowing to study the effect of therapies specifically designed against metastatic dissemination and growth (C. Mas, pers. comm.).

Here it is interesting to note that at the preclinical level, the *in vivo* antiangiogenic activity of Sunitinib (see "New anti-angiogenesis therapies" section before) was evaluated in sub-cutaneous xenograft tumor models derived from HT29 and Colo205 human colon carcinoma cell lines implanted in athymic mice [71-72]. However, thereafter no advantage in anti-tumor efficacy could be shown in Phase III trial. Although the reasons for this failure are not clearly established, the genetic heterogeneity observed in primary CRC patient tumors could explain this lack of efficacy: *in vitro* selected cell lines are not enough representative of CRC patient's tumors. This observation suggests that new models including large tumor panels able to recapitulate the biological heterogeneity of patient's populations appear necessary for an accurate evaluation of molecular targeted agents.

3.4.2. Orthotopic xenografts

A number of observations suggest that the behavior of tumor cells can be significantly different when implanted as a subcutaneous xenograft, compared to their behavior when grown into the tissue of origin. For these reasons, orthotopic models are thought to be better predictors of drug efficacy and are more clinically relevant. To this purpose, intracolonic xenografts have been developed. Technically, a small incision is made in the abdomen of the immunodeficient mouse, directly over the colon, and CRC cells are implanted under the serosa of the colon. Local tumor growth on the colon is then monitored. Although more realistic, the use of orthotopic xenograft models does not guarantee success. The efficacy of Semaxanib, an antiangiogenic molecule, has been tested in preclinical stages using an intracolonic Xenograft [73] but compound development was stopped after negative results from Phase III. Again, representation of patient heterogeneity should be taken into account at the preclinical level.

Finally, if the use of selected tumor lines and the value of the mouse as a host could be questionable in xenograft models, the response end points, survival end points, and tumor cell killing end points that are usually used during *in vivo* efficacy studies remain in line with clinical investigations.

3.4.3. Patient-derived xenograft models (PDXs)

In order to circumvent the difficulties of establishing new cell lines, as well as to establish an *in vivo* model preserving the histopathological characteristics of the original tumor, investigators have developed a new xenograft system based on the direct grafting of human tumor fragment into immunodeficient mice (Figure 4). Several CRC patient-derived xenograft collections (PDX) have been reported, with an average tumor take rate of over 60% [56, 74-75]. They can be cryopreserved and re-established in mice as needed, or maintained as xenografts from mice to mice. Intensive characterization has demonstrated that the architecture of PDX tumors, their gene expression profile and their chromosomal instability remains very similar to the parental tumor, even after successive passages [75-76]. Importantly, high correlation between drug activity in PDX and clinical outcome has been reported, making this model a valuable pharmacological tool for drug development [74-75]. Moreover, because they are derived from tumor fragment, PDX tumors retains the genetic heterogeneity existing in the original human tumor and are therefore useful for studies exploring acquired drug resistance mechanisms [75, 77]. The use of PDX as a model for tumor-stroma interaction is however less obvious since by the fourth passages human tumor stroma is replaced by the murine host [75]. All together, the above considerations highlight the potential of the PDX model to accelerate drug development and predictive biomarker discovery in CRC.

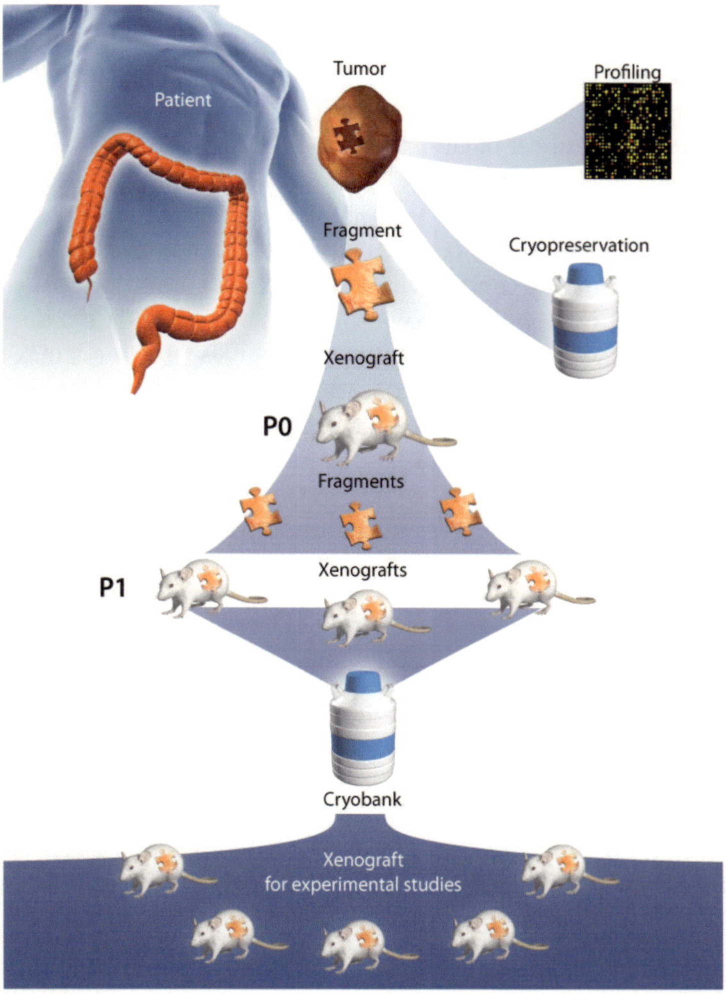

Figure 4. The PDX model. Sequential steps leading to the establishment of a CRC primary Patient-Derived Tumor Xenograft collection. Briefly, a CRC tumor fragment coming from surgical waste is directly xenografted in an immunodeficient mouse (Passage 0). After successful engraftment, new fragments are taken from the mouse hosted human tumor and xenografted again in multiple immunodeficient mice (Passage 1). A collection of fragments from the resulting tumors can then be cryopreserved in a tissue bank for subsequent experiments or directly re-engrafted in mice for expansion (P2, P3, etc...). At any step, tumor fragments can be analyzed and compared to the parental tumor in terms of gene expression, genetic mutations, genomic stability or histopathological features.

3.5. *Ex-Vivo* Organotypic Culture models (EVOCs)

As previously mentionned, current 2D monolayer culture systems are not enough predictive of *in vivo* tumor behavior. Indeed, 3D environement is required to provide essential signaling necessary for establishing and maintaining tumor specific morphogenic programs. Thus, an *ex vivo* methodology which can recapitulate physiological processes and generate multiple experimental replicates from a single tumor, saving at the same time animals involved in *in vivo* experiments will be of great benefit. *Ex vivo* organotypic cultures (EVOCs), by preserving the original cancer microenvironement (e.g. epithelial-stromal interaction) fulfill this requirement. Recently, a number of culture methods have been perfected leading to the development of breast, lung, liver and colon EVOC tumor models [78-81]. EVOCs allow the evaluation of tumor morphology, proliferation, viability and resistance to therapy *in vitro*. Moreover, differential gene-expression profiling across tumor and stroma compartments can be performed, without any contamination coming from a murine host as seen in xenograft models [78]. Recent observations have shown that CRC EVOCs mimic closely the *in vivo* situation, at the immunohistochemical level [81], but also in term of oncogenic pathway fonctionallity and pharmacodynamic properties [78]. Importantly, dose-response experiments with the PIK3 inhibitor LY294002 demonstrate that CRC EVOCs may be used to predit tumor sensitivity to drugs in a patient-specific manner [78]. EVOCs represent therefore a highly promising *in vitro* tumor model, when combined with automated medium-throughput analyses, has the potential to significantly enhance preclinical drug evaluation studies.

4. Conclusion

The development of relevant and predictive models is key to increase the quality of preclinical researches and to increase the success rate of new drugs. Many progresses have been made in this area to get as closer as possible to *in vivo* situations of human CRC cancers. Even though cell lines and animal models are still indispensable, the Xenograft Models, EVOCs as well as the 3D culture of CRC cancer cells hold the promises for the development of new, more efficient and safer drugs.

Author details

Samuel Constant, Song Huang, Ludovic Wiszniewski and Christophe Mas*

*Address all correspondence to: christophe.mas@oncotheis.com

OncoTheis, 14 Chemin des aulx, CH-1228 Plan-les-Ouates, Geneva, Switzerland

References

[1] Scannell, J. W., Blanckley, A., Boldon, H., & Warrington, B. (2012). Diagnosing the decline in pharmaceutical R&D efficiency. *Nat Rev Drug Discov*, 11, 191-200.

[2] Arrowsmith, J. (2011a). Trial watch: Phase II failures: 2008-2010. *Nat Rev Drug Discov*, 10, 328-9.

[3] Arrowsmith, J. (2011b). Trial watch: phase III and submission failures: 2007-2010. *Nat Rev Drug Discov*, 10, 87.

[4] Mayr, L. M., & Fuerst, P. (2008). The future of high-throughput screening. J Biomol Screen.; , 13, 443-8.

[5] Groden, J., Thliveris, A., Samowitz, W., Carlson, M., Gelbert, L., Albertsen, H., Joslyn, G., Stevens, J., Spirio, L., Robertson, M., et al. (1991). Identification and characterization of the familial adenomatous polyposis coli gene. *Cell*, 66, 589-600.

[6] Powell, S. M., Zilz, N., Beazer-Barclay, Y., Bryan, T. M., Hamilton, S. R., Thibodeau, S. N., Vogelstein, B., & Kinzler, K. W. (1992). APC mutations occur early during colorectal tumorigenesis. *Nature*, 359, 235-7.

[7] Clevers, H., & Nusse, R. (2012). Wnt/β-catenin signaling and disease. *Cell*, 149, 1192-205.

[8] Morin, P. J., Sparks, A. B., Korinek, V., Barker, N., Clevers, H., Vogelstein, B., & Kinzler, K. W. (1997). Activation of beta-catenin-Tcf signaling in colon cancer by mutations in beta-catenin or APC. *Science*, 275, 1787-90.

[9] Howlader, N., Noone, A. M., Krapcho, M., Neyman, N., Aminou, R., Altekruse, S. F., Kosary, C. L., Ruhl, J., Tatalovich, Z., Cho, H., Mariotto, A., Eisner, M. P., Lewis, D. R., Chen, H. S., Feuer, E. J., & Cronin, K. A. (2012). SEER Cancer Statistics Review, 1975Vintage 2009 Populations). *National Cancer Institute*.

[10] Zavoral, M., Suchanek, S., Zavada, F., Dusek, L., Muzik, J., Seifert, B., & Fric, P. (2009). Colorectal cancer screening in Europe. *World J Gastroenterol*, 15, 5907-5915.

[11] Gaya, A., & Tse, V. (2012). A preclinical and clinical review of aflibercept for the management of cancer. *Cancer Treat Rev*, 38, 484-93.

[12] Merlos, Suárez., et al. (2011). The Intestinal Stem Cell Signature Identifies Colorectal Cancer Stem Cells and Predicts Disease Relapse. *Cell Stem Cell*, 8, 511-24.

[13] He, B., You, L., Uematsu, K., Xu, Z., Lee, A. Y., Matsangou, M., Mc Cormick, F., & Jablons, D. M. (2004). A monoclonal antibody against Wnt-1 induces apoptosis in human cancer cells. *Neoplasia*, 6, 7-14.

[14] You, L., He, B., Xu, Z., Uematsu, K., Mazieres, J., Fujii, N., Mikami, I., Reguart, N., Mc Intosh, J. K., Kashani-Sabet, M., Mc Cormick, F., & Jablons, D. M. An anti-Wnt-2 monoclonal antibody induces apoptosis in malignant melanoma cells and inhibits tumor growth. *Cancer Res*, 64(15), 5385-9.

[15] De Almeida, V. I., Miao, L., Ernst, J. A., Koeppen, H., Polakis, P., & Rubinfeld, B. (2007). The soluble wnt receptor Frizzled8CRD-hFc inhibits the growth of teratocarcinomas in vivo. *Cancer Res*, 67, 5371-9, Taniguchi H, Yamamoto H, Hirata T, Miyamoto N, Oki M, Nosho K, Adachi Y, Endo T, Imai K, Shinomura Y. '05 Frequent epigenetic inactivation of Wnt inhibitory factor-1 in human gastrointestinal cancers. Oncogene.; 24:7946-52.

[16] Morin, P. J., Sparks, A. B., Korinek, V., Barker, N., Clevers, H., Vogelstein, B., & Kinzler, K. W. (1997). Activation of beta-catenin-Tcf signaling in colon cancer by mutations in beta-catenin or APC. *Science*, 275(5307), 1787-90.

[17] Van de Wetering, M., Sancho, E., Verweij, C., de Lau, W., Oving, I., Hurlstone, A., van der Horn, K., Batlle, E., Coudreuse, D., Haramis, A. P., et al. (2002). The β-catenin/TCF-4 complex imposes a crypt progenitor phenotype on colorectal cancer cells. *Cell*, 111, 241-250.

[18] Verma, U. N., Surabhi, R. M., Schmaltieg, A., Becerra, C., & Gaynor, R. B. (2003). Small interfering RNAs directed against beta-catenin inhibit the in vitro and in vivo growth of colon cancer cells. *Clin Cancer Res*, 9, 1291-300.

[19] Scholer-Dahirel, A., Schlabach, M. R., Loo, A., Bagdasarian, L., Meyer, R., Guo, R., Woolfenden, S., Yu, K. K., Markovits, J., Killary, K., Sonkin, D., Yao, Y. M., Warmuth, M., Sellers, W. R., Schlegel, R., Stegmeier, F., Mosher, R. E., & Mc Laughlin, M. E. (2011). Maintenance of adenomatous polyposis coli (APC)-mutant colorectal cancer is dependent on Wnt/beta-catenin signaling. *Proc Natl Acad Sci U S A*, 108, 17135-40.

[20] Van der Flier, L. G., & Clevers, H. (2009). Stem cells self-renewal, and differentiation in the intestinal epithelium. *Annu Rev Physiol*, 71, 241-60.

[21] Mas, C., Ruiz, i., & Altaba, A. Small molecule modulation of HH-GLI signaling: current leads, trials and tribulations. *Biochem Pharmacol*, 80, 712-23.

[22] Takahashi-Yanaga, F., & Kahn, M. Targeting Wnt signaling: can we safely eradicate cancer stem cells? *Clin Cancer Res*, 6(12), 3153-62, 2010 Jun 8.

[23] Vaze, M. B., Wu, T. S., Shaguna, Templin. M., & Polisky, B. Engineering of trans kingdom RNAi (tkRNAi) against gastrointestinal polyps. *Cancer Research*, 72(8, 1).

[24] Zhang, N., Zhang, J., Shuai, L., Zha, L., He, M., Huang, Z., & Wang, Z. Krüppel-like factor 4 negatively regulates β-catenin expression and inhibits the proliferation, invasion and metastasis of gastric cancer. *Int J Oncol*, 40(6), 2038-48.

[25] Cukier, H., Peralta, R. , Hongnan, J. , Huesca, M., Yoon, L., & Aiping, Y. (2012). Preclinical dose scheduling studies of LOR-253, a novel anticancer drug, in combination with chemotherapeutics in lung and colon cancers. *Annual Meeting of the American Association for Cancer Research; Chicago, IL. Philadelphia (PA): AACR; Cancer Res*, 72(8), Abstract nr 3710.

[26] Forber, S. A., et al. (2011). COSMIC: mining complete cancer genomes in the Catalogue of Somatic Mutations in Cancer. *Nucleic Acids Res*, 39, D945-50.

[27] Sartore, Bianchi., et al. (2009). PIK3CA mutations in colorectal cancer are associated with clinical resistance to EGFR-targeted monoclonal antibodies. *Cancer Res*, 69, 1851-7.

[28] De Roock, W., De Vriendt, V., Normanno, N., Ciardiello, F., & Tejpar, S. (2011). KRAS, BRAF, PIK3CA, and PTEN mutations: implications for targeted therapies in metastatic colorectal cancer. *Lancet Oncol*, 12, 594-603.

[29] Mueller, A., Bachmann, E., Linnig, M., Khillimberger, K., Schimanski, C. C., Galle, P. R., & Moehler, M. (2012). Selective PI3K inhibition by BKM120 and BEZ235 alone or in combination with chemotherapy in wild-type and mutated human gastrointestinal cancer cell lines. *Cancer Chemother Pharmacol*, 69, 1601-15.

[30] Misale, , et al. (2012). Emergence of KRAS mutations and acquired resistance to anti-EGFR therapy in colorectal cancer. *Nature*, 486, 532-6.

[31] Munshi, N., Jeay, S., Li, Y., Chen, C. R., France, Ashwell. DS, et al. (2010). ARQ 197, a novel and selective inhibitor of the human c-Met receptor tyrosine kinase with anti-tumor activity. *Mol Cancer Ther*, 9, 1544-53.

[32] Tenbaum, S. P., et al. (2012). β-catenin confers resistance to PI3K and AKT inhibitors and subverts FOXO3a to promote metastasis in colon cancer. *Nat Med*, 18, 892-901.

[33] Prahallad, A., Sun, C., Huang, S., Di Nicolantonio, F., Salazar, R., Zecchin, D., Beijersbergen, R. L., Bardelli, A., & Bernards, R. (2012). Unresponsiveness of colon cancer to BRAF(V600E) inhibition through feedback activation of EGFR. *Nature*, 483(7387), 100-3.

[34] Holash, J., Davis, S., Papadopoulos, N., Croll, S. D., Ho, L., Russell, M., Boland, P., Leidich, R., Hylton, D., Burova, E., Ioffe, E., Huang, T., Radziejewski, C., Bailey, K., Fandl, J. P., Daly, T., Wiegand, S. J., Yancopoulos, G. D., & Rudge, J. S. (2002). VEGF-Trap: a VEGF blocker with potent antitumor effects. *Proc Natl Acad Sci*, 99, 11393-11398.

[35] Ferrarotto, R., & Hoff, P. M. (2012). Antiangiogenic Drugs for Colorectal Cancer: Exploring New Possibilities. *Clin Colorectal Cancer*, in press.

[36] Spratlin, J. L., Cohen, R. B., Eadens, M., et al. (2010). Phase I pharmacologic and biologic study of ramucirumab (IMC-1121B), a fully human immunoglobulin G1 monoclonal antibody targeting the vascular endothelial growth factor receptor-2. *J Clin Oncol*, 28, 780-7.

[37] Schwartz, J. D., Rowinsky, E. K., Youssoufian, H., Pytowski, B., & Wu, Y. (2010). Vascular endothelial growth factor receptor-1 in human cancer: concise review and rationale for development of IMC-18F1 (Human antibody targeting vascular endothelial growth factor receptor-1). *Cancer*, 116(4), 1027-32.

[38] Grothey, A., Sobrero, A. F., Siena, S., et al. (2012). Results of a phase III randomized, double-blind, placebo-controlled, multicenter trial (CORRECT) of regorafenib plus best supportive care (BSC) versus placebo plus BSC in patients (pts) with metastatic colorectal cancer (mCRC) who have progressed after standard therapies. *J Clin Oncol*, 30(4), abstract LBA385.

[39] Hecht, J. R., Trarbach, T., Hainsworth, J. D., Major, P., Jäger, E., Wolff, R. A., Lloyd-Salvant, K., Bodoky, G., Pendergrass, K., Berg, W., Chen, B. L., Jalava, T., Meinhardt, G., Laurent, D., Lebwohl, D., & Kerr, D. (2011). Randomized, placebo-controlled, phase III study of first-line oxaliplatin-based chemotherapy plus PTK787/ZK 222584, an oral vascular endothelial growth factor receptor inhibitor, in patients with metastatic colorectal adenocarcinoma. *J Clin Oncol*, 29, 1997-2003.

[40] Van Cutsem, E., Bajetta, E., Valle, J., Köhne, C. H., Hecht, J. R., Moore, M., Germond, C., Berg, W., Chen, B. L., Jalava, T., Lebwohl, D., Meinhardt, G., Laurent, D., & Lin, E. (2011). Randomized, placebo-controlled, phase III study of oxaliplatin, fluorouracil, and leucovorin with or without PTK787/ZK 222584 in patients with previously treated metastatic colorectal adenocarcinoma. *J Clin Oncol*, 29, 004-10.

[41] Neal, J., & Wakelee, H. (2010). AMG-386, a selective angiopoietin-1/-2-neutralizing peptibody for the potential treatment of cancer. *Curr Opin Mol Ther*, 12, 487-95.

[42] Temmink, O. H., Emura, T., de Bruin, M., Fukushima, M., & Peters, G. J. (2007). Therapeutic potential of the dual-targeted TAS-102 formulation in the treatment of gastrointestinal malignancies. *Cancer Sci*, 98, 779-89.

[43] Mandl-Weber, S., Meinel, F. G., Jankowsky, R., Oduncu, F., Schmidmaier, R., & Baumann, P. (2010). The novel inhibitor of histone deacetylase resminostat (RAS2410) inhibits proliferation and induces apoptosis in multiple myeloma (MM) cells. *Br J Haematol*, 149, 518-28.

[44] Russell, S. J., Peng, K. W., & Bell, J. C. (2012). Oncolytic virotherapy. *Nat Biotechnol*, 30, 658-670.

[45] Kuhn, I., Harden, P., Bauzon, M., Chartier, C., Nye, J., Thorne, S., Reid, T., Ni, S., Lieber, A., Fisher, K., Seymour, L., Rubanyi, G. M., Harkins, R. N., & Hermiston, T. W. (2008). Directed evolution generates a novel oncolytic virus for the treatment of colon cancer. *PLoS One*, 3, e2409.

[46] Geevarghese, S. K., Geller, D. A., de Haan, H. A., Hörer, M., Knoll, A. E., Mescheder, A., Nemunaitis, J., Reid, T. R., Sze, D. Y., Tanabe, K. K., & Tawfik, H. (2010). Phase I/II study of oncolytic herpes simplex virus NV1020 in patients with extensively pretreated refractory colorectal cancer metastatic to the liver. *Hum Gene Ther*, 21, 1119-28.

[47] Stoeckel, J., & Hay, J. G. (2006). Drug evaluation: Reolysin--wild-type reovirus as a cancer therapeutic. *Curr Opin Mol Ther*, 8, 249-60.

[48] Park, B. H., Hwang, T., Liu, T. C., Sze, D. Y., Kim, J. S., Kwon, H. C., Oh, S. Y., Han, S. Y., Yoon, J. H., Hong, S. H., Moon, A., Speth, K., Park, C., Ahn, Y. J., Daneshmand, M., Rhee, B. G., Pinedo, H. M., Bell, J. C., & Kirn, D. H. (2008). Use of a targeted oncolytic poxvirus, JX-594, in patients with refractory primary or metastatic liver cancer: a phase I trial. *Lancet Oncol*, 9, 533-42.

[49] Pedersen, J. V., Karapanagiotou, E. M., Biondo, A., Tunariu, N., Puglisi, M., Denholm, K. A., Sassi, S., Mansfield, D., Yap, T. A., De Bono, J. S., & Harrington, K. J. (2011). A phase I clinical trial of a genetically modified and imageable oncolytic vaccinia virus GL-ONC1 with clinical green fluorescent protein (GFP) imaging. *J Clin Oncol*, 29, abstr 2577.

[50] Minchinton, A. I., & Tannock, I. F. (2006). Drug penetration in solid tumours. *Nature Rev Cancer*, 6, 583-92.

[51] Pipiya, T., Sauthoff, H., Huang, Y. Q., et al. (2005). Hypoxia reduces adenoviral replication in cancer cells by downregulation of viral protein expression. *Gene Ther*, 12, 911-17.

[52] Cappellani, A., Zanghi, A., Di Vita, M., Zanet, E., Veroux, P., Cacopardo, B., Cavallero, A., Piccolo, G., Lo, Menzo. E., Merabito, P., et al. (2010). Clinical and biological markers in gastric cancer: update and perspectives. *Front Biosci*, 2, 403-412.

[53] García-Bilbao, A., Armañanzas, R., Ispizua, Z., Calvo, B., Alonso-Varona, A., Inza, I., Larrañaga, P., López-Vivanco, G., Suárez-Merino, B., & Betanzos, M. Identification of a biomarker panel for colorectal cancer diagnosis. *BMC Cancer*, 12, 43.

[54] Ascierto, M. L., Worschech, A., Yu, Z., Adams, S., Reinboth, J., Chen, N. G., Pos, Z., Roychoudhuri, R., Di Pasquale, G., Bedognetti, D., Uccellini, L., Rossano, F., Ascierto, P. A., Stroncek, D. F., Restifo, N. P., Wang, E., Szalay, AA, & Marincola, F. M. (2011). Permissivity of the NCI-60 cancer cell lines to oncolytic Vaccinia Virus GLV-1h68. *BMC Cancer*, 11, 451.

[55] Barretina, , et al. (2012). The Cancer Cell Line Encyclopedia enables predictive modelling of anticancer drug sensitivity. *Nature*, 483, 603-7.

[56] Dangles-Marie, V., Pocard, M., Richon, S., Weiswald, L. B., Assayag, F., Saulnier, P., Judde, J. G., Janneau, J. L., Auger, N., Validire, P., Dutrillaux, B., Praz, F., Bellet, D., & Poupon, M. F. (2007). Establishment of human colon cancer cell lines from fresh tumors versus xenografts: comparison of success rate and cell line features. *Cancer Res*, 67, 398-407.

[57] Rehfeldt, F., Engler, A. J., Eckhardt, A., Ahmed, F., & Discher, D. E. (2007). Cell responses to the mechanochemical microenvironment--implications for regenerative medicine and drug delivery. *Adv Drug Deliv Rev*, 59, 1329-1339.

[58] Kanwar, S. S., Yu, Y., Nautiyal, J., Patel, B. B., & Majumdar, A. P. (2010). The Wnt/beta-catenin pathway regulates growth and maintenance of colonospheres. *Mol Cancer*, 9, 212.

[59] Kunz-Schughart, L. A., Freyer, J. P., Hofstaedter, F., & Ebner, R. The use of 3-D cultures for high-throughput screening: the multicellular spheroid model. *J Biomol Screen*, 9(4), 273-85.

[60] Gaedtke, L., Thoenes, L., Culmsee, C., Mayer, B., & Wagner, E. (2007). Proteomic Analysis Reveals Differences in Protein Expression in Spheroid versus Monolayer

Cultures of Low-Passage Colon Carcinoma Cells. *Journal of Proteome Research*, 6, 4111-4118.

[61] Herrmann, R., Fayad, W., Schwarz, S., Berndtsson, M., & Linder, S. J Screening for Compounds That Induce Apoptosis of Cancer Cells Grown as Multicellular Spheroids. *Biomol Screen*, 13(1), 1-8.

[62] Tung, , et al. (2011). High-throughput 3D spheroid culture and drug testing using 384 hanging drop array. *Analyst*, 136, 473-478.

[63] Drewitz, M., Helbling, M., Fried, N., Bieri, M., Moritz, W., Lichtenberg, J., & Kelm, J. M. (2011). Towards automated production and drug sensitivity testing using scaffold-free spherical tumor microtissues. *Biotechnol. J*, 6, 1488-1496.

[64] Karlssona, H., Fryknäsa, M., Larssona, R., & Nygren, P. (2012). Loss of cancer drug activity in colon cancer HCT-116 cells during spheroid formation in a new 3-D spheroid cell culture system. *Exp Cell Res*, 318(13), 1577-85.

[65] Fan, X., Ouyang, N., Teng, H., & Yao, H. (2011). Isolation and characterization of spheroid cells from the HT29 colon cancer cell line. *Int J Colorectal Dis*, 26, 1279-1285.

[66] Rosenberg, D. W., Giardina, C., & Tanaka, T. (2009). Mouse models for the study of colon carcinogenesis. *Carcinogenesis*, Feb, 30(2), 183-96.

[67] Moser, A. R., Pitot, H. C., & Dove, W. F. (1990). A dominant mutation that predisposes to multiple intestinal neoplasia in the mouse. *Science*, 247, 322-324.

[68] Mc Cart, A. E., Vickaryous, N. K., & Silver, A. (2008). Apc mice: models, modifiers and mutants. *Pathol Res Pract*, 204(7), 479-90.

[69] Zbinden, M., Duquet, A., Lorente-Trigos, A., Ngwabyt, S. N., Borges, I., Ruiz, i., & Altaba, A. (2010). NANOG regulates glioma stem cells and is essential in vivo acting in a cross-functional network with GLI1 and P53. *EMBO J*, 29, 2659-74.

[70] Rong, S., Bodescot, M., Blair, D., Dunn, J., Nakamura, T., Mizuno, K., Park, M., Chan, A., Aaronson, S., & Vande, Woude. G. F. (1992). Tumorigenicity of the met proto-oncogene and the gene for hepatocyte growth factor. *Mol Cell Biol*, 12, 5152-8.

[71] Mendel, D. B., Laird, A. D., Xin, X., Louie, S. G., Christensen, J. G., Li, G., Schreck, R. E., Abrams, T. J., Ngai, T. J., Lee, L. B., Murray, L. J., Carver, J., Chan, E., Moss, K. G., Haznedar, J. O., Sukbuntherng, J., Blake, R. A., Sun, L., Tang, C., Miller, T., Shirazian, S., Mc Mahon, G., & Cherrington, J. M. (2003). In vivo antitumor activity of SU11248, a novel tyrosine kinase inhibitor targeting vascular endothelial growth factor and platelet-derived growth factor receptors: determination of a pharmacokinetic/pharmacodynamic relationship. *Clin Cancer Res*, 9, 327-37.

[72] Marzola, P., Degrassi, A., Calderan, L., Farace, P., Nicolato, E., Crescimanno, C., Sandri, M., Giusti, A., Pesenti, E., Terron, A., Sbarbati, A., & Osculati, F. (2005). Early antiangiogenic activity of SU11248 evaluated in vivo by dynamic contrast-enhanced

magnetic resonance imaging in an experimental model of colon carcinoma. *Clin Cancer Res*, 11, 5827-32.

[73] Fong, T. A., Shawver, L. K., Sun, L., Tang, C., App, H., Powell, T. J., Kim, Y. H., Schreck, R., Wang, X., Risau, W., Ullrich, A., Hirth, K. P., & Mc Mahon, G. (1999). SU5416 is a potent and selective inhibitor of the vascular endothelial growth factor receptor (Flk-1/KDR) that inhibits tyrosine kinase catalysis, tumor vascularization, and growth of multiple tumor types. *Cancer Res*, 59, 99-106.

[74] Fichtner, I., et al. (2004). Anticancer drug response and expression of molecular markers in early-passage xenotransplanted colon carcinomas. *Eur. J. Cancer*, 40, 298-307.

[75] Julien, S., Merino-Trigo, A., Lacroix, L., Pocard, M., Goere, D., Mariani, P., Landron, S., Bigot, L., Nemati, F., Cuilliere-Dartigues, P., Weiswald, L. B., Lantuas, D., Morgand, L., Pham, E., Gonin, P., Dangles-Marie, V., Job, B., Dessen, P., Bruno, A., Pierre, A., De The, H., Soliman, H., Nunes, M., Lardier, G., Calvet, L., Demers, B., Prevost, G., Vrignaud, P., Roman-Roman, S., Duchamp, O., & Berthet, C. (2012). Characterization of a large panel of patient-derived tumor xenografts representing the clinical heterogeneity of human colorectal cancer. *Clin Cancer Res*, In Press.

[76] Guenot, D., et al. (2006). Primary tumour genetic alterations and intra-tumoral heterogeneity are maintained in xenografts of human colon cancers showing chromosome instability. *J. Pathol*, 208, 643-652.

[77] Krumbach, R., et al. (2011). Primary resistance to cetuximab in a panel of patient-derived tumour xenograft models: activation of MET as one mechanism for drug resistance. *Eur. J. Cancer*, 47, 1231-1243.

[78] Vaira, V., Fedele, G., Pyne, S., Fasoli, E., Zadra, G., Bailey, D., Snyder, E., Faversani, A., Coggi, G., Flavin, R., Bosari, S., & Loda, M. (2010). Preclinical model of organotypic culture for pharmacodynamic profiling of human tumors. *Proc Natl Acad Sci U S A*, 107, 8352-6.

[79] Buchsbaum, D. J., Zhou, T., Grizzle, W. E., Oliver, P. G., Hammond, C. J., Zhang, S., Carpenter, M., & Lo, Buglio. A. F. (2003). Antitumor efficacy of TRA-8 anti-DR5 monoclonal antibody alone or in combination with chemotherapy and/or radiation therapy in a human breast cancer model. *Clin Cancer Res*, 9, 3731-41.

[80] Kern, M. A., Haugg, A. M., Eiteneuer, E., Konze, E., Drebber, U., Dienes, H. P., Breuhahn, K., Schirmacher, P., & Kasper, H. U. (2006). Ex vivo analysis of antineoplastic agents in precision-cut tissue slices of human origin: effects of cyclooxygenase-2 inhibition in hepatocellular carcinoma. *Liver Int*, 26, 604-12.

[81] Dame, M. K., Bhagavathula, N., Mankey, C., Da, Silva. M., Paruchuri, T., Aslam, M. N., & Varani, J. (2010). Human colon tissue in organ culture: preservation of normal and neoplastic characteristics. *In vitro Cell Dev Biol Anim*, 46, 114-22.

Chapter 16

Applications of Snake Venom Proline-Rich Oligopeptides (Bj-PROs) in Disease Conditions Resulting from Deficient Nitric Oxide Production

Claudiana Lameu and Henning Ulrich

Additional information is available at the end of the chapter

http://dx.doi.org/10.5772/52509

1. Introduction

Snake venoms contain a complex mixture of proteins and biologically active peptides [1, 2]. Some of these bioactive peptides are derived from precursor proteins that through proteolytic processing generate mature active polypeptides [3]. As an example, the protein precursor of natriuretic peptide type-C (CNP) from the Brazilian pit viper *Bothrops jararaca* venom and brain originates CNP, a hormone present in several animal species as well as various isoforms of proline-rich oligopeptides (*Bj*-PROs) [4, 5]. *Bj*-PROs were the first natural inhibitors of angiotensin I-converting enzyme (ACE) described [6]. The metalloproteinase ACE, the key enzyme of the renin-angiotensin system, displays two homologous active sites, one at the C-terminal and the other at the N-terminal of the protein [7]. While both active sites convert angiotensin I into angiotensin II and cleave bradykinin (BK) into BK1-5 and BK1-7, the C-terminal is more effective in hydrolysis of these vasoactive peptides [8].

Bj-PROs are molecules of 5 to 14 amino acids residues with a pyroglutamyl residue (<E) at the N-terminus and a proline residue at the C-terminus. *Bj*-PROs longer than seven amino acids share similar features, including a high content of proline residues and a C-terminal tripeptide sequence Ile–Pro–Pro [13]. Since *Bj*-PROs are ACE inhibitors, they potentiate some pharmacological activities of BK, such as induction of contractile action of smooth muscles of guinea-pig ileum *in vitro* as well as *in vivo* BK-induced effects on central nervous, cardiovascular and anti-nociceptive systems [6, 9, 10]. For this reason, these peptides were initially named bradykinin-potentiating peptides (BPPs). The ability of some *Bj*-PROs inhibiting ACE turned them in structural models to develop the first non-peptide site directed inhibitor of this enzyme. The development of Captopril in the early 1980s became a paradigm

for "rational drug design", a concept much heralded today and made possible by computer imaging and genome science [11].

Many studies on structure–activity of *Bj*-PROs showed that a simple analogous structure to Ala–Pro was optimal for binding to the active site of ACE. Replacement of the carboxyl by a sulfhydryl group enhanced the inhibitory activity of the analogue by 1,000-fold. This compound proved to be one of the most potent competitive inhibitors of ACE and, therefore, turned into a useful drug to treat human hypertension (reviewed by [12]). Captopril was a blockbuster drug and inspired the creation of several generations of similar antihypertensive compounds.

However, due to structural diversity of *Bj*-PROs [13] other mechanisms besides inhibiting ACE were proposed. In fact, some of these peptides augmenting argininosuccinate synthase (AS) activity *in vitro* and *in vivo,* can also induce rises in free intracellular calcium concentration ($[Ca^{2+}]_i$) by acting on muscarinic acetylcholine, BK or yet unidentified receptors [15-18] or reversal inhibition of nicotinic acetylcholine receptor [19]. These novel mechanisms of action, recently identified for *Bj*-PROs explain their anti-hypertensive effects [14-17, 20, 21]. Therefore, investigation of *Bj*-PRO-induced effects through acting on different targets opens possibilities of applications for these peptides in the treatment of several pathologies lacking efficient treatment options.

Here, we describe the targets of various *Bj*-PROs and their potential use to treat different target-related pathologies, as well as discuss chemical properties of these peptides for obtaining an oral pharmaceutical formulation.

2. Targets of proline-rich oligopeptides from Bothrops jararaca

Recently, argininosuccinate synthase (AS) was identified as another target for the *Bj*-PROs, which both *in vitro* and *in vivo* positively modulates the activity of this enzyme [14] which leads to L-arginine synthesis [22]. L-arginine is a nonessential amino acid under normal conditions as it is obtained from the breakdown of proteins or synthesized de novo from citrulline in the kidneys by AS (EC 6.3.4.5) and argininosuccinate lyase (ASL, EC 4.3.2.1). AS catalyses the reversible condensation of citrulline with aspartate with consumption of ATP to form argininosuccinate; ASL catalyzes the conversion of the argininosuccinate to fumarate and L-arginine, which is released into the circulation [22].

In the liver, enzymes involved in the anabolism of L-arginine, AS and ASL are present; however, there is not a net production of L-arginine due to arginase activity (EC 3.5.3.1) as part of the urea cycle, catalyzes the hydrolysis of L-arginine into L-ornithine and urea. The urea is then excreted in the urine and L-ornithine is recycled back into the cycle [23]. Furthermore, AS is the rate-limiting enzyme of the citrulline-nitric oxide (NO) cycle for the supply of L-arginine which is then metabolized by NO synthase (NOS) to form NO and citrulline [24-26]. Citrulline, through the reactions catalyzed by AS and ASL may cycle back to arginine, constituting the citrulline-NO cycle [27, 28]. In summary, AS activity contributes to three major different functions in the adult organism depending on the cell/tissue considered: (i) ammonia detoxification in the liver, (ii) L-arginine production for the whole organism by kidney and (iii) L-arginine synthesis for NO production in many other cells [22].

Three isoforms of NOS catalyze the reaction: the endothelial constitutive NOS (eNOS), the neuronal constitutive NOS (nNOS) and the inducible NOS (iNOS), reviewed in [29, 30]. NO is a gaseous molecule capable of interacting with many intracellular targets for triggering a series of signal transduction pathways, resulting in a stimulatory and inhibitory signals. NO plays roles in cardiovascular, immune and neuronal control. It is directly involved in arterial tension control since it regulates the local and systemic resistance of vascular walls, as well as the sodium balance [31]. The NO produced by endothelial cells reaches neighboring smooth muscle cells where it activates two types of K^+ channels, ATP-sensitive and Ca^{2+}-dependent [32, 33], and thereby induces the relaxation of blood vessels and brings about vascular dilation leading direct consequences in processes like erection, arterial pressure systemic or organ-specific [34].

Due to the great physiological importance of the NO, compounds revealing properties aspotential NO donors have been protected by patents. They are based on the fact that there are many pathological states related to NO deficiency (reviewed by [35]). However, a major problem of NO donors is to achieve a therapeutic dose without reaching a threshold of toxicity. Mostly, if NO is produced in excess around of cells in a pro-oxidant state, NO could react with reactive oxygen species (ROS) such as superoxide and hydrogen peroxide forming peroxynitrite and nitrogen oxide III, which has been linked to pathogenesis of neurodegenerative disorders [35].

The superoxide anion is produced by uncoupling of NOS due to the lack of its natural substrate L-arginine or tetrahydrobiopterin (BH_4) [36], an important cofactor for NOS. Excessive production of superoxide is explained by increased activity and expression of the enzyme arginase, which competes with eNOS for its substrate L-arginine [37]. Other possible sources for elevated concentrations of ROS include increased expression and activity of NADPH and reduced superoxide dismutase activity [38, 39].

In order to compensate for the deficiency of NO production without induction of toxicity, addition of exogenous L-arginine in the maintenance of NO production has been investigated. The inefficiency of swallowed L-arginine in promoting increase of NO can be explained by its low availability, due to the first pass effect, since the viability of L-arginine as substrate for NOS is reduced by the activity of arginase in the liver. Several studies have shown that induction or activation of arginase may lead to impaired NO production and endothelial dysfunction (reviewed by [35]).

Thus, NO presents challenges and opportunities to intervene and promote human health. The study of regulation of NO production becomes important for understanding the mechanisms which maintain NO levels in a safe range and not injurious to the body.

An important mechanism for control and maintenance of NO levels is achieved by its recycling via the NO-citrulline cycle. The obtained L-arginine provided by the citrulline-NO cycle is then directed to sustain NO production, sparing bulk intracellular L-arginine for other metabolic roles [24]. In view of that, compounds that increase AS activity and sustain tightly NO production avoiding an excess production will ensure adequate bioavailability for proper physiological functioning. Guerreiro and colleagues demonstrated that a *Bj*-PRO promotes activation of AS, assayed in the presence of the substrates ATP, citrulline, and aspartate, thus leading to NO production by endothelial cells [14]. More recently, we have demonstrated that other *Bj*-PROs induce NO production by activation of AS or kinin-B2 receptors as well as by M1 muscarinic acetylcholine activation, thereby inducing vasodilatation *in vivo* [16, 17].

The patent entitled "Proline-Rich Peptides, Pharmaceutical Composition, use of one or more peptides and method of treatment" was deposited to protect the use and application of *Bj*-PROs and analogous molecules [patent: BR2007/ 000003]. All applications contemplated by patent BR2007/ 000003 are consistent with the use of PROs as prototype molecules for the development of new drugs aiming to treat a range of pathological states related to deficiency in NO production and AS activity, e.g. lung hypertension, preeclampsia, essential hypertension, coagulopathies and citrullinemia. Some of these applications will be discussed below.

3. Pulmonary hypertension

Pulmonary hypertension (PH) is an increase in blood pressure in the pulmonary artery, vein or capillaries, together known as the lung vasculature. In fetus life, PH is a normal state essential for survival. Since the placenta, not the lung, serves as the organ of gas exchange during embryonic development, most of the right ventricular output crosses from the ductus arteriosus to the aorta, and only 5–10% of the combined ventricular output is directed to the pulmonary vascular bed. Pulmonary vascular constriction plays a key role in maintaining high pulmonary vascular tone during fetal life. At the same time, the fetal lung and pulmonary vasculature must prepare for the dramatic adaptation to air breathing at the time of birth [40].

However, PH can continue even after the birth, called persistent pulmonary hypertension that develops when pulmonary vascular resistance remains elevated, resulting in right-to-left shunting of blood through fetal circulatory pathways. The pulmonary vascular resistance may remain elevated due to pulmonary hypoplasia and cause disease states, like congenital diaphragmatic hernia, as well as impaired development of the pulmonary arteries, resulting in the meconium aspiration syndrome, or failing adaption of the pulmonary vascular bed as occurs with perinatal asphyxia [41]. Moreover, PH has more than one etiological factor, thus it can be classified as idiopathic PH when there is no identifiable cause of this disease; familial PH with a previous disease history; and associated PH when an underlying cause of PH such as connective tissue disease is present [42].

PH has been reported in patients with chronic hemolytic anemias, including sickle cell disease, thalassemia, paroxysmal nocturnal hemoglobinuria, hereditary spherocytosis, malaria, among other disease states [43, 44]. The exact mechanism(s) involved in the development of

PH in these patients is unclear. Hemolysis may result in a nitric oxide deficient state through free hemoglobin scavenging of nitric oxide and release of erythrocyte arginase, which limits L-arginine, a substrate for nitric oxide synthesis [45].

Nitric oxide is synthesized from terminal nitrogen of L-arginine by NOS. All three NOS isoforms are expressed in the lung and are distinguished by regulation of their activities, as well as by specific sites and developmental patterns of expression [46]. The isoform eNOS is expressed in vascular endothelial cells and is believed to be the predominant source of NO production in pulmonary circulation [40]. This hypothesis is corroborated by the fact that NO inhalation in premature newborns with severe respiratory failure due to PH provides improvement of symptoms, accompanied by marked increase in oxygenation [34].

Although large well-designed studies paved the way to Food and Drug Administration (FDA) approval of therapeutic NO inhalation, it is equally important to note that inhaled NO did not reduce the mortality, length of hospitalization, or the risk of significant neurodevelopmental impairment associated with persistent PH in newborn children [40]. It is known that at excessive levels NO can react with reactive oxygen species (ROS) such as superoxide and hydrogen peroxide. Such increase in ROS was observed in the smooth muscle and adventitia of pulmonary arteries from lambs with chronic intrauterine PH [47, 48], forming peroxynitrite, an anion with deleterious tissue-oxidant effects [49].

Inhaled NO is usually delivered with high concentrations of oxygen. Whereas hyperoxic ventilation continues to be a mainstay in the treatment of PH, little is known about the side effects of oxygen supply together with NO. The extreme hyperoxia routinely used in PH management may in fact be toxic to the developing lung due to ROS formation [39, 50, 51]. Superoxide may react with arachidonic acid to increase concentrations of isoprostanes and may also combine with NO to form peroxynitrite [52] with possible induction of vasoconstriction, cytotoxicity, and damage to surfactant proteins and lipids. Moreover, peroxynitrite has been shown to directly induce NOS uncoupling. New data indicate that even brief (30 min) periods of exposure to 100% O_2 are sufficient to increase reactivity of pulmonary vessels in healthy lambs [53, 54], to diminish the response of the pulmonary vasculature to endogenous and exogenous nitric oxide [54], and to increase the activity of cGMP-specific phosphodiesterases [51]. Inhaled NO would theoretically benefit patients with chronic primary or secondary pulmonary hypertension, but its therapeutic application in this setting has been limited by the risk of causing rebound pulmonary hypertension, if it is inadvertently discontinued, and the lack of practical home-based continuous delivery devices.

Therefore, we have proposed an alternative approach for controlled induction of NO production. We believe that cytosolic L-arginine provides a major NO donor. Arginine concentrations subject to metabolic fine-tuning controls will assure that the amino acid is kept in a homeostatic concentration range. These effects could be achieved by the action of *Bj*-PRO on AS, a target unexplored by the pharmaceutical industry. Compounds inducing an increase in AS expression and activity are promising for the treatment of diseases related with deficient NO production.

4. Preeclampsia

Preeclampsia, a pregnancy-specific syndrome characterized by hypertension, proteinuria and edema, causes fetal and maternal morbidity and mortality with high incidence in developing countries [55]. Symptoms of preeclampsia are currently combated by sodium restriction, rest and medication for blood pressure control to avoid complications for the mother and prolong the pregnancy for fetal maturation [56-58]. However, this attempt is rather unspecific with possible side effects for the developing fetus [59, 60]. Currently, the only therapy of preeclamsia involves placenta removal resulting in pre-term birth [61]. Therefore, novel drug development for pregnancy-specific conditions remains a challenge [59].

The pathology of preeclampsia involves systemic inflammation, oxidative stress, alterations in the levels of angiogenic factors, and vascular reactivity leading to hypertension of the mother and metabolic alterations in the fetus [61, 62]. A number of evidence suggests that clinical manifestations are caused by endothelial malfunction including insufficient production of NO [63, 64]. Levels of eNOS, the enzyme responsible for NO synthesis in the endothelium from L-arginine, are decreased in human umbilical vein endothelial cells from pregnant women suffering from preeclampsia [62] together with impaired AS expression [65]. The low availability of L-arginine uncouples eNOS activity, decreases NO production and increases eNOS-dependent superoxide generation [62, 66], consequently resulting in reduced vasodilatation or in inflammatory processes observed in preeclampsia [66, 67]. Therefore, it is expected that the sustained concentration of L-arginine in endothelial cells is likely to play a critical role not only in the control of systemic blood pressure, but also in inhibition of inflammatory processes [68].

Recently, we have reported that a *Bj*-PRO containing ten amino acid residues (*Bj*-PRO-10c), activating AS, is able to correct dysfunction of human umbilical vein endothelial cells from pregnant women suffering from preeclampsia [65] (Figure 1).

Bj-PRO-10c, besides augmenting the activity of AS both *in vitro* and *in vivo* [14] increases significantly eNOS expression of human umbilical vein endothelial cells obtained from pregnant women suffering from preeclampsia [65]. It was observed that the increase in NO levels induced by *Bj*-PRO-10c diminished the oxidative stress of the endothelial cells of preeclamptic women, shown as a 50% reduction in superoxide levels [65] (Figure 1).

Most importantly, *Bj*-PRO-10c promoted NO production only in endothelial cells from patients suffering from the disorder and not in normotensive pregnant women. In agreement, *Bj*-PRO-10c is a molecule endowed with antihypertensive activity that reduced blood pressure in hypertensive but not in normotensive rats [69]. These observations led to suggest that *Bj*-PRO-10c promotes its anti-hypertensive effect in mothers with preeclampsia without any effect on the blood pressure of the fetus, a problem with drugs currently used for minimizing health problems arising from preeclampsia. Taken together, *Bj*-PRO-10c becomes a potential tool for the development of an efficient drug for preeclampsia treatment.

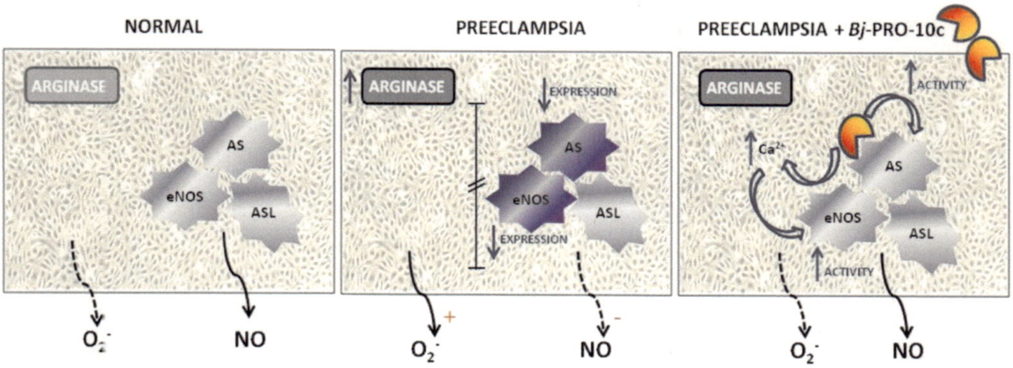

Figure 1. *Bj*-PRO-10c-induced effects on endothelial cell from healthy and pregnant women suffering from preeclampsia. In endothelial cells from normotensive pregnant women (NORMAL), NO production is adequate to maintain normal gestation. In cells from patients with the disease (PREECLAMPSIA) both decreased NO production and increased superoxide (O_2^-) production are observed together with enhanced activity of the enzyme arginase, reduced expression of eNOS and AS and uncoupled eNOS. When endothelial cells from pregnant women suffering from preeclampsia are exposed to *Bj*-PRO-10c (PREECLAMPSIA + *Bj*-PRO-10c), production of NO and superoxide return to normal ranges, since *Bj*-PRO-10c initiates a signaling cascade including increases of cytosolic calcium concentration activating eNOS and augmenting AS activity.

5. Citrullinemia

Citrullinemia, a disorder causing serious episodes of neurological symptoms associated with hyperammonemia involving disorientation, abnormal behaviors (aggression, irritability, and hyperactivity), seizures, coma, and potentially death from brain edema [70], occurs in two variants: CTLN1 (MIM#215700) or classical neonatal onset, and CTLN2 (MIM#603471) or adult-onset [71-74]. Classical citrullinemia in children is associated with a mutation in the AS gene [75]. However, in CTLN2 the enzyme reveals normal kinetic properties and is quantitatively deficient only in the liver of adult-onset citrullinemia patients [71-74]. The most successful therapy of CTLN2 has been liver transplantation [76, 77] because this treatment prevents hyperammonemic crises and corrects consequent metabolic disturbances [70].

It has been reported that administration of L-arginine to CTLN2 patients is effective in decreasing blood ammonia concentration [78, 79]. For ammonia detoxification, arginine needs to enter the liver via the portal vein where is metabolized by mitochondrial arginase to provide ornithine for citrulline and aspartate synthesis and for the priming of the urea cycle [80]. However, care must be taken when administering L-arginine, as fatal cases caused by L-arginine hydrochloride overdose have been reported [81]. In general, the dose of L-arginine supplementation used in the treatment of hyperammoaemia is in the high range between 100 and 700 mg/kg body weight per day [82-85]. In animal models the effects of hyperargininaemia can be observed, reflecting toxic effects of high L-arginine concentration and making it possible to predict side effects of L-arginine supplementation including cognitive deficits, epilepsy and a progressive spastic diplegia [86]. Therefore, drugs augmenting AS activity, the step-limiting enzyme of urea cycle, may be a promising strategy for CTLN2 therapy, since AS is the step-limiting enzyme of the urea cycle. A consequence of increased AS activity, a final common pathway is triggered resulting in the excretion of waste nitrogen as urea [87].

As previously mentioned, CTLN2 is not associated with genetic mutation of the AS gene; however, Saheki et al. identified the SLC25A13 gene as being defective in CTLN2 patients. This gene encodes for a Ca^{2+}-dependent mitochondrial solute carrier, designated citrin [88]. According to Saheki et al., it is difficult to predict disease-causing effects of citrin deficiency in CTLN2, since children carrying citrin gene mutations may suffer from CTLN2 after more than 10 years or several decades of being asymptomatic [70]. In view of that, an option to prevent CLTN2 in infants with mutation of the citrin gen is being sought, having in mind that the nutritional management with appropriate intake of proteins only avoids accumulation of nitrogen [70].

Based on information discussed here, the strategy to increase AS activity in the liver could be an effective treatment for CTLN2 as well to prevent that children diagnosed as carrying SLC25A13 mutations from developing CTLN2 in the future [89]. We believed that direct pharmacological and clinical studies with *Bj*-PROs for these proposals, could turn them into a powerful therapeutic tool. The efficiency of *Bj*-PRO action can yet be improved by the rational design of a compound which in the liver accelerates the urea cycle for eliminating ammonia or even preventing its accumulation.

6. Conclusion

AS as molecular target for drug development will be important for the treatment of a wide variety of diseases associated with deficiency of NO production, and also could transform *Bj*-PROs or their synthetic analogous into blockbuster medicine, as happened in the 80s with Captopril [90, 91]. The properties of *Bj*-PROs enhancing AS activity [14, 17], provides a precise pharmacological tool for controlling pathophysiological mechanisms with advantages of uncontrolled application of exogenous L-arginine or NO donors [92]. For instance, the effect of exogenous NO donors is not subject to physiological control, thus being more susceptible of generating undesired ROS [93, 94]. For all these reasons, keeping NO production in a safe level, so that a deleterious threshold would not be reached, is of particular interest. In this way, *Bj*-PROs should serve as structural models for the development of therapeutic agents for the treatment of various diseases related to NO deficiency, as cause or effect, as well AS deficiency.

Chemical properties of *Bj*-PROs make these peptides even more attractive potential lead compounds for drug development. For instance, *Bj*-PRO-10c is able to penetrate cells, where it remains as an intact molecule for hours [14]. Moreover, *Bj*-PROs contain a notable high proline content [13], which gives them some resistance to hydrolysis by aminopeptidases, carboxypeptidases and endopeptidases [95]. Nevertheless, cyclodextrins or nanocompounds could provide carriers for *Bj*-PROs, since drug release could be controlled in accordance with therapeutic propose [96, 97].

Acknowlegments

H.U. acknowledges grant support from Fundação de Amparo à Pesquisa do Estado de São Paulo (FAPESP) and (Conselho Nacional de Desenvolvimento Científico e Tecnológico (CNPq), Brazil. C.L. is grateful for a postdoctoral fellowship awarded by FAPESP.

Author details

Claudiana Lameu and Henning Ulrich

Department of Biochemistry, Institute of Chemistry, University of São Paulo, São Paulo, Brazil

References

[1] Tanen DA, Ruha AM, Graeme KA, Curry SC, Fischione MA. Rattlesnake envenomations: unusual case presentations. Arch Intern Med. 2001 Feb 12;161(3):474-9.

[2] Walter FG, Bilden EF, Gibly RL. Envenomations. Crit Care Clin. 1999 Apr;15(2): 353-86, ix.

[3] Kini RM. Molecular moulds with multiple missions: functional sites in three-finger toxins. Clinical and experimental pharmacology & physiology. 2002 Sep;29(9):815-22.

[4] Hayashi MA, Murbach AF, Ianzer D, Portaro FC, Prezoto BC, Fernandes BL, et al. The C-type natriuretic peptide precursor of snake brain contains highly specific inhibitors of the angiotensin-converting enzyme. J Neurochem. 2003 May;85(4):969-77.

[5] Murayama N, Hayashi MA, Ohi H, Ferreira LA, Hermann VV, Saito H, et al. Cloning and sequence analysis of a Bothrops jararaca cDNA encoding a precursor of seven bradykinin-potentiating peptides and a C-type natriuretic peptide. Proceedings of the National Academy of Sciences of the United States of America. 1997 Feb 18;94(4): 1189-93.

[6] Ferreira SH. A Bradykinin-Potentiating Factor (Bpf) Present in the Venom of Bothrops jararca. Br J Pharmacol Chemother. 1965 Feb;24:163-9.

[7] Wei L, Alhenc-Gelas F, Corvol P, Clauser E. The two homologous domains of human angiotensin I-converting enzyme are both catalytically active. The Journal of biological chemistry. 1991 May 15;266(14):9002-8.

[8] Jaspard E, Wei L, Alhenc-Gelas F. Differences in the properties and enzymatic specificities of the two active sites of angiotensin I-converting enzyme (kininase II). Studies with bradykinin and other natural peptides. The Journal of biological chemistry. 1993 May 5;268(13):9496-503.

[9] Camargo AC, Graeff FG. Subcellular distribution and properties of the bradykinin inactivation system in rabbit brain homogenates. Biochemical pharmacology. 1969 Feb;18(2):548-9.

[10] Ribeiro SA, Corrado AP, Graeff FG. Antinociceptive action of intraventricular bradykinin. Neuropharmacology. 1971 Nov;10(6):725-31.

[11] van Dongen M, Weigelt J, Uppenberg J, Schultz J, Wikstrom M. Structure-based screening and design in drug discovery. Drug discovery today. 2002 Apr 15;7(8): 471-8.

[12] Camargo AC, Ianzer D, Guerreiro JR, Serrano SM. Bradykinin-potentiating peptides: beyond captopril. Toxicon. 2012 Mar 15;59(4):516-23.

[13] Ianzer D, Konno K, Marques-Porto R, Vieira Portaro FC, Stocklin R, Martins de Camargo AC, et al. Identification of five new bradykinin potentiating peptides (BPPs) from Bothrops jararaca crude venom by using electrospray ionization tandem mass spectrometry after a two-step liquid chromatography. Peptides. 2004 Jul;25(7): 1085-92.

[14] Guerreiro JR, Lameu C, Oliveira EF, Klitzke CF, Melo RL, Linares E, et al. Argininosuccinate synthetase is a functional target for a snake venom anti-hypertensive peptide: role in arginine and nitric oxide production. The Journal of biological chemistry. 2009 Jul 24;284(30):20022-33.

[15] Lameu C, Hayashi MA, Guerreiro JR, Oliveira EF, Lebrun I, Pontieri V, et al. The central nervous system as target for antihypertensive actions of a proline-rich peptide from Bothrops jararaca venom. Cytometry A. 2010 Mar;77(3):220-30.

[16] Morais KL, Hayashi MA, Bruni FM, Lopes-Ferreira M, Camargo AC, Ulrich H, et al. Bj-PRO-5a, a natural angiotensin-converting enzyme inhibitor, promotes vasodilatation mediated by both bradykinin B(2)and M1 muscarinic acetylcholine receptors. Biochemical pharmacology. 2011 Mar 15;81(6):736-42.

[17] Morais KLP, Ianzer D, Santos RAS, Miranda JRR, Melo RL, Guerreiro JR, et al. The structural diversity of proline-rich oligopeptides from Bothrops jararaca (Bj-PROs) provides synergistic cardiovascular actions Submitted.

[18] Negraes PD, Lameu C, Hayashi MA, Melo RL, Camargo AC, Ulrich H. The snake venom peptide Bj-PRO-7a is a M1 muscarinic acetylcholine receptor agonist. Cytometry A. 2011 Jan;79(1):77-83.

[19] Nery AA, Trujillo CA, Lameu C, Konno K, Oliveira V, Camargo AC, et al. A novel physiological property of snake bradykinin-potentiating peptides-reversion of

MK-801 inhibition of nicotinic acetylcholine receptors. Peptides. 2008 Oct;29(10): 1708-15.

[20] Ianzer D, Xavier CH, Fraga FC, Lautner RQ, Guerreiro JR, Machado LT, et al. BPP-5a produces a potent and long-lasting NO-dependent antihypertensive effect. Therapeutic advances in cardiovascular disease. 2011 Dec;5(6):281-95.

[21] Lameu C, Pontieri V, Guerreiro JR, Oliveira EF, da Silva CA, Giglio JM, et al. Brain nitric oxide production by a proline-rich decapeptide from Bothrops jararaca venom improves baroreflex sensitivity of spontaneously hypertensive rats. Hypertens Res. 2010 Dec;33(12):1283-8.

[22] Husson A, Brasse-Lagnel C, Fairand A, Renouf S, Lavoinne A. Argininosuccinate synthetase from the urea cycle to the citrulline-NO cycle. European journal of biochemistry / FEBS. 2003 May;270(9):1887-99.

[23] Aminlari M, Shahbazkia HR, Esfandiari A. Distribution of arginase in tissues of cat (Felis catus). Journal of feline medicine and surgery. 2007 Apr;9(2):133-9.

[24] Flam BR, Eichler DC, Solomonson LP. Endothelial nitric oxide production is tightly coupled to the citrulline-NO cycle. Nitric Oxide. 2007 Nov-Dec;17(3-4):115-21.

[25] Shen LJ, Beloussow K, Shen WC. Accessibility of endothelial and inducible nitric oxide synthase to the intracellular citrulline-arginine regeneration pathway. Biochemical pharmacology. 2005 Jan 1;69(1):97-104.

[26] Xie L, Gross SS. Argininosuccinate synthetase overexpression in vascular smooth muscle cells potentiates immunostimulant-induced NO production. The Journal of biological chemistry. 1997 Jun 27;272(26):16624-30.

[27] Hattori Y, Campbell EB, Gross SS. Argininosuccinate synthetase mRNA and activity are induced by immunostimulants in vascular smooth muscle. Role in the regeneration or arginine for nitric oxide synthesis. The Journal of biological chemistry. 1994 Apr 1;269(13):9405-8.

[28] Hecker M, Sessa WC, Harris HJ, Anggard EE, Vane JR. The metabolism of L-arginine and its significance for the biosynthesis of endothelium-derived relaxing factor: cultured endothelial cells recycle L-citrulline to L-arginine. Proceedings of the National Academy of Sciences of the United States of America. 1990 Nov;87(21):8612-6.

[29] Alderton WK, Cooper CE, Knowles RG. Nitric oxide synthases: structure, function and inhibition. The Biochemical journal. 2001 Aug 1;357(Pt 3):593-615.

[30] Knowles RG, Moncada S. Nitric oxide synthases in mammals. The Biochemical journal. 1994 Mar 1;298 (Pt 2):249-58.

[31] Umans JG, Levi R. Nitric oxide in the regulation of blood flow and arterial pressure. Annual review of physiology. 1995;57:771-90.

[32] Bolotina VM, Najibi S, Palacino JJ, Pagano PJ, Cohen RA. Nitric oxide directly activates calcium-dependent potassium channels in vascular smooth muscle. Nature. 1994 Apr 28;368(6474):850-3.

[33] Murphy ME, Brayden JE. Nitric oxide hyperpolarizes rabbit mesenteric arteries via ATP-sensitive potassium channels. J Physiol. 1995 Jul 1;486 (Pt 1):47-58.

[34] McCurnin DC, Pierce RA, Chang LY, Gibson LL, Osborne-Lawrence S, Yoder BA, et al. Inhaled NO improves early pulmonary function and modifies lung growth and elastin deposition in a baboon model of neonatal chronic lung disease. American journal of physiology. 2005 Mar;288(3):L450-9.

[35] Lameu C, de Camargo AC, Faria M. L-arginine signalling potential in the brain: the peripheral gets central. Recent patents on CNS drug discovery. 2009 Jun;4(2):137-42.

[36] Mata-Greenwood E, Jenkins C, Farrow KN, Konduri GG, Russell JA, Lakshminrusimha S, et al. eNOS function is developmentally regulated: uncoupling of eNOS occurs postnatally. American journal of physiology. 2006 Feb;290(2):L232-41.

[37] Sankaralingam S, Xu H, Davidge ST. Arginase contributes to endothelial cell oxidative stress in response to plasma from women with preeclampsia. Cardiovascular research. 2010 Jan 1;85(1):194-203.

[38] Brennan LA, Steinhorn RH, Wedgwood S, Mata-Greenwood E, Roark EA, Russell JA, et al. Increased superoxide generation is associated with pulmonary hypertension in fetal lambs: a role for NADPH oxidase. Circulation research. 2003 Apr 4;92(6):683-91.

[39] Wedgwood S, Lakshminrusimha S, Fukai T, Russell JA, Schumacker PT, Steinhorn RH. Hydrogen peroxide regulates extracellular superoxide dismutase activity and expression in neonatal pulmonary hypertension. Antioxidants & redox signaling. 2011 Sep 15;15(6):1497-506.

[40] Steinhorn RH. Therapeutic approaches using nitric oxide in infants and children. Free radical biology & medicine. 2011 Sep 1;51(5):1027-34.

[41] Stayer SA, Liu Y. Pulmonary hypertension of the newborn. Best practice & research. 2010 Sep;24(3):375-86.

[42] Simonneau G, Galie N, Rubin LJ, Langleben D, Seeger W, Domenighetti G, et al. Clinical classification of pulmonary hypertension. Journal of the American College of Cardiology. 2004 Jun 16;43(12 Suppl S):5S-12S.

[43] Barnett CF, Hsue PY, Machado RF. Pulmonary hypertension: an increasingly recognized complication of hereditary hemolytic anemias and HIV infection. Jama. 2008 Jan 23;299(3):324-31.

[44] Machado RF, Gladwin MT. Pulmonary hypertension in hemolytic disorders: pulmonary vascular disease: the global perspective. Chest. 2010 Jun;137(6 Suppl):30S-8S.

[45] Morris CR, Kuypers FA, Kato GJ, Lavrisha L, Larkin S, Singer T, et al. Hemolysis-associated pulmonary hypertension in thalassemia. Annals of the New York Academy of Sciences. 2005;1054:481-5.

[46] Shaul PW. Regulation of endothelial nitric oxide synthase: location, location, location. Annual review of physiology. 2002;64:749-74.

[47] Barr FE, Tirona RG, Taylor MB, Rice G, Arnold J, Cunningham G, et al. Pharmacokinetics and safety of intravenously administered citrulline in children undergoing congenital heart surgery: potential therapy for postoperative pulmonary hypertension. The Journal of thoracic and cardiovascular surgery. 2007 Aug;134(2):319-26.

[48] Smith HA, Canter JA, Christian KG, Drinkwater DC, Scholl FG, Christman BW, et al. Nitric oxide precursors and congenital heart surgery: a randomized controlled trial of oral citrulline. The Journal of thoracic and cardiovascular surgery. 2006 Jul;132(1): 58-65.

[49] Lopez BL, Liu GL, Christopher TA, Ma XL. Peroxynitrite, the product of nitric oxide and superoxide, causes myocardial injury in the isolated perfused rat heart. Coronary artery disease. 1997 Mar-Apr;8(3-4):149-53.

[50] Farrow KN, Lakshminrusimha S, Reda WJ, Wedgwood S, Czech L, Gugino SF, et al. Superoxide dismutase restores eNOS expression and function in resistance pulmonary arteries from neonatal lambs with persistent pulmonary hypertension. American journal of physiology. 2008 Dec;295(6):L979-87.

[51] Farrow KN, Groh BS, Schumacker PT, Lakshminrusimha S, Czech L, Gugino SF, et al. Hyperoxia increases phosphodiesterase 5 expression and activity in ovine fetal pulmonary artery smooth muscle cells. Circulation research. 2008 Feb 1;102(2):226-33.

[52] Lakshminrusimha S, Russell JA, Wedgwood S, Gugino SF, Kazzaz JA, Davis JM, et al. Superoxide dismutase improves oxygenation and reduces oxidation in neonatal pulmonary hypertension. American journal of respiratory and critical care medicine. 2006 Dec 15;174(12):1370-7.

[53] Lakshminrusimha S, Russell JA, Steinhorn RH, Ryan RM, Gugino SF, Morin FC, 3rd, et al. Pulmonary arterial contractility in neonatal lambs increases with 100% oxygen resuscitation. Pediatric research. 2006 Jan;59(1):137-41.

[54] Lakshminrusimha S, Russell JA, Steinhorn RH, Swartz DD, Ryan RM, Gugino SF, et al. Pulmonary hemodynamics in neonatal lambs resuscitated with 21%, 50%, and 100% oxygen. Pediatric research. 2007 Sep;62(3):313-8.

[55] Sibai B, Dekker G, Kupferminc M. Pre-eclampsia. Lancet. 2005 Feb 26-Mar 4;365(9461):785-99.

[56] Khalil A, Muttukrishna S, Harrington K, Jauniaux E. Effect of antihypertensive therapy with alpha methyldopa on levels of angiogenic factors in pregnancies with hypertensive disorders. PloS one. 2008;3(7):e2766.

[57] Podymow T, August P. Update on the use of antihypertensive drugs in pregnancy. Hypertension. 2008 Apr;51(4):960-9.

[58] Lindheimer MD, Taler SJ, Cunningham FG. Hypertension in pregnancy. J Am Soc Hypertens. 2010 Mar-Apr;4(2):68-78.

[59] Thadhani R. Inching towards a targeted therapy for preeclampsia. Hypertension. 2010 Feb;55(2):238-40.

[60] Sachdeva P, Patel BG, Patel BK. Drug use in pregnancy; a point to ponder! Indian journal of pharmaceutical sciences. 2009 Jan;71(1):1-7.

[61] Myatt L, Webster RP. Vascular biology of preeclampsia. J Thromb Haemost. 2009 Mar;7(3):375-84.

[62] Escudero C, Sobrevia L. A hypothesis for preeclampsia: adenosine and inducible nitric oxide synthase in human placental microvascular endothelium. Placenta. 2008 Jun;29(6):469-83.

[63] Lopez-Jaramillo P, Arenas WD, Garcia RG, Rincon MY, Lopez M. The role of the L-arginine-nitric oxide pathway in preeclampsia. Therapeutic advances in cardiovascular disease. 2008 Aug;2(4):261-75.

[64] Rytlewski K, Olszanecki R, Korbut R, Zdebski Z. Effects of prolonged oral supplementation with l-arginine on blood pressure and nitric oxide synthesis in preeclampsia. European journal of clinical investigation. 2005 Jan;35(1):32-7.

[65] Benedetti G, Morais KL, Guerreiro JR, de Oliveira EF, Hoshida MS, Oliveira L, et al. Bothrops jararaca peptide with anti-hypertensive action normalizes endothelium dysfunction involved in physiopathology of preeclampsia. PloS one. 2011;6(8):e23680.

[66] Lowe DT. Nitric oxide dysfunction in the pathophysiology of preeclampsia. Nitric Oxide. 2000 Aug;4(4):441-58.

[67] Schulz E, Jansen T, Wenzel P, Daiber A, Munzel T. Nitric oxide, tetrahydrobiopterin, oxidative stress, and endothelial dysfunction in hypertension. Antioxidants & redox signaling. 2008 Jun;10(6):1115-26.

[68] Noris M, Todeschini M, Cassis P, Pasta F, Cappellini A, Bonazzola S, et al. L-arginine depletion in preeclampsia orients nitric oxide synthase toward oxidant species. Hypertension. 2004 Mar;43(3):614-22.

[69] Ianzer D, Santos RA, Etelvino GM, Xavier CH, de Almeida Santos J, Mendes EP, et al. Do the cardiovascular effects of angiotensin-converting enzyme (ACE) I involve ACE-independent mechanisms? new insights from proline-rich peptides of Bothrops jararaca. J Pharmacol Exp Ther. 2007 Aug;322(2):795-805.

[70] Saheki T, Kobayashi K, Iijima M, Horiuchi M, Begum L, Jalil MA, et al. Adult-onset type II citrullinemia and idiopathic neonatal hepatitis caused by citrin deficiency: in-

volvement of the aspartate glutamate carrier for urea synthesis and maintenance of the urea cycle. Molecular genetics and metabolism. 2004 Apr;81 Suppl 1:S20-6.

[71] Saheki T, Nakano K, Kobayashi K, Imamura Y, Itakura Y, Sase M, et al. Analysis of the enzyme abnormality in eight cases of neonatal and infantile citrullinaemia in Japan. Journal of inherited metabolic disease. 1985;8(3):155-6.

[72] Saheki T, Ueda A, Hosoya M, Kusumi K, Takada S, Tsuda M, et al. Qualitative and quantitative abnormalities of argininosuccinate synthetase in citrullinemia. Clinica chimica acta; international journal of clinical chemistry. 1981 Feb 5;109(3):325-35.

[73] Saheki T, Ueda A, Iizima K, Yamada N, Kobayashi K, Takahashi K, et al. Argininosuccinate synthetase activity in cultured skin fibroblasts of citrullinemic patients. Clinica chimica acta; international journal of clinical chemistry. 1982 Jan 5;118(1):93-7.

[74] Saheki T, Kobayashi K, Inoue I. Hereditary disorders of the urea cycle in man: biochemical and molecular approaches. Reviews of physiology, biochemistry and pharmacology. 1987;108:21-68.

[75] Gao HZ, Kobayashi K, Tabata A, Tsuge H, Iijima M, Yasuda T, et al. Identification of 16 novel mutations in the argininosuccinate synthetase gene and genotype-phenotype correlation in 38 classical citrullinemia patients. Human mutation. 2003 Jul; 22(1):24-34.

[76] Kawamoto S, Strong RW, Kerlin P, Lynch SV, Steadman C, Kobayashi K, et al. Orthotopic liver transplantation for adult-onset type II citrullinaemia. Clinical transplantation. 1997 Oct;11(5 Pt 1):453-8.

[77] Todo S, Starzl TE, Tzakis A, Benkov KJ, Kalousek F, Saheki T, et al. Orthotopic liver transplantation for urea cycle enzyme deficiency. Hepatology (Baltimore, Md. 1992 Mar;15(3):419-22.

[78] Hoshi N, Mukai S, Oishi M, Takano M, Shinzawa J, Watanabe S, et al. A case of hepatic angiosarcoma supplied by both hepatic artery and portal vein. Fukushima journal of medical science. 2006 Jun;52(1):13-9.

[79] Imamura Y, Kobayashi K, Shibatou T, Aburada S, Tahara K, Kubozono O, et al. Effectiveness of carbohydrate-restricted diet and arginine granules therapy for adult-onset type II citrullinemia: a case report of siblings showing homozygous SLC25A13 mutation with and without the disease. Hepatol Res. 2003 May;26(1):68-72.

[80] Nissim I, Luhovyy B, Horyn O, Daikhin Y, Nissim I, Yudkoff M. The role of mitochondrially bound arginase in the regulation of urea synthesis: studies with [U-15N4]arginine, isolated mitochondria, and perfused rat liver. The Journal of biological chemistry. 2005 May 6;280(18):17715-24.

[81] Gerard JM, Luisiri A. A fatal overdose of arginine hydrochloride. Journal of toxicology. 1997;35(6):621-5.

[82] Batshaw ML, Wachtel RC, Thomas GH, Starrett A, Brusilow SW. Arginine-responsive asymptomatic hyperammonemia in the premature infant. The Journal of pediatrics. 1984 Jul;105(1):86-91.

[83] Walser M, Batshaw M, Sherwood G, Robinson B, Brusilow S. Nitrogen metabolism in neonatal citrullinaemia. Clinical science and molecular medicine. 1977 Aug;53(2): 173-81.

[84] Brusilow SW, Valle DL, Batshaw M. New pathways of nitrogen excretion in inborn errors of urea synthesis. Lancet. 1979 Sep 1;2(8140):452-4.

[85] Summar M. Current strategies for the management of neonatal urea cycle disorders. The Journal of pediatrics. 2001 Jan;138(1 Suppl):S30-9.

[86] Iyer R, Jenkinson CP, Vockley JG, Kern RM, Grody WW, Cederbaum S. The human arginases and arginase deficiency. Journal of inherited metabolic disease. 1998;21 Suppl 1:86-100.

[87] Coman D, Yaplito-Lee J, Boneh A. New indications and controversies in arginine therapy. Clinical nutrition (Edinburgh, Scotland). 2008 Aug;27(4):489-96.

[88] Kobayashi K, Sinasac DS, Iijima M, Boright AP, Begum L, Lee JR, et al. The gene mutated in adult-onset type II citrullinaemia encodes a putative mitochondrial carrier protein. Nature genetics. 1999 Jun;22(2):159-63.

[89] Closs EI. Expression, regulation and function of carrier proteins for cationic amino acids. Current opinion in nephrology and hypertension. 2002 Jan;11(1):99-107.

[90] Smith CG, Vane JR. The discovery of captopril. Faseb J. 2003 May;17(8):788-9.

[91] Smith CG, Vane JR. The discovery of captopril: a reply. Faseb J. 2004 Jun;18(9):935.

[92] Angus DC, Linde-Zwirble WT, Tam SW, Ghali JK, Sabolinski ML, Villagra VG, et al. Cost-effectiveness of fixed-dose combination of isosorbide dinitrate and hydralazine therapy for blacks with heart failure. Circulation. 2005 Dec 13;112(24):3745-53.

[93] Beckman JS. Ischaemic injury mediator. Nature. 1990 May 3;345(6270):27-8.

[94] Lipton SA, Choi YB, Pan ZH, Lei SZ, Chen HS, Sucher NJ, et al. A redox-based mechanism for the neuroprotective and neurodestructive effects of nitric oxide and related nitroso-compounds. Nature. 1993 Aug 12;364(6438):626-32.

[95] Cheung HS, Cushman DW. Inhibition of homogeneous angiotensin-converting enzyme of rabbit lung by synthetic venom peptides of Bothrops jararaca. Biochim Biophys Acta. 1973 Feb 15;293(2):451-63.

[96] Shen TT, Bogdanov A, Jr., Bogdanova A, Poss K, Brady TJ, Weissleder R. Magnetically labeled secretin retains receptor affinity to pancreas acinar cells. Bioconjugate chemistry. 1996 May-Jun;7(3):311-6.

[97] Uekama K, Hirayama F, Irie T. Cyclodextrin Drug Carrier Systems. Chemical reviews. 1998 Jul 30;98(5):2045-76.

Chapter 17

Introduction to Biochemical Pharmacology and Drug Discovery

Gabriel Magoma

Additional information is available at the end of the chapter

http://dx.doi.org/10.5772/52014

1. Introduction

This chapter introduces biochemical pharmacology and highlights drug absorption and drug transformation reactions and a general introduction to pharmacology, drug discovery and clinical trials for new drug candidates. It also introduces the concept of individualization of drug therapies. After studying this chapter, one is expected to demonstrate understanding the following: (i) Linkage between the various pharmacological processes (ii) Routes of drug administration, (iii) Mechanisms of drug absorption (iv) The kinetics of drug disposition and concepts, such as volume of distribution, initial dose and half-life, (v) The biotransformation and excretion of drugs.(vi) The role of biochemical knowledge in the discovery and development of candidate drug compounds into useful drugs (vii) Basic design of clinical trials of new drugs and the drug approval process.(viii) The linkage between genetic variations and varied drug responses in different individuals (ix) The various adverse drug reactions in different patients (x) How different dosage regimens are calculated with respect to the prevailing health status of individuals and how adjustments are carried out in old patients or geriatrics.

2. Pharmacology

Pharmacology is the science that deals with drugs, their properties, actions and fate in the body. It embraces the sciences of pharmaceutics (preparation of drugs), therapeutics (treatment of diseases by use of drugs) and toxicosis or adverse side-effects that arise from the therapeutic interventions. Pharmacology can be divided into the following processes:-

i. The pharmaceutical process of drugs; deals with chemical synthesis, formulation and distribution of drugs.

ii. Pharmacokinetic process; deals with the time course of drug concentration in the body.This process can be further subdivided into; absorption, distribution, biotransformation and excretion of the drug.

iii. The pharmacodynamic process; deals with the mechanism of drug action: that is interaction of drugs with the molecular structures in the body.

iv. The therapeutic process; deals with the clinical response arising from the pharmacodynamic process.

v. Toxicologic process; deals with adverse effects of drugs arising from either over dosage or interference of biochemical pathways unrelated to the intended drug target. The five processes are related as exemplified in Figure1.

3. Biochemical pharmacology

Biochemical pharmacology is concerned with the effects of drugs on biochemical pathways underlying the pharmacokinetic and pharmacodynamic processes and the subsequent therapeutic and the toxicological processes. The pharmaceutical process is, however, outside the realms of biochemical pharmacology.

4. Routes of drug administration and systemic availability

This depends on the actual biochemical characteristics of the drug and the interaction of drug molecules with body fluids and tissues. The main routes of drug administration are the topical application, parenteral, and enteral routes.

The route of drug application determines how quickly the drug reaches its site of action. The choice of the route of administration of a drug, therefore, depends on the therapeutic objectives of the treatment. For instance, intravenous injection or inhalation may be selected to produce intense, but rather short-lived effects, whereas oral dosing may be better and more convenient for long lasting effects and even intensity. The various types of drug administration include;

4.1. Topical application

This is the most direct and easiest mode of drug administration. It involves local application of a drug to the site of action e.g. eye drop solutions, sprays and lotions for oral, rectal, vaginal and urethral use. These drugs are absorbed through the cell membranes. Absorption of drugs through the skin is proportional to their lipid solubility since the epidermis behaves like a hydrophilic barrier. Lipid insoluble drugs are therefore suspended in oily vehicles to enhance solubility and hence absorption.

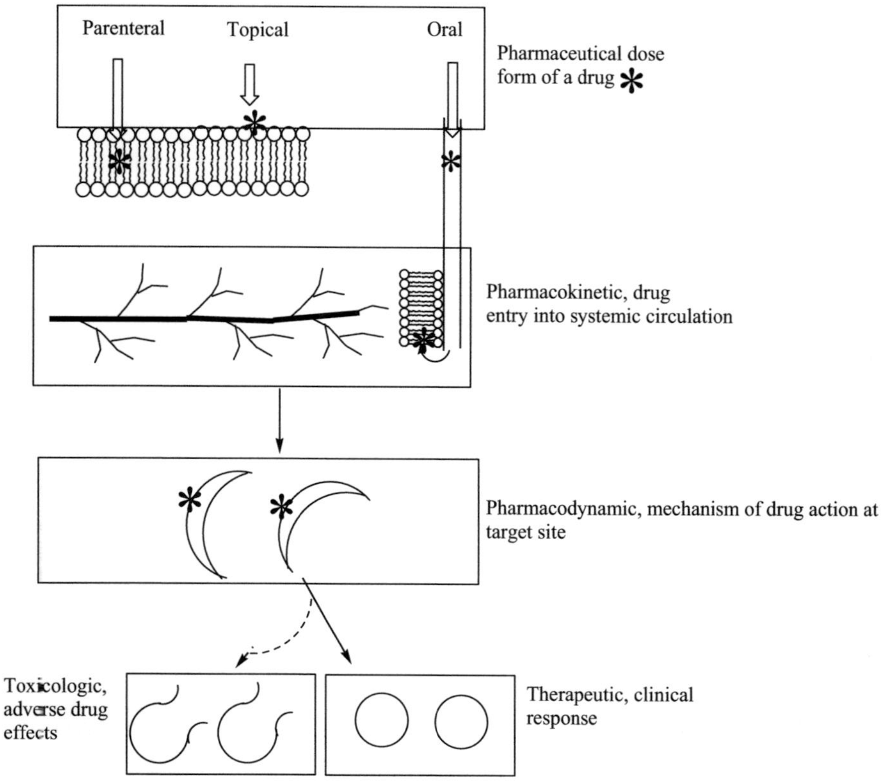

Figure 1. Relationships between the five pharmacological processes starting with the entry of the drug and ending with the clinical response and/or the toxic effects

4.2. Oral administration

The drugs administered orally are absorbed at different sites along the gastrointestinal tract (GIT):

4.2.1. Oral mucosal or sublingual

Drug absorption is generally rapid because of the rich vascular supply to the mucosa and the absence of a stratum corneum. Drugs delivered using this route are not exposed to gastric and intestinal digestive juices and are not subjected to immediate passage through the liver. Therefore there is no prior biotransformation or first-effect before the drugs enter the systemic circulation.

4.2.2. Stomach and intestine

Absorption depends on different factors such as pH, gastric emptying, intestinal motility and solubility of solid drugs. The rapidity with which a drug reaches the small intestine is enhanced when a drug is taken with water and when the stomach is relatively empty. However drugs absorbed in the stomach and intestine are subjected to first-pass effect.

4.3. Rectal administration

This is the preferred route when the oral route is unsuitable because of nausea or if the drugs have objectionable taste or odor. This route also protects susceptible drugs from the biotransformation reactions in the liver. However, absorption by this route is often irregular and incomplete. Formulations such as suppositories or enemas are applied via rectal route.

4.4. Parenteral administration

This mode of administration is also known as injection. It is generally more rapid and enables more accurate dose selection and predictable absorption. Parenteral routes include;

4.4.1. Subcutaneous injection

This mode of administration is mainly used for non-irritating drugs. It provides even and slows absorption producing sustained drug effects. Vasoconstrictor agents such as epinephrine can be added to the drug solution to decrease the rate of absorption.

Large volumes of drugs may, however, be painful because of tissue distention.

4.4.2. Intramuscular injection

This method of drug delivery ensures rapid absorption of the drug in aqueous solutions. Slow and even absorption is possible when drugs are suspended in oily vehicles.

4.4.3. Intravenous administration

This route ensures rapid delivery of the desired blood concentration of the drug to be obtained accurately and immediately and is the preferred route of delivery in emergency situations. Irritating drugs are delivered intravenously because the veins have low sensitivity to pain. This mode of delivery is also preferred for drug such as the barbiturates and phenytoin, anti-seizure drugs which dissolve only in rather strong alkaline solution and therefore need the blood to buffer the pH of the drug solution for better solubility. Drugs such as ethylene diamine tetra acetic acid (EDTA) for treatment of heavy-metal poisoning are given by intravenous injection or through an infusion because they are poorly absorbed in the gut. The other advantage of this mode of delivery is the avoidance of the hepatic and pulmonary first-pass effect. Generally, the properties of the drug may determine the route that must be used for reasonable efficacy.

5. Mechanisms of drug absorption across membranes

In order for drugs to elicit their pharmacological effects, they have to cross the biological membranes into systemic circulation and reach the site of action. Therefore an insight into the structure and function of the membrane leads to a better understanding of drug absorption.

http://dx.doi.org/10.5772/52014

Membranes are phospholipid bi-layers with interspersed integral and peripheral proteins which behave either as molecular 'gates' or 'pumps'. Molecular gates are non-specific. The intake of molecules into the cell depends on the charged groups in the pore and the size of molecule to be transported across the membrane. Molecular pumps, however, are highly specific and require energy for molecular transport. There are several mechanisms by which drugs traverse membranes to reach their intended target site and they include the following:

5.1. Simple diffusion

This involves is the passage of polar but uncharged substances across water filled channels in response to the concentration gradient. Simple diffusion is the mechanism of choice for water soluble drugs and those with low molecular weight such as the an aesthetic nitrous oxide (44kD) and ethanol (46 KDa). The majority of lipid-soluble drugs permeate cell membranes by passive diffusion between the lipid molecules of the membrane. The permeation rate of a lipid soluble drug depends on the concentration of the drug, its lipid/water partition coefficient concentration of protons and the surface area of the absorbing membrane. The lipid/water partition coefficient of a drug is the principal factor determining its absorption.

The higher the value of lipid/water partition coefficient of a drug, the more rapidly it will be absorbed and vice versa. The chemical force that causes lipid-soluble drugs to move readily across membranes is termed the hydrophobic force since water molecules repels the lipid-soluble drugs. In most cases, drug absorption can be enhanced by absorption enhancers, such as fatty acids, phospholipids and muco-adhesive polymers. These compounds disrupt the lipid bilayer making it more permeable and also increase the solubility of insoluble drugs.

5.2. Facilitated diffusion

This type of diffusion is achieved by carrier molecules which combine with the drug in question to form complexes that can diffuse more rapidly across the membrane than free-drug could do alone. An example is the transport of nucleotide antimetabolites used in viral or cancer chemotherapy.

5.3. Active transport of drugs

This is the transport which is linked to a source of energy. Examples of specific active transport systems are the sodium pump, which maintains high potassium and low sodium ions inside the cell relative to the external medium and the calcium pump that maintains a high concentration of calcium inside the sarcoplasmic reticulum and a low concentration around the myofibrils. Active transport of drugs across membranes have been discovered and an example is the uptake of pentazocine (a narcotic antagonist) by leukocytes which is dependent upon energy supply (glucose) and can be inhibited by cyclazocine, which competes for the same transport mechanism.

5.4. Pinocytosis and phagocytosis of drugs

Proteins, bacterial toxins and drugs with high molecular weights, (1000 KDa or more) enter cells by means of pinocytosis and endocytosis. These substances finally enter the lysosomal system.

6. Factors affecting absorption of drugs

6.1. Surface area

For any substance that can penetrate the GIT in measurable amounts, the small intestine represents the greatest area of absorption. For instance, ethanol can be absorbed by the stomach, but it is absorbed eight times faster from the small intestine because of the large surface area provided by the villi. The rate at which the stomach empties its contents into the small intestine also markedly affects the overall rate at which drugs reach general circulation after oral administration. For this reason many agents are administered on an empty stomach with sufficient water to ensure their rapid passage to the small intestine.

6.2. Tissue pH

Drugs can be classified either as organic amines or organic acids and therefore their absorption is markedly affected by pH. Tertiary amines are not charged at high pH and have a high lipid/water partition coefficient and hence readily penetrate membranes.

At low pH, the tertiary amine is protonated and has low lipid/water partition coefficient thus lower rate of permeation.

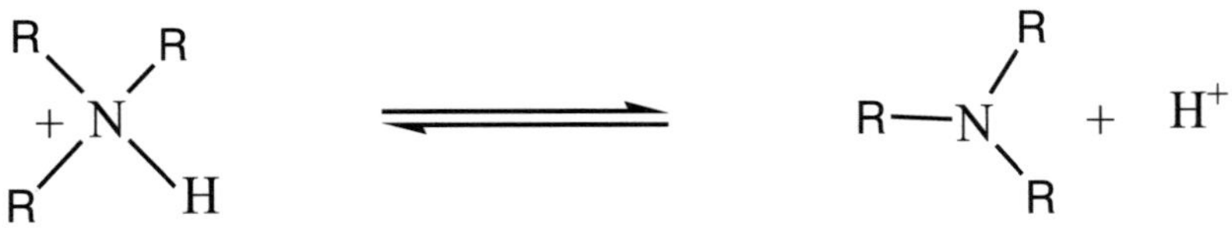

Stomach	Small intestines
Low pH	High pH
(protonated form)	(unprotonated form)
Lower absorption	Higher absorption.

In case of an organic acid, the same general principle applies. The unprotonated organic acid at low pH permeates the tissues more readily as compared to the charged form of the drug at high pH.

Low pH		High pH
R-COOH	$\rightleftharpoons$	$R-COO^{-} + H^{+}$
Stomach		Intestine

Therefore organic acids such as barbiturates and acetyl salicylic acid (aspirin) have a higher absorption rate in the stomach.

The degree of ionization of the drug when in the GIT or other body fluids is the main determinant of the amount of the drug found in an uncharged form and this depends upon the relation between pH of the fluid and the pKa of the drug:

Acidic drugs:

$$RCOOH \overset{Ka}{\rightleftharpoons} RCOO^{-} + H^{+}$$

Basic drugs:

$$R - {}^{+}NH_3 \overset{Ka}{\rightleftharpoons} RNH_2 + H^{+}$$

If the pH of the fluid is low, the ionization of acidic drugs is less while the ionization of basic drugs will be high.When the pKa of a drug is equal to the pH of the surrounding fluid, there is 50% ionization.

7. Types of tissue barriers to drugs

Most of these barriers are typically the same systems that animals use for defense against invasion by foreign agents. These barriers include the skin, the GIT membranes, blood-brain barrier and placenta.

7.1. Skin

The superficial layer of the skin, stratum corneum is particularly impermeable to most drugs. The skin permeability for the drugs is enhanced by using a co-solvent system such as ethanol/water which increases drug partition into the skin. The lipid domains of the buccal and nasal mucosa also restrict drug entry and the drugs which permeate are able to do so through passive diffusion using the hydrophilic trans-cellular spaces and direct permeation through the membrane.

7.2. Tight junctions

The gap junctions between cells in different cell types within a tissue can form channels for the passage of drugs between epithelial, endothelial, and mesothelial cells of the same tissue. These channels comprise of a group of proteins known as connexin. Cells in different tissues are however connected by tight junctions and these can impair transport between cells in different tissues. The tight junctions are dynamic structures, which normally regulate the trafficking of nutrients, medium sized compounds between cells, and form a regulated barrier in spaces between cells. There is need therefore to use drug absorption enhancers such as bile salts and long chain acyl-carnitines which act as Ca^{2+}chelatorsand disrupt the tight junctions thereby improving transport across the junctions. Tight junctions are shown in Figure 2.

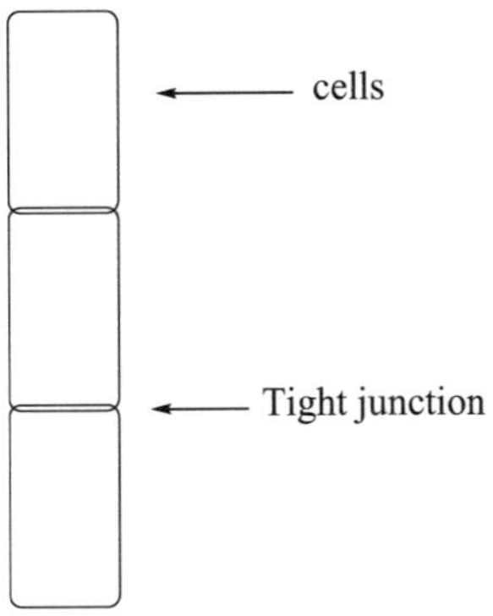

Figure 2. Arrangement of epithelial cells with tight junctions

7.3. Cerebrospinal fluid barrier (CSF)

Epithelial cells which are in contact with the brain ventricular spaces form a barrier to the movement of drugs. These epithelial cells are connected by occluding zonulae (blood- brain barrier) as shown in Figure 3. The zonulae severely restrict the passage of most molecules between the bloodstream and the parenchyma of the central nervous system. Drug entry across this barrier is through either passive diffusion or carrier mediated transport. Only the lipid soluble drugs cross into the CSF from blood.

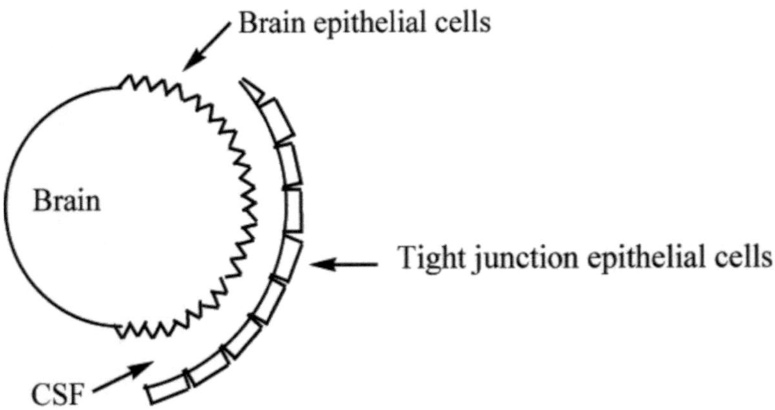

Figure 3. Epithelial cells with tight junctions as part of the blood brain barrier

Epithelial cells that separate the CSF from the brain are connected with tight junctions and are characterized by marked scarcity of pinocytic vesicles. However, the epithelial cells that lines the brain are not connected by occluding zonulae and therefore, there is unrestricted passage of drug molecules from CSF to the brain. Drugs like penicillin which are not much lipid-soluble and required in high concentrations for the treatment of brain abscesses are administered through intrathecal injections directly into the CFS.

http://dx.doi.org/10.5772/52014

7.4. Placental barrier

The placental membrane limits the amount of maternal blood following through the placenta to the foetus and passive diffusion is the main mechanism of drug entry from the maternal blood to the foetus. The shortest time required for equilibration of a drug between mother and foetus is about ten minutes and this delay is useful as it can allow a mother to be anaesthetized during final stages of labour.

8. Systemic availability of drugs

A drug will reach systemic arterial circulation only if it is absorbed from the GIT and if it escapes metabolism in the gut, liver, and lungs. When the concentration of the drug in plasma is measured at specified time intervals, it is possible to construct concentration versus time graph and hence be able to determine the extent of drug availability as shown in Figure 4.

The availability depends on both the extent of absorption and the extent of presystemic metabolism and comprises three aspects; Peak concentration (C_{max}), Time taken to reach the peak (T_{max}) and area under the curve (AUC)as shown in Figure 4. The C_{max} and T_{max} are measures of the rate of availability while AUC is a measure of the extent of availability (i.e. proportion of the administered drug which reaches systemic circulation intact). For the three curves shown for the formulations a, b, and c; the AUC is the same, but the rate of availability is different in each case; a, has the lowest rate of availability followed by b, while c has the highest rate of availability.

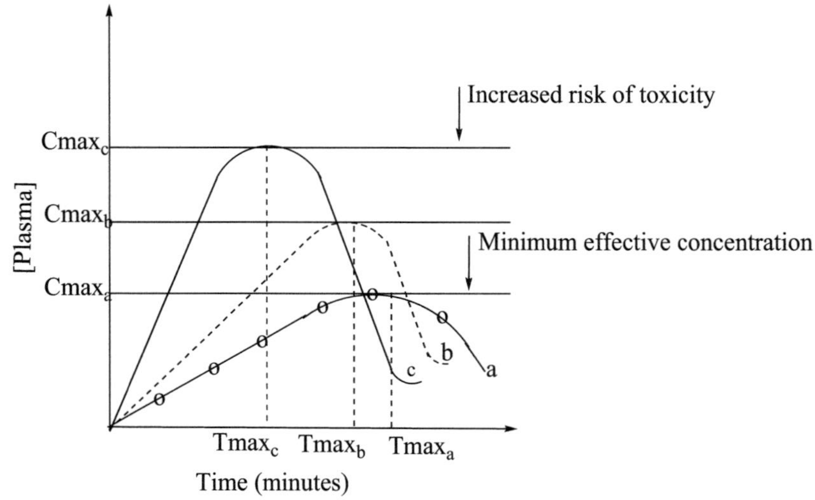

Figure 4. Plasma concentration versus time curves for different drug formulations

The speed at which a particular drug is needed to reach the site of action will determine the type of formulation to use. Drugs with the same relative bioavailability and can be used to treat the same condition using either the same routes or dosages are known as bioequivalent drugs.

9. Dosage and effect

A particular dose of an administered drug is subject to the biochemical processes in the body as shown in Figure 5. The desired effect of a drug is proportional to the concentration of the drug at its site of action which is described by the following kinetic parameters: (i) The apparent volume of distribution (V_d) which is the volume of the hydrophilic and hydrophobic spaces in the body that the drug is distributed in. It is obtained by dividing the injected dose (D_o) by the initial concentration (C_o) in blood plasma. Drugs that bind to tissues extensively exhibit low concentrations in the plasma and therefore, have higher a V_d compared to those that are mainly bound by blood plasma proteins. An average 70kg person has a total body water volume of ~ 50L of which ~ 10L occupy extra-cellular space.

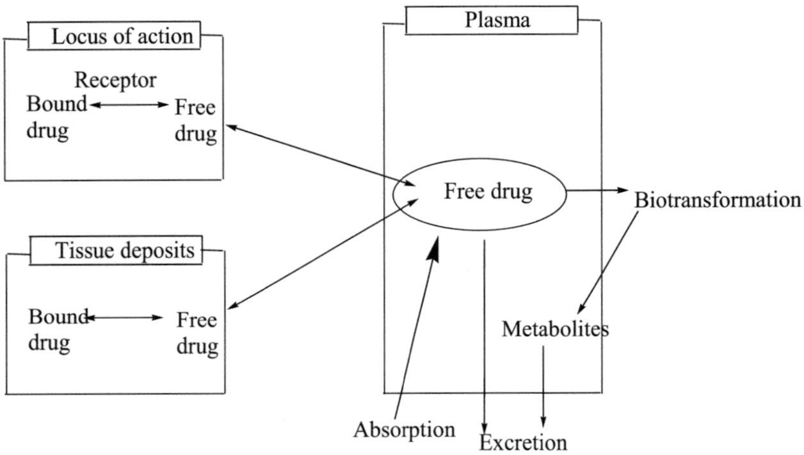

Figure 5. Drug disposition routes from absorption to excretion

The apparent volume of distribution cannot tell us where in the body the drug really is. The (C_{tox}) is the maximum drug concentration beyond which there would be toxic effects in the body, while the (C_{ther}) is the plasma concentration of a drug that would achieve a therapeutic effect or effective clinical response. The steady state concentration (C_{ss}) is that concentration that should be maintained between any two drug administration intervals. These pharmacokinetic data are important in that they characterize the fate of drugs in the body and are required by pharmacologists to calculate doses and frequencies of drug administration. However, in some clinical responses, the intensity of pharmacological action correlates better with the concentration of free drug in plasma, while in other responses there is no direct relationship between drug concentration and clinical response. The main variations of the drug response effects include;

i. Drugs which combine with their receptors as quickly as they dissociate from them; for this category of drugs, the pharmacological effect increases or reduces in tandem with the plasma drug concentration.

ii. Drugs which do not readily dissociate from their receptors. In this case the pharmacological effect persists despite the falling plasma concentration.

iii. Drugs which combine with receptors and irrespective of their rates of association/dissociation sets in motion a cascade of events which runs on despite falling plasma concentrations.

10. Kinetics of drug disposition process

Drug disposition process most of the times follows the 1st order kinetics in which disposition is proportional to the concentration of the drug at any given time. Therefore, the concentration of a drug in plasma will decrease at a rate that is proportional at all times to the concentration itself. Therefore;

$$\frac{-d[C]}{dt} = K[C]$$

$$\int \frac{-d[C]}{[C]} = \int K dt$$

$$\left[In[C] \right]_{C_o}^{ct} = Kt$$

$$In[C]_t - In[C]_o = Kt \text{ or } InC = InC_o - Kt$$

$$e^{In} \frac{[C]_t}{[C]_o} = e^{-Kt}$$

$$[C_t] = [C_o] e^{-Kt}$$

A more convenient form of this equation is obtained by taking $\log_{10}$

Since

$$\ln x = 2.303 \log_{10} x \quad (1)$$

It follows that;

$$2.303 \log_{10} C = 2.30.3 \log_{10} C_0 - Kt$$

and $\log_{10} C = \log_{10} C_0 - \frac{Kt}{2.303}$

A linear relationship is obtained when the logarithm of concentrations ($\log_{10}C$) is plotted against (t). times of observation (Figure 6).

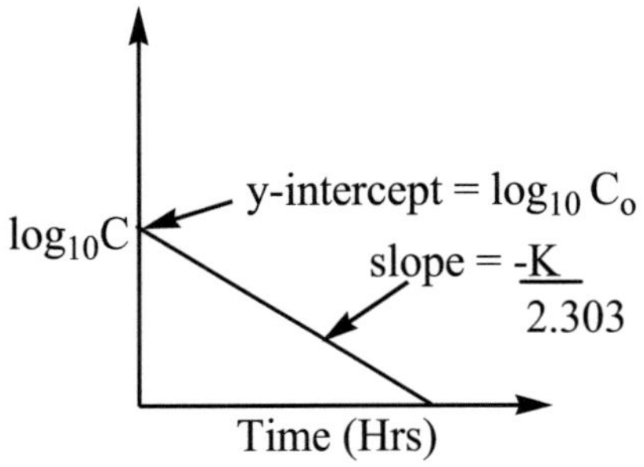

Figure 6. Logarithmic time course of drug concentration

Half-life ($t_{1/2}$) of a drug: this is the time period during which the concentration decreases to one- half of its previous value. $T_{1/2}$ can be evaluated from the elimination rate constant.

When $t = t_{1/2}$, $C_t = \frac{C_0}{2}$

therefore,

$$\frac{C_0}{2} = C_0 e^{-K t_{1/2}}$$

$$\frac{1}{2} = e^{-K t_{1/2}} \quad \text{but,} \quad K t_{1/2} = \log_e 2$$

$$t_{1/2} = \log_e \frac{2}{K} = \frac{0.693}{K}$$

11. Drug biotransformation reactions

Drugs and other foreign substances (xenobiotics) undergo series of biotransformation reactions in the body. The biotransformation reactions act as first line defense strategy against these xenobiotics. It is armed with a battery of enzymes which convert the lipid-soluble xenobiotics into more water-soluble metabolites to allow more efficient excretion of the drugs in a limited volume of water in urine or bile.

The enzymes involved in the biotransformation of endogenous chemicals are the same ones that are used in the biotransformation of xenobiotics. There is, therefore, a close relationship between drug biotransformation and fundamental homeostatic processes.

The drug biotransformation reaction may result in the following potential effects with respect to pharmacological activity:

11.1. Activation

An inactive precursor may be converted into a pharmacologically active drug. For instance, the nucleoside analogue used as an anti-HIV drug, have to undergo *in vivo* phosphorylation to form the active triphosphates which functions to inhibit the enzyme reverse transcriptase, while L– dopa (inactive), which is used in the treatment of parkinsons disease, is converted into dopamine (active) in the basal ganglia. Futamide, a drug used in the treatment of prostate cancer, undergoes hydroxylation at the alkyl side chain to form hydroxyflutamide, a metabolite that is more active and has a longer duration of action compared to the parent drug.

11.2. Maintenance of activity

An active drug is converted into another form which is also active, for instance diazepam, a sedative hypnotic, is metabolized to an equally active metabolite, oxazepam.

11.3. Inactivation

An active drug is converted to inactive products, for example, pentobarbital is hydroxylated to forminactive metabolites.

11.4. Phase I reactions

These include oxidation, reduction and hydrolytic reactions and such reactions generally introduce or unmask a functional group (hydroxyl, amine, sulfhydryl etc) that make the drug more polar.

11.5. Phase II reactions

Consist of synthetic/conjugation reactions in which an endogenous substance such as glucuronic acid or glutathione combines with the functional group derived from phase I reactions to produce a highly polar drug conjugate. All tissues have some ability to carry out drug biotransformation reactions but the most important organs of biotransformation include; the liver, GIT, lungs, skin, and kidneys in that order and most phase II reactions result in a decrease in the pharmacological activity of the drug. The fact that the GIT and liver are the major sites of drug biotransformation means that drugs which are administered orally will be extensively bio-transformed before they eventually reach systemic circulation. This first-pass effect can severely limit the oral bio- availability of some drugs. In addition, intestinal micro-organisms are capable of catalyzing drug biotransformation reactions e.g. a glucuronide conjugate of a drug may be excreted through the intestine via the bile where gut bacteria may convert the conjugate back into free drug. The free drug is then reabsorbed and re-enters the liver via the portal vein where the conjugation process is repeated. This leads to a phenomenon known as entero-hepaticcirculation.

At sub-cellular level, enzymes of drug biotransformation are located in the endoplasmic reticulum, mitochondria, cytosol and lysosome. The major site of drug biotransformation within the hepatocytes and other cells is the membrane of the smooth endoplasmic reticulum. The smooth endoplasmic reticulum constitutes the microsome fraction during differential centrifugation of whole blood. The microsome fraction can be used to carry out many drug biotransformation reactions *in vitro.*

11.6. Mechanisms of phase I reactions

11.6.1. Oxidation

Is the most important category of the microsomal drug oxidizing systems and requires participation of two distinct proteins in endoplasmic reticulum; cytochromes P_{450} (which functions as a terminal oxidase) and cytochrome P_{450} reductase. The name Cyt_{450} is derived from the fact that the reduced form of this hemoprotein complexes with carbon monoxide to form a complex that has a unique absorption spectrum with a maximum at 450nm.Cytochrome P_{450} reductase serves to transfer reducing equivalent from NADPH to the cytochrome P_{450} oxidase:

$$DrugRH + O_2 + NADPH + H^+ \rightarrow DrugROH\ (hydroxylated\ product) + H_2O + NADP^+$$

The sequence of reactions that transform a drug to its hydroxylated product is shown below (Figure 7).

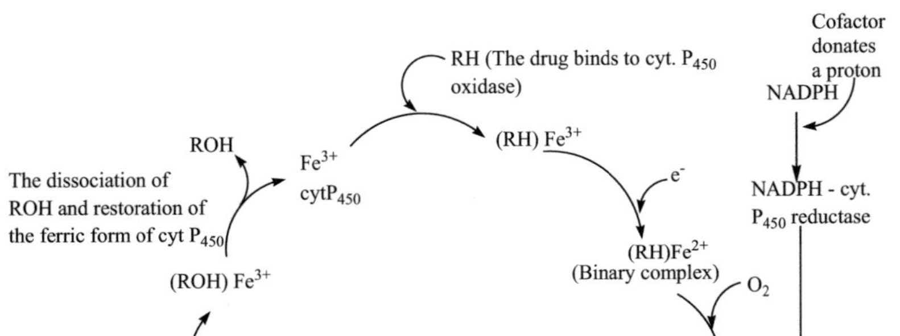

Figure 7. Phase 1 drug biotransformation reactions in the liver microsomal fraction in which the drug is converted to a more polar form.

http://dx.doi.org/10.5772/52014

The phospholipids of the endoplasmic reticulum are required for substrate binding, electron transfer, and facilitating the interaction between $CytP_{450}$ and its reductase. However, cytochrome P_{450} does not catalyze all Oxidation reactions. The microsomal flavin– containing monooxygenases (FMOs) catalyze NADPH – dependent oxygenation of nucleophilic phosphorous, nitrogen and sulfur atoms. These atoms are present in a wide variety of xenobiotics including the carbamate containing pesticides and therapeutic agents such as phenothiazines, ephedrine and N-methylamphetamine. Another important drug–oxidizing system is the prostaglandin synthetase–dependent co-oxidation.

$$\text{Prostaglandin } G_2 \text{ reduced} \xrightleftharpoons[\text{synthetase}]{} \text{prostaglandin } H_2$$

prostaglandin
synthetase

Many xenobiotics including phenytoin can be co-oxidized along with the above reduction reaction. This pathway is of considerable toxicological importance as it often leads to generation of toxic reactive metabolites. Other enzymes that catalyze oxidation of xenobiotic include alcohol dehydrogenase, aldehyde dehydrogenase, xanthine oxidase and monoamine oxidase.

11.6.2. Reduction

Some drugs with azo-linkages (RN=NR, e.g. prontosil) and nitrogen groups (RNO_2, such as chloramphenicol) are transformed by reductive pathways. The Cyt P_{450} and NADPH–cyt P_{450}reductase enzymes that catalyze oxidation reactions are also involved in reduction reactions for drugs containing quinine moieties. These transformation results in the formation of semiquinone free radicals illustrated in Figure 8. The free radicals that are generated cause oxidative stress, lipid peroxidation, DNA damage, and hence cytotoxicity. These effects are particularly responsible for the antitumor property of a drug like doxorubicin.

11.6.3. Hydrolysis

Drugs containing ester functions (R_1COOR_2) such as procaine are hydrolyzed by a variety of non-specific esterases in liver, and plasma while drugs with amide bonds are hydrolyzed by amidases in the liver. The polypeptide drugs such as insulin and growth hormones are hydrolyzed by peptidases in the plasma and erythrocytes. The metabolites resulting from hydrolysis reactions are subjected to phase II biotransformation reactions before excretion in the bile or urine.

11.7. Mechanisms of phase II reactions

The phase II reactions generally involve coupling of drug/drug metabolite with an endogenous substance to enhance their removal from the body. They require participation of specific transferase enzymes and high energy activated endogenous substances.

Most of the conjugation reactions result in detoxification of the drug although in some cases conjugation reactions result in bioactivation of drugs. The following is a summary of the different types of phase II biotransformation reactions;

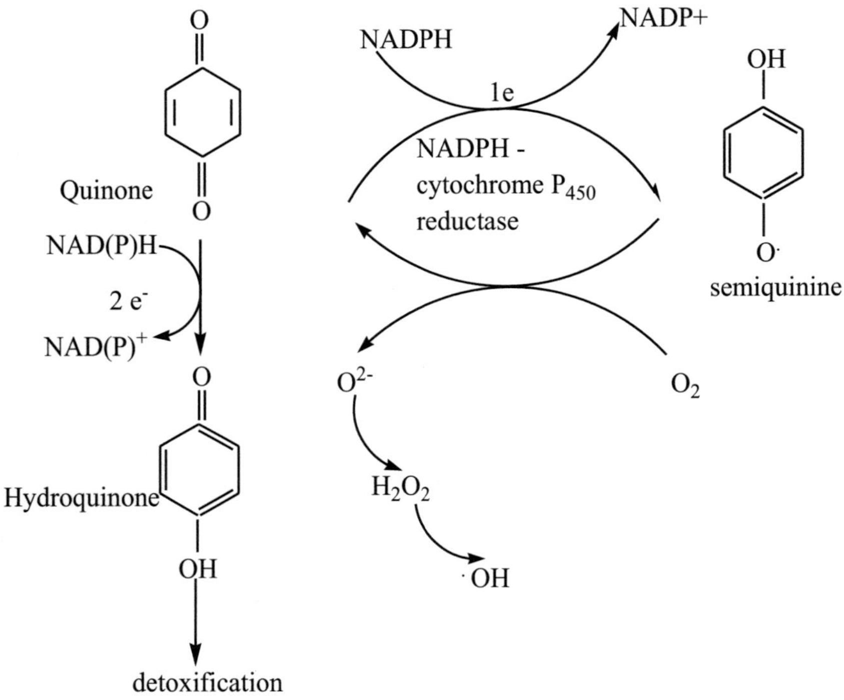

Figure 8. The transformation pathways for drugs with quinine moieties to generate free radicals.

11.7.1. Glutathione conjugation

Glutathione-S-transferases catalyze the enzymatic conjugation of xenobiotics with the endogenous tripeptide glutathione, glutamylcystenylglycine (GSH). The xenobiotics with suitable electrophilic centres such as the epoxides and nitro groups can be subjected to nucleophilic attack by glutathione (Figure 9). The final product, mercapturic acid is easily excreted from the body.

http://dx.doi.org/10.5772/52014

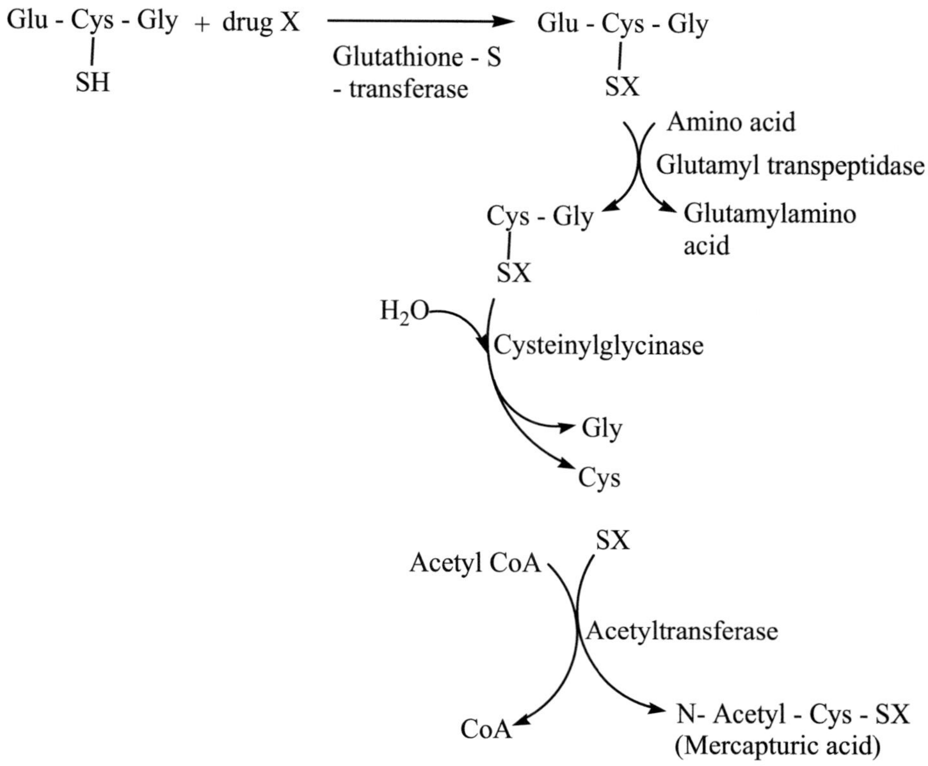

Figure 9. Glutathione conjugation reactions for a drug with a suitable nucleophilic centre leads to the formation of mercapturic acid which is easily excreted from the body

11.7.2. Glucuronidation

This is the conjugation of a drug or xenobiotic with glucuronic acid. Many functional groups are subject to glucuronidation. The benzoyl group in morphine, (an analgesic) and the amine group in meprobamate (a sedative) can undergo glucuronidation. A drug with a benzoyl group can undergo glucoronidation by a transferase as shown below:

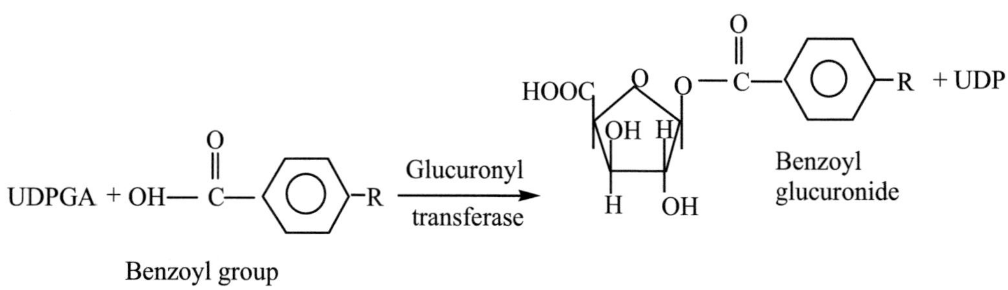

11.7.3. Epoxide hydration

A number of aromatic compounds are transformed by phase I reactions to form epoxide intermediates. The epoxides are reactive electrophilic species that can bind covalently to proteins and nucleic acids to bring about toxic effects. These epoxides are detoxified via the nucleophilic attack of water molecule on one of the electron deficient carbon atoms of the oxizane ring as shown below:

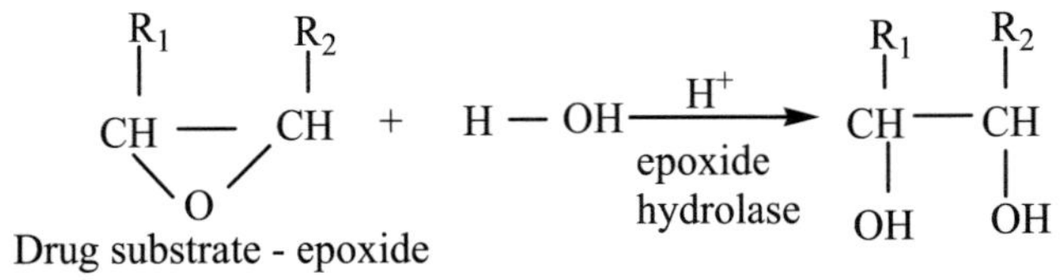

The glucuronide conjugates can be excreted via the bile or urine.

11.7.4. Acetylation

Acetylation is achieved by cytosolic enzymes known as N-acetyl transferases which catalyze transfer of acetate from acetyl co-enzyme A to primary aromatic amine or hydrazides (figure 10)

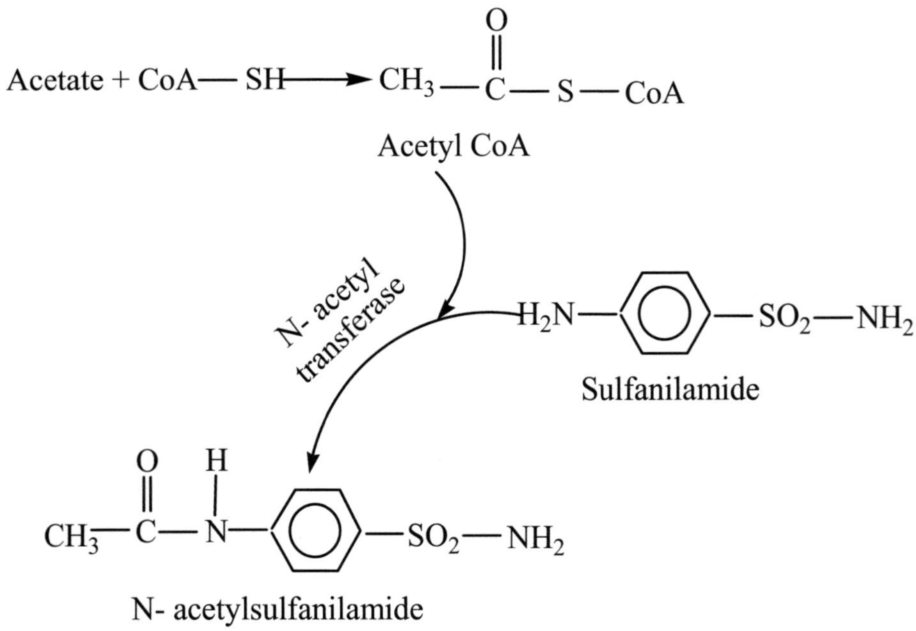

Figure 10. Acetylation reations leading to the formation of N– Acetylsulfanilamide, the final metabolite of the antimicrobial agent sulfanilamide which is secreted from the body.

http://dx.doi.org/10.5772/52014

11.7.5. Methylation

Most of the methyl transferases are cytosolic enzymes. They utilize S-adenosyl methionine (SAM) as the methyl donor. The final metabolite, thiopurine, has antineoplastic properties and is used as an anticancer agent (Figure 11)

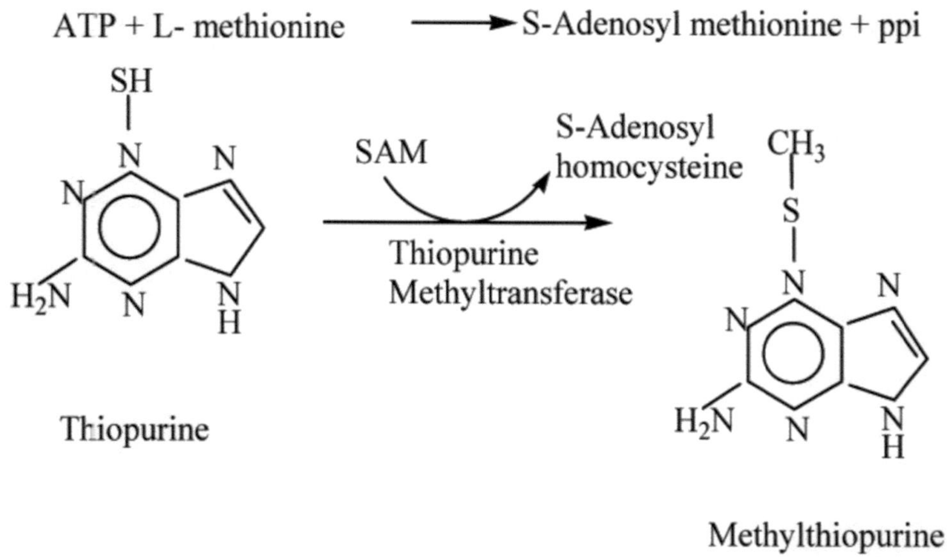

Figure 11. Methylation reactions leading to the formation of methylthiopurine

12. Adverse drug reactions associated with drug biotransformation reactions

Many adverse drug reactions can be traced to an improper balance between bioactivation and detoxification reactions. For example, when the analgesic acetaminophen is given at normal therapeutic doses, it undergoes glucuronidation and sulfation reactions that terminate the action of the drug and hasten its elimination. However, some of the drug is bioactivated via Cyt P_{450} to form N-acetylbenzoquinimine, a reactive intermediate that can be detoxified by conjugation with glutathione (GSH). When excessive doses of the drug are given, glucuronidation and sulfation reactions become saturated and more acetaminophen is bioactivated via Cyt P_{450}. This imbalance leads to high concentrations of N-acetylbenzoqunonine which cannot be sufficiently eliminated by the limited concentrations of gluthathione. This metabolite binds covalently to cellular protein thiols and initiates hepatotoxicity leading to hepatic necrosis.

12.1. Revision exercise 1

1. Discuss the absorption of ά-D- Ribose-5-phosphate, given that the two ionizable hydroxyl groups of the monophosphate ester ribose have pKa values of 1.2. and 6.6. The fully protonated form of ά-D-ribose 5-phosphate has the following structure;

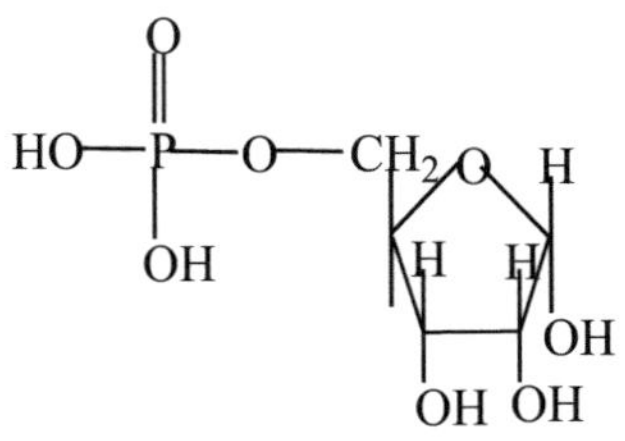

2. Using specific examples of drugs, justify their various routes of administration.

12.2. Revision exercise 2

If the concentration of a drug in plasma decreases at a rate that is proportional to its initial concentration, give an expression that describes this relationship and hence show that $[C_t] = [C_o].e^{-kt}$

12.3. Worked examples

Problem 1: Describe how you can determine the partition coefficient of a labeled drug

Solution: The partition coefficient of a drug is its differential distribution between the hydrophobic and hydrophilic phases. The distribution of the drug between these two phases can be determined by allowing equilibration of a radioactively labeled drug between aqueous buffer containing the drug and a cell membrane preparation obtained by homogenization and fractionation of a tissue sample. The ratio of drug concentration in the membrane to the concentration in the aqueous phase gives the partition coefficient.

Problem 2: Describe how you can demonstrate transport across membranes

Solution: Erythrocyte 'ghosts' or self sealing micelles formed when the erythrocytes release cytoplasmic contents upon exposure into a hypotonic solution can be used to study the uptake or release of labeled molecules across erythrocytes. When the ghosts are prepared in ^{14}C glucose, it will be possible to monitor the rate of release or uptake of the labeled ^{14}C glucose from the membranes into the aqueous environment. These 'ghosts' can also be used to study the uptake of various molecules at various concentrations under different conditions of temperatures and the presence of inhibitors for specific molecular uptake.

Problem 3: A 120mg per kg dose of a drug was injected intravenously and its concentration (mg/L) monitored regularly over time. When $\log_{10} C$ was plotted vs time (h) a linear response was obtained with a slope of – 0.08 and an extrapolated y-intercept of 1.3. Calculate the following pharmacokinetic parameters;

http://dx.doi.org/10.5772/52014

i. elimination rate constant (k)

ii. initial concentration of the drug in blood plasma (C_o)

iii. volume of distribution (V_d)

iv. half-life of drug elimination ($t_{½}$).

Solution:

i. Slope = - k/2.303, therefore, k = -2.303x -0.08 = 0.184

ii. C_o = Antilog of 1.3 = $10^{1.3}$ = 20 mg/L

iii. Volume of distribution (V_d) = Do/Co = 120/20 = 6 L

iv. The half-life of elimination $t_{1/2}$ = 0.693/k = 0.693/0.184 = 3.7 hours.

Once the apparent volume of distribution is known for a particular drug the amount of drug that must be given to achieve a desired concentration can be determined from

Do = Co.V_d

Problem 4: You have been given the following data based on a 65 kg patient; $t_{1/2}$ of drug X = 4.5hrs, V_d = 0.56L/kg, C_{min} the = 5mg/L, C_{tox} = 20mg/L and C_{ss} = 10mg/L; calculate:-

i. Drug clearance from the body

ii. Average rate of drug intake (Dosing rate)

iii. Maintenance dose

iv. Maintenance interval

v. Initial loading dose

vi. Loading dose at steady state concentration

Solution

Since $t_{1/2}$ = 0.693/ k; k= 0.693/ $t_{1/2}$ i.e. 0.693/4.5=0.154, and V= 0.56 x 65 = 36.4.

i. Total drug clearance = kV = 0.154 x 36.4 = 5.6L/h = 93.3ml/min.

ii. Average rate of drug intake = rate elimination constant

= kxVxCss

= 0.154 x 36.4 x 10

= 56 mg/h

iii. Maintenance dose

= (C_{tox} - C_{ther}). V

= (20 – 5) x 36.4 = 546 mg

iv. Maintenance interval = maintenance dose/ rate of elimination

= 546/56

= 9.75 hrs

For a practical loading schedule, the maintenance interval should be lowered to say 8.0 hrs and the maintenance dose reduced proportionately: = 546 x 8/9.75 ~ 437 mg.

v. The initial loading dose

= $C_{tox.}V$

= 36.4 x 20

= 728 mg

vi. The loading dose at steady state

= C_{ss} x V

= 36.4 x 10 = 364 mg

Practical problem 1

The analytical method of assaying paracetamol relies on the introduction of a nitro group into the molecule after the removal of plasma proteins through precipitation. The resultant nitrophenol compound which is formed has a deep yellow colour in an alkaline medium and absorbs at 430nm Figure 12.

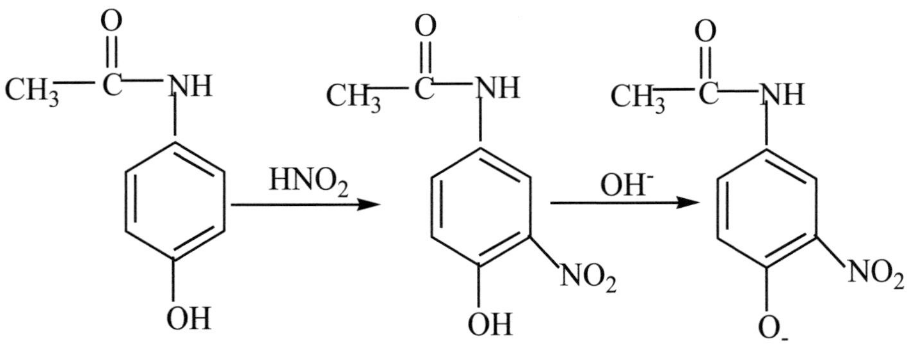

Figure 12. Formation of a chromogenic nitro compound from an analgesic Acetaminophen

i. Describe how you would construct the standard curve for determination of paracetamol concentration.

$$K = \ln \frac{\frac{x_1}{x}}{t1-t2}$$

2. Design an experiment that would enable you to determine the $t_{1/2}$ of paracetamol

http://dx.doi.org/10.5772/52014

Practical problem 2

Liver damage can be induced by 20% w/v carbon tetrachloride. Given 10mg/ml pentobarbitone and 10mg/ml Phenolbarbitone, design an experiment that demonstrates that the duration of action of short acting barbiturates are dependent on the integrity of the liver.

13. Drug discovery and preclinical trials

The development of new drugs over the past 30 years has revolutionalized the practice of medicine and has for instance seen the increased use of new anti-hypertensives and drugs that reduce cholesterol synthesis or dissolve blood clots which led to a 50% reduction in the number of deaths from cardio-vascular diseases and stroke among other diseases.

13.1. Conventional approaches to drug discovery

These are the classical approaches to drug discovery that do not initially involve detailed scientific study they include the following;

Traditional knowledge approach

This is the discovery of drugs based on traditional medical knowledge. The best example is the documented analgesic effects of extracts from opium poppy that led to the isolation of morphine from the plant and the subsequent synthesis of related analgesics.

Discovery through serendipity

This is the accidental discovery of novel drugs based on the ingenuity of a scientist investigating a problem initially unrelated to the observed phenomenon; examples of such discoveries include the observation by Alexander Flemmings that penicilliummould could inhibit the growth of bacteria. This finding led to the discovery of antibiotics.

Discovery of therapeutic usefulness of a side effect e.g. clonidine originally used as a nasal decongestant was found to have antihypertensive properties while, the hypoglycemic effects of sulphonamides used in the treatment of typhoid fever led to the development of structurally related sulphonylureas as oral hypoglycemic drugs.

Discovery from effects of endogenous agents in test animals

An example of discovery arising from studies of endogenous agents in test animals is the anticoagulant action of the venom from the Malayan viper that led to the identification of the anticoagulant ancrod.

Modern approaches to drug discovery

These are those approaches that form a basis for the rational design of drugs and include the following;

Bioprospecting

This is the screening of a large number of natural products, chemical entities, large libraries of peptides, nucleic acids and other organic molecules for biological activity. This approach may lead to identification and development of new drug molecules.

Metabolomics

This is the profiling of natural products of related plant species screening using either liquid or gas chromatography mass spectrometry to determine active metabolites that may be present in novel crude herbal medical preparations.

In silico screening

This is the most advanced technique for drug discovery. It entails virtual screening or docking of compounds on the 3-D- structure of a known receptor based on homologies of the test drug molecules with a known test parent drug. *In silico* screening can form a basis for the modification of a known drug molecule to determine possible therapeutic applications and may lead to the development of putative drugs against new targets.

13.2. Screening of putative drug molecules

Selection of molecules for further study is usually conducted in animal models of human disease and the pharmacological tests include both the *in vitro* and *in vivo* studies after the initial screening for biological activity. For instance, antibacterial activity of drugs is assessed by their ability to inhibit growth of a variety of micro-organisms, while hypoglycemic drugs are tested for their ability to lower blood pressure.

The *in vitro* methods include incubation of a parent compound with various subcellular fractions such as microsomes, individual recombinant drug metabolizing enzymes from cells or tissue slices. The *in vivo* studies involve working on typical animal models such as dogs or rats. Some of the *invitro* and *invivo* studies that may be performed are shown in tables 1 and 2 below;

	Target	Specific or tissue in vitro studies	Biochemical measurement
a.	(i) Receptor binding	Cell membrane fraction / cloned receptors	Receptor affinity
	(ii) Receptor activity	Sympathetic nerves	Inhibition of nerve activity
	(iii) Enzyme activity e.g. tyrosine hydroxylase	Purified enzymes from adrenal glands	Inhibition of enzyme activity
b.	Cellular function	Cultured cells	Cell viability
c.	Isolated tissue	Blood vessels, heart lung or ileum from rat	Effects on vascular contraction and relaxation

Table 1. Screening of drugs for specific inhibitory effects on enzymes and isolated tissues.

	Disease model	Animal model	Route of administration	Physiological measurements
a.	Blood pressure	Hypertensive rat (conscious)	Parenteral	Systolic/diastolic
b.	Cardiac effects	Dog (conscious) Dog (anesthetized)	Oral Parenteral	Electrocardiography (cardiac output)
c.	CNS	Mouse, rat	Parenteral	Degree of sedation
d.	Respiratory effects	Dog/guinea pig	Parenteral	Respiratory rate and amplitude
e.	GIT effects	Rat	Oral	GIT motility and secretions

Table 2. Putative animal models used in studying effects of drugs

If an agent possesses useful activity it would be further studied for possible adverse effects on other major organs. These studies might suggest the need for further chemical modification to achieve desirable pharmacokinetic/pharmacodynamic properties.

13.3. Preclinical trials

The data from animal studies form a basis for the calculation of the initial or starting doses to be used in the subsequent clinical studies. The human equivalent dose calculations for the maximum recommended dose are normally based on either the body surface area or body weight. The candidate drugs that survive initial screening and profiling must be carefully evaluated for potential risks before and during clinical testing. The main types of evaluation needed from safety and toxicity studies include:-

Acute toxicity

This involves looking at the effects of large single doses of therapeutic agent. Acute toxicity studies are usually performed in animal models such as mice and rats. These studies enable investigators to correlate any observed effects with the systemic level of the drug.

Sub-acute toxicity

This is similar to acute toxicity but measures the effects of multiple doses based on expected duration of clinical usage. It entails haematological, histology and electron microscope studies to identify organs which might be affected by toxicity. It usually lasts between one to three months. This enables the selection of putative compounds for subsequent studies.

Chronic toxicity testing

These studies are required when the drug is intended to be used in humans for prolonged periods. The goals of this investigation are mostly similar to those of sub-acute toxicity.

The reproductive performance

These are measurements intended to determine the effects of the drug agents on; mating behaviour, reproduction, parturition, progeny birth defects, and postnatal development.

Carcinogenicity studies

These studies are required to determine the effects of prolonged usage of the drug under investigation. They involve hematological and histological autopsy analysis.

Mutagenicity studies

These studies look at the genetic stability and mutations of bacterial or mammalian cells in culture. These studies are at the academic research level and are intended to provide data for future research.

Investigative toxicology

The main purpose of toxicology is to discover the pathways that are involved in toxic action. It includes studies on mechanisms of toxic action of drugs which may lead to the development of safer drugs.

14. Evaluation of new drugs and drug approval process

Toxicity testing is time consuming and expensive and may require two to five years to collect and analyze data before the drug can be considered ready for testing in humans.

Large numbers of animals are needed to obtain valid preclinical data.

Extrapolation of toxicity data from animals to humans may not be completely reliable.

The safety or efficacy of a drug must be thoroughly understood before the drug is administered to any group of individuals. Therefore regulations governing the development of new drugs have evolved to assure safety and efficacy of new medications. The clinical trials during drug development and post marketing experience form the scientific basis of patient response to a drug.

Once a drug is judged ready to be studied in humans, a notice of clinical investigational exemption for a new drug (IND) must be filled with the government body concerned with the regulation and registration of drugs. The IND includes manufacturing information, all data from animal studies, clinical plans and protocols and the names and credentials of physicians who will conduct the clinical trials.

14.1. Phase I clinical trials

The main goal in phase I is to determine whether test animals and humans show significant different responses to the drug and to establish limits of the safe clinical dosage range. The measurements carried out in phase I include, the rate of absorption, $t_{1/2}$ and metabolism of the candidate drug compound. The effects of the drug as a function of dosage are established in a small number 25 – 50 of healthy volunteers. When the drug is expected to have significant toxicity, as often the case with cancer and AIDS therapy, volunteer patients with the disease are used instead of the healthy volunteers. The requirements of clinical trials include the following:

i. Homogenous populations of patients must be selected.

ii. Appropriate controls for the investigation must be included.

iii. Meaningful and sensitive indices for drug effects must be used i.e. well defined end-points such as survival or pain relief should be used rather than surrogate or intermediate markers e.g. levels of enzymes involved in the process of survival/pain relief.

iv. The experimental observations must be converted to data and then into valid conclusions.

v. The accuracy of diagnosis and severity of the disease must be comparable between the groups being contrasted.

vi. The dosages of the drugs must be chosen and individualized in a manner that allows relative efficacy to be compared at equivalent toxicities.

vii. Compliance with experimental regimens should be assessed before subjects are assigned to experimental or control groups. Non-compliance may cause false estimates of the true potential benefits or toxicity of a particular treatment.

viii. Ethical considerations. These may be the major determinants of the types of controls that can be used e.g. for therapeutic trials that involve life threatening diseases for which there is already in-effective therapy, the use of a placebo is considered unethical. In such cases, new treatments must be compared with standard therapies.

14.2. Study design of phase I trials

For clinical trials to have validity they must be based on a sound statistical basis. Some of the of the criteria that must be met include;

Randomization

Randomization is a design which ensures that there is no bias in allocation of treatments among the different groups. The purpose of randomization is to minimize the possibility that an observed treatment effect is due to inherent differences between groups. Randomization eliminates bias by avoiding recruiting patients who have a particular characteristic to one group and not the other e.g. only women/men and smokers/alcoholics. Randomization should not be carried out until immediately before treatment. The delay allows a patient to have second thoughts about taking part or the investigator to have to re-consider about admitting patients to the study. Simple methods of randomization can be designed using published tables of random numbers, where treatments are in a form of a square in which each treatment is contained only once in each row and column and the order of treatment is different in each group (Table 3).The presence of other diseases or risk factors should be taken into consideration i.e. need for careful selection and assignment of patients to each of the study groups.

		Group Treatment		
1	A	B	C	D
2	C	D	A	B
3	D	C	B	A
4	B	A	D	C

Table 3. A random number table array for assignment of various treatment regimes to various groups of patients in clinical trials

This approach eliminates systematic variation between groups since the patients are allocated at random order to group 1, 2, 3, or 4. A code list should be drawn up so that the main investigators may be kept blind to the treatment an individual is receiving but also so that it is possible to know the treatment by breaking the code. Coding should be such that when broken, it does not yield information about the treatments other patients are getting. The treatment information about all the patients should be left to one person preferably the pharmacist or trial co-ordinator.

Blindness

Blinding is a design which does not allow the investigator to know what treatment the patient is receiving. The purpose of blinding is to eliminate bias in reporting the outcome of the treatment since if an investigator knows what treatment the patient is taking, he/she may in some way influence a measurement or an outcome thus shifting the outcome in one direction or another consciously or unconsciously. The ideal trial should be double blind where neither the investigator nor the patient knows what treatment the patient is taking. Placebos or dummies are used in order to achieve blindness. The placebos should match the active treatment as closely as possible in terms of size, shape, color, texture, weight, taste and smell with the active formulation.

Number of testing centers

Clinical trial should be carried out in a defined centre so as to minimize variations in the population and in the investigators techniques. This also avoids problems of data collection, communication and follows up. Multi-centre trials may become necessary when studying a rare disease hence scarcity of patients or when the effect being investigated is small one e.g. when one is looking out for an interaction effect between a major condition and a minor condition.

Clinical trials designed to evaluate efficacy of new drugs should always be prospective i.e. the characteristics of the population to be studied should be identified before the study begins. For example, if one randomized all patients with heart failure to treatment with either digoxin or a new drug X and then studied the outcome over six months that would be a prospective trial. In case of control study the outcome is first identified and then comparisons are made retrospectively between the characteristics of patients who did or did not have the outcome. Such a study for instance has shown that oral anticoagulants can reduce incidences of re-infarction in patients who have already had a myocardial infarction. The case control studies may be carried out some time, after the introduction of a drug therapy in order to get some idea of its place in the overall management of the disease since the results of a case control study may prompt formal prospective trials in order to confirm original findings.

14.3. Molecular markers in drug development

In vitro predictive efficacy and toxico-genomics should be carried out after phase 1 clinical trials in order to validate the results of the phase 1 clinical trials. This is achieved by using animal cell lines in which gene expression profiling and patterns of protein production are used to identity candidate biomarkers for the disease. The utilization of markers that are associated with the disease or those that indicate a known response to a therapeutic intervention or reflect a clinical outcome may yield information on efficacy or toxicity of a test drug. An example of a biological readout that has traditionally been used to determine efficacy during the treatment of diabetics is the determination of glucose in the urine of a diabetic patient. Reliable and specific biomarkers that act as predictors of efficacy or long-term toxicity are useful because they reduce the time, size and cost of clinical trials.

14.4. Phase II clinical trials

These are studies that recruit willing and informed patients and are designed to assess long term safety, refine pharmacokinetic data, determine optimal dose. The purpose of phase II studies is to determine efficacy. Typically, phase II trials require 100-150 subjects and take 9-12 months. An assessment of no effect or no worthwhile effect of a given drug demonstrates that it is futile to proceed with further clinical testing of the drug. It is therefore important to minimize type I errors or false negatives in the study design in order to minimize the risk of discontinuing a potentially effective drug. The data from well designed phase I and phase II trials are therefore critical in planning the subsequent trials. The phase III trials are large trials intended to determine whether a treatment is effective and to establish safety data.

Phase II clinical trials include inert placebos as negative controls and older active drugs as positive controls alongside the investigative compound. These studies are done in special clinical centers such as University Hospitals. A broader range of toxicities may be detected at this phase

14.5. Phase III clinical trials

The drug is evaluated in a much larger number of patients (thousands) to further establish safety and efficacy. Phase III trials are performed in settings similar to those anticipated for the ultimate use of the drug. After successful phase III trials, the next step is the application for review of the new drug to seek approval to use the drug for clinical management of the disease condition.

14.6. Phase IV clinical trials

This phase is concerned with post-marketing surveillance and the main goal is to assess adverse reactions, patterns of drug utilization, discovery of additional indications. The interrelationships between the various studies in drug development are illustrated in Fig 13 below;

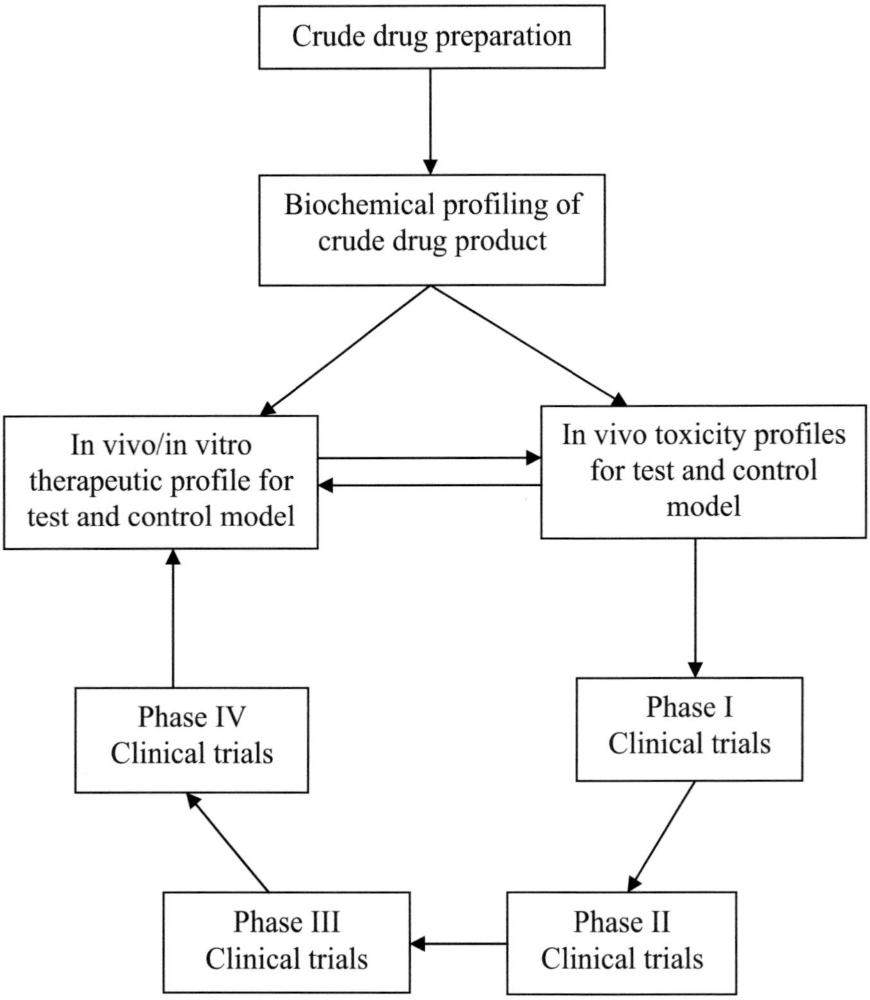

Figure 13. Illustration of the key steps in the development of a drug from a putative drug candidate extract

14.7. Pharmacogenomics and drug development

The personalized medication which takes into account the genetic make-up of individuals is known as pharmacogenomics. The pharmacogenomic differences that determine individualized therapy include genetic polymorphisms of drug transporters, drug receptors, and drug metabolizing enzymes. For example, genetic variation in Cyt P_{450} enzymes that are largely responsible for drug metabolism shows that different individuals respond differently to drug efficacy or toxicity. Genetic variants in the drug target, the disease pathway, genes or drug metabolizing enzymes could all be used as predictors of drug efficacy or toxicity. For example, drug monitoring using perpherazine, a Cyt P_{450} substrate, shows that there are three main categories of individuals; the efficient metabolizers obtained from the heterozygotes, the poor metabolizers from the homozygotes and the ultra-rapid metabolizers which carry two or more active genes in the same chromosome, a phenomenon known as gene duplication.

The information obtained from pharmacogenetic studies can be used to design new drugs that take the persons' genetic profile into consideration. The most common type of genetic variation are single nucleotide polymorphisms, therefore, a high resolution of single nucleotide map may expedite the identification of genes for various diseases. The molecular profiles of patients identified in phase I and II clinical trials as likely non-responders to the putative drug under investigation might present an opportunity to initiate new discovery programs for other pharmaceutical compounds.

14.8. Individualized drug therapy

Clinical usage of drugs requires a basic understanding of the pharmacokinetic and pharmacodynamic drug processes and an appreciation that a relationship does exist between the pharmacological effect or toxic response to a drug and the concentration of the drug. The interpatient and intrapatient variation in disposition of a drug must be taken into account in choosing a drug regimen.

A drug dosage regimen therefore is a recipe for the administration of a drug so as to produce a desired therapeutic effect with minimum toxic effects.

The regimen is described in terms of the following:

i. Dose of the drug to be used and the formulation.

ii. Frequency with which it is administered.

iii. Route of drug administration.

The factors that determine the relationship between the prescribed drug dosage and drug effect operate at three levels; prescription level, drug administration level and at the physiological level of patient (Figure 14).

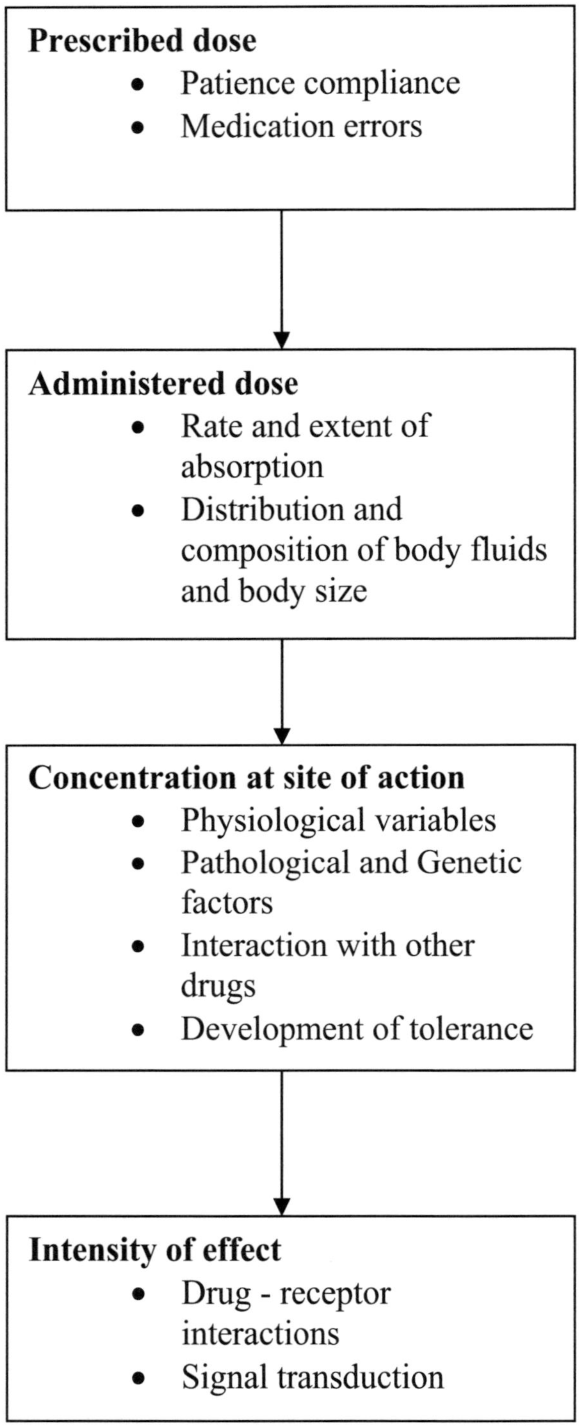

Figure 14. The operational levels that determine the relationship between prescribed drug dosage and the drug effect.

http://dx.doi.org/10.5772/52014

Drugs that are excreted primarily unchanged by the kidneys tend to have low variation among patients with similar renal function than do drugs which are inactivated by metabolism. For the extensively metabolized drugs, those with high metabolic clearance and large first pass elimination have marked difference in bioavailability, whereas those with low biotransformation tend to have largest variation in elimination rates among individuals.

14.9. Determination of drug dosage

The simplest way of determining a drug dosage regimen is to base it on the published recommended dosage. These are derived from the pharmacokinetics studies of the drug and the general procedure in using the published recommendations is to start at the lower end of the recommended dosage range and monitor the therapeutic effect. If the desired effect does not occur, the dosage can be increased gradually until one reaches the upper limit of the range. In certain conditions it may be necessary a sufficiently high dose for the drug to accumulate in the body to a satisfactory degree. This dose is known as the loading dose and is equal to the volume of distribution multiplied by the target concentration in the plasma. The reason for giving a loading dose is to circumvent the sometimes unacceptable time lag preceding the steady state levels. Once the correct loading dose is given, a steady-state concentration can be achieved rapidly and then maintained by giving a smaller maintenance dose.

Adjustment of dosage in individual patients is often as a result of the modification of pharmacokinetic parameters of which the three most important include; the bioavailability or the fraction of a drug that is absorbed into systemic circulation, its clearance and the volume of distribution.

For drugs with a high toxicity to therapeutic ratio, the loading dose can be given as a single dose and for drugs with a low toxicity: therapeutic ratio and a long half-life, the loading dose can be divided into several portions and given at intervals long enough to allow detection of adverse effects, but short enough to ensure that the loading dose is a true loading dose i.e. relatively little amounts of the drug is eliminated from the body during the period of loading.

14.10. Systemic drug availability

The extent of availability of a drug after oral administration is expressed as a percentage of the dose. The fractional availability (F) varies from 0 to 1. The extent of availability is more important parameter to measure rather than the rate of availability.

A true decrease in bioavailability could be due to several reasons including, a poorly administered dosage form that fails to disintegrate or dissolve in the GIT, interaction with other drugs in the GIT, metabolism of the drug in the GIT and/or first pass hepatic metabolism or biliary excretion.

Hepatic disease may in particular cause high availability because the metabolic capacity decreases or development of vascular shunts in the liver. Significantly high availability requires dosage adjustment by a factor of two, while significantly low in availability requires dosage adjustment by a factor of half.

14.11. Maintenance dose

In most clinical situations drugs are administered in such a way as to maintain a steady concentration i.e. just enough drug is given in each dose to replace the drug eliminated since the preceding dose. Therefore, clearance is the most important pharmacokinetic term to be considered in defining a rational steady-state drug dosage regimen.

The rate of elimination = Cl x Tc

Where, Cl is the rate of clearance and Tc is the target concentration of the drug.

The Dosing rate = Rate of elimination = Cl x Tc.

Therefore, if the target concentration is known, the prevailing clearance in that patient will determine the dosing rate and if the drug is given by a route that has a bio availability of less than 100%, then the dosing rate above can be modified using the formula:

$$\text{Dosing rate oral} = \frac{\text{Dosing rate}}{\text{Fractional availability}}$$

If intermitted doses are given, then maintenance dose = Dosing rate x Dosing interval.

14.12. Alteration of maintenance dose

The maintenance dose is usually altered when the clearance of the drug changes. For example, during renal impairment, the clearance of drugs which are predominantly cleared by the kidney is greatly reduced and therefore, the desired steady state concentration can only be achieved either through altering the dose or altering the dosing interval. Therefore, when a drug is cleared almost completely via kidneys, the dosage interval should be changed in proportion to renal clearance as follows:

The % eliminated in dosing interval should be proportional to creatinine clearance by a published constant to yield the percentage excreted in one dosage interval.

The quantities required for this adjustment are:

i. Fraction of normal function remaining, and the

ii. Fraction of drug usually excreted unchanged in urine.

The fraction of normal function remaining is equal to the ratio of patient's creatinine clearance to a normal value (120 ml/min/70kg).

The following equation is for adjustment of renal clearance

$$rf_{pt} = 1 - fe_{nl}(1 - rfx_{pt})$$

Where;

rf_{pt} = the adjusted total clearance of the patient,

fe_{nl} = fraction of drug excreted unchanged in normal individuals,

rfx_{pt} = fraction of renal clearance of the normal individual.

http://dx.doi.org/10.5772/52014

Clearance should also be adjusted for the size of the patient and for convenience, the published values are normalized to the metabolic rate = weight $^{0.75}$.

When clearance is low, $t_{1/2}$ is similarly high and when the volume of distribution is high, the $t_{1/2}$ is also high. Therefore, by using parameters for the individual patient, the dosing rate = Tc x Cl/F where, Tc = target concentration, Cl = clearance and F = fractional availability of the drug.

If a drug is relatively non toxic then the maximum loading strategy can be employed so that the dosing interval is much longer than $t_{1/2}$.. For example t½, of penicillin is less than one hour but it is usually given in very large doses every six to twelve hours since it is non-toxic. The normal steady-state theophylline concentration can be determined using the equation:

$$Css,\ max = \frac{F.dose/V_{ss}}{1 - \exp^{(-KT)}}$$

$$Css,\ min = \frac{F.dose/V_{ss}.\ (\exp^{-KT})}{1 - \exp^{(-KT)}}$$

Where, Css, max and Css min are the maximum and minimum steady state concentrations,

$$T = \text{dosage interval and } K = \frac{0.693}{t½}$$

14.13. Drug dosage adjustment in old patients (geriatrics)

Drug absorption in the elderly is slightly different from the normal patients and therefore adjustment of the dosage should be taken into consideration during drug therapy. The rate of transdermal drug absorption may be diminished in elderly because of reduced tissue blood perfusion. Compounds that permeate the intestinal epithelium by carrier mediated transport mechanisms may be absorbed at lower rates in the elderly.

14.14. Drug distribution

In geriatrics the 'body mass' declines with age and the total body water content falls by between 10 – 15%. The volume of distribution of hydrophilic drugs will therefore decrease while plasma concentration will increase and the likelihood of toxic drug effects will also increase. When geriatric patients use diuretics, the extracellular space reduces even further leading to a higher likelihood of drug toxicity. The total body fat in the elderly increases by 12 – 18%, therefore, for hydrophobic drugs, the higher volume of distribution implies an increase in half life of distribution and the time needed to reach steady-state serum concentration. Therefore, for geriatrics a once or twice daily drug administration is optimal. This can be achieved though delayed release or fixed drug combinations.

14.15. Patient compliance and rational use of drugs

Drug treatment of any kind is often compromised by lack of full compliance by the patient. The common errors of compliance to a regimen by a patient include; omission in taking the drug, wrong timing of dosages, premature termination of therapy or using additional medications. In order to improve patient compliance, the patient should be made to understand the nature and prognosis of the illness and what to expect from the medication by detailing both the acceptable and undesirable unwanted effects as well as signs of efficacy that may help enforce compliances.

Patients frequently discontinue taking a medication such as septrin because they have not been told the necessity of continuing with the drug after the acute symptoms have subsided.

The effectiveness of physician-patient communication is inversely related to the error rate in the taking of drugs. A physician might prescribe a drug to be taken three times a day with meals for a patient who either eats only twice a day or sleeps all day and works at night. Therefore, an exploration of the patients eating, sleeping and working habits is necessary before a prescription is given.

The educational level of a patient may also require that the prescription is carefully worded and oral instructions given in the primary language of the patient since when such patients take three or more medications they are less likely to use them properly. It is therefore important to provide identifying symbols for each medication e.g. "Heart pill" or "sugar pill"and to reduce the doses into once or twice daily regimens.

14.16. Adverse drug reactions

Pharmacological formulations are potentially harmful to the individuals taking the drugs. There is need to ascertain the safety of new drugs before allowing them to be marketed. The following figures highlight the magnitude of the problem: ~ 10 – 20% of hospitalized patients suffer adverse drug reactions, while 0.3 – 5.0% inpatients admissions and ~ 0.3% deaths in hospital are due to adverse drug reactions. Adverse drug reactions can be classified into two main categories: They may be dose related or non dose related with each being short-term or long-term.

14.17. Dose related adverse reactions

Adverse drug reactions can occur because of the changes in the systemic availability of a formulation. For instance, the change of excipients in phenytoin capsules from $CaSO_4$ to lactose leads to high availability and hence adverse drug reactions. Sometimes, adverse drug reactions can occur due to the presence of contaminants like bacteria if quality control breaks down. Out-of-date formulations may also cause adverse drug reactions because of degradation products arising from the drug e.g. outdated tetracycline may cause Faconis Syndrome (a type of rickets) because of the transformation product,epiandrotetracycline. Dose related adverse reactions may also arise from pharmacokinetic variations in the individuals taking the drug. Pharmacokinetic variations may also arise due to hepatic disease like advanced cirrhosis which lowers the clearance of drugs such as phenytoin and morphine. The pharmacological variations could be environmental such as diet or smoking, while others are genetic.

http://dx.doi.org/10.5772/52014

14.18. Non-dose related adverse drug reactions

These include immunologic reactions and are related to the surface proteins present on β-humans lymphocytes (HLA antigens) which are important in the function of T-lymphocytes. The association of HLA antigens with foreign antigens stimulates T-lymphocytes. Some of these antigens expressed by major histocompatibility complex (MHC) genes have been associated with an increased risk of adverse drugs e.g. nephrotoxicity from penicillamine is increased in patients with HLA types B8 and DR 3 while patients with HLA- DR, 7 are protected against adverse drug effects.

14.19. Types of drug allergies

Drug allergies can be classified into five categories:

Type I

This anaphylaxis or immediate hypersensitivity reactions; the body reacts within five to thirty minutes. The IgE molecules fixed to mast cells and basophil leucocytes release histamine and other pharmacological mediators such as kinins. Drugs likely to cause are anaphylactic shock include;-penicillins, streptomycin, local anaesthetics etc.

Type II

In these reactions, the circulating antibody of 1gG, 1gM or 1gA interacts with the drug combined with a cell membrane protein to form a hapten-protein/antigen-Ab complex. This leads to the activation of the complement leading to cell lysis of phagocytic attack of the cell with the complex. Drugs such as the cephalosporins, penicillins, quinine and transfusion of improperly matched blood can yield this type of reactions.

Type III

In this type of allergy, the immune complex reactions initiate an inflammatory response due to the combination of the excess drug- protein complex with the IgG in circulation. The complex thus formed is deposited in the tissues and causes activation of the complement and damage of capillary endothelium. This type of reaction is manifested mostly as fever, arthritis, and/or enlarged lymph nodes. Penicillins, sulphonamides and streptomycin may elicit type III allergic reactions.

Type IV

This is the cell-mediated or delayed hypersensitivity reactions in which the T - lymphocytes are sensitized by a hapten to form protein-antigenic complex such that when the lymphocytes come into contact with the antigen, an inflammatory response ensues. Type IV reactions are exemplified by contact dermatitis caused by local anaesthetic areas, antihistamine areas, topical antibiotics and antifungal drugs.

Type V

These are pseudo allergic reactions, that resemble allergic reactions clinically, but for which no immunological basis can be found, e.g. asthma and skin rashes caused by aspirin. Administration of ampicillin or amoxicillin causes a skin rash which resembles the one caused by penicillin hypersensitivity. The ampicillin-caused rash can be distinguished from penicillin hypersensitivity on the basis of two features; it has a later onset, typically ten to fourteen days, compared to penicillin sensitivity which comes between seven to ten days. Furthermore, the sensitivity does not recur following re-exposure to ampicillin and is not as serious as the one caused by penicillin.

14.20. Clinical evaluation of adverse drug reactions

The two basic approaches for clinical evaluation of adverse drug reactions include the cohort studies (or follow-up studies) of patients taking the drug and the case control studies which record the incidences of adverse drug effects retrospectively.

Cohort or prospective studies

In cohort studies, drugs are identified and incidences of adverse effects recorded. The weaknesses of these studies include; the relatively small number of patients likely to be recruited, and lack of suitable control groups to assess the background incidence of any apparent adverse reaction noted.

Case control or retrospective studies

The approach here is to start with the incidence of adverse reaction(s) and then look for the drug and the individuals with symptoms which could be due to an adverse drug reaction. These individuals are screened to see if they had taken the drug. The prevalence of drug taking in the group is then compared with the prevalence in a reference population which did not take the drug. This approach is excellent for validation and assessment of adverse drug effects, but it may not detect new adverse effects. Furthermore, it requires a very large number of patients and is very expensive to undertake hence difficult to justify and organize for every new product.

14.21. Worked examples

Problem 5

Drug clearance must always be adjusted for alterations of renal function using the formula: $rf_{pt} = 1 - fe_{nl}(1 - rfx_{pt})$, where fe_{nl} = fraction of the drug excreted unchanged in normal individuals, rf_{pt} = adjustment factor for total clearance in patient, rfx_{pt} = patients' clearance as a fraction of normal clearance and Cl_{nl}= normal clearance.

Given that an asthmatic patient has a creatinine clearance of $40 ml min^{-1}\ 70 kg^{-1}$ and that the fraction of terbutaline excreted unchanged, fe_{nl}= 0.56, the normal clearance,Cl_{nl} = 3.4 ml/min/kg, calculate the clearance of the drug in the patient.

Solution

The patient has depressed renal function: rfx_{pt} = (40 ml/min)/ (120 ml/min) = 0.33

$rf_{pt} = 1 - fe_{nl}(1 - rfx_{pt})$

inline formula $rf_{pt} = 1 - 0.56\ (1 - 0.33) = 0.62$

$$Cl_{pt} = Cl_{nl} \cdot rf_{pt}$$

inline formula $= 3.4 ml.min^{-1}kg^{-1} x\ 0.62$

$= 2.1 ml.min^{-1}kg^{-1}$

Problem 6

Given the following characteristics of drug A; $t_{½} = 8h$, given at a dosage of 450mg every 12h, has $V_{ss} = 0.5$ L/kg, effective concentration is 12mg/L and that

$$C_{ss} min = \frac{F\ x\ dose / V_{ss}(exp^{-kt})}{1 - exp^{(-KT)}}$$

$$C_{ss}, max = \frac{F\ x\ dose/V_{ss}}{1 - exp^{(-kT)}}$$

Determine the C_{ss}min and C_{ss}max for a 60 kg patientif F = 1 and $exp^{KT} = 0.35$. Explain how changing of the dosage interval to 6 hours would affect C_{ss}min.

Solution

The term $exp^{(-KT)}$ is the fraction of the last dose that remains in the body at the end of a dosing interval and is equal to 0.35 and C_{ss} min = C_{ss} max.exp($^{-kt}$). Therefore,

$$C_{ss}min = \frac{450/30\ x\ 0.35}{1 - 0.35} = 15/0.65\ x\ 0.35 \sim 8.0\ mg/L \text{ while } C_{ss}max = 15/0.65 = 23\ mg/L$$

The predicted minimum of 8.0mg/L is below the effective concentration to achieve efficacy. Therefore the dosing interval should be reduced. A reduction of the interval to, say, six hours, increases denominator and therefore causes an increase of C_{ss}min. Since $t_{1/2} = 0.693/K$, K = 0.086 i.e. $1 - e^{-KT} = 1 - 2.71^{-0.086 \times 6} = 1 - 0.596 = 0.4$.

The new C_{ss} minimum becomes; = 450/30 x 0.4 = 15 mg/L which is within the required therapeutic concentration.

Review exercise

1. Write an essay on statistical considerations that guide clinical evaluation of new drug agents

2. Write an essay on bioprospecting for new antimicrobial agents.

3. Drug clearance must always be adjusted for alterations of renal function using the formula: $rf_{pt} = 1 - fe_{nl}\ (1 - rfx_{pt})$, explain what each term in the above equation represents. Consequently, calculate the clearance of acetaminophen (panadol) in a 70 kg patient with depressed renal function given the following; normal clearance = 350 ml min $^{-1}$70 kg; f_{enl} = 0.56. The patient creatinine clearance = 80 mlmin^{-1} 70 kg. Normal creatinine clearance = 120 ml min^{-1} 70 kg. What effect would the impaired renal function have on dosing interval?

4. Given that fe_{nl} for drug X = 0.42, and the normal creatinine clearance is 120 ml/min/70 kg, calculate the clearance rate of the drug by a patient with creatinine clearance of 75 ml/min/70 kg.

5. Write an essay on adverse drug reactions associated with the use of macrolide antimicrobial agents.

Author details

Gabriel Magoma

Department of Biochemistry, Jomo Kenyatta University of Agriculture and Technology. Nairobi, Kenya

References

[1] Christoph & F., Heike Brotz-Oesterhelt (2005). Functional genomics in antibacterial drug discovery. *Today Targets* DD. 10

[2] David, A. L. and Michael P. W. (2004). Molecular biomarkers in drug development. *Research Focus* DDT. 9, 22

[3] Di Bernardo, A.B. and Cudkowicz, M.E. (2006). Translating preclinical insights into effective human trials in ALS. *Biochemicaet Biophysica Acta*1762, 1139 -1149.

[4] Harvey A, L. (2007). Natural products as screening source. *Current Opinions in Chemical Biology*.11, 480 - 484.

[5] Jaennefer M. F., Paul, A. L. (2000) Emerging novel antifungal agents. *Therapeutic focus*. DD. 5, 1 January 2000

[6] Iris, R. (2008). PK/PD Modelling and simulations: utility in drug development. *Drug Discovery Today*.348, 1 - 6.

[7] Klaus, T. (2003).When drug therapy gets old: pharmacokinetics and pharmacodynamics in the elderly. *Experimental Gerontology*38 843-853.

[8] Kieran, F. R., Eric S. and Philip H. W. (2001).Modelling and simulation in clinical drug development. *Research Focus* DD Vol. 6, 15

[9] Lindpaintner, K. (2002). The Impact of pharmacogenetics and pharmagenomics on drug discovery. *Naure Review on Drug Discovery*.1, 463 - 469.

[10] Sundbergh, M. I. (2001). Genetic susceptibility to adverse effects of drugs and environmental toxicants. The role of the CYP family of enzymes *Mutants Researh* 482. 11-19

[11] Timothy, D. R., Steven R.G., Herve, T., Brian A.D. (2001). Finding drug targets in microbial genomes. *Drug Discovery Today*6, (17): 887-892.

[12] Tim, R. C. and Marc L. (2007). Pharmacogenitics of antiretroviral drugs for the treatment of HIV-infected patients: An update. Infection, Genetics and Evolution 7, 333-342

[13] Turnheim, K. (2003). Why drug therapy gets old Pharmacokinetics and pharmacodynamics in the eldery. *Experimental Gerontology* 38 843-853.

[14] Paul, B. (2003). Toxicokinetics in preclinical evaluation. *Research Focus* DD Vol. 8

[15] Ulrich, R., Friend, S. H. (2000). Toxicogenomics and drug discovery: Will new technologies help us produce better drugs? *Nat. Rev. Drug Discov.* 1, 84 – 88.

[16] Werbovetz, K. A. (2000). Target based drug discovery for Malaria, Leishmania and Trypanosomiasis. *Current medicinal Chemistry* 7 (8) 835 – 860.

[17] Aungst B. (2000). Intestinal permeation enhancers. *Journal of Pharmacological Sciences*,89 (4), 429-442.

[18] Salama, N.N. Eddington N.D. Fasano, A. (2006).Tight junction modulation and its relationship with drug delivery. *Advanced Drug Delivery Reviews*.58: 15-28.

[19] Guengerich F. P. (2001). Common and uncommon cytochrome P_{450} reactions related to metabolism and chemical toxicity. *Chemical Research and Toxicology*.14: 611 - 650.

[20] Blanka R., (1998). Receptor-mediated targeted drug or toxin delivery. *Advanced Drug Delivery Reviews* 29: 273-289.

[21] John R. C. (2005). Some distinctions between flavin-containing and cytochrome P_{450}monooxygenases.*Biochemical and Biophysical Research Communications* 338: 599-604.

[22] Xiaoling L. William K. C. (1999). Transport, metabolism and elimination mechanisms of anti-HIV agents. *Advanced Drug Delivery Reviews*29: 273-289 39, 81-103.

[23] Brown, M.J., Bennet, P.N., Lawrence, D.R. (1997). Clinical pharmacology (8th Edition) Wesley, Longman China Ltd.

[24] Hardman J.G., Gilman A.G., Limbird L. E.(1996). *The pharmacological basis of therapeutics* (9thEdition) McGraw-Hill.

[25] Katzung B. G.,(2004). *Basic and clinical pharmacology* (9th Edition) Mcgraw Hill Inc.